Evidence Based Color Atlas of OBSTETRICS & GYNECOLOGY
Diagnosis and Management

Richa Saxena MBBS, MD

Obstetrician and Gynecologist
New Delhi, India

Foreword
PK Shah

JAYPEE BROTHERS MEDICAL PUBLISHERS (P) LTD

New Delhi • London • Philadelphia • Panama

Jaypee Brothers Medical Publishers (P) Ltd

Headquarters

Jaypee Brothers Medical Publishers (P) Ltd
4838/24, Ansari Road, Daryaganj
New Delhi 110 002, India
Phone: +91-11-43574357
Fax: +91-11-43574314
Email: jaypee@jaypeebrothers.com

Overseas Offices

J.P. Medical Ltd
83 Victoria Street, London
SW1H 0HW (UK)
Phone: +44-2031708910
Fax: +02-03-0086180
Email: info@jpmedpub.com

Jaypee-Highlights Medical Publishers Inc.
City of Knowledge, Bld. 237, Clayton
Panama City, Panama
Phone: + 507-301-0496
Fax: + 507-301-0499
Email: cservice@jphmedical.com

Jaypee Brothers Medical Publishers Ltd
The Bourse
111 South Independence Mall East
Suite 835, Philadelphia, PA 19106, USA
Phone: + 267-519-9789
Email: joe.rusko@jaypeebrothers.com

Jaypee Brothers Medical Publishers (P) Ltd
17/1-B Babar Road, Block-B, Shaymali
Mohammadpur, Dhaka-1207
Bangladesh
Mobile: +08801912003485
Email: jaypeedhaka@gmail.com

Jaypee Brothers Medical Publishers (P) Ltd
Shorakhute, Kathmandu
Nepal
Phone: +00977-9841528578
Email: jaypee.nepal@gmail.com

Website: www.jaypeebrothers.com
Website: www.jaypeedigital.com

Inquiries for bulk sales may be solicited at: jaypee@jaypeebrothers.com

This book has been published in good faith that the contents provided by the contributors contained herein are original, and is intended for educational purposes only. While every effort is made to ensure accuracy of information, the publisher and the author specifically disclaim any damage, liability, or loss incurred, directly or indirectly, from the use or application of any of the contents of this work. If not specifically stated, all figures and tables are courtesy of the author. Where appropriate, the readers should consult with a specialist or contact the manufacturer of the drug or device.

Evidence Based Color Atlas of Obstetrics & Gynecology Diagnosis and Management

First Edition: **2013**

ISBN 978-93-5090-431-2

Printed at Ajanta Offset & Packagings Ltd., New Delhi.

"My mom is a never-ending song in my heart of comfort, happiness and being. I may sometimes forget the words but I always remember the tune."

— Graycie Harmon

Dedicated to

My mother, Mrs Bharati Saxena
And all the mothers
"I always remember my mother, she is my bridge and my good luck charm"

Special Acknowledgments

Ankit Kaushik MD Pathology (Std)
Vardhman Mahavir Medical College
and Safdarjung Hospital
New Delhi, India
For interpretation of histopathology figures

Rekha Khandelwal MS (Obstetrics and Gynecology)
Director and Consultant Obstetrician and Gynecologist
Vardaan Health Care Hospital and Senior Citizen Home
Malviya Nagar, New Delhi, India
For providing figures for Section 2

Rajiv Khandelwal MD (Pediatrics)
Director and Consultant Pediatrician
Vardaan Health Care Hospital and Senior Citizen Home
Malviya Nagar, New Delhi, India
For providing figures for Sections 4 and 6

AP Manjunath
Department of Obstetrics and Gynecology
Kasturba Medical College and Hospital,
Manipal, Karnataka, India
For providing figures for Section 12: Abdominal Hysterectomy

Ritsuko K Pooh
Department of Obstetrics and Maternal Fetal Medicine
Center for Maternal Fetal and Neonatal Medicine
Kagawa National Children's Hospital
Zentsuji, Japan
For providing figures for Section 7

KyongHon Pooh
Department of Neurosurgery
Kagawa National Children's Hospital
Zentsuji, Japan
For providing figures for Section 7

Foreword

It gives me great pleasure to write foreword for the book titled *"Evidence Based Color Atlas of Obstetrics & Gynecology: Diagnosis and Management"*. It is like a ready reckoner for practicing obstetricians and gynecologists. The formatting of all the chapters of the book makes it a very interesting reading material.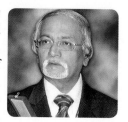

A distinctive feature of the book is the inclusion of "Evidence-based breakthrough facts" at the end of each chapter describing the latest evidence and research. The illustrations are very clear and informative. I am sure that the information provided in this book will tremendously help Federation of Obstetric and Gynaecological Societies of India (FOGSI) members, all postgraduate students, consultants and researchers to know as well as understand various topics related to obstetrics and gynecology.

I congratulate Dr Richa Saxena from Delhi, the author of this book, for her wonderful efforts.

PK Shah
President FOGSI

Preface

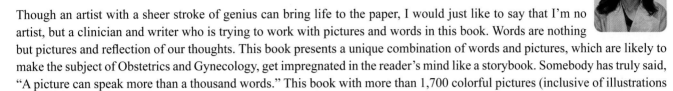

"The combination of picture and words together can be really effective and I began to realize in my career that unless I wrote my own words, my message was diluted."

— ***Galen Rowell***

Though an artist with a sheer stroke of genius can bring life to the paper, I would just like to say that I'm no artist, but a clinician and writer who is trying to work with pictures and words in this book. Words are nothing but pictures and reflection of our thoughts. This book presents a unique combination of words and pictures, which are likely to make the subject of Obstetrics and Gynecology, get impregnated in the reader's mind like a storybook. Somebody has truly said, "A picture can speak more than a thousand words." This book with more than 1,700 colorful pictures (inclusive of illustrations and photographs) is likely to be a testimony to the above statement.

In today's era of evidence-based medicine, it is important for every clinician to be aware of the recent evidence-based management options. It is difficult for clinicians with a busy practice to keep abreast with the latest evidence-based developments in any field of medicine. To help the consultant obstetricians and gynecologists get acquainted with recent research studies, a special heading titled as "Evidence-Based Breakthrough Facts" has been added at the end of each chapter. Very brief description of the new clinical guidelines or new research discoveries (over the past decade) have been highlighted. In case the reader wants to know about further details, the exact source (journal) details have also been provided.

The book has been divided into two parts: Obstetrics and Gynecology, which have been further divided into a total of 15 sections. Not a textbook, but an atlas, this book would prove to be useful to the postgraduate students and consultants in practice. Each topic has been explained with the help of pictures. Each picture is accompanied by its medical description and diagnosis as well as management (surgical as well as medical). Places where required, clinical highlights have also been elaborated. This information would facilitate rapid diagnosis and accurate management of various obstetric and gynecological conditions and would therefore serve as a ready source of reference as well as a ready reckoner.

"Lord, I commit my failures as well as my successes into your hands, and I bring for your healing the people and the situations, the wrongs and the hurts of the past.

Lead me always to be positive as I entrust the past to your mercy, the present to your love, and the future to your providence."

— ***St Augustine***

Although a prayer going at the end of preface may appear very odd, I wanted to end this preface with a prayer because I truly believe that writing a book is a mammoth task, which cannot be accomplished without His divine intervention. Therefore, I would sincerely like to thank the "Almighty" for the conception, initiation and completion of this book. I would like to extend my thanks and appreciation to all the related authors and publishers whose references have been used in this book. Book creation is teamwork, and I acknowledge the way the entire staff of M/s Jaypee Brothers Medical Publishers (P) Ltd., New Delhi, India, worked hard on this manuscript to give it a final shape. I would like to thank Shri Jitendar P Vij (Group Chairman), Jaypee Brothers Medical Publishers, for being the guiding beacon, and source of inspiration and motivation behind this book. I would also like to thank Mr Ankit Vij (Managing Director) and Mr Tarun Duneja (Director-Publishing). Last but not the least, I would like to thank the entire staff of Jaypee Brothers, especially Dr Anchal Kaushik, Ms Jagriti Kundu, Mr Nitish Kumar Dubey and Mr Amit Rai (Medical Editors) for editing the manuscript and coordinating the process of publication; Mr Gopal Sharma (DTP Operator) for formatting the book; Mr Manoj Pahuja and Mr Vijay Singh (for making beautiful four-colored illustrations); Mr Rajesh Sharma (for coordinating the production team) and Ms Seema Dogra (for cover designing). May God bless them all!

I would also like to thank my teachers, professors and colleagues at Maulana Azad Medical College and Leighton Hospital (Cheshire, UK) for their support and encouragement in writing this book. I am simply overwhelmed with gratitude for their commendable help.

Richa Saxena

Contents

Part 1: Obstetrics

Section 5: Medical Conditions During Pregnancy

Section 6: Postnatal Period

Section 7: Imaging in Obstetrics

Part 2: Gynecology

Section 8: General Gynecology

Section 9: Menstrual Disorders

Section 10: Benign Tumors of Genital Tract

Section 11: Malignancies of Genital Tract

Section 12: Uterus

Section 13: Abnormalities in Conception

Section 14: Infections of the Genital Tract

Section 15: Contraception

EVIDENCE BASED COLOR ATLAS OF OBSTETRICS & GYNECOLOGY DIAGNOSIS AND MANAGEMENT

Abbreviations

A & E	Accident and Emergency		FL	Femur Length
A-A	Artery-to-Artery		FNAC	Fine Needle Aspiration Cytology
AC	Abdominal Circumference		FSH	Follicle Stimulating Hormone
ACOG	American College of Obstetricians and Gynecologists		GA	General Anesthesia
AFI	Amniotic Fluid Index		GCT	Glucose Challenge Test
AFP	Alpha Fetoprotein		GDM	Gestational Diabetes Mellitus
AFS	American Fertility Society		GFR	Glomerular Filtration Rate
AIGA	American Institute of Graphic Arts		GnRH	Gonadotropin-Releasing Hormone
ANC	Antenatal Care		GTD	Gestational Trophoblastic Disease
APAS	Antiphospholipid Antibody Syndrome		GTT	Glucose Tolerance Test
APGAR	Activity, Pulse, Grimace, Appearance and Respiration		HbS	Hemoglobin S
APH	Antepartum Hemorrhage		HC	Head Circumference
APLA	Antiphospholipid Antibody		hCG	Human Chorionic Gonadotropin
APTT	Activated Partial Thromboplastin Time		HELLP	Hemolysis, Elevated Liver Enzymes, Low Platelets
ART	Assisted Reproductive Technology		HIE	Hypoxic-Ischemic Encephalopathy
ASRM	American Society of Reproductive Medicine		HIV	Human Immunodeficiency Virus
AUB	Abnormal Uterine Bleeding		HPE	Histopathology Examination
BBT	Basal Body Temperature		HPV	Human Papillomavirus
BMI	Body Mass Index		HRT	Hormone Replacement Therapy
BPD	Biparietal Diameter		HSG	Hysterosalpingogram
BPP	Biophysical Profile		ICSI	Intracytoplasmic Sperm Injection
BSO	Bilateral Salpingo-Oophorectomy		ICU	Intensive Care Unit
CA-MRSA	Community-Acquired Methicillin-Resistant Staphylococcus aureus		IUCD	Intrauterine Contraceptive Device
			IUD	Intrauterine Death
CC	Clomiphene Citrate		IUGR	Intrauterine Growth Retardation
CDC	Centers for Disease Control and Prevention		IUI	Intrauterine Insemination
CHM	Complete Hydatidiform Mole		IVF	In Vitro Fertilization
CL	Corpus Luteum		IVH	Intraventricular Hemorrhage
CNS	Central Nervous System		IVIG	Intravenous Immunoglobulin
COCP	Combined Oral Contraceptive Pills		KEEPS	Kronos Early Estrogen Prevention Study
CPD	Cephalopelvic Disproportion		KFT	Kidney Function Test
CPP	Central Precocious Puberty		LA	Local Anesthesia
CRL	Crown-Rump Length		LAVH	Laparoscopic-Assisted Vaginal Hysterectomy
CST	Contraction Stress Test		LGA	Large for Gestational Age
CT	Computerized Tomography		LH	Luteinizing Hormone
CTG	Cardiotocography		LHRH	Luteinizing Hormone-Releasing Hormone
D&C	Dilatation and Curettage		LMA	Left Mentoanterior
DFMC	Daily Fetal Movement Count		LMP	Left Mentoposterior
DHEA	Dehydroepiandrosterone		LMT	Left Mentotransverse
DHEAS	Dehydroepiandrosterone Sulfate		LMWH	Low-Molecular-Weight Heparin
DIC	Disseminated Intravascular Coagulation		LNG-IUS	Levonorgestrel-Intrauterine System
DMPA	Depot Medroxyprogesterone Acetate		LOA	Left Occiput Anterior
DUB	Dysfunctional Uterine Bleeding		LOD	Laparoscopic Ovarian Drilling
DV	Ductus Venosus		LOP	Left Occiput Posterior
DVT	Deep Vein Thrombosis		LOT	Left Occiput Transverse
EB	Endometrial Biopsy		LSA	Left Sacroanterior
ECV	External Cephalic Version		LSCS	Lower Segment Cesarean Section
EDD	Expected Date of Delivery		LSH	Laparoscopic Supracervical Hysterectomy
EFW	Expected Fetal Weight		LSP	Left Sacroposterior
ER	Extended Release		LST	Left Sacrotransverse
ESHRE	European Society of Human Reproduction and Embryology		MCA	Middle Cerebral Artery
FBS	Fasting Blood Sugar		MCH	Mean Corpuscular Hemoglobin
FDA	Fetal Descending Aorta		MCHC	Mean Corpuscular Hemoglobin Concentration
FDP	Fibrinogen Degradation Product		MCV	Mean Corpuscular Volume
FHR	Fetal Heart Rate		MFPR	Multifetal Pregnancy Reduction
FHS	Fetal Heart Sound		MRI	Magnetic Resonance Imaging

MSAFP	Maternal Serum Alpha Fetoprotein	ROT	Right Occiput Transverse
MTP	Medical Termination of Pregnancy	RSA	Right Sacroanterior
NAAT	Nucleic Acid Amplification Test	RSP	Right Sacroposterior
NICU	Neonatal Intensive Care Unit	RST	Right Sacrotransverse
NSAID	Nonsteroidal Anti-Inflammatory Drug	rT3	Reverse T3
NST	Nonstress Test	SERM	Selective Estrogen Receptor Modulator
NYHA	New York Heart Association	SFH	Symphysis-Fundal Height
OCP	Oral Contraceptive Pill	SGA	Small for Gestational Age
OFD	Occipitofrontal Diameter	SHBG	Serum Hormone Binding Globulin
OGTT	Oral Glucose Tolerance Test	SIS	Saline Infusion Sonography
OHSS	Ovarian Hyperstimulation Syndrome	SOGC	Society of Obstetricians and Gynaecologists of Canada
OPD	Out-Patient Department	STD	Sexually Transmitted Disease
PCOD	Polycystic Ovarian Disease	STI	Sexually Transmitted Infection
PCOS	Polycystic Ovarian Syndrome	SUI	Stress Urinary Incontinence
PEFR	Peak Expiratory Flow Rate	TAH	Total Abdominal Hysterectomy
PHM	Partial Hydatidiform Mole	TAS	Transabdominal Sonography
PID	Pelvic Inflammatory Disease	TBG	Thyroid Binding Globulin
PMS	Premenstrual Syndrome	TCD	Transverse Cerebellar Diameter
PNDT	Prenatal Diagnostic Techniques	TCRE	Transcervical Resection of Endometrium
POC	Products of Conception	TNF	Tumor Necrosis Factor
POG	Period of Gestation	TNM	Tumor, Node, Metastases
POI	Progestogen Only Injectable	TOA	Tubo-ovarian Abscess
POP	Progestogen Only Pill	TORCH	Toxoplasma, Other viruses, Rubella, Cytomegalovirus, Herpes virus
PP	Postprandial		
PPH	Postpartum Hemorrhage	TRAP	Twin Reversed Arterial Perfusion
PROM	Premature Rupture of Membranes	TRH	Thyroid Releasing Hormone
PSTT	Placental Site Trophoblastic Tumor	TSH	Thyroid Stimulating Hormone
PUBS	Percutaneous Umbilical Cord Blood Sampling	TTTS	Twin-to-Twin Transfusion Syndrome
RCOG	Royal College of Obstetricians and Gynaecologists	TVS	Transvaginal Sonography
RDW	Red Cell Distribution Width	UGF	Urogenital Fistula
REM	Rapid Eye Movement	USDA	United States Department of Agriculture
RMA	Right Mentoanterior	USPTF	United States Preventive Task Force
RMP	Right Mentoposterior	UTI	Urinary Tract Infection
RMT	Right Mentotransverse	VBAC	Vaginal Birth after Cesarean (Section)
ROA	Right Occiput Anterior	V-V	Vein-to-Vein
ROM	Rupture of Membranes	VVC	Vulvovaginal Candidiasis
ROP	Right Occiput Posterior	VVF	Vesicovaginal Fistula

Section 1

General Obstetrics

Obstetrics

1.1: REPRODUCTIVE SYSTEM

1.1.1: Reproductive Organs

1.1.1.1: Male Reproductive System

Picture	Medical/Surgical Description	Management/Clinical Highlights
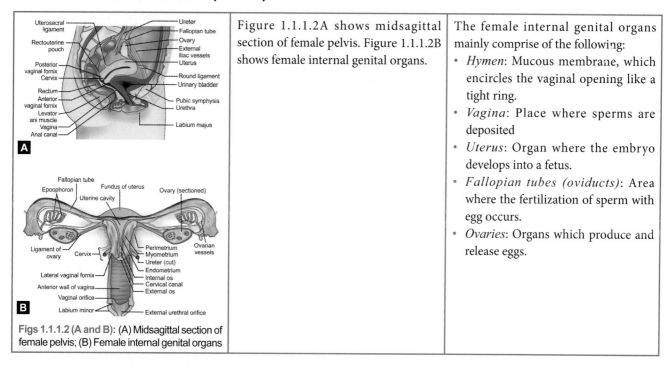Fig. 1.1.1.1: Male reproductive system	The adjacent figure shows male reproductive system.	Male genital system comprises of male internal sex organs which are testes and male external genital organs (penis and scrotal sac containing one testicle each). The testes are organs where spermatogenesis occurs. The sperms and secretions from various sexual organs such as seminal vesicles, prostate, bulbourethral glands, etc. form the semen.

1.1.1.2: Female Internal Genitalia (A and B)

	Medical/Surgical Description	Management/Clinical Highlights
Figs 1.1.1.2 (A and B): (A) Midsagittal section of female pelvis; (B) Female internal genital organs	Figure 1.1.1.2A shows midsagittal section of female pelvis. Figure 1.1.1.2B shows female internal genital organs.	The female internal genital organs mainly comprise of the following: • *Hymen*: Mucous membrane, which encircles the vaginal opening like a tight ring. • *Vagina*: Place where sperms are deposited • *Uterus*: Organ where the embryo develops into a fetus. • *Fallopian tubes (oviducts)*: Area where the fertilization of sperm with egg occurs. • *Ovaries*: Organs which produce and release eggs.

1.1.1.3: Female External Genitalia

Picture	Medical/Surgical Description	Management/Clinical Highlights
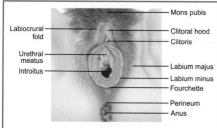Figs 1.1.1.3 : Diagrammatic representation of female external genital organs	The external genital organs include structures such as mons pubis, labia majora, labia minora, Bartholin's glands and clitoris. An ill-defined area containing these external genital organs along with the perineum is known as the vulva. Anteriorly the vulva is bound by mons pubis, posteriorly by the perineum and on the two sides by the labia majora.	The female external genital organs have three main functions: enabling sperm to enter the cervical canal, protecting the internal genital organs from infectious organisms and provision of sexual pleasure.

1.1.1.4: Different Types of Hymens

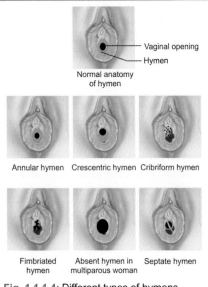

Annular hymen | Crescentric hymen | Cribriform hymen

Fimbriated hymen | Absent hymen in multiparous woman | Septate hymen

Fig. 1.1.1.4: Different types of hymens

At the beginning of the genital tract, just inside the opening of the vagina, is the hymen, a mucous membrane. In virgins, the hymen usually encircles the vaginal opening like a tight ring. Figure 1.1.1.4 illustrates different types of hymens, which can be of the following types: annular, crescentic, imperforate, fimbriated, cribriform and septate. Normal anatomy of hymen in a nulliparous woman is shown in the topmost figure. Imperforate hymen and its management have been described in details in 9.9.1C.

Septate hymen has a thin hymenal membrane with extra band of tissue in the middle. Minor surgery may be done to remove this. In cribriform hymen, the hymen is fenestrated, resulting in a sieve-like vaginal opening. Surgical resection of the tissues around the openings may be required to create a single opening.

Annular hymen forms a circumferential ring around the vaginal opening. It a natural variant of hymen commonly observed amongst newborns. Fimbriated hymen imparts irregular edges to the hymenal orifice. Crescentic hymen is semilunar in shape. It has attachments at 10'O clock to 11'O clock and 1'O clock to 2'O clock positions with no hymenal tissue at 12'O clock position. For all these types of natural variants of hymen, no treatment is required.

1.1.2: Blood Supply

1.1.2.1: Blood Supply to the Uterus

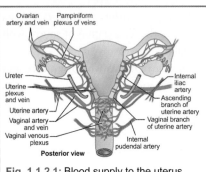

Fig. 1.1.2.1: Blood supply to the uterus

Blood supply to the uterus is mainly by the uterine arteries with the collateral supply from the ovarian arteries. Uterine arteries are main branches of the internal iliac arteries.

The uterine artery passes inferiorly from its origin into the pelvic fascia. It runs medially in the base of broad ligament to reach the uterus. After reaching the internal os, it then ascends along the lateral margin of the uterus within the broad ligament. It continues to move along the lower border of the fallopian tubes where it ends by anastomosing with the ovarian artery, which is a direct branch from the abdominal aorta.

1.1.2.2: Blood Supply to the Ovaries

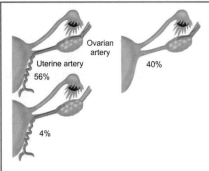

Fig. 1.1.2.2: Blood supply to the ovaries

In maximum number of cases (i.e. approximately 56% of cases), blood supply to the ovaries is both from the uterine arteries and ovarian arteries.

In 40% of cases, the blood supply is from the ovarian artery only, while in the remainder 4% of cases, it is only from the uterine artery.

Picture	Medical/Surgical Description	Management/Clinical Highlights

1.1.2.3: Blood Supply to the Female Breasts (A and B)

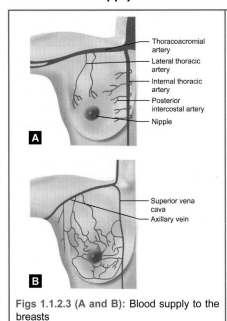

A

B

Figs 1.1.2.3 (A and B): Blood supply to the breasts

Figure 1.1.2.3A shows arterial supply to the breasts. Figure 1.1.2.3B shows venous supply to the breasts.

Blood supply to the breasts is mainly derived from the perforating branches (second to fifth perforators) of internal mammary arteries derived from internal thoracic arteries. Other blood vessels which supply the breast tissues include thoracoacromial artery and lateral thoracic artery.

Venous drainage of breasts is mainly by axillary vein. Other veins draining the breast tissues include subclavian, intercostal and internal thoracic veins.

1.1.2.4: Blood Supply to the Pelvic Structures

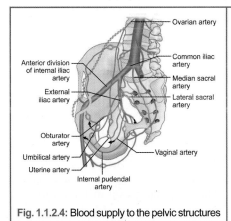

Fig. 1.1.2.4: Blood supply to the pelvic structures

As shown in Figure 1.1.2.4, blood supply to the pelvis is mainly by the internal iliac artery.

Internal iliac artery, also known as the hypogastric artery, is a branch of the common iliac artery at the level of sacroiliac joint.

1.1.2.5: Relationship of Uterine Artery to Ureters

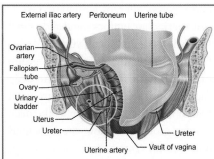

Fig. 1.1.2.5: Relationship of the uterine artery to ureters

The uterine artery, once it originates from internal iliac vessel, runs medially in the base of broad ligament to reach the uterus. It then reaches the junction of the body and cervix of the uterus (internal os) by passing superiorly. Here, the uterine artery is closely related to the ureter. It is important for the gynecologist to know this relationship so that the ureter does not inadvertently get injured while clamping, cutting and ligating the uterine arteries.

While moving toward the internal os, uterine artery passes above the ureter at right angles. It then ascends along the lateral margin of the uterus within the broad ligament. It continues to move along the lower border of the fallopian tubes where it ends by anastomosing with the ovarian artery, which is a direct branch from the abdominal aorta.

1.1.3: Lymphatic Drainage

1.1.3.1: Lymphatic Drainage of Pelvis (A and B)

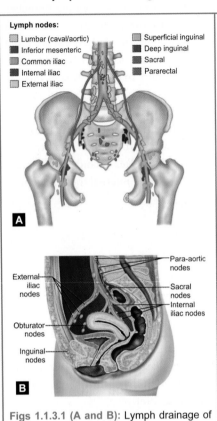

Figs 1.1.3.1 (A and B): Lymph drainage of pelvis: (A) Frontal view; (B) Lateral view

Lymph nodes of the pelvic region, which drain the female genital organs comprise of the groups as shown in the Figures 1.1.3.1 (A and B). These lymph node groups include the inguinal group, hypogastric group, external iliac group, internal iliac group, sacral group, common iliac group, pararectal group of lymph nodes and the lumbar group.

The cervix drains primarily into the external and internal iliac group of lymph nodes, whereas the body of the uterus drains mainly into the external iliac and lumbar nodes. These drain into the common iliac group, which in turn drain into paraaortic group of lymph nodes. Lymphatic drainage of ovaries is into the paraaortic group of lymph nodes.

1.1.3.2: Lymphatics of Perineum

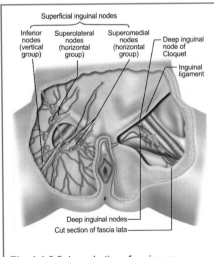

Fig. 1.1.3.2: Lymphatics of perineum

Lymphatic drainage of perineum is shown in the Figure 1.1.3.2 and is primarily into the inguinal group of lymph nodes.

The inguinal group of lymph nodes comprises of a vertical and a horizontal group. The horizontal group is also known as the superficial inguinal group and receives afferent lymphatic vessels from perineum, buttocks, and abdominal wall below the umbilicus, vulva and anus (below the pectinate line). This group of lymph nodes drains into the deep inguinal group. The vertical group of lymph nodes is also known as the deep femoral group and follows the saphenous and femoral veins.

| Picture | Medical/Surgical Description | Management/Clinical Highlights |

1.1.3.3: Lymphatic Drainage of the Breasts

Picture	Medical/Surgical Description	Management/Clinical Highlights
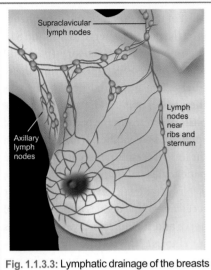 **Fig. 1.1.3.3:** Lymphatic drainage of the breasts	Lymphatic drainage of the breast is described in Figure 1.1.3.3.	Nearly three-fourths of the breast tissue drains into the ipsilateral axillary group of lymph nodes. The drainage is mainly into the pectoral, subscapular and humeral groups of axillary nodes. These eventually drain into the apical and central groups of axillary nodes. The remaining 25% of the breast tissue drains into the parasternal group of lymph nodes. These drain into the lymph nodes of contralateral breast and abdomen.

1.1.4: Nerve Supply

1.1.4.1: Nerve Supply to Pelvis (A and B)

Picture	Medical/Surgical Description	Management/Clinical Highlights
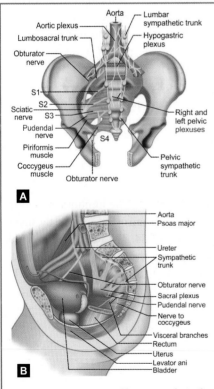 **Figs 1.1.4.1 (A and B):** Nerve supply to the pelvis: (A) Frontal view; (B) Lateral view	The pelvis is innervated mainly by the sacral and coccygeal spinal nerves, and the pelvic part of the autonomic nervous system (Hypogastric plexus). *Hypogastric plexus*: Sympathetic fibers reach the pelvis by downward continuations of the sympathetic trunk and of the aortic plexus. In front of the sacrum, the sympathetic trunks consist largely of preganglionic fibers and present three or four ganglia each. This forms the hypogastric plexus of nerves, which supplies the viscera of pelvic cavity. It is formed by the presacral nerve, which lies in front of sacral promontory and divides into two hypogastric nerves which pass downward and laterally along the pelvic wall. They help to form the inferior hypogastric plexus, which is a diffuse plexus, lying in the region of uterosacral ligaments. This plexus also receives fibers from parasympathetic system comprising of sacral fibers(S2 to S4). The hypogastric plexus divides into two lateral portions called the pelvic plexus. These are situated at the sides of rectum and vagina in females and supply the viscera of pelvis.	The piriformis and coccygeus muscles form a bed for the sacral and coccygeal nerve plexuses. The anterior rami of the S2 and S3 nerves emerge between the digitations of these muscles.

1.1.4.2: Nerve Supply to the Pelvic Floor

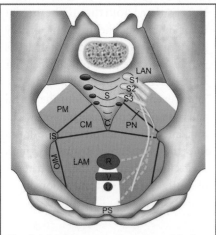

Fig. 1.1.4.2: Nerve supply to the pelvic floor (C, coccyx; CM, coccygeus muscle; IS, ischial spine; LAM, levator ani muscle; OIM, obturator internus muscle; PM, piriformis muscle; PS, pubic symphysis; R, rectum; S, sacrum; U, uterus; V, vagina; LAN levator ani nerve; PN, pudendal nerve)

Figure 1.1.4.2 presents schematic illustration of the pelvic floor, containing the pelvic floor muscles, the levator ani nerve (LAN, light yellow) and the pudendal nerves (PN, dark yellow).

Most of the innervation of the perineum is by the pudendal nerve (S2, S3 and S4). It contains motor, sensory (pain and reflex), and postganglionic sympathetic fibers. The pudendal nerve traverses the greater sciatic foramen below the piriformis, crosses the back of the ischial spine, and enters the perineum through the lesser sciatic foramen. It traverses the pudendal canal in the lateral wall of the ischiorectal fossa, gives off the inferior rectal nerve, and divides into the perineal nerve and the dorsal nerve of the penis (or clitoris). The perineal nerve divides into a deep branch, which supplies the perineal muscles and a superficial branch, which supplies the labium majus in females (or scrotum in males). The pudendal nerve also supplies the external urethral sphincter, whereas the internal urethral sphincter is innervated by the pelvic nerve (part of parasympathetic system). An abnormality in the neuroanatomical integrity of the pelvic floor and its muscles is likely to result in urinary and/or fecal incontinence as well as pelvic organ prolapse.

1.1.4.3: Sacral Plexus

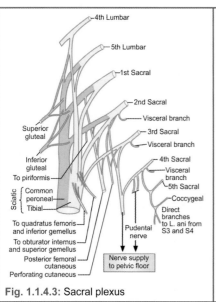

Fig. 1.1.4.3: Sacral plexus

The sacral plexus (Figure 1.1.4.3), which lies in the front of piriformis, supplies most of the pelvic structures, buttocks and lower limbs. It lies on the back of the pelvis between the piriformis muscle and the pelvic fascia.

It is formed by the lumbosacral trunk, the ventral rami of S1 to S3 and the upper division of S4. The lumbosacral trunk comprises the whole of the anterior division of the V and a part of the IV lumbar nerve.

1.2: EMBRYOLOGY

1.2.1: Development of Human Embryo

1.2.1.1: Structure of Male Gamete

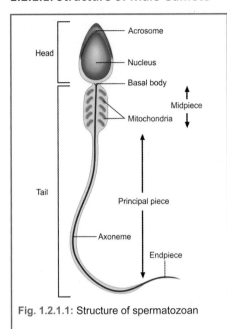

Fig. 1.2.1.1: Structure of spermatozoan

Figure 1.2.1.1 demonstrates the structure of a human spermatozoan, which comprises of four main parts: head, neck, middle piece and tail.

Head: Head is a conical structure containing an acrosome and nucleus enclosed by a thin membrane. Acrosome releases tissue dissolving lytic enzymes, such as hyaluronidase, which help in penetrating the ovum. The nucleus contains closely packed DNA and proteins.

Neck: The short neck contains two centrioles: proximal and distal. Proximal centriole is introduced into the egg during fertilization and helps in initiating cleavage of the zygote. The distal centriole helps in providing attachment to the axial filament of sperm tail.

Middle piece: Middle piece comprises of tightly-coiled mitochondrion which contains oxidative enzymes and helps in providing motility to the sperms.

Tail or flagellum: It comprises of a central axial filament (made up of nine pairs of longitudinal fibers, extending up to the tip of axial filament).

1.2.1.2: Internal Structure of Testes

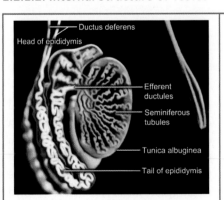

Fig. 1.2.1.2: Internal structure of testes

The testes are male gonads, responsible for producing sperms and male hormone, mainly testosterone. Internal structure of testes is shown in the Figure 1.2.1.2. In males two testes are present, one in each scrotal sac.

Each testis is surrounded by a fibrous capsule or tunica albuginea and comprises of numerous lobules. Each lobule contains one or more convoluted tubule known as the seminiferous tubule, where the sperms are formed. Spermatogenesis occurs under the effect of hormone testosterone, which is produced by interstitial cells of Leydig. Various seminiferous tubules join to form approximately 20 small ducts, which pierce the fibrous capsule to enter the head of epididymis. These ducts eventually join up and become continuous with ductus deferens, which begins at the lower end of epididymis.

1.2.1.3: Male Gametogenesis

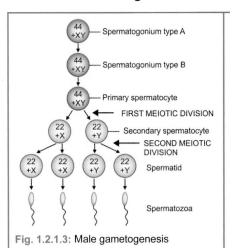

Fig. 1.2.1.3: Male gametogenesis

The process in which spermatogonia gets transformed into spermatozoon is known as spermatogenesis and is primarily under the control of follicle stimulating hormone (FSH) and testosterone. It involves the production of sperms. Initial process of spermatogenesis involves mitotic division, which is responsible for converting spermatogonia to primary spermatocytes. The spermatozoa then develop through a process of meiosis so that eventually diploid spermatocytes get converted into four haploid spermatids. Stages of spermatogenesis are described in the adjacent figure.

The spermatids eventually transform into spermatozoa by a process known as spermiogenesis. Testosterone, which plays an important role in the facilitation of spermatogenesis, is synthesized in the interstitial Leydig cells from where it diffuses into the seminiferous tubules.

1.2.1.4: Structure of Female Gamete

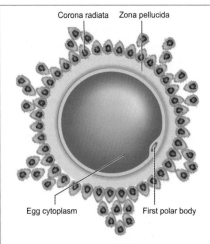

Fig. 1.2.1.4: Structure of female gamete (ovum)

An ovum is a haploid cell, containing a nucleus (germinal vesicle) and cytoplasm (ooplasm or yolk). The ovum is surrounded by a thick envelope called zona pellucida, which is radially striated. Zona pellucida may persist for some time postfertilization, following which it disappears. It provides protection to the zygote during the early stages of cell division. Present on the outer surface of ovum are several layers of cells (derived from the follicle), which continue to stick on the surface of ovum as it is extruded out of the follicle.

A mature human ovum is released as a result of the rupture of a follicle at the time of ovulation. It is conveyed via the fallopian tubes into the uterine cavity where it may be fertilized by the sperm. If fertilization does not occur, the ovum does not undergo further maturation and degenerates. In case of fertilization, the ovum fuses with a sperm resulting in formation of a zygote, which develops into an embryo in future.

1.2.1.5: Internal Structure of Ovary

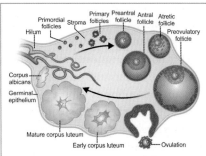

Fig. 1.2.1.5: Internal structure of the ovary

Inside the ovary, various follicles are present in different stages of development (as shown in Figure 1.2.1.5). This may include primordial follicle, primary follicle, preantral follicle, antral follicle, preovulatory follicle, etc. Following ovulation and the extrusion of ovum, the ovarian follicle gets converted into corpus luteum. If pregnancy does not occur, corpus luteum eventually becomes atretic and forms atretic follicle.

During the follicular phase of menstrual cycle, FSH takes control and stimulates a cohort of follicles encouraging them to develop up to the preantral stage. Out of the various developing follicles, only one single (preovulatory) follicle is destined to develop into a dominant follicle, which eventually undergoes ovulation.

Picture	Medical/Surgical Description	Management/Clinical Highlights

1.2.1.6: Ovulation from the Dominant Follicle

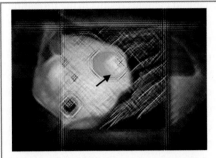 Fig. 1.2.1.6: Ovulation from dominant follicle (indicated by arrow)	Ovulation takes place as the ovarian follicle ruptures and the discharged oocyte is carried into the peritoneal cavity via the uterine tube. Once the oocyte has been extruded out, the cells of the empty ovarian follicle get converted into the corpus luteum. Corpus luteum produces progesterone for about 14 days, in absence of fertilization and for 3–4 months if fertilization has taken place, after which it eventually dies off.	Just prior to ovulation, a surge of luteinizing hormone (LH) occurs. The presence of LH in the follicle prior to ovulation is important for optimal follicular development, which in due course results in the formation of a healthy oocyte. LH initiates luteinization and progesterone production in the granulosa layer of ruptured follicle which ultimately results in the formation of corpus luteum.

1.2.1.7: Female Gametogenesis

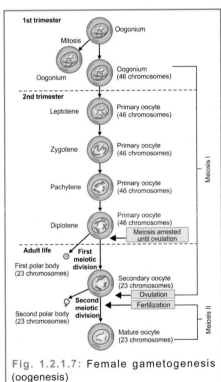 Fig. 1.2.1.7: Female gametogenesis (oogenesis)	Various stages of oogenesis have been described in Figure 1.2.1.7. The primordial germ cells, after arriving in the female gonad, differentiate into oogonia by around 9th week of gestation. These enter the first meiotic division and are converted into primary oocytes.	Progression of meiosis to the diplotene stage is accomplished throughout the pregnancy and is completed by birth. In the last week before birth, all the primary oocytes get arrested in the diplotene stage of prophase. The primary oocytes remain arrested at this stage and do not undergo the completion of first meiotic division till the age of puberty, when the completion of first meiotic division occurs at the time of ovulation. Second meiotic division starts, but gets arrested in the metaphase, which is completed only at the time of fertilization.

1.2.1.8: Fertilization (A to D)

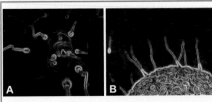 Figs 1.2.1.8 (A and B):(A) Sperms entering the cervical canal; (B) Sperms approaching the ovum	Figure 1.2.1.8 A shows numerous sperms entering the cervical canal. From here they swim up and reach the uterine cavity and ultimately move to the ampulla of fallopian tube. Here, the numerous sperms which have arrived approach the ovum (as shown in the Figure 1.2.1.8B).	While the sperms arrive at the ampulla of fallopian tube, simultaneously the oocyte also moves from the ovary to the uterine tube. It may or may not get fertilized by one of the numerous male gametes approaching it in the ampulla of fallopian tube.

Picture	Medical/Surgical Description	Management/Clinical Highlights

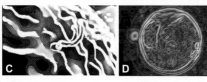

Figs 1.2.1.8 (C and D): (C) Fertilization of the ovum with sperms; (D) Formation of zygote containing the male and female pronuclei (*Source*: Computerized generation of images)

Even though many spermatozoa may approach the oocyte, only one spermatozoon is allowed to enter the oocyte.

It passes the zona pellucida by capacitation and acrosome reaction. Fertilization results in the formation of zygote, which is formed due to the fusion between the male and female pronuclei.

The process of fertilization between two haploid gametes results in the formation of a diploid zygote, thereby restoring the number of chromosomes to that of the normal somatic cell. On fertilization, the chromosomal configuration can be of two types, either 44(XY), i.e. a male child or 44(XX), i.e. a female child. In case fertilization does not occur between the male and female gamete, both the ovum and sperms die off and the uterine endometrium sloughs off, resulting in menstruation.

1.2.1.9: Development of Embryo until the Morula Stage (A to D)

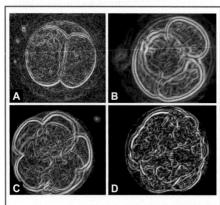

Figs 1.2.1.9 (A to D): (A) Division of the zygote to form a two-celled embryo; (B) Formation of a four-celled embryo; (C) Formation of an eight-celled embryo; (D) Formation of morula (*Source*: Computerized generation of images)

The zygote, a diploid cell with 46 chromosomes, forms as a result of fertilization of the mature egg with a sperm. The zygote then undergoes numerous cleavage divisions to produce cells known as blastomeres as shown in the Figures 1.2.9 (A to D).

At this stage the zygote is present inside the fallopian tube and is surrounded by a thick zona pellucida. For 3 days as the blastomeres continue to divide; they produce a solid, mulberry-like ball of cells. This 16-celled ball is called morula.

The morula enters the uterine cavity approximately 3 days after fertilization and floats around in the cavity for a few more days. During this time, fluid gradually accumulates between the morula's cells, transforming the morula into a blastocyst.

1.2.1.10: Development of Embryo (until Implantation) (A to C)

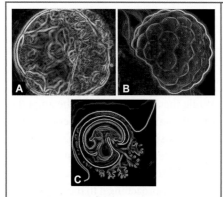

Figs 1.2.1.10 (A to C): (A) Formation of inner cell mass; (B) Implantation of embryo; (C) Internal view of implanted embryo (*Source*: Computerized generation of images)

Once the morula is formed, fluid gradually accumulates between the morula's cells, transforming the morula into a blastocyst. When the blastocyst reaches 58-celled stage at about 4th–5th day of fertilization, it gets transformed into two types of cells: (1) trophoblast cells and (2) an inner cell mass. Implantation begins with the burrowing of the blastocyst into the endometrium, which occurs by about 6–7 days after fertilization.

The inner cell mass (consisting of blastomeres) is destined to form the various tissues of the embryo. The trophoblast comprises of outer single layer of flattened cells, which later get converted into the future placenta. The cavity of the blastocyst is called the blastocele.

Picture	Medical/Surgical Description	Management/Clinical Highlights

1.2.1.11: Development of Embryo from Implantation up to Day Eight (A to D)

Picture	Medical/Surgical Description	Management/Clinical Highlights
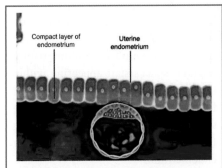 Fig. 1.2.1.11A: Attachment of blastocyst to the surface endometrium [*Source (A to D)*: Computerized generation of images]	Prior to implantation, the blastocyst starts getting attached to the surface endometrium.	Attachment of the blastocyst to the surface endometrium occurs by 5th–6th day postfertilization.
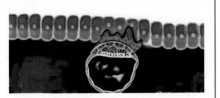 Fig. 1.2.1.11B: Penetration of the blastocyst	Implantation begins with the burrowing and penetration of the blastocyst into the endometrium, which occurs by about 6–7 days after fertilization.	The most common site of implantation is upper posterior wall of the uterine cavity
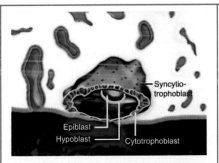 Fig. 1.2.1.11C: Fourth to fifth day of implantation	By fourth to fifth day of implantation, the trophoblast gets differentiated into an outer multinucleated syncytium known as syncytiotrophoblast and an inner layer of cytotrophoblasts. As the trophoblastic cells invade deeper into the endometrium, by 10th day postfertilization the blastocyst gets totally embedded within the endometrium. The inner cell mass gets differentiated into a top layer: ectoderm (epiblast) and an underlying layer of endoderm (hypoblast). Later, there is appearance of mesodermal cells between the ectoderm and endoderm.	As the blastocyst implants into the uterine wall, simultaneously it also prepares its cells and surrounding endometrium to develop into a placenta.
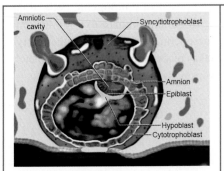 Fig. 1.2.1.11D: Eighth day of implantation	By eighth day of implantation, small cells appear between the embryonic disc and trophoblast enclosing a space that later gets transformed into amniotic cavity.	The ectoderm forms the floor of the amniotic cavity while the roof is formed by aminogenic cells. As the amniotic fluid accumulates in the amniotic cavity, it enlarges.

Picture	Medical/Surgical Description	Management/Clinical Highlights

1.2.1.12: Development of Embryo From Day 9 up to Day 13 of Implantation (A to D)

Picture	Medical/Surgical Description	Management/Clinical Highlights
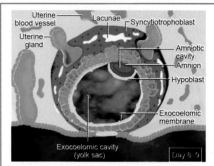 Fig. 1.2.1.12A: Ninth day of implantation	By 9th day of implantation, the endodermal germ layer produces additional cells which form a new cavity, known as the primary umbilical vesicle or definitive yolk sac.	By 9th day of implantation, the syncytiotrophoblast continues to expand into the surrounding endometrium. Lacunar spaces start appearing within the syncytiotrophoblast and these start filling with maternal blood. Also, during this period, primary villi start extending from the trophoblast into the surrounding endometrium.
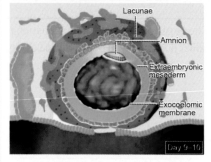 Fig. 1.2.1.12B: Tenth day of implantation	By 10th day of implantation, small embryonic mesenchymal cells appear as isolated cells within the cavity of blastocyst. They soon line the cavity of blastocyst. When the blastocyst is completely lined with mesoderm, it is termed as chorionic vesicle.	By the 10th day of implantation, the blastocyst completely penetrates below the surface of decidua. The part of decidua at the site of the fetal portion gets transformed into chorion frondosum (the fetal precursor of mature placenta), whereas the maternal part is known as decidua basalis.
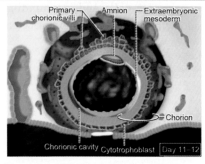 Fig. 1.2.1.12C: Eleventh to twelfth day of implantation	By 12th day of implantation, numerous small cavities appear within the extraembryonic mesoderm. These cavities soon become confluent and form the extraembryonic coelom.	The presence of extraembryonic coelom splits the extraembryonic mesoderm into two layers: (1) the extraembryonic somatopleuric mesoderm, lining the trophoblast and amnion and (2) the extraembryonic splanchnopleuric mesoderm, covering the yolk sac.
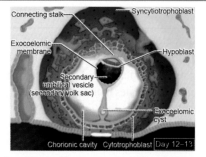 Fig. 1.2.1.12D: Twelfth to thirteenth day of implantation	With the development of extraembryonic coelom, the yolk sac becomes much smaller and is known as the secondary yolk sac.	The membrane called amnion is composed of amniogenic cells along with somatopleuric extraembryonic mesoderm. As the folding of the embryo takes place, amniotic cavity completely surrounds the embryo.

| Picture | Medical/Surgical Description | Management/Clinical Highlights |

1.2.1.13: Stages of Further Embryo Development (A to D)

Picture	Medical/Surgical Description	Management/Clinical Highlights
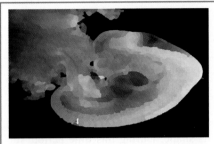 Fig. 1.2.1.13A: Third to fourth week of embryo development	As the embryo grows, there is enlargement of the amniotic cavity, resulting in progressive reduction in the size of extraembryonic coelom. Eventually the extraembryonic coelom completely disappears, causing the amnion to come in contact with chorion and fuse with it to form the chorioamniotic membrane.	On the dorsal side of embryo, contours of first four to twelve somites can be recognized. At the same time, there occurs development of abdominal wall and first two pharyngeal arches (mandibular and hyoid arches). Cervical and caudal flexures appear which give it a characteristic C-shape.
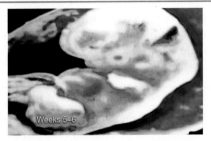 Fig. 1.2.1.13B: Fifth to sixth week of embryo development	In the early stages, the embryo acquires the form of a three-layered disc. These three layers are also called as germ layers, from outside to inward are: ectoderm (outer layer), mesoderm (middle layer) and endoderm (inner layer). These three layers of embryo are responsible for the formation of different organ systems and tissues giving the embryo more "human-like" appearance.	During the 5th week of life, there is development of neural tube from ectoderm, which results in the formation of brain, spinal cord and nerves. The ectoderm also results in the formation of nails, tooth, enamel, skin and hair. Mesoderm forms the heart and circulatory system. Mesoderm also results in the formation of cartilage, bone, etc. Endoderm forms the various organ systems in the body.
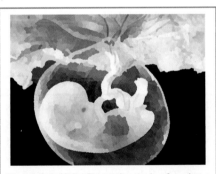 Fig. 1.2.1.13C: Seventh week of embryo development	By 7th week of development, the limb buds start growing, the mouth opening appears and the inner ear is formed.	During the 7th week of development, the digestive tract starts developing and the organs such as lungs, liver, pancreas and thyroid glands are formed. The heart starts beating, but there is only one chamber at that time.
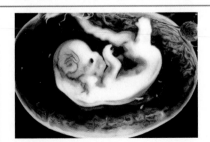 Fig. 1.2.1.13D: Eighth week of embryo development [*Source (A to D)*: Computerized generation of images]	During the 8th week of development, the limbs have grown to full length, and the hands and feet buds start appearing. The stomach is also formed.	At 8 weeks of development, the baby's face begins to take a more definite shape because baby's mouth and nostrils have developed. Teeth begin to develop under the gums. Eyes develop in form of small hollows on each side of the head.

1.2.1.14: Stages of Embryo Development as Observed Through Ultrasound Examination

This has been discussed in details in Section 7.

1.2.1.15: Fetal Development up to Six Months of Pregnancy (A to D)

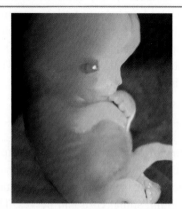

Fig. 1.2.1.15A: Ten-weeks-old fetus

When the embryo becomes about 10 weeks old, it is known as a "fetus". During this period, the development of upper and lower limbs is almost complete. Development of upper limbs occurs faster than that of lower limbs. By the end of 9th week, formation of fingers and toes is almost complete.

Physiological midgut herniation occurs, which becomes normal by 10th week. Nipples and hair follicles begin to form during this time. The neck begins to take its shape. During this time period, the fetus starts moving because the muscles also have developed by this time. The internal sex organs such as ovaries and testes have developed. The head of the fetus is still much larger in comparison to the chest.

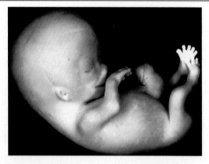

Fig. 1.2.1.15B: Twelve-weeks-old fetus

During the 12th week of gestation, the fetus becomes about 6 cm in size and starts moving spontaneously. By 12 weeks of gestation, fetal sex can also be distinguished. The fetus now starts resembling the baby's face. The fetal heart can be heard using a Doppler ultrasound.

By 12 weeks, the number of fetal fingers and toes can be counted. The baby's fingers and toe nails also appear during this time. The pancreas start functioning and producing insulin. Since the baby's brain has started developing during this time, it can feel pain.

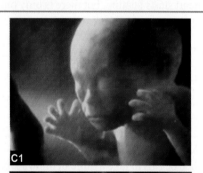

C1

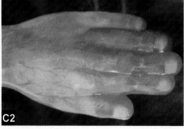

C2

Figs 1.2.1.15 (C1 and C2): Twenty-weeks-old fetus

By 20 weeks of pregnancy, the growth of hair begins on the rest of the body. The skin starts getting thicker and development of various sense organs starts occurring.

By 20 weeks of gestation, the baby is able to hear and recognize mother's voice. The mother is likely to start perceiving the fetal movements by this time. The baby's heart rate can now be heard with a stethoscope. Until 20 weeks of gestation, the baby's crown rump length is measured, following which the baby's crown heel length is measured.

Picture	Medical/Surgical Description	Management/Clinical Highlights
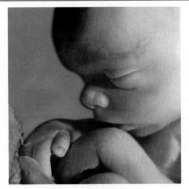 Fig. 1.2.1.15D: Twenty-four-weeks-old fetus	By 24 weeks of gestation, the baby's eyelids can be seen clearly. The baby starts gaining weight at the rate of 3 ounces per week mainly due to an increase in the bone/muscle mass. The baby's body gets covered with fine lanugo hair. The development of taste buds and appearance of creases on the palms occur during this time.	Twenty weeks can be considered as the period of gestation when the baby becomes clinically viable and is likely to survive if born. Development of the surfactant producing cells in the lungs starts occurring during this period. The baby starts breathing and may start inhaling the amniotic fluid. The fetal activities which had appeared at 20 weeks of gestation (1.2.1.15C) become even more defined at 24 weeks.

1.2.1.16: Fetal Development from Eight Months of Pregnancy till Term (A to D)

Picture	Medical/Surgical Description	Management/Clinical Highlights
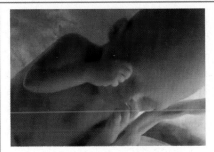 Fig. 1.2.1.16A: Thirty-two-weeks-old fetus	At 32 weeks of gestation, the fetal weight is about 1.7−1.8 kg and fetal length is about 42−44 cm. The nails of the toes have formed completely and the hair on the head continues to grow. During this time, the baby's reproductive development continues to occur. In boys, the testes start descending from their location near the kidneys in the abdomen into scrotal sacs. In girls, the clitoris becomes prominent.	During this time, there is accumulation of subcutaneous fat in the body. Since the baby has grown larger in size by this time, its movements inside the uterine cavity may slightly decrease due to a reduction in space.
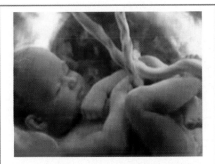 Fig. 1.2.1.16B: Thirty-six-weeks-old fetus	At 35 weeks of gestation, further accumulation of fat occurs on the arms and legs to help the baby regulate its temperature. The baby's face becomes chubbier due to the accumulation of subcutaneous fat. Creases begin to form on baby's neck and palms. The baby's weight is about 2.3–2.5 kg and the length is about 45−48 cm. In the male babies, by 35 weeks of gestation, the testes have completely descended into the scrotum.	During this phase, the baby may start growing at the rate of 1 ounce per day. The mother may experience lightening during this stage. This refers to a slight reduction in the fundal height due to the engagement of baby's head inside the pelvis in case of vertex presentation. The baby is able to recognize the mother's voice and may respond to loud noises by kicking its limbs.
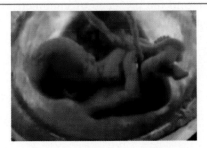 Fig. 1.2.1.16C: Forty-weeks-old fetus	By 39–40 weeks of gestation, most of the lanugo hair has disappeared, with a little amount remaining over the shoulders, arms and legs. During this period, the lungs are maturing and the amount of surfactant is increasing.	The baby's length becomes about 50−52 cm and weight becomes about 3.0−3.2 kg. Accumulation of fat (particularly that of brown fat, required for thermogenesis) continues to occur during this phase.

Picture	Medical/Surgical Description	Management/Clinical Highlights
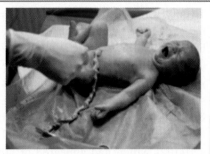 Fig. 1.2.1.16D: Full term fetus at the time of delivery	Full term fetus is ready for life outside the uterine cavity. At birth, the length of a full term fetus is about 20 inches and the weight is about 2.7–4.0 kg. The health "term baby" is capable of independent survival outside the uterine cavity.	After birth as the placenta detaches from the uterine cavity and the umbilical circulation ceases to work, the baby takes its first breath of fresh air in the outside world. Changes in the circulatory system take place and the deoxygenated blood now starts moving toward the lungs.

1.2.2: Development of Placenta

1.2.2.1: Placental Structure

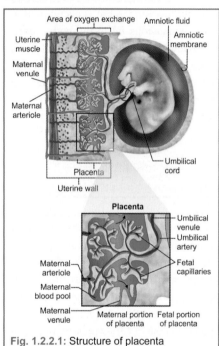 Fig. 1.2.2.1: Structure of placenta	The placenta is an organ with dual origin from both fetus and mother. A part of placenta develops from fetal chorion, and the rest develops from maternal endometrium.	The human placenta is rounded and discoidal in shape; the average diameter of the placenta being about 15–20 cm and weight about 500 g. Despite the small size of a placenta, the surface area available for maternal-fetal exchange is greatly large due to the presence of villi.

1.2.2.2: Surfaces of Placenta (A and B)

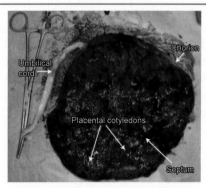 Fig. 1.2.2.2A:Maternal surface of placenta	Figure 1.2.2.2A shows maternal surface of placenta. The placental cotyledons are visible on the maternal side of the placenta.	The placental cotyledons are formed due to the presence of endometrial projections called septa.

Picture	Medical/Surgical Description	Management/Clinical Highlights
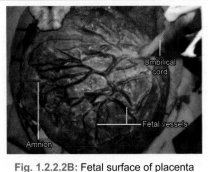 **Fig. 1.2.2.2B:** Fetal surface of placenta	Figure 1.2.2.2B shows fetal surface of placenta. On the fetal side, the placenta shows a flat surface due to the presence of a smooth chorion.	The umbilical cord is attached at the center of the fetal surface of placenta.

1.2.2.3: Functions of Placenta

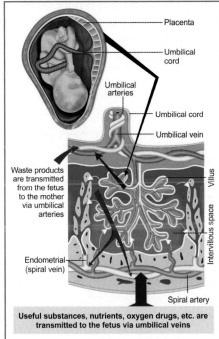 **Fig. 1.2.2.3:** Various functions performed by the placenta	Functions of the placenta: • *Transportation*: Placenta plays an important role in facilitating transport of various substances between the mother and the fetus. • *Endocrine functions*: Placenta is also a major endocrine organ. In almost all mammals, the placenta synthesizes and secretes the hormones progestins and estrogens, chorionic gonadotropins, relaxin, and placental lactogens. Placental hormones have profound effects on both fetal and maternal physiology. • *Immunological functions*	Substances transferred to fetal umbilical veins from maternal endometrial arteries include nutrients (such as oxygen, water, glucose, amino acids, lipids, minerals, etc.), drugs (medicines taken by the mother), harmful substances of abuse (nicotine, alcohol, cocaine, etc.) and infections [such as rubella, cytomegalovirus (CMV)], etc. Waste products such as CO_2, uric acid, bilirubin, etc. move from fetal umbilical arteries to the mother via endometrial veins and are excreted from mother's lungs and kidneys.

1.2.2.4: Placental Development

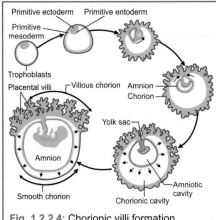 **Fig. 1.2.2.4:** Chorionic villi formation	As the blastocyst with its surrounding trophoblasts grows and expands into the decidua, the outer pole of the mass expands outward towards the endometrial cavity. The chorionic villi over this part gradually disappear, resulting in the formation of chorion laeve. The villi over the opposite, innermost pole proliferate. This results in the formation of placenta comprising of villous trophoblasts and anchoring cytotrophoblasts.	Each primary chorionic villus divides at least five times, forming villous trees. This leads to the formation of extremely large number of terminal villi, resulting in a large surface area, all of which is bathed in the uterine blood. Blood present in the intervillous spaces comes through the maternal endometrial arteries. The chorionic villi comprises of fetal blood as it contains branches of umbilical vein and umbilical arteries.

1.2.2.5: Decidualization

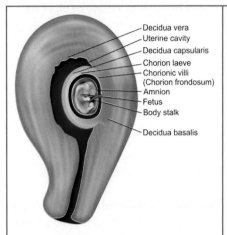

Fig. 1.2.2.5: Process of decidua formation

Following implantation, the syncytio-trophoblast starts secreting the hormone hCG. Under the influence of this hormone, secretory changes taking place in the endometrial lining are further intensified resulting in conversion of endometrial lining into specialized cells which are known as the decidua. This reaction is known as decidual reaction and endometrium is known as decidua. By the 10th day of implantation, the blastocyst completely penetrates below the surface of decidua.

The part of decidua at the site of the fetal portion gets transformed into chorion frondosum (the fetal precursor of mature placenta), whereas the maternal part is known as decidua basalis. The decidua at this stage can be classified into three portions. The side lying in contact with the blastocyst at the site of implantation is the decidua basalis; the decidua lying over the surface of the implanted blastocyst is the decidua capsularis; and the remainder of the decidua lining the inside of the uterus is the decidua vera.

1.2.2.6: Placental Villus Formation

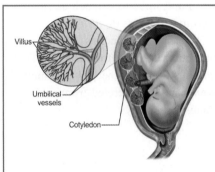

Fig. 1.2.2.6: Formation of placental villi

The chorionic villi are the finger-like projections arising from chorion and serve as precursors of human placenta. In the early pregnancy, the villi are distributed over the entire periphery of the chorionic membrane. The chorionic villi in contact with decidua basalis, proliferate to form chorion frondosum, the fetal component of the placenta.

Chorionic villi of the placenta primarily function to transfer oxygen and other important nutrients between mother and fetus.

1.2.2.7: Circulation in the Umbilical Cord

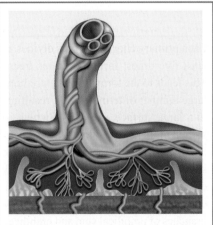

Fig. 1.2.2.7: Blood circulation in the umbilical cord

Blood circulation in the umbilical cord is described in Figure 1.2.2.7. The umbilical cord contains two umbilical arteries and one umbilical vein. Umbilical arteries carry deoxygenated blood from the fetus to the mother. On the other hand, umbilical veins supply oxygenated blood from the mother to the fetus.

Umbilical arteries are the only arteries in the body which carry deoxygenated blood and umbilical veins are the only veins in the body carrying oxygenated blood.

Picture	Medical/Surgical Description	Management/Clinical Highlights

1.2.2.8: Stages of Development of Placental Villi (A to C)

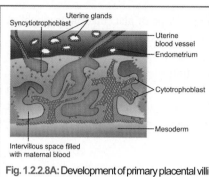 **Fig. 1.2.2.8A:** Development of primary placental villi	The development of chorionic villi passes through three stages: primary, secondary and finally tertiary. Figure 1.2.2.8A illustrates development of primary villi.	Primary villi comprises of solid villi composed of cytotrophoblast core, which is surrounded by syncytium.
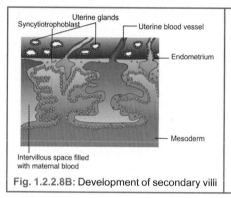 **Fig. 1.2.2.8B:** Development of secondary villi	Figure 1.2.2.8B shows the development of secondary villi, which progresses from the primary villi.	Secondary villi are formed when embryonic mesoderm has invaded the solid trophoblast columns of primary villi.
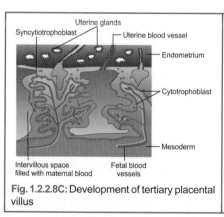 **Fig. 1.2.2.8C:** Development of tertiary placental villus	Figure 1.2.2.8B shows the development of tertiary villi, which progresses from the secondary villi.	In tertiary villi, there is occurrence of angiogenesis in the mesenchymal core of secondary villi.

1.2.2.9: Cytotrophoblastic Shell

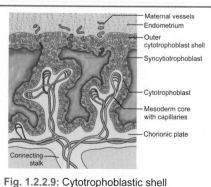 **Fig. 1.2.2.9:** Cytotrophoblastic shell	With increasing gestation, the cells of the cytotrophoblast in the tertiary villi proliferate and pass through the syncytiotrophoblast at the tip of the villi resulting in the formation of a continuous layer of cytotrophoblasts on the surface of decidua which is known as the cytotrophoblastic shell.	Cytotrophoblastic shell helps in attaching the maternal and fetal components to one another. This helps in fixing the chorionic villi to the decidua. Thus, the tertiary villi at one end are continuous with fetal component (chorion) and to the maternal component (decidua) at the other end.

1.2.2.10: Different Types of Placenta (A to C)

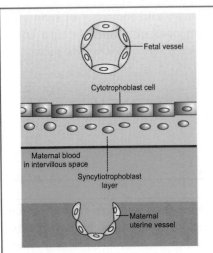

Fig. 1.2.2.10A: Hemochorial placenta

In hemochorial placenta, the word "hemo" stands for maternal blood, which directly bathes the lacunae present in syncytiotrophoblast. On the other hand, the word "chorio" stands for chorion placenta, which in turn is separated from fetal blood by the endothelial lining of fetal capillaries that traverse the villous core.

In this type of placentation, trophoblast cells causing rupture and release of blood into the intervillous space infiltrate maternal uterine blood vessels. Hemochorial placenta is present in humans, monkeys, rodents and most primates.

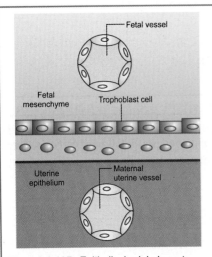

Fig. 1.2.2.10B: Epitheliochorial placenta

In epitheliochorial placenta, the trophoblast cells of the placenta are in direct apposition with the surface epithelial cells of the uterus but there is no trophoblast cell invasion beyond this layer.

Epitheliochorial placenta is commonly present in ruminants such as cattle, sheep, goats, etc.

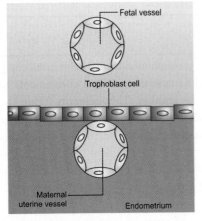

Fig. 1.2.2.10C: Endotheliochorial placenta

In endotheliochorial placenta, the uterine epithelium is breached and trophoblast cells are in direct contact with endothelial cells of maternal uterine blood vessels.

This type of placenta is most commonly present in carnivores such as dog, cat, etc.

Picture	Medical/Surgical Description	Management/Clinical Highlights

1.2.2.11: Trophoblastic Invasion of Spiral Vessels During Pregnancy

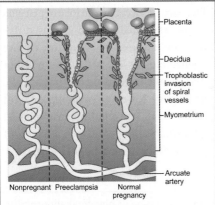Fig. 1.2.2.11: Trophoblastic invasion of spiral vessels during pregnancy	Due to trophoblastic invasion of maternal spiral vessels, there occurs a significant increase in placental intervillous oxygen tension, and hence maternal perfusion of the placenta, between 8 weeks and 12 weeks of gestation. Coincident with this increased perfusion and oxygen tension within the placenta between 8 weeks and 12 weeks, there is a corresponding increase in antioxidant systems, presumably to counteract the oxidative stress of the increased intervillous perfusion and oxygen tension.	The process of decidualization (as described previously) helps in protecting the mother from excessive invasion by the trophoblasts. This not only restricts the movement of invasive trophoblasts by forming a physical barrier, it also helps in local production of cytokines that acts as inhibitor of invasion and helps in promoting trophoblast attachment rather than invasion.

1.2.2.12: Normal Placental Implantation

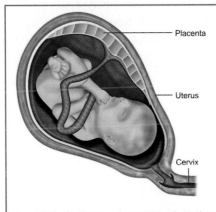Fig. 1.2.2.12: Normal placental implantation	Figure 1.2.2.12 shows normal placental implantation.	Implantation most commonly occurs on the upper wall of the uterine cavity, with posterior wall being more commonly involved in comparison to the anterior wall.

1.2.2.13: Abnormal Implantation of Placenta into the Lower Uterine Segment

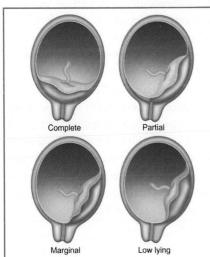Fig. 1.2.2.13: Abnormal implantation of placenta into the lower uterine segment	Figure 1.2.2.13 shows abnormal implantation of the placenta in the lower uterine segment. Another type of abnormal implantation can be extrauterine implantation, which may take place at an extrauterine site, commonly the fallopian tube, resulting in the development of ectopic pregnancy.	If the blastocyst gets implanted in the lower uterine segment, it results in a condition called placenta previa. In this condition the placenta may cover the internal os partially or completely. Management of placenta previa has been discussed in Section 4.

Picture	Medical/Surgical Description	Management/Clinical Highlights

1.2.2.14: Placental Abnormalities (A to C)

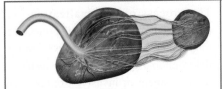 Fig. 1.2.2.14A: Succenturiate lobe of placenta	As shown in the adjacent diagram, succenturiate lobe of placenta is a morphological anomaly where the main part of placenta is connected to one or more accessory lobes through blood vessels.	Presence of succenturiate lobe of placenta is not associated with an increased risk of fetal anomalies. Rupture of the connecting vessels at the time of labor may result in fetal death. In case the accessory lobes of placenta are not recognized, placental material can be retained, resulting in an increased risk of postpartum hemorrhage (PPH).
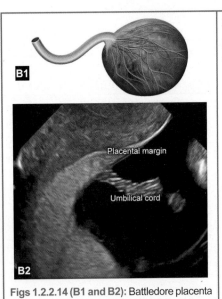 B1 / Placental margin / Umbilical cord / B2 / Figs 1.2.2.14 (B1 and B2): Battledore placenta	This is a morphological anomaly of placenta where the umbilical cord is attached to the placental edge.	It is a rare type of placental abnormality which is not associated with coincidental fetal anomalies. It does not affect the functioning of placenta in any way. The condition is commonly discovered at the time of delivery. This condition is usually associated with an increased risk of cord rupture at the time of delivery, resulting in massive PPH.
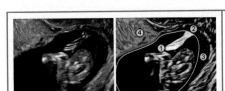 C1 / C2 / Figs 1.2.2.14 (C1 and C2): Velamentous insertion of the cord: (C1) Transvaginal ultrasound image showing umbilical cord attached to the amnion; (C2) Diagrammatic representation of the same 1:Umbilical cord; 2: Cord insertion into the amnion; 3: Placenta; 4: amnion (*Source:* Computerized generation of image C2)	In case of velamentous insertion of cord, the umbilical cord inserts into the fetal membranes (chorion levae) and then travels within the membranes (amnion and chorion) to the placenta. Since the exposed vessels are not surrounded by Wharton's jelly, they are prone to rupture. If the umbilical vessels are present near the cervical os, this condition is known as vasa previa (see Section 4). These vessels are more likely to rupture during labor.	Velamentous insertion of cord is commonly present in the cases of monochorionic twins or triplets. Ultrasound is able to accurately diagnose these cases in the second trimester, with a specificity of 100%. In these cases, presence of vasa previa must be ruled out. Careful fetal monitoring must be done in the third trimester. In case of velamentous cord insertion in the lower segment or vasa previa, the baby must be delivered by an elective cesarean section in order to prevent fetal death.

1.2.3: Development of Fetal Circulation

1.2.3.1: Fetal Circulation Just Before Birth (A to C)

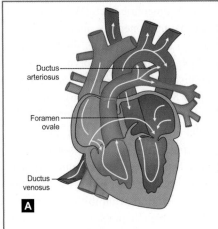

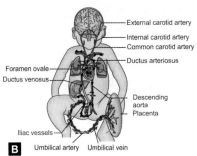

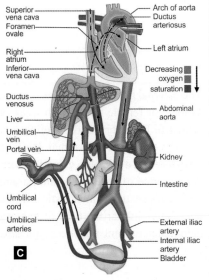

Figs 1.2.3.1 (A to C): Fetal circulation just before birth

Fetal circulation is characterized by presence of three shunts: ductus venosus, foramen ovale and ductus arteriosus. These shunts permit the blood to bypass the liver and lungs, and shunt the most oxygenated blood from the right to the left side of the heart.

These shunts disappear following the birth of the baby. Also, in the fetus the lungs are not fully developed, therefore exchange between the oxygenated and deoxygenated blood does not take place in the lungs. Rather it takes place in the placenta. Therefore the fetal circulation differs from adult circulation in many ways. In the normal adult heart, all the blood from right atrium moves into the right ventricle and from there through pulmonary arteries to the lungs. On the other hand, in the fetal heart, some but not all blood flows from the right atrium to the right ventricle and then through the pulmonary artery to the lungs. Since the lungs of the fetus are not functioning to oxygenate, only a small amount of blood is required to go there for its adequate growth and development. There is high resistance in the pulmonary vessels that forces most of this blood to flow through the shunt called ductus arteriosus into the descending aorta.

In fetal circulation, the deoxygenated blood from the hypogastric arteries moves into the two umbilical arteries. The umbilical arteries carry the deoxygenated blood from the fetus to the placenta. These arteries on reaching the placenta form numerous branches and enter the chorionic villi, where the exchange with oxygenated blood carried by maternal endometrial arteries takes place. The accompanying branches of umbilical veins in the chorionic villi, which carry the oxygenated blood, drain into umbilical vein, which carries the oxygenated blood to the fetus from placenta. As this oxygenated blood bypasses a shunt called ductus venosus, some of the oxygenated blood goes to the liver, but most of it bypasses the liver and empties directly into the inferior vena cava (IVC). In the IVC, oxygenated blood from umbilical veins mixes with deoxygenated blood returning from the lower extremities, pelvis and kidneys.

As the blood from the inferior vena cava enters the right atrium, a large proportion of it is shunted directly into the left atrium through an opening called the foramen ovale. A small valve called the septum primum, located at the atrial septum, prevents blood from moving in the reverse direction. The oxygenated blood in the left atrium mixes with a small amount of deoxygenated blood returning from the lungs (by means of pulmonary veins), and then enters the left ventricle and ascending aorta. From here the oxygenated blood is supplied to the brain, heart and other parts of the body.

SECTION 1 ❖ GENERAL OBSTETRICS

1.2.4: Development of Reproductive Organs

1.2.4.1: Development of Male and Female Internal Genitalia (A and B)

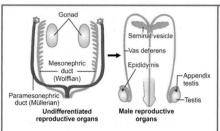

Fig. 1.2.4.1A: Development of male internal genitalia from Wolffian ducts

Gonadal sex is determined by the genetic sex, which is determined by the presence or absence of Y chromosome. Gonadal sex is dependent on the presence of gonads: testes in males and ovaries in females. Gonadal sex controls the development of both internal and external genitalia. Internal genitalia in males comprise of testes, epididymis and vas deferens.

The mesonephric ducts (Wolffian ducts) and paramesonephric ducts (Müllerian ducts) are two discreet duct systems, which coexist in all embryos during the ambisexual period of development (i.e. up to 8 weeks of gestation). Under the influence of testosterone from the Leydig cells of testes, the Wolffian ducts form the epididymis, vas deferens and seminal vesicles (male internal genitalia). The Sertoli cells of testis produce a substance called Müllerian inhibiting substance (MIS), which suppresses the development of Müllerian ducts.

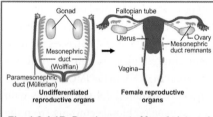

Fig. 1.2.4.1B: Development of female internal genitalia from paramesonephric ducts

Internal genitalia in females comprises of fallopian tubes, uterus and cervix. In the absence of MIS, a substance produced by the Sertoli cells of testis, Müllerian ducts develop passively to form fallopian tubes, uterus and upper vagina as shown in the adjacent picture.

Differentiation of Müllerian ducts occurs in a cephalocaudal direction to form the female internal genital organs.

1.2.4.2: Development of Male and Female External Genitalia (A and B)

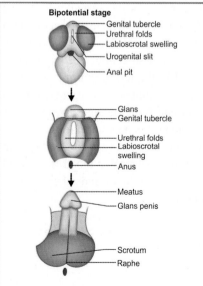

Fig. 1.2.4.2A: Development of male external genitalia

External genitalia persists in bipotential state until 9 weeks of gestation at which time it consists of a genital tubercle, urogenital sinus (UGS) and lateral labioscrotal folds or swellings. Dihydrotestosterone, produced by the testes, determine the development of male external genitalia.

Under the influence of testosterone, the genital tubercle forms the penis; the edges of the UGS fuse to form the penile urethra and the labioscrotal folds fuse to form the scrotum. This process is complete by 12–14 weeks of gestation.

The external genitalia can be recognized as male or female by the 16th week of fetal life by ultrasound examination. The development of external genitalia is controlled by the gonadal sex. Appearance of external genitalia and secondary sexual characteristics, which become visible at the time of puberty help in determining the phenotypic sex.

Picture	Medical/Surgical Description	Management/Clinical Highlights
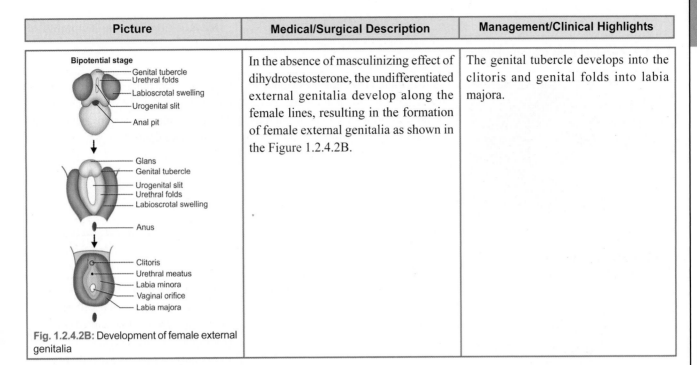 **Fig. 1.2.4.2B:** Development of female external genitalia	In the absence of masculinizing effect of dihydrotestosterone, the undifferentiated external genitalia develop along the female lines, resulting in the formation of female external genitalia as shown in the Figure 1.2.4.2B.	The genital tubercle develops into the clitoris and genital folds into labia majora.

1.2.4.3: Development of Vagina (A to D)

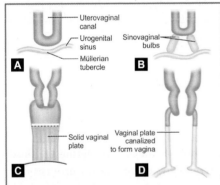 **Figs 1.2.4.3 (A to D):** Development of vagina (Part derived from mesoderm is brown; part derived from endoderm is yellow)	Figures 1.2.4.3 (A to D) show the development of vagina. Figure 1.2.4.3A demonstrates the mesoderm of uterovaginal canal pressing on the posterior wall of the endodermal UGS forming Müllerian tubercle. Proliferation of the endoderm of UGS results in the formation of sinovaginal bulbs (Fig. 1.2.4.3B). Solid vaginal plate is formed due to fusion of mesoderm of uterovaginal canal and endoderm of sinovaginal bulbs (Fig. 1.2.4.3C). Vagina is eventually formed by canalization of this vaginal plate (Fig. 1.2.4.3D).	The UGS, which is of endodermal origin, is derived from the cloaca and it gives rise to caudal two thirds of vagina in females. In males, this may be responsible for the formation of prostate, bulbourethral glands and urethra.

1.3: ANATOMICAL CHANGES DURING PREGNANCY

1.3.1: Changes in Pelvic Organs

1.3.1.1: Jacquemier's Sign

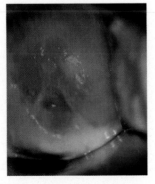 **Fig. 1.3.1.1:** Jacquemier's sign	Jacquemier's sign, also known as Chadwick's sign, is shown in Figure 1.3.1.1. It is sign of pregnancy and can be observed on vaginal or cervical mucosa.	In this sign the vaginal walls show a bluish discoloration as a result of congestion of pelvic blood vessels during pregnancy. This sign can be observed by 8–10 weeks of gestation.

Picture	Medical/Surgical Description	Management/Clinical Highlights

1.3.1.2: Cervical Sign (Goodell's Sign)

	Cervical sign, also known as Goodell's sign, usually is shown in Figure 1.3.1.2. This sign becomes apparent by 6th week of gestation in a primipara and even earlier in a multipara.	In this sign, softening of the cervix causes it to become like lips of the mouth. On the other hand, the nonpregnant cervix may feel like tip of the nose.
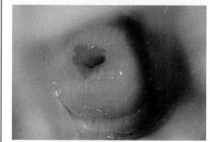 Fig. 1.3.1.2: Cervical sign (Goodell's Sign)		

1.3.1.3: Hegar's Sign in the Uterus

	Figure 1.3.1.3 demonstrates Hegar's sign, which can be elicited in the first trimester of pregnancy.	At 6–8 weeks of gestation, the cervix is firm in contrast to the soft isthmus and fundus. Due to the marked softness of uterine isthmus, cervix and body of uterus may appear as separate organs. As a result, the isthmus of the uterus can be compressed between the fingers palpating vagina and abdomen, which is known as Hegar's sign.
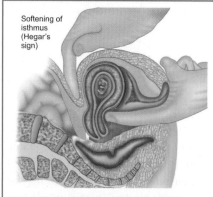 Softening of isthmus (Hegar's sign) Fig. 1.3.1.3: Hegar's sign in the uterus		

1.3.1.4: Development of Uterus During Various Stages of Pregnancy

	As shown in Figure 1.3.1.4, with the advancement of pregnancy, progressive enlargement of the lower abdomen occurs due to the growing uterus.	In normal pregnancy, during the third trimester, there occurs progressive enlargement of the abdomen, which can result in development of symptoms of mechanical discomfort such as palpitations and dyspnea.
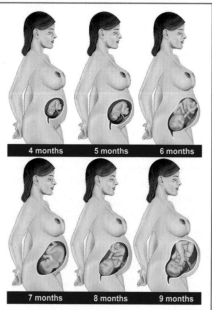 4 months 5 months 6 months 7 months 8 months 9 months Fig. 1.3.1.4: Development of uterus during various stages of pregnancy		

Picture	Medical/Surgical Description	Management/Clinical Highlights

1.3.1.5: Changes in Fundal Height with Period of Gestation

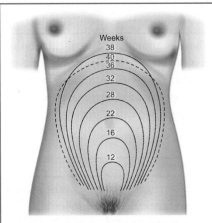 **Fig. 1.3.1.5:** Changes in fundal height with the period of gestation	The rough estimation of fundal height with increasing period of gestation is shown in Figure 1.3.1.5.	In the first few weeks of pregnancy, there is primarily an increase in the anterior-posterior diameter of the uterus. By 12 weeks, the uterus becomes globular and attains a size of approximately 8 cm. From the second trimester onward, the uterine height starts corresponding to the period of gestation.

1.3.1.6: Changes in the Amniotic Fluid Volume with Increasing Gestation

Kindly refer to Section 4 (4.5.1.5).

1.3.1.7: External Ballottement

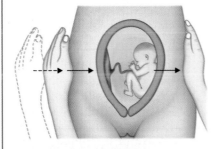 **Fig. 1.3.1.7:** External ballottement	Nowadays external ballottement is rarely used for diagnosing pregnancy. A sharp tap is given with the forefingers of clinician's right hand on the left side of patient's abdominal wall. The presence of fetus can be felt by the return impact of the tossing fetus on the clinician's left hand placed on the patient's right abdominal wall.	External ballottement can be elicited as early as 20th week of gestation because the size of fetus is relatively smaller in comparison to the amount of amniotic fluid. It may be difficult to elicit this sign in woman who are obese or who have a reduced volume of amniotic fluid.

1.3.1.8: Internal Ballottement

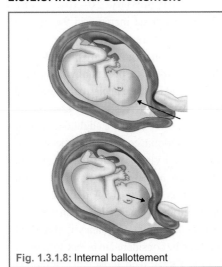 **Fig. 1.3.1.8:** Internal ballottement	This has now become an obsolete method for diagnosis of pregnancy. Forefingers of the clinician's right hand are placed in the patient's anterior fornix of vagina. Using these fingers a sharp tap is made against the lower segment of the uterus. If the fetus is present, it gets tossed upward and as it falls back it can be observed to strike against the wall of uterus, if the fingers are in the vagina.	Internal ballottement can be elicited between 16 weeks and 28 weeks of gestation.

Picture	Medical/Surgical Description	Management/Clinical Highlights

1.3.2: Changes in the Breast

1.3.2.1: Breast Changes During Pregnancy (A and B)

Picture	Medical/Surgical Description	Management/Clinical Highlights
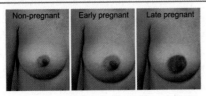 **Fig. 1.3.2.1A:** Changes in the breasts, occurring during pregnancy	Figure 1.3.2.1 demonstrates various changes, which occur in the breasts of a woman during pregnancy. Changes in the breasts are best evident in the primigravida in comparison to multigravida as shown in this figure.	There is pronounced pigmentation of areola and nipples. There also occurs appearance of secondary areola, development of Montgomery's tubercles and increased vascularity.
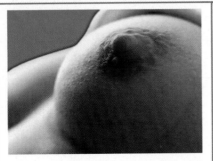 **Fig. 1.3.2.1B:** Breast of a woman during full-term pregnancy	Figure 1.3.2.1B shows breast of a pregnant woman with full-term pregnancy. During pregnancy, there occurs marked proliferation and hypertrophy of mammary ducts and alveoli. Increased vascularity of the tissues results in the appearance of bluish veins under the breast skin. The nipples become larger, erectile and pigmented. There occurs hypertrophy of the sebaceous glands in the areola resulting in the formation of Montgomery's tubercles.	Other changes occurring in the breasts during pregnancy are as follows: • Hypertrophy of the connective tissue stroma • Formation of secondary areola during the second trimester • Production of sticky, thick, yellowish secretions from the breasts after about 12th week of pregnancy.

1.4: PHYSIOLOGICAL CHANGES DURING PREGNANCY

1.4.1: Hematological Changes During Pregnancy

Picture	Medical/Surgical Description	Management/Clinical Highlights
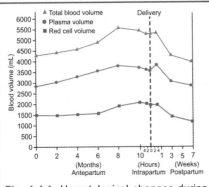 **Fig. 1.4.1:** Hematological changes during pregnancy	The following hematological changes occur during pregnancy: • Increase in the blood volume starts from 6th week of pregnancy. By 30–32 weeks, the blood volume may have increased by 40–50% above the nonpregnant level. • Due to hemodilution, there is an actual decrease in the concentration of plasma proteins from 7 g% to 6 g%. • Pregnancy is a hypercoagulable state. There is an increase in the fibrinogen levels from 200 mg% to 400 mg% in the nonpregnant state to 300–600 mg% during pregnancy.	The increase in the blood volume during pregnancy is due to an increase in the plasma volume (by 50%) and RBC volume (by 20–30%). The disproportionate increase in the plasma and RBC volume is likely to cause hemodilution, resulting in a physiological hemodilution of pregnancy. Due to a substantial increase in plasma volume and only a slight increase in the erythrocyte volume, there occurs a slight decrease in the hemoglobin concentration, hematocrit and blood viscosity during pregnancy. Average hemoglobin concentration at term is 12.5 g/dL. A decline in the hemoglobin value of less than 11 g/dL especially late in pregnancy is abnormal and can be considered to be due to anemia (most likely iron deficiency anemia) rather than hypervolemia of pregnancy.

1.4.2: Changes in Hematological Parameters During Pregnancy

	Pregnant	Nonpregnant
Hemoglobin	13–15 g/dL	11.5–12.5 g/dL
Packed cell volume	37–47%	33–38%
RBC count	4.2–5.4 million/mm³	3.8–4.4 million/mm³
Mean corpuscular volume	80–100 μm³/cell	70–90 μm³/cell
Mean corpuscular hemoglobin	27–34 pg/cell	23–31 pg/cell
Mean corpuscular hemoglobin concentration	31–36 g/dL	Unchanged
Reticulocyte count	0.5–1.0%	1–2%

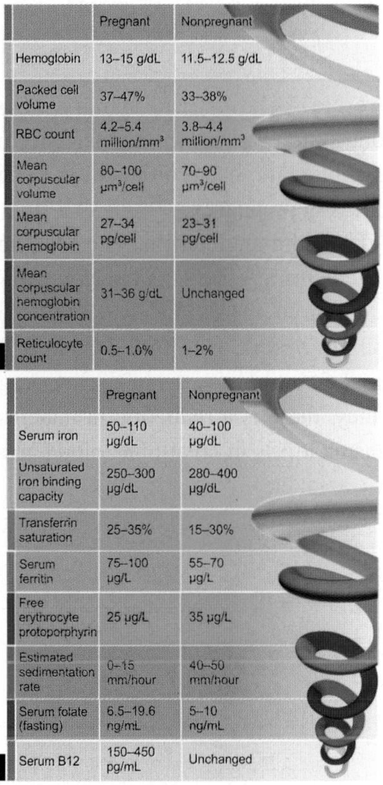

A

	Pregnant	Nonpregnant
Serum iron	50–110 μg/dL	40–100 μg/dL
Unsaturated iron binding capacity	250–300 μg/dL	280–400 μg/dL
Transferrin saturation	25–35%	15–30%
Serum ferritin	75–100 μg/L	55–70 μg/L
Free erythrocyte protoporphyrin	25 μg/L	35 μg/L
Estimated sedimentation rate	0–15 mm/hour	40–50 mm/hour
Serum folate (fasting)	6.5–19.6 ng/mL	5–10 ng/mL
Serum B12	150–450 pg/mL	Unchanged

B

Figs 1.4.2 (A and B): Changes in hematological parameters during pregnancy

Figures 1.4.2 (A and B) illustrates the changes in hematological parameters occurring during pregnancy in comparison to the nonpregnant women. As previously described, due to physiological hemodilution during pregnancy, there is a slight decrease in hemoglobin concentration, hematocrit, blood viscosity and the blood indices (except for mean corpuscular hemoglobin concentration, which remain unchanged during pregnancy). Due to extra demand of approximately 980–1,000 mg of iron during pregnancy, there is also slight reduction in the serum iron concentration, transferring saturation and serum ferritin levels. There is a slight increase in the unsaturated iron binding capacity, free erythrocyte protoporphyrin and erythrocyte sedimentation rate. While the serum B12 levels remain unchanged, serum folate levels are reduced during pregnancy.

Management of iron deficiency anemia during pregnancy is described in Section 5.

1.4.3: Changes in the Blood Flow of Various Organs During Pregnancy

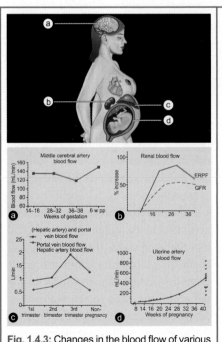

Fig. 1.4.3: Changes in the blood flow of various organs during pregnancy

Figure 1.4.3 illustrates changes in blood flow of various organs during pregnancy. There is incredible increase in the blood flow of some organs at the expense of others.

During pregnancy, there is a tremendous increase in the blood flow to the uterus by almost 350 mL/minute in order to support the growing fetus and the placenta. There is also an increase in blood volume and cardiac output for increasing the blood flow to various body organs. The blood flow to the brain also sharply increases by middle of pregnancy, whereas via a compensatory mechanism there is reduction in the blood flow to the liver, extremities and kidneys during the second half of pregnancy.

SECTION 1 ❖ GENERAL OBSTETRICS

33

1.4.4: Cardiovascular Changes During Pregnancy

Kindly refer to Section 5 [5.4.1 (A and B)].

1.4.5: Changes in the Kidneys (A and B)

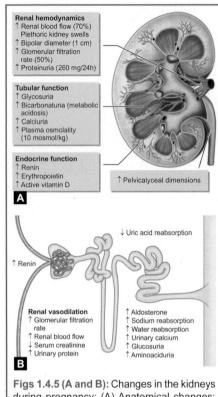

Figs 1.4.5 (A and B): Changes in the kidneys during pregnancy: (A) Anatomical changes; (B) Changes in renal function

Anatomic Changes

During pregnancy, kidney size increases by about 1 cm. In the remaining part of the urinary tract, there is dilatation of the calyces, renal pelvis and ureters. The dilation is more marked on the right side than the left and is apparent as early as the first trimester.

Changes in Renal Function

- There is an increase in GFR by 50% and RPF by 50–75% by 16 weeks of pregnancy and is maintained until 34 weeks. While the GFR remains elevated throughout pregnancy, RPF falls after 34 weeks of pregnancy.
- There is failure of complete absorption of substances, such as glucose, uric acid, amino acid, etc., from the renal tubules, resulting in an increased excretion of proteins, amino acids and glucose.
- Serum creatinine levels decrease during normal gestation to levels less than 0.8 mg/dL.
- Serum bicarbonate levels decrease by 4–5 mEq/L.
- Serum osmolality decreases.

Ureteral dilation and urinary stasis contribute to an increased incidence of asymptomatic bacteriuria and pyelonephritis in pregnancy.

The renin-angiotensin system is stimulated during gestation, and cumulative retention of approximately 950 mEq of sodium occurs. Due to the changes in renal function occurring during pregnancy, there is a reduction in maternal plasma levels of creatinine, blood urea, uric acid, etc.

1.4.6: Changes in the Gastrointestinal Tract

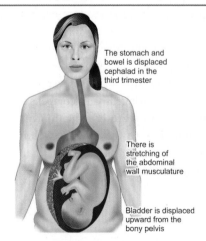

Fig. 1.4.6: Changes in the gastrointestinal tract during pregnancy

The physiological changes occurring in the gastrointestinal tract at the time of pregnancy include the following:
- Reduced gastric motility and emptying, resulting in constipation
- Cephalad displacement of the bowel in the third trimester
- Stretching of the abdominal wall musculature and peritoneum
- Displacement of bladder from the bony pelvis.

The physiological changes occurring in the gastrointestinal tract at the time of pregnancy are likely to result in an increased risk of aspiration, increased risk of injury to the bowel and bladder, and reduced sensitivity of abdominal examination.

Relaxation of the cardiac sphincter may result in regurgitation of gastric acid into the esophagus, thereby producing chemical esophagitis and heart burns. Gastric secretions are also reduced and the emptying time of the stomach is delayed. This results in reduced risk for the development of peptic ulcer disease.

Picture	Medical/Surgical Description	Management/Clinical Highlights

1.4.7: Changes in Carbohydrate Metabolism (A and B)

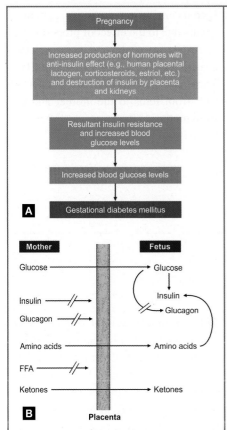

A

B

Figs 1.4.7 (A and B): (A) Changes in carbohydrate metabolism during pregnancy; (B) Exchange of various nutrients and hormones across the placenta (FFA, Free fatty acid)

Changes related with carbohydrate metabolism during pregnancy are as follows:

• There is transfer of increased amount of glucose from the mother to the fetus throughout the pregnancy.

• There is mild fasting hypoglycemia, postprandial hyperglycemia and hyperinsulinemia as well as greater suppression of glucagon

• When fasting is prolonged in pregnant women, ketonemia rapidly results in the postprandial state.

These changes in carbohydrate metabolism help in ensuring continuous supply of glucose to the fetus.

Pregnancy is a diabetogenic state, resulting in development of insulin resistance. In the first half of pregnancy there is an increased sensitivity to insulin and therefore a tendency toward development of hypoglycemia. On the other hand, the second half of pregnancy (especially after 24 weeks of gestation) is related with development of insulin resistance.

Movement of nutrients such as glucose, amino acids and ketones can occur freely in the fetal circulation. On the other hand, movement of substances such as insulin, glucagon and free fatty acids (FFA) cannot occur freely. Therefore, maternal hyperglycemia and ketonemia is also manifested by the fetus.

1.4.8: Changes in the Thyroid Glands

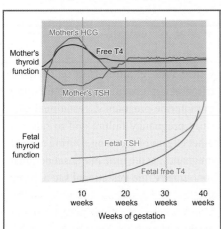

Fig. 1.4.8: Changes in the thyroid glands during pregnancy

Changes occurring in the thyroid glands during pregnancy are as follows:

• Moderate enlargement of thyroid glands is caused by glandular hyperplasia and increased vascularity.

• There is a marked and early increase in hepatic production of thyroid binding globulins (TBG) and placental production of hCG.

• Increase in TBG increases serum thyroxine concentrations, whereas hCG has thyrotropin-like activity which stimulates maternal T4 production.

There is an increased production of thyroid hormones by 40–100% in order to meet the maternal and fetal requirements. Levels of TBG start increasing from first trimester. They peak at 20 weeks of pregnancy and plateau during the remainder part of pregnancy.

Levels of thyroid releasing hormone are not increased during normal pregnancy. However, this hormone can cross the placenta and stimulates the fetal pituitary to secrete thyrotropin. This causes on increase in fetal TSH and free T4 concentration with increasing period of gestation during pregnancy.

Picture	Medical/Surgical Description	Management/Clinical Highlights

1.4.9: Changes in Respiratory Function

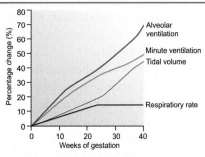 **Fig. 1.4.9:** Changes in respiratory function during pregnancy	The following changes in respiratory function occur during pregnancy: • State of hyperventilation, resulting in an increase in tidal volume and respiratory minute volume by 40%. This hyperventilation causes changes in acid-base balance. • Fall in the arterial $PaCO_2$ from 38 mm Hg to 32 mm Hg and a rise in PaO_2 from 95 mm Hg to 105 mm Hg. • There is an overall rise in the pH and a base excess of 2 mEq/L. This results in respiratory alkalosis.	Hyperventilation during pregnancy occurs due to the effect of progesterone on respiratory center and increase in the sensitivity of respiratory center to CO_2. These changes facilitate the transfer of CO_2 from fetus to the mother and O_2 from mother to the fetus.

1.5: ANTENATAL ASSESSMENT

1.5.1: Diagnosis of Pregnancy

1.5.1.1: Urine Pregnancy Test

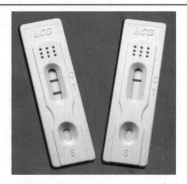 **Fig. 1.5.1.1:** Urine pregnancy test for the diagnosis of pregnancy. The test strip on the right side shows a positive result whereas that on the left side shows a negative result with only the control line	Urine pregnancy tests help in detecting the presence of hCG in the urine samples. Appearance of a line on the test strip after putting a drop of urine is indicative of a positive test. No colored line appears in case of a negative result. The control line is present in both the cases.	The laboratory test for pregnancy is based on the identification of hCG, which can be detected as early as 7–9 days after fertilization by highly sensitive techniques. The samples may be blood or urine. Most current pregnancy tests have sensitivity to detect hCG levels of approximately 25 mIU/mL and involve the use of antibodies, which are highly specific for β-subunit of hCG.

1.5.1.2: Transabdominal Ultrasound for Diagnosis of Pregnancy

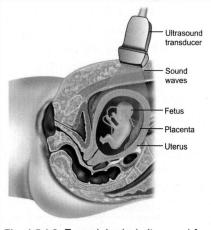 Ultrasound transducer Sound waves Fetus Placenta Uterus **Fig. 1.5.1.2:** Transabdominal ultrasound for diagnosis of pregnancy	The technique of transabdominal sonography for the diagnosis of intrauterine pregnancy is shown in Figure 1.5.1.2 and has been described in details in Section 7.	Ultrasound examination in the first trimester is essential in establishing intrauterine pregnancy, gestational age, early pregnancy failure and to rule out other causes of bleeding. During normal pregnancy, at the time of transabdominal sonography, the gestational sac appears first by 5–5.5 weeks; the yolk sac by 5.5–6 weeks; the fetal pole by 6–6.5 weeks and fetal heartbeat by 6–7 weeks.

1.5.1.3: Transvaginal Ultrasound for Diagnosis of Pregnancy

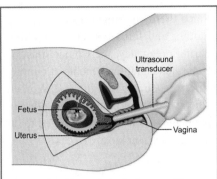

Fig. 1.5.1.3: Transvaginal ultrasound for diagnosis of pregnancy

The technique of transvaginal sonography for the diagnosis of intrauterine pregnancy is shown in Figure 1.5.1.3 and has been described in details in Section 7.

During normal pregnancy, at the time of transvaginal sonography, the gestational sac appears first by 4.5–5 weeks; the yolk sac by 5–5.5 weeks; the fetal pole by 5.5–6 weeks and fetal heartbeat by 6 weeks. All these findings are likely to appear 1 week later on the transabdominal scan.

1.5.2: Antenatal Care

1.5.2.1: Antenatal Schedule

5–10 Wk	16 Wk	18 Wk	20 Wk
Booking	Amniocentesis (if required)	Blood test	Ultrasound scan

24 Wk	28 Wk	32 Wk	34 Wk
Follow-up	Ultrasound scan	Follow-up	Follow-up

36 Wk	37 Wk	38 Wk	39 Wk	40 Wk
Follow-up	Follow-up	Vaginal exam	Follow-up	Delivery

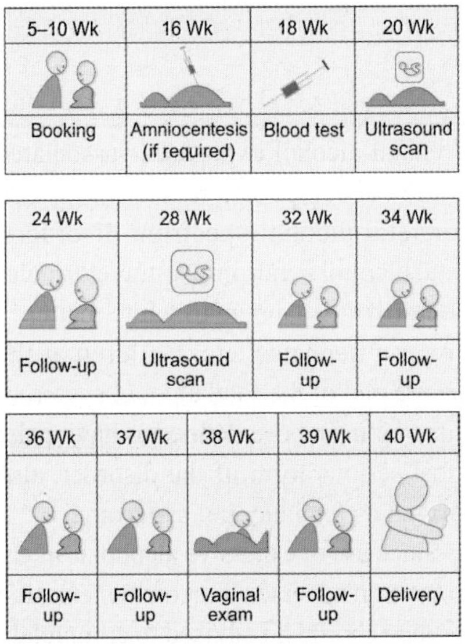

Fig. 1.5.2.1: Antenatal schedule

Routine antenatal care schedule is illustrated in Figure 1.5.2.1 and comprises of the following:

- *Pregnancy dating*: This can be done using Naegele's rule and ultrasonographic dating during the first visit.
- *Nutrition*: Woman with a singleton pregnancy must be advised to consume approximately 100–300 kcal more per day along with iron and calcium supplements. Supplementation with folic acid (500 µg daily) must be started before conception and continued up to 12 weeks of gestation.
- *Frequency of antenatal visits*: The antenatal visits should be at every 4-weekly up to 28 weeks; at every 2-weekly up to 36 weeks and thereafter weekly till the expected date of delivery.
- *Weight gain*: The total weight gain recommended for pregnancy based on the prepregnancy body mass index
- *Exercise and employment*: In the absence of obstetric or medical complications, most patients are able to work throughout the entire pregnancy.
- *Immunizations*: For unimmunized women, tetanus toxoid must be administered intramuscularly in the dosage of 0.5 mL at 6-weekly intervals, with the first dose being administered at 16–24 weeks.
- *Sexual intercourse*: No restriction of sexual activity is necessary.

Using Naegele's rule, the estimated date of delivery is calculated by adding 9 calendar months and 7 days to the 1st day of the last menstrual (28-day cycle) period.

Ultrasound examination for dating of pregnancy must be performed early in gestation (commonly at 7–11 weeks of pregnancy).

Iron supplements containing 30 mg of elemental iron is prescribed daily starting from second trimester onward. For calcium, the prenatal daily requirement is 1,200 mg.

A minimum of four visits during the antenatal period are mandatory: first at 16 weeks; second at 24–28 weeks; third at 32 weeks and fourth at 36 weeks.

Addition of nuchal translucency to the biochemical markers helps in improving the accuracy of detection rate by 80%. Lifting of heavy weights and excessive physical activity should be avoided during pregnancy.

Varicella zoster immune globulin should be administered to any newborn whose mother has developed chickenpox within 5 days before or 2 days after delivery. Avoidance of sexual activity must be recommended for women at risk of preterm labor, placenta previa or women with previous history of pregnancy loss.

1.5.2.2: Smoking During Pregnancy

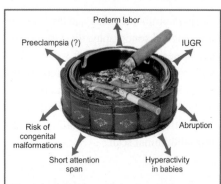

Fig. 1.5.2.2: Adverse effects of smoking tobacco during pregnancy

Maternal smoking during pregnancy can result in numerous adverse effects for both the mother and fetus such as:
- *Maternal*: Preeclampsia, abruption placentae, ectopic pregnancy, abnormal placental attachment, resulting in placenta previa, vaginal bleeding, etc.
- *Fetal*: Low birth weight babies (preterm and intrauterine growth retardation), risk of congenital anomalies, developmental and behavioral abnormities in the child, short attention span and hyperactivity, reduced IQ and cognitive performance, suppression of lactation, etc.

Since there are numerous risks to the mother and fetus related to smoking during pregnancy, the woman must be counseled about the benefits of quitting smoking during pregnancy. Women who are unable to quit smoking during pregnancy should be encouraged to at least reduce smoking.

1.5.2.3: Alcohol Use During Pregnancy (A to C)

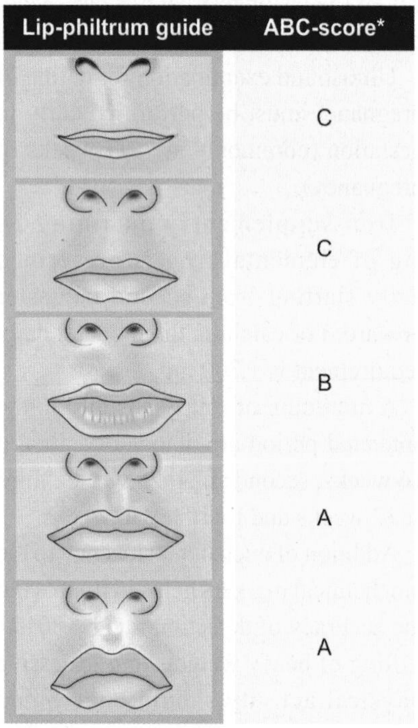

Lip-philtrum guide	ABC-score*
	C
	C
	B
	A
	A

Figs 1.5.2.3A: Lip-philtrum guide
[*ABC score*: A (score of 1 or 2) > 10th centile; B (score of 3) > 3rd and ≤ 10th centile; C (score of 4 or 5) ≤ 3rd centile]

The individual to be diagnosed with fetal alcohol syndrome must exhibit all three characteristic facial dysmorphic features: smooth philtrum, thin vermillion upper lip border, and small palpebral fissures. Smooth philtrum or thin vermillion border is defined as a measurement equivalent to 4 or 5 on Lip-Philtrum Guide (as shown in Figure 1.5.2.3A).

Prenatal alcohol exposure is associated with fetal complications such as the risk for fetal alcohol spectrum disorders, fetal alcohol syndrome, intraventricular hemorrhage, damage to white matter in preterm neonates, etc. Children at the severe end of the fetal alcohol spectrum disorder have been defined as having the most serious form of the disorder, also termed as fetal alcohol syndrome.

Since use of excessive alcohol is likely to have an adverse effect on the fetus, the woman should be advised to completely stop or at least limit alcohol consumption to no more than one standard unit per day during her pregnancy.

Picture	Medical/Surgical Description	Management/Clinical Highlights
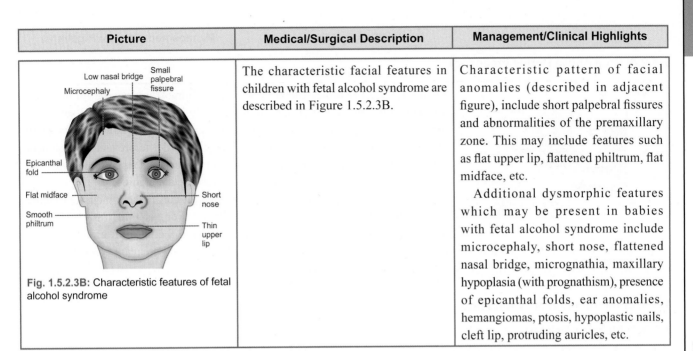 **Fig. 1.5.2.3B:** Characteristic features of fetal alcohol syndrome	The characteristic facial features in children with fetal alcohol syndrome are described in Figure 1.5.2.3B.	Characteristic pattern of facial anomalies (described in adjacent figure), include short palpebral fissures and abnormalities of the premaxillary zone. This may include features such as flat upper lip, flattened philtrum, flat midface, etc. Additional dysmorphic features which may be present in babies with fetal alcohol syndrome include microcephaly, short nose, flattened nasal bridge, micrognathia, maxillary hypoplasia (with prognathism), presence of epicanthal folds, ear anomalies, hemangiomas, ptosis, hypoplastic nails, cleft lip, protruding auricles, etc.
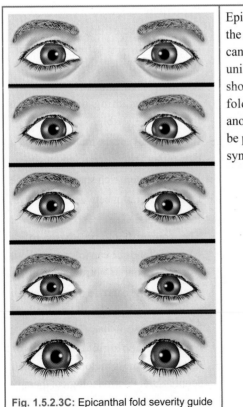 **Fig. 1.5.2.3C:** Epicanthal fold severity guide	Epicanthal fold is the lateral extension of the skin of nasal bridge along the medial canthus of the eye. These folds can be unilateral or bilateral. Figure 1.5.2.4C shows the severity index for epicanthal folds. Presence of epicanthal folds is another dysmorphic feature which may be present in children with fetal alcohol syndrome.	The set of lowermost pair of eyes in this figure are normal eyes having no epicanthal fold. As we move upward the severity and extension of epicanthal folds gradually increases with the uppermost pair of eyes showing the most prominent epicanthal folds bilaterally. The epicanthal folds are likely to become more prominent with increasing saverity of fetal alcohol spectrum disorders.

1.5.2.4: Drug Abuse During Pregnancy

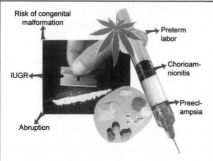

Fig. 1.5.2.4: Adverse effects of drug abuse during pregnancy

Figure 1.5.2.5 illustrates the adverse effects due to drug abuse during pregnancy. Fetal complications due to drug abuse during pregnancy include IUGR, intrauterine death, malpresentation (breech presentation), neural tube defects, etc. Maternal complications due to drug abuse during pregnancy include miscarriage, preterm rupture of membranes, preterm labor, chorioamnionitis, preeclampsia, abruption, etc.

It is of utmost importance for the clinicians to identify and prevent substance abuse during pregnancy in its early stages in order to prevent development of pregnancy related complications and adverse fetal outcomes.

It is the duty of the clinician to increase the awareness and understanding regarding the harmful effects of drug abuse among pregnant women.

1.5.3: Common Pregnancy Ailments

1.5.3.1: Morning Sickness

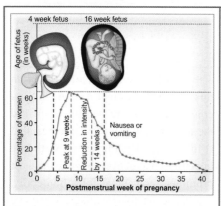

Fig. 1.5.3.1: Pattern of morning sickness during pregnancy

Nausea and vomiting of pregnancy, commonly known as "morning sickness", is generally a mild, self-limited condition, commonly encountered between 4th to 7th week of pregnancy, peaking at approximately 9th week and diminishing greatly in intensity by 14–16 weeks of pregnancy. It may be controlled with conservative measures. It usually subsides or greatly diminishes in intensity by the time the woman approaches the second trimester.

Emotional and psychological support from family, especially the spouse helps the women in effectively dealing with the condition.

The following dietary and lifestyle changes must be advised to the women in order to reduce the discomfort associated with morning sickness:

- Eating a piece of dry, toasted bread or biscuits before getting out of bed (even before brushing one's teeth).
- Avoiding fatty and spicy foods and instead consuming more of fresh foods and vegetables
- Eating small meals multiple times a day, rather than three fixed meals
- Eating a protein rich snack at bedtime
- Drinking fluids in between, rather than with meals
- The women should be advised to eat whatever food she can tolerate without worrying about its nutritional value.
- Sucking some candy, a piece of lemon or drinking small sips of lemonade in between meals helps.
- Nonpharmacological therapy for morning sickness includes ginger and acupressure. Pharmacological therapy includes use of antihistaminic agents.

Picture	Medical/Surgical Description	Management/Clinical Highlights

1.5.3.2: Constipation During Pregnancy

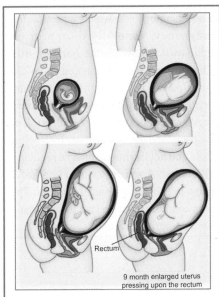

Fig. 1.5.3.2: Development of constipation during pregnancy

Constipation is defined as having bowel movements fewer than three times per week. Chronic constipation is a highly prevalent problem, especially in women at the time of pregnancy. Causes of constipation in pregnancy are as follows:

- Increase in the levels of circulating progesterone, which acts as a smooth muscle relaxant
- Decreased physical activity
- In the later stages of pregnancy the enlarged uterus may also press upon rectum resulting in constipation.

Management of constipation during pregnancy comprises of the following steps:

- *High fiber diet*: The recommended dietary fiber intake during pregnancy is about 28 g of fiber everyday. Dietary supplements of fiber in the form of bran or wheat fiber are also likely to help the women.
- *Laxatives*: If the problem fails to resolve with dietary and lifestyle modifications, laxatives need to be prescribed. Initially, the bulk laxatives, which are the safest, like cellulose and hemi-cellulose, psyllium seed, flax seed, ispaghula or osmotic laxatives like lactose, etc. can be advised. If bulk laxatives do not appear to be useful and the woman's constipation keeps worsening, stimulant laxatives may be prescribed.

1.5.3.3: Varicose Veins During Pregnancy

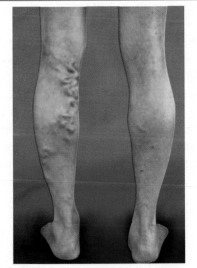

Fig. 1.5.3.3: Development of varicose veins during pregnancy

During pregnancy, varicosities of the veins in calf, thighs and vulva can commonly develop due to pressure on the pelvic veins and IVC by the gravid uterus. Figure 1.5.3.3 shows development of varicosities in the veins of legs (popliteal veins) during pregnancy.

The varicosities, which appear during pregnancy, generally disappear on their own following the baby's birth. In order to prevent the development of varicosities, the woman must be asked to do regular daily exercises during her pregnancy and elevate her legs and foot whenever possible. She should be advised not to sit or stand in the same position for a long time. Use of graded compression stockings also help.

Picture	Medical/Surgical Description	Management/Clinical Highlights

1.5.3.4: Hemorrhoids During Pregnancy (A and B)

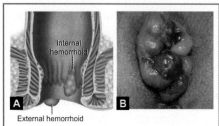 **Figs 1.5.3.4 (A and B):** Development of hemorrhoids during pregnancy	Hemorrhoids are varicosities of the veins in the rectum, which develop due to pressure on the pelvic veins and IVC by the gravid uterus. These can commonly occur in pregnancy during the third trimester, during labor and early postpartum period.	These hemorrhoids, which appear during pregnancy, generally disappear on their own following the baby's birth. The woman must be asked to avoid constipation by eating high fiber diet, drinking plenty of fluids and doing regular Kegel exercises. Application of ice packs and use of warm sitz bath helps. Cold and hot treatment must be regularly alternated. Application of witch hazel helps in providing relief from pain. The woman must be advised not to sit or stand for long periods of time.

1.5.4: Clinical Assessment During Pregnancy

For details regarding clinical assessment during pregnancy, kindly refer to Section 2

1.5.5: Investigations During Pregnancy

1.5.5.1: Blood Group Determination

Fig. 1.5.5.1: Blood group determination during pregnancy	Two main blood group classification systems are as follows: *ABO System* • *Blood type A:* Erythrocytes have type A surface antigen and anti-B antibodies are present in the plasma • *Blood type B*: Erythrocytes have type B surface antigen and anti-A antibodes are present in the plasma. • *Blood type AB*: Erythrocytes have both type A and B surface antigens and there are neither anti-A nor anti-B antibodies in the plasma. • *Blood type O*: Erythrocytes have neither antigen A nor antigen B and there are both anti-A and anti-B antibodies in the plasma. *Rh System* • *Rh-positive individuals:* They have D antigen on their erythrocytes and no anti-D antibody in their plasma. • *Rh-negative individuals:* They do not have D antigen on their erythrocytes or anti-D antibodies in their plasma. Anti-D antibodies appear in the plasma, only if there has been an exposure to Rh positive blood.	It is important to know blood groups of the pregnant woman because there can be a requirement for blood transfusion during pregnancy. All pregnant women must be offered testing for ABO blood group and RhD status in early pregnancy. If a pregnant woman is RhD-negative, her partner must be also tested to determine if the administration of anti-D prophylaxis would be necessary. National Institute of Clinical Excellence (2002) recommends that routine antenatal anti-D prophylaxis should be offered to all nonsensitized pregnant women who are RhD negative.

Picture	Medical/Surgical Description	Management/Clinical Highlights

1.5.5.2: Hemoglobin Estimation (A and B)

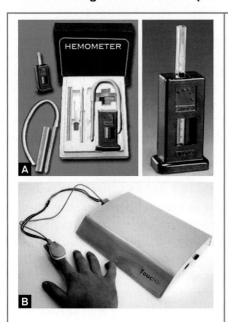

Figs 1.5.5.2 (A and B): Hemoglobin estimation

Figure 1.5.5.2A shows estimation of hemoglobin using Sahli's apparatus while Figure 1.5.5.2B estimation of hemoglobin using a nonpricking method (ToucHb)

Iron deficiency anemia is one of the most prevalent nutritional deficiencies in the world and affects billions of people worldwide. Nearly 40% of maternal deaths are directly and indirectly attributed to anemia. Mortality related to anemia can be prevented by early diagnosis with the help of hemoglobin estimation. Conventional method for hemoglobin estimation involves the use of Sahli's apparatus. Mumbai based company Biosense Technologies has developed a new product, ToucHb, which is a noninvasive method for hemoglobin estimation in cases of severe anemia during pregnancy. ToucHb can prove to be a significant diagnostic procedure for anemia screening and monitoring.

1.5.5.3: Urine Test for Proteins and Glucose

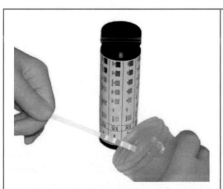

Fig. 1.5.5.3: Urine dipstick test for detection of proteins and glucose

The glucose and protein dipstick are respectively used for detection of glucose and protein in the urine. The test strip is dipped in urine, following which the color of strip is compared with the color on the bottle to evaluate the amount of protein or glucose which could be present in the urine.

Presence of glucose in the urine is indicative of gestational diabetes, while the presence of protein in the urine could be indicative of preeclampsia. Management of both preeclampsia and gestational diabetes has been described in Section 5.

1.5.5.4: Screening for HIV

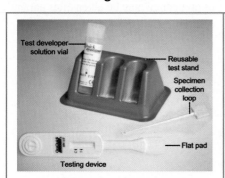

Fig. 1.5.5.4: Rapid HIV antibody testing kits

Rapid HIV test (as shown in the Figure 1.5.5.4) usually provides results within 20 minutes. In this test, samples of saliva obtained using the specimen collection loop are placed in the developer solution vial to detect the presence of anti-HIV antibodies. Then the sample is placed on the testing device for 20–40 minutes. If a single line shows up, it is considered as a negative result, whereas if double lines show up, it is considered as positive result.

Positive test results on rapid tests must be followed up with confirmatory tests. Pregnant women should be offered screening for HIV infection early in antenatal period. Prophylaxis with antiretroviral therapy can be given to prevent mother-to-child transmission during pregnancy, delivery and breastfeeding. Lifelong antiretroviral therapy can be prescribed to HIV-infected women, requiring treatment.

1.5.6: Antenatal Screening

1.5.6.1: Screening for Thalassemia (A and B)

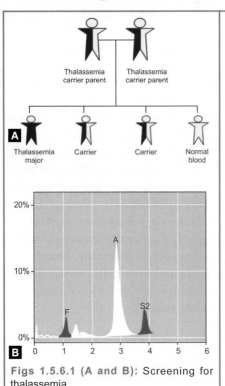 Figs 1.5.6.1 (A and B): Screening for thalassemia	Thalassemia is a genetic disorder associated with reduced production of specific globin chains of the hemoglobin molecule. Figure 1.5.6.1A shows autosomal recessive pattern of inheritance of thalassemia. Thalassemia major would be manifested only if the woman inherits the defective genes from each of the parents. Heterozygote individuals, who have inherited only one defective gene from either of the parents, are carriers. Figure 1.5.6.1B demonstrates serum electrophoresis pattern in case of thalassemia showing an increase in the levels of minor hemoglobins such as hbF ($\alpha_2\gamma_2$) and hbA2 ($\alpha_2\delta_2$), which may be respectively present in an amount greater than 1% and 3.5% of total hemoglobin.	Women belonging to ethnic groups whose members are at higher risk of being carriers are usually offered screening comprising of a complete blood count, as well as hemoglobin electrophoresis or hemoglobin high performance liquid chromatography. This investigation should include quantitation of HbA2 and HbF. If both partners are found to be carriers of thalassemia, they should be referred to genetic counseling. Prenatal diagnosis (DNA analysis on cells obtained by chorionic villus sampling or amniocentesis) should be offered to the pregnant women who are at a risk for having a fetus affected with clinically significant thalassemia. In case an abnormality is detected, the woman must be referred to a tertiary care center for further assessment and counseling.

1.5.6.2: Screening for Structural Anomalies

Kindly refer to Section 7 for details.

1.5.6.3: Screening for Down's Syndrome

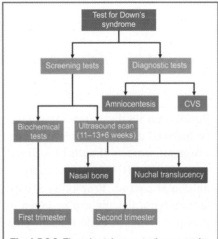 Fig. 1.5.6.3: Flow chart demonstrating screening for Down's syndrome	*Screening tests for Down's syndrome from 11 weeks to 14 weeks include ultrasound scan:* • Nuchal translucency (NT) • Absence of nasal bone Ultrasound features for diagnosis of Down's syndrome have been described in Section 7 (7.8.1). *Screening tests for Down's syndrome from 14 weeks to 20 weeks include biochemical tests:* • The triple test [hCG, alpha fetoprotein (AFP) and estriol] • The quadruple test (hCG, AFP, estrial and, inhibin A)	Diagnostic tests for Down's syndrome include amniocentesis (refer to 1.5.7.1) and CVS (refer to 1.5.7.2). In case of diagnosis of Down's syndrome on either of these tests, decision for termination of pregnancy may be taken after patient counseling and consent.

Picture	Medical/Surgical Description	Management/Clinical Highlights

1.5.6.4: Screening for Infection (A to C)

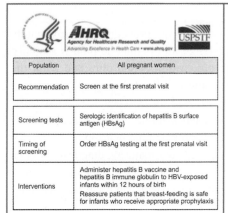

Fig. 1.5.6.4A: Screening for hepatitis B
Source: US Preventive Service Task Force Recommondation statement. (2004). Screening for hepatitis B virus infection

Serological screening for hepatitis B virus (HBV) should be offered to all pregnant women at the time of first prenatal visit so that effective postnatal intervention can be offered to infected women to reduce the risk of mother-to-child-transmission

Infants of mothers who are found to be positive for HbsAg must be administered hepatitis B vaccine and hepatitis B immune globulins (100 IU of HBIg) within 72 hours of birth. Engerix-B vaccine in the dosage of 0.5 mL is administered three times each (at birth, 1–4 months and 6–18 months). This helps in significantly reducing the baby's risk for acquiring HBV infection.

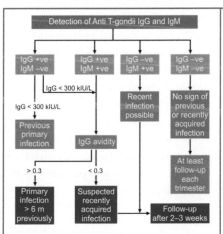

Fig. 1.5.6.4B: Screening for TORCH/toxoplasmosis

The available evidence does not support routine antenatal serological screening for toxoplasmosis because the harms of screening may outweigh the potential benefits. Serological screening test for Toxoplasma gondii involves the quantification and detection of *T. gondii* IgG and IgM antibodies in the pregnant women during the first trimester. Interpretation of negative and positive results for both the antibodies has been described in the adjacent Figure.

In oder to prevent this disease, pregnant women should be advised about avoiding contact with cat feces in cat litter or in soil.

In case of pregnant woman, who has acquired the infection during pregnancy, if the period of gestation is less than 18 weeks, spiramycin is administered and fetal ultrasound is performed. Amniotic fluid PCR should also be done at 18 weeks (not before or later). After 18 weeks of gestation, the risk of the procedure should be carefully weighed against the benefits of diagnosing fetal infection. In case of negative findings on PCR, spiramycin must be continued. In case of positive findings on PCR or ultrasound, pyrimethamine, sulphadiazine and folinic acid must be administered.

Fig. 1.5.6.4C: Screening for chlamydial infections (*Source*: US Preventive Services Task Force Recommendation, Statement. Screening for chlamydial infection: Ann Intern Med. 2007;147(2):128-34)

Women, 24 years of age or younger are at the highest risk of acquiring chlamydial infection. Screening is done using the test nucleic acid amplification test (NAAT), which can identify chlamydial infection in asymptomatic pregnant women. This test has a high specificity and sensitivity and can be used with urine and vaginal swabs.

Screening must be done during the first prenatal visit in women who are 24 years or younger and older women who are at an increased risk. For patients at continuing risk or who are newly at risk, screening must be done in the third trimester. Treatment of chlamydial infections involves the use of antibiotics such as azithromycin, doxycycline, erythromycin and ofloxacin. For details kindly refer to Section 15 (15.2.1).

Picture	Medical/Surgical Description	Management/Clinical Highlights

1.5.7: Prenatal Diagnosis

1.5.7.1: Amniocentesis

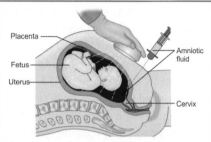

Fig. 1.5.7.1: The procedure of amniocentesis

Amniocentesis is a prenatal diagnostic procedure, which involves the use of ultrasound-guided, needle-insertion technique for aspiration and sampling of amniotic fluid. This procedure is usually performed between 16 to 18 weeks of gestation and has been demonstrated in Figure 1.5.7.1.

During the procedure, approximately 15–20 ml of amniotic fluid is aspirated out. Amniocytes, obtained from the amniotic fluid during the procedure are used for cytogenetic and molecular genetics studies. Biochemical analysis of amniotic fluid helps in assessment of pulmonary maturity, diagnosis of open neural tube defects and for the assessment of various viral and bacterial infections.

1.5.7.2: Chorionic Villus Sampling (A and B)

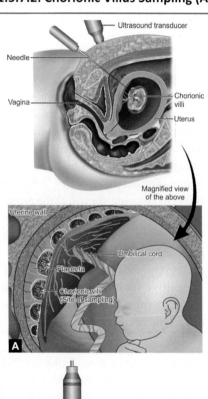

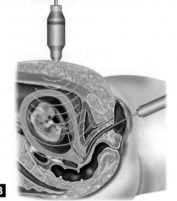

Figs 1.5.7.2 (A and B): Procedure of chorionic villus sampling: (A) Transabdominal approach; (B) Transvaginal approach

Chorionic villus sampling is a prenatal diagnostic technique in which a sample of fetal chorionic tissue is obtained from the chorion frondosum (future placenta) between 10 to 14 weeks of gestation. CVS is performed either with the help of a catheter inserted transcervically (transcervical CVS) or a needle inserted transabdominally (transabdominal CVS) under the guidance of ultrasonography. The third type of CVS procedure (transvaginal CVS) is rarely done nowadays.

The decision regarding whether CVS is to be performed transabdominally or transcervically is usually made by the obstetrician based on the placental localization. Fundal placenta or that located within upper two-thirds of the uterine walls is better approached with transabdominal route as compared to transcervical route. On the other hand, placenta located in the lower one third of the uterine walls is better approached by transcervical route. Majority of CVS procedures are performed by transabdominal route.

Picture	Medical/Surgical Description	Management/Clinical Highlights

1.5.7.3: Cordocentesis

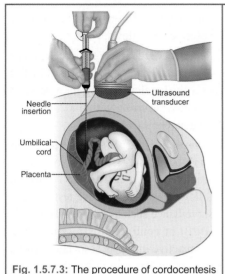

Fig. 1.5.7.3: The procedure of cordocentesis

Cordocentesis, also sometimes called percutaneous umbilical cord blood sampling (PUBS), is a diagnostic test, which aims at detection of fetal anomalies (e.g. chromosomal anomalies like Down's syndrome; blood disorders like hemolytic anemia, etc.) through direct examination of fetal blood.

Cordocentesis is usually performed during 18–24 weeks of pregnancy. In cases of fetal anemia, such as Rh negative immunized women, and cases of nonimmune hydrops, the procedure of cordocentesis helps in estimating the fetal hemoglobin and hematocrit levels. It can be used for the diagnosis of hematological disorders such as thrombocytopenia; diagnosis of congenital infections such as rubella, CMV, toxoplasmosis, etc., for fetal blood gas analysis and for therapeutic purposes such as intrauterine transfusion, drug therapy and stem cell transplantation.

1.5.8: Antepartum Fetal Surveillance
1.5.8.1: Daily Fetal Movement Count

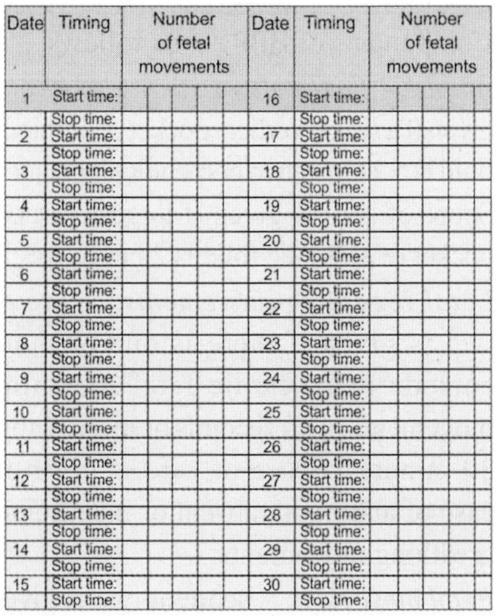

Fig. 1.5.8.1: Daily fetal movement count

While performing the kick count, the mother must lie on her left side in comfortable location and is asked to report the time it takes for her to feel 10 movements, no matter how small and is instructed to record them in the form of a chart. Whenever she feels a fetal movement, she is instructed to mark each movement on the chart shown in Figure 1.5.8.1 until she has marked 10 movements in all. Then she must note the time it has taken her to do so. As a general rule, a baby is doing well if he/she moves at least 10 times during three different time periods each day.

If the women can feel about 10 movements in an hour, it is considered as a normal test. If she is not able to feel adequate movements, she should have something to eat or drink and lie in left lateral position. She must also concentrate a little more to feel the fetal movements. If she is not able to count 10 movements in about an hour at this second attempt, she should contact her midwife or doctor. Adequate fetal movements ensure the integrity of uteroplacental circulation and imply that placenta is supplying the fetus with an adequate amount of oxygen and nutrients.

1.5.8.2: Contraction Stress Test (CST)

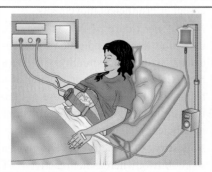

Fig. 1.5.8.2: Contraction stress test

While performing a CST, the mother is placed in dorsal supine position with a leftward tilt, and external monitors are applied. Contractions are induced either through nipple stimulation or through infusion of a dilute solution of oxytocin. An IV infusion of dilute oxytocin may be initiated at a rate of 0.5 mU/minute until there are at least three contractions, within a 10-minute period, each lasting for 40 seconds or more.

Interpretation of CST is as follows:

Negative: No decelerations with the three contractions in the 10-minute window

Suspicious: Presence of intermittent late decelerations or severe variable decelerations.

Positive: Late decelerations with 50% or more of the contractions. Even though CST is rarely performed nowadays, a positive CST is an indication for cesarean delivery.

1.5.8.3: Nonstress Test (A and B)

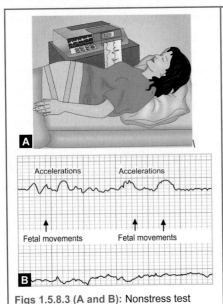

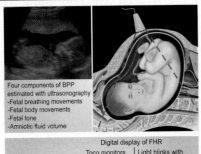

Figs 1.5.8.3 (A and B): Nonstress test

Nonstress test (NTS) involves attaching one belt of an external tocodynamometer to the mother's abdomen to measure fetal heart rate and another belt to measure uterine contractions. Fetal movement, heart rate and "reactivity" of fetal heart are measured for 20–30 minutes. The NST is classified as reactive (normal or indicative of fetal well-being) or nonreactive (abnormal or may be indicative of fetal compromise). The NST is based on principle that the heart rate of a well-oxygenated, non acidic, neurologically intact fetus normally acccelerates with fetal movements.

The results of nonstress test can be described as follows:

Reactive NST: If there are accelerations of the fetal heart rate of at least 15 BPM over the baseline, lasting for at least 15 seconds, occurring within a 20 minutes time block.

Nonreactive NST: If these accelerations don't occur, the test is said to be nonreactive. A nonreactive NST must be followed by an alternative test for fetal surveillance such as biophysical profile (BPP) or contraction stress test. The nonreactive group is associated with a significant increase in the overall rate of cesarean delivery and a high rate of perinatal mortality.

1.5.8.4: Biophysical Profile

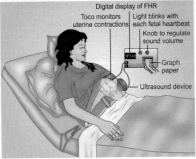

Fig. 1.5.8.4: Biophysical profile (TOCO: Toco dynamometer)

The biophysical profile (BPP) has five components altogether, each scored 0 or 2 for a maximum score of 10. A BPP test score of at least 8 out of 10 is considered reassuring. A score of 6 or 7 out of 10 is equivocal, and must be repeated within 24 hours. A score of 4 or less out of 10 is nonreassuring and strongly suggests preparing the patient for delivery.

Components of BPP are as follows:

Amniotic fluid volume: Score of two is given if a single vertical pocket of amniotic fluid is > 2 cm in two perpendicular planes. Score of zero is given if largest vertical pocket of amniotic fluid is 2 cm or less.

Fetal breathing movements: Score of two is given if there is one or more episode of rhythmic fetal breathing movements of 30 seconds or more within 30 minutes. Score of zero is given in case of abnormal, absent or insufficient breathing movements.

Fetal movement: A score of two is given in case of three or more discreet body or limb movements within 30 minutes. Score of zero is given in case of abnormal, absent or insufficient movements.

Fetal tone: Score of two is given in case of at least one episode of flexion-extension of a fetal extremity with return to flexion, or opening or closing of a hand within 30 minutes. Score of zero is given in case of abnormal, absent or insufficient fetal tone.

Nonstress test: Reactive NST is given a score of two, whereas nonreactive NST is given a score of zero.

Picture	Medical/Surgical Description	Management/Clinical Highlights

1.5.8.5: Doppler Velocimetry

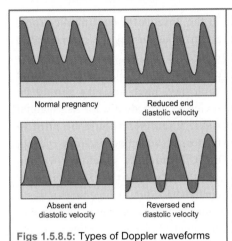

Figs 1.5.8.5: Types of Doppler waveforms

Doppler velocimetry is a noninvasive method for assessing fetal vascular impedance. Description of various Doppler indices has been done in Section 7. Some of important Doppler indices, which help in evaluating the blood flow through uterine and umbilical blood vessels, include the S/D ratio, pulsatility index and the resistance index. In normal pregnancy, S/D ratio and pulsatility index decreases with an increase in the gestational age. Various types of Doppler waveforms are discribed in adjacent Figure.

Doppler velocimetry helps in assessing fetal-placental unit by detecting the movement of blood flow through the maternal and fetal vessels. In normal pregnancy, there is an increase in the end-diastolic velocity with an increase in the gestational age. Absent and reversed end-diastolic flows are the more extreme examples of abnormal S/D ratio and may prompt delivery in some situations.

1.6: LIFESTYLE CHANGES DURING PREGNANCY

1.6.1: Diet/Nutrition During Pregnancy (A and B)

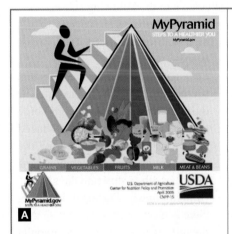

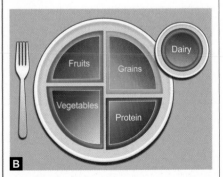

Figs 1.6.1 (A and B): (A) My pyramid: Steps to a healthier you; (B) My plate: components of a healthy diet
Source: US Department of Agriculture, www.mypyramid.org

In 2005, the US department of Agriculture (USDA) created "My Pyramid", demonstrating the various components of a healthy diet (Fig. 1.6.1A). The health pyramid demonstrates that healthy dietary choices must be balanced with appropriate activities (person on stairs). USDA's "My pyramid" was replaced in 2011 by "USDA's my plate" (Fig. 1.6.1B). The pregnant woman must try to consume 6–7 ounces of grain, two to three cups of fruits and vegetables, at least three cups of milk and 5–6 ounces of beans and meat every day. In the absence of any complications, the woman must try to do moderate-intensity physical activity for at least 30 minutes or more every day.

In this pyramid, the food is grouped into six categories on the basis of their similar nutrient content, i.e. grains, fruits, vegetables, milk, meat, beans and fish. For example, food in milk group includes those foods, which are high in calcium, riboflavin and proteins. Each food group supplies some but not all the essential nutrients, thus some food form belonging to each group must be consumed daily. The pregnant woman must avoid consuming too much sugary or fatty food. She must try to obtain most of the fats from fish, nuts and vegetable oils.

1.6.2: Exercise During Pregnancy (A and B)

Picture	Medical/Surgical Description	Management/Clinical Highlights
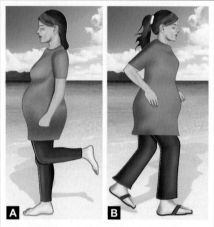 **Figs 1.6.2 (A and B):** Exercise during pregnancy	Figures 1.6.2 (A and B) shows a woman performing exercises during pregnancy. It is the duty of the clinician to emphasize the importance of exercising and activity during pregnancy. Brisk walking and swimming are two exercises, which are acceptable to most women. The obstetrician should help devise an exercise program for the women who want to remain active during pregnancy and alleviate their myths and doubts related to adverse effects of exercise during pregnancy.	In the absence of contraindications, pregnant lady should be encouraged to engage in regular, moderate-intensity physical activity 30 minutes or more each day. Each activity should be reviewed individually for its potential risks. Exercises should be mild to moderate (swimming, walking, cycling, etc.). Previously sedentary women should begin with 15 minutes of continuous exercise three times a week, which should be gradually increased to 30-minutes sessions, four times a week.

1.7: LACTATION

1.7.1: Endocrine Mechanism of Milk Ejection

Picture	Medical/Surgical Description	Management/Clinical Highlights
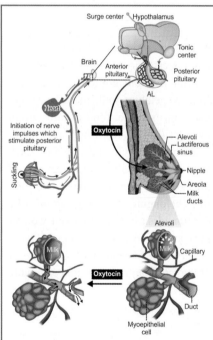 **Fig. 1.7.1:** Endocrine mechanism of milk ejection	Lactation is the process of milk production, which occurs from the mammary glands. The endocrine mechanism of milk ejection is illustrated in Figure 1.7.1. These are exocrine glands, whose function is to nourish the neonate. Prolactin is the most important hormone, which is responsible for galactopoiesis. Sucking is essential for maintenance of effective lactation. It helps in removal of milk produced by the glands as well as causes release of prolactin.	The endocrine control of lactation can be divided into the following stages: • *Mammogenesis*: This stage is associated with preparation of the breast tissues. • *Lactogenesis*: There is synthesis and secretion of milk by breast alveoli during this phase. Although some amount of secretions are produced from the breasts throughout the pregnancy, actual milk secretion starts by 3rd or 4th postpartum days. • *Galactokinesis*: During this phase, there is ejection of milk. Due to this, the milk is forced down the ampulla of lactiferous ducts from where it can be sucked by the infant. • *Galactopoiesis*: This phase is associated with maintenance of lactation.

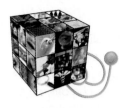

EVIDENCE-BASED BREAKTHROUGH FACTS

1. USE OF HERBAL SUPPLEMENTS IN PREGNANCY

According to a multicentric, retrospective, cohort study, use of herbal supplements is quite common in pregnancy, with almond oil, chamomile and fennel being the most commonly used herbs. These drugs are commonly consumed without taking physician's advice. Both length of gestation and birthweight are adversely affected by herb consumption. Use of almond oil during pregnancy is significantly associated with an increased incidence of preterm birth. Therefore it is important for the healthcare providers to counsel patients against the use of these drugs. However larger studies are required in future in order to clarify the causality of this relationship.

Source: Facchinetti F, Pedrielli G, Benoni G, et al. Herbal supplements in pregnancy: unexpected results from a multicentre study. Hum Reprod. 2012. [Epub ahead of print]

2. USE OF VITAMINS AND MINERALS DURING PREGNANCY

Upon the review of literature, related to the effect of supplementation with various minerals and vitamins during pregnancy, it has been found that maternal iron deficiency is likely to directly influence the neonatal iron stores and birthweight. Iron deficiency may also cause cognitive and behavioral problems in childhood. Therefore, iron supplementation is recommended to all low-income pregnant women, especially in the developing countries or in areas where iron deficiency is documented. However, since iron overload can result in toxicity, overtreatment should be avoided. Deficiency of calcium in the diet is also associated with the development of preeclampsia and intrauterine growth restriction. Supplementation of pregnant women with calcium is likely to reduce the risk of both low birthweight and the severity of preeclampsia. Deficiency of magnesium during pregnancy may cause hematological and teratogenic damage. Supplementation with zinc during pregnancy is likely to improve poor gastrointestinal function, and increase birthweight and head circumference. Selenium is an antioxidant, which is essential for the development of humoral and cell-mediated immunity. Low levels of selenium during pregnancy is likely to cause recurrent abortion, preeclampsia and IUGR. Though beneficial effects of selenium supplementation have been described, presently no evidence-based recommendation for selenium supplementation during pregnancy is available. Deficiency of vitamin B6 is associated with preeclampsia, gestational carbohydrate intolerance, hyperemesis gravidarum and neurologic disease of infants. Deficiency of folic acid may cause congenital malformations (neural tube damage, orofacial clefts, cardiac anomalies.), anemia, etc. spontaneous abortions, preeclampsia, IUGR and abruption placentae. Supplementation with folic acid (in the dose of 400 µg/day) during the preconceptional and periconceptional period helps in preventing neural tube defects. An insufficient supply of vitamin B12 is common in the developing countries, especially amongst the vegetarians. Deficiency of vitamin B12 may cause reduced fetal growth. Therefore, supplementation of vitamin B12, especially amongst vegetarian women may be required. Deficiency of vitamin A is also prevalent in the developing world. The recommended upper limit for intake of retinol supplements during pregnancy is 3,000 IU/day. Supplementation with vitamin A helps in improving birthweight and growth in infants born to HIV-infected women. Overdosage must be avoided as it causes toxicity. Deficiency of vitamin C may increase the risk for the development of pre-eclampsia, and supplementation may be useful. Supplementation with vitamin D in the third trimester in vitamin D deficient women also seems to be beneficial.

Source: Hovdenak N, Haram K. Influence of mineral and vitamin supplements on pregnancy outcome. Eur J Obstet Gynecol Reprod Biol. 2012;164(2):127-32.

3. PREVENTION OF VARICELLA-ZOSTER INFECTION AFTER EXPOSURE

VariZIG (Cangene Corporation, Winnipeg, Canada) is the only varicella zoster immune globulin preparation available in the United States for postexposure prophylaxis of varicella in persons at high risk for severe disease who lack evidence of immunity to varicella and are ineligible for varicella vaccine. When postexposure prophylaxis is indicated and active immunization is contraindicated, passive immunization with VariZIG should be offered as soon as possible. The US food and drug administration has extended the window of passive immunization after varicella exposure from 4 days (96 hours) in the past to 10 days, now. VariZIG should be administered as soon as possible after exposure.

Source: Centers for Disease Control and Prevention (CDC). FDA approval of an extended period for administering VariZIG for postexposure prophylaxis of varicella. MMWR. 2012;61(12):212.

4. HYPERIMMUNE GLOBULIN FOR TREATMENT OF PRIMARY CMV INFECTION IN PREGNANCY

Cytomegalovirus infection early in gestation is likely to be associated with a high risk of adverse neonatal outcomes such as sensorineural hearing loss or neurological deficits. Administration of intravenous hyperimmune globulin to pregnant women with primary CMV infection in early pregnancy is likely to be associated with a significant reduction in the rate of poor neonatal outcome (13% with maternal treatment versus 43% without maternal treatment). Although this therapy appears to be a promising approach for reducing poor neonatal outcomes associated with congenital CMV infection, presently there is insufficient evidence to recommend routine treatment of pregnant women with primary CMV infection in early pregnancy.

Source: Visentin S, Manara R, Milanese L, et al. Early primary cytomegalovirus infection in pregnancy: maternal hyperimmunoglobulin therapy improves outcomes among infants at 1 year of age. Clin Infect Dis. 2012;55(4):497.

5. VITAMIN D SUPPLEMENTATION FOR TERM NEONATES

Deficiency of vitamin D is likely to result in rickets in children. There is also likely to be an association between vitamin D insufficiency and development of type 1 diabetes mellitus as well as inflammatory diseases amongst the infants. The Institute of Medicine of the National Academies, the American Academy of Paediatrics, the Drug and Therapeutics Committee of the Lawson Wilkins Paediatric Endocrine Society, the Canadian Paediatric Society and the European Society for Paediatric Endocrinology have recommended daily supplementation with 400 IU/day of vitamin D for term infants to help maintain the serum levels greater than 50 nmol/L.

Source: Onwuneme C, Carroll A, McCarthy R, et al. What is the ideal dose of vitamin d supplementation for term neonates? Arch Dis Child. 2012;97(4):387-9.

Section 2

Labor and Delivery

2.1: FEMALE PELVIS

2.1.1: Ventral/Anterior View of Pelvis (A and B)

Picture	Clinical Description	Management/Clinical Features
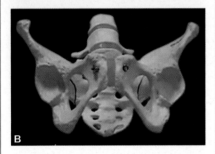 **Figs 2.1.1 (A and B):** Ventral/anterior view of pelvis	The human pelvis comprises of four bones: two innominate bones, one sacrum (which forms the rear of the pelvis and articulates with the innominate bones on the two sides) and the other coccyx (which forms the base of the spine and pelvis). Together, all these bones help in forming the true pelvis. This helps in forming the bony canal through which the fetus passes during the normal vaginal mechanism of childbirth. The true pelvis is composed of an inlet, cavity and the outlet.	The four bones of the pelvis connect at four joints: two sacroiliac joints, one pubic symphysis between the two innominate bone and one sacrococcygeal joint. Each of the innominate bones is composed of three parts: ilium, ischium and pubis.

2.1.2: Superior View of Inlet (A and B)

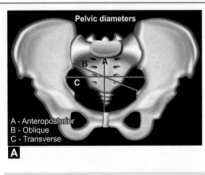 **Figs 2.1.2 (A and B):** Superior view of inlet	Superior border of the inlet or the pelvic brim helps in separating false pelvis on above from the true pelvis below. The superior border of the inlet is round in shape except for the sacral promontory which protrudes into it posteriorly. No muscle normally crosses the pelvic brim. The boundaries of pelvic inlet are described in 2.1.10.	The anterior-posterior (AP) diameters of pelvic inlet have been described in Figure 2.1.5. The transverse diameter of the inlet is the distance between the farthest two points on the iliopectineal line and is the largest diameter of the pelvis. It measures about 13 cm (4 cm anterior to the promontory and 7 cm behind the symphysis). Right and left oblique diameters of the inlet extend from right and left sacroiliac joints to the left and right iliopectineal eminences respectively.

Picture	Clinical Description	Management/Clinical Features

2.1.3: View of Pelvic Outlet (A and B)

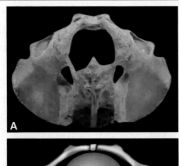

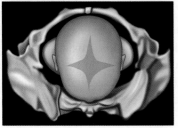

Figs 2.1.3 (A and B): View of pelvic outlet

The pelvic outlet as shown in Figures 2.1.3 (A and B) is lozenge-shaped and is bounded by lower border of pubic symphysis, pubic arch, ischial tuberosities, sacrotuberous and sacrospinous ligaments, and tip of coccyx.

Diameters of pelvic outlet are as follows:
Anterior-posterior diameter: Anatomical AP diameter (11 cm) extends from tip of coccyx to the lower border of pubic symphysis. Obstetric AP diameter (13 cm) extends from the tip of sacrum to the lower border of symphysis pubis as the coccyx moves backward during the second stage of labor.
Transverse diameter: This extends between the two ischial tuberosities and measures 11 cm.

2.1.4: Posterior/Dorsal View of Pelvis

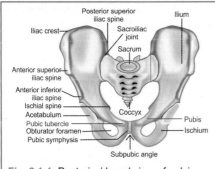

Fig. 2.1.4: Posterior/dorsal view of pelvis

Figure 2.1.4 shows bony landmarks of the pelvis as visualized from posterior aspect.

The structures on the back of pelvis include sacrum (with the posterior sacral foramina), coccyx, iliac crest, posterior superior iliac spines, acetabulum (where the greater trochanter of femur articulate), ischiopubic ramus, ischial spine, obturator foramen, etc.

2.1.5: Medial View of Pelvis

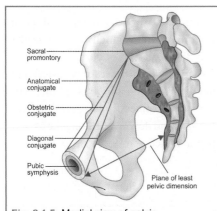

Fig. 2.1.5: Medial view of pelvis

Figure 2.1.5 shows the medial view of pelvis from left, illustrating various diameters of the pelvic inlet.

Various AP diameters of pelvic inlet are as follows:
- *True conjugate or anatomical conjugate (11 cm)*: This is measured from the midpoint of sacral promontory to the upper border of pubic symphysis.
- *Obstetric conjugate (10.5 cm)*: This is measured from the midpoint of sacral promontory to the most bulging point on the back of symphysis pubic.
- *Diagonal conjugate (12.5 cm)*: It is measured from the tip of sacral promontory to the lower border of pubic symphysis.

2.1.6: Ventral/Anterior View of Sacrum

Picture	Clinical Description	Management/Clinical Features
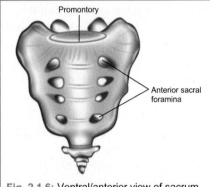 Fig. 2.1.6: Ventral/anterior view of sacrum	Figure 2.1.6 shows ventral/anterior view of the sacrum.	Sacrum is a triangular bone at the base of the spine, which connects with the lumbar vertebra in the upper part and coccyx in the lower part. The base of sacrum in the upper part projects outward to form the sacral promontory. This articulates with the last lumbar vertebra. The two lateral projections of sacrum are known as the alae and articulate with the iliac bones on either side forming the sacroiliac joints. Ventral sacral foramen can be located on the anterior side of sacrum. At the tip of the sacrum is present the coccyx.

2.1.7: Dorsal/Posterior View of Sacrum

Picture	Clinical Description	Management/Clinical Features
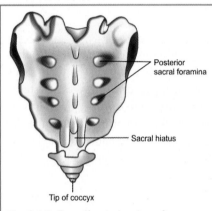 Fig. 2.1.7: Dorsal/posterior view of sacrum	Figure 2.1.7 shows dorsal or posterior view of sacrum.	Ala of sacrum can be seen on the two sides. There is a midline bony projection termed as the median sacral crest at the top of which is the sacral canal and below is the sacral hiatus. Dorsal sacral foramina can be visualized from the posterior side of sacrum. On the top can be visualized the two superior articular processes or facets which articulate with the lumbar bone.

2.1.8: Pelvic Axis

Picture	Clinical Description	Management/Clinical Features
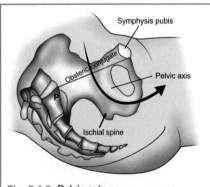 Fig. 2.1.8: Pelvic axis	Pelvic axis or the curve of Carus is an imaginary line joining the center points of the plane of inlet, cavity and outlet. It is C-shaped with concavity directed forward and has no obstetric significance.	Obstetric axis, on the other hand, is an imaginary line, which represents the way the head moves during labor. It is J-shaped which passes downward and backward along the axis of inlet till the ischial spines from where it passes forward and downward along the axis of pelvic outlet.

Picture	Clinical Description	Management/Clinical Features

2.1.9: Pelvic Assessment (A to F)

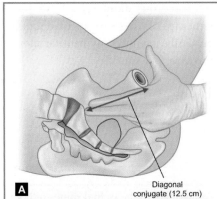

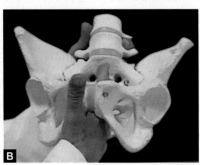

Figs 2.1.9 (A and B): Measurement of diagonal conjugate

The method of measuring diagonal conjugate is as follows:
- After placing the patient in dorsal position and taking all aseptic precautions two fingers are introduced into vagina. The clinician tries to feel the anterior sacral curvature with these fingers.
- The point at which the bone recedes from the finger is sacral promontory.
- A marking is placed over the clinician's gloved index finger with the index finger of the other hand. After removing the fingers from the vagina, the distance between the marking and the tip of the middle finger is measured in order to obtain the measurement of diagonal conjugate.

If the pelvis is adequate, middle finger will not reach the sacral promontory. The clinician may be required to depress the elbow and wrist while mobilizing the fingers upward in order to reach the promontory. In normal cases, it will be difficult to feel the sacral promontory.

In clinical situations if the middle finger fails to reach the sacral promontory or reaches it with difficulty, the diagonal conjugate can be considered as adequate.

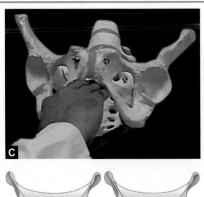

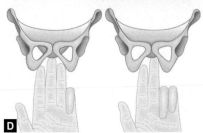

Figs 2.1.9 (C and D): Assessment of subpubic angle

After separating the labia with left hand, two fingers of the right hand are gently introduced inside the vaginal introitus. To measure the subpubic angle, while withdrawing the hand out, the clinician's examining fingers are turned so that the palm of the hand faces downward. At the same time, the third finger is also held out at the vaginal introitus and the angle under the pubis is felt.

Subpubic angle is the angle between two pubic rami. It varies from 85° ± 5°. Normal subpubic angle allows the placement of three to four fingers in the subpubic space. If at least three fingers can be placed under the pubis, the subpubic angle is approximately 90°, which can be considered as adequate. If the subpubic angle allows only two fingers, the subpubic angle is about 60°, which is indicative of an inadequate pelvis.

Picture	Clinical Description	Management/Clinical Features
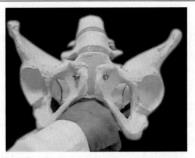 **Fig. 2.1.9E:** Measurement of transverse diameter of the outlet	For assessment of the pelvic outlet, the subpubic angle, intertuberous diameter (transverse diameter of the outlet) and mobility of the coccyx are determined. After measuring the subpubic angle, as the obstetrician's hand is withdrawn from the vaginal introitus, the intertuberous diameter is measured with the knuckles of the closed fist of the hand placed between the ischial tuberosities.	If the pelvis is adequate, the intertuberous diameter allows four knuckles. In case of an inadequate pelvis, the intertuberous diameter allows less than four knuckles.
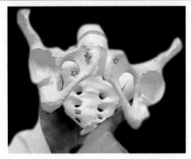 **Fig. 2.1.9F:** Assessment of ischial spines	Ischial spines are palpated for the assessment of midpelvis. After assessing the sacrum, the obstetrician must move his/her fingers lateral to the midsacrum where the sacrospinous ligaments can be felt. If these ligaments are followed laterally, the ischial spines can be palpated.	Assessment of the ischial spines of both the sides can help in the evaluation of interischial diameter, which is also known as the plane of least pelvic dimensions. The plane of least pelvic dimensions should not be less than 9.5 cm. Also, in case of inadequate pelvis, the ischial spines may appear sharp and prominent.

2.1.10: Boundaries of Pelvic Brim

Picture	Clinical Description	Management/Clinical Features
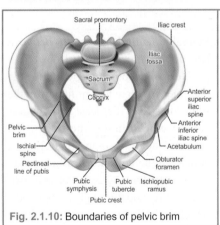 **Fig. 2.1.10:** Boundaries of pelvic brim	Figure 2.1.10 shows margins of pelvic brim, which can be considered as the boundary line of pelvic inlet and divides the pelvis anatomically into false pelvis and true pelvis.	The boundaries of pelvic brim are sacral promontory, alae of sacrum, sacroiliac joints, iliopectineal line, iliopectineal eminence, upper border of superior pubic rami, pubic tubercle, pubic crest and upper border of symphysis pubis.

2.1.11: Entry of Fetal Head into Maternal Pelvis (A to D)

Picture	Clinical Description	Management/Clinical Features
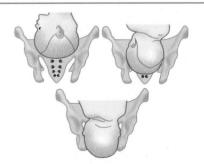 **Fig. 2.1.11A:** Diagram showing rotation of fetal head by 90° as it descends into the pelvis	At the time of entry of fetal head into the maternal pelvis, the occipitofrontal diameter engages through the superior pelvic aperture in transverse diameter of the inlet.	With further descent, the fetal head undergoes 90° rotation so that longest diameter of the fetal head engages in AP diameter of the outlet, which is its largest diameter. This rotation facilitates the passage of fetal head, which is the least compressible part of fetal body, easily through the pelvic inlet and then through the outlet to the outside world.

Picture	Clinical Description	Management/Clinical Features
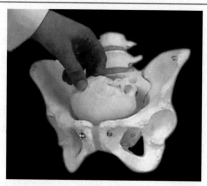 Fig. 2.1.11B: The engaging diameter of fetal head engages in the transverse diameter of the inlet	At the time of entry of fetal head into the maternal pelvis, the occipitofrontal diameter engages through the superior pelvic aperture in transverse diameter because it is the longest diameter of the pelvic inlet.	Dimensions of fetal head are most important because it is the least compressible part of the fetus. Therefore, the fetal head engages in the longest available pelvic dimension.
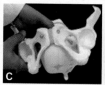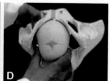 Figs 2.1.11 (C and D): The fetal head undergoes internal rotation by 90° inside the pelvic cavity	As the fetal head descents downward, it undergoes rotation by 90° so that the longest diameter of fetal head engages in AP diameter of the outlet, which is its largest diameter.	Rotation of the fetal head by 90° is facilitated by contractions of levator ani muscles of pelvic diaphragm.

2.1.12: Different Planes and Axis of the Pelvis

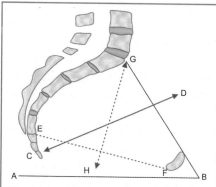

Fig. 2.1.12: Different planes and axis of the pelvis (AB, Horizontal line; GB, Plane of inlet; FE, Plane of obstetric outlet; DC, Axis of the inlet; GH, Axis of obstetrical outlet)

The plane of the pelvic inlet (also known as superior strait) is not horizontal, but is tilted forward. It makes an angle of 55° with the horizontal. This angle is known as the angle of inclination. Radiographically this angle can be measured by measuring the angle between the front of the vertebra L5 and plane of inlet, and subtracting this from 180°. Increase in the angle of inclination has obstetric significance as this may result in delayed engagement of the fetal head and delay in descent of fetal head. Increase in the angle of inclination also favors occipitoposterior position. On the other hand, the reduction in the angle of inclination may not have any obstetric significance.

The axis of the pelvic inlet is a line drawn perpendicular to the plane of inlet in the midline. It is in downward and backward direction. Upon extension, this line passes through the umbilicus anteriorly and through the coccyx posteriorly.

In a typical female pelvis, widest diameter of the inlet is the transverse diameter, whereas the widest diameter of the outlet is AP diameter. For the proper descent and engagement of fetal head, it is important that the uterine axis coincides with the axis of inlet.

Picture	Clinical Description	Management/Clinical Features

2.1.13: Waste Space of Morris

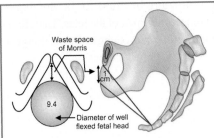

Fig. 2.1.13: Waste space of Morris

Normally the width of the pubic arch is such that a round disc of 9.4 cm (diameter of a well flexed head) can pass through the pubic arch at a distance of 1 cm from the midpoint of the inferior border of the symphysis pubis. This distance is known as the "waste space of Morris".

In case of an inadequate pelvis with narrow pubic arch, the fetal head would be pushed backward and the waste space of Morris would increase. As a result, reduced space would be available for fetal head to pass through, due to which the fetal head would be forced to pass through a smaller diameter termed as the "available anterior-posterior diameter". This is likely to injure the perineum or sometimes cause the arrest of fetal head.

2.1.14: Different Types of Pelvis

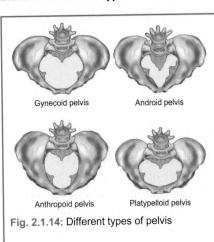

Fig. 2.1.14: Different types of pelvis

Using the "Caldwell-Moloy" system, the pelvic shape can be classified into four basic types:
- Gynecoid (50%)
- Android (20%)
- Anthropoid (25%)
- Platypelloid (5%)

Of these various types of pelvis, gynecoid pelvis is the classical female pelvis, which is most favorable for delivery.

Gynecoid pelvis is oval at the inlet with AP diameter being just slightly less than the transverse diameter. In gynecoid pelvis, the sacrum is wide with an average concavity and inclination. Sidewalls are straight with blunt ischial spines. Sacrosciatic notch is wide and subpubic angle is 90−100°.

Anthropoid pelvis is oval, long and narrow. The AP diameter of the inlet exceeds the transverse diameter giving it an oval shape. Sacrum is long and narrow. Sacrosciatic notch is wide and subpubic angle is narrow.

Android pelvis is heart shaped/triangular shaped male type of pelvis with the base toward the sacrum. As a result, posterior segment is short, and anterior segment is narrow. The pelvic sidewalls are convergent with projecting ischial spines. Both the sacrosciatic notch and subpubic angles are narrow (< 90°).

In platypelloid pelvis, pelvic brim is flat and transverse, kidney shaped. Transverse diameter is much larger than the AP diameter.

Picture	Clinical Description	Management/Clinical Features

2.2: FETAL SKULL

2.2.1: Bones of Fetal Skull (A and B)

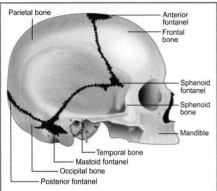

Fig. 2.2.1A: Important bones of fetal skull as seen from the side

The skull is made up of two frontal, two parietal and two temporal bones, along with the upper portion of the occipital bone and the wings of the sphenoid. The bones are not united rigidly but are separated by membranous spaces, the sutures.

Obstetrically, the head of fetus is the most important part, since an essential feature of labor is an adaptation between the fetal head and the maternal bony pelvis. Only a comparatively small part of the head of the fetus at term is represented by the face; the rest is composed of the firm skull.

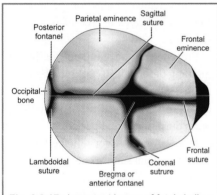

Fig. 2.2.1B: Important bones of fetal skull as seen from the top

Figure 2.2.1B shows fetal skull as seen from top. Many fetal bones, sutures and fontanels can be observed.

The fetal bones as seen from the top include parts of unossified frontal bone showing frontal eminence; two parietal bones showing parietal eminence each; and part of the occipital bone. Anterior fontanel between two parietal bones and two parts of unossified frontal bone, and posterior fontanel between the occipital bone and the parietal bones can be seen. The sutures which can be seen include sagittal suture, coronal sutures and lambdoid sutures.

2.2.2: Fontanels of Fetal Skull (A to G)

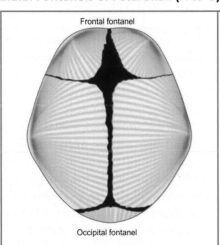

Fig. 2.2.2A: Fontanels of fetal skull as seen from the top

The place where several sutures meet, an irregular space is formed, which is enclosed by a membrane and is designated as a fontanel. Figure 2.2.2A shows fontanels of fetal skull as seen from the top.

The two main fontanels of fetal skull as seen from the top include the anterior and posterior fontanel. The greater or anterior fontanel is a lozenge-shaped space situated at the junction of the sagittal and coronal sutures. The lesser, or posterior fontanel is represented by a small triangular area at the intersection of the sagittal and lambdoid sutures.

Picture	Clinical Description	Management/Clinical Features
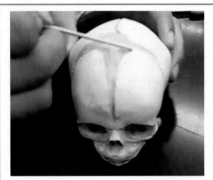 **Fig. 2.2.2B:** Fontanels of fetal skull as seen from the side Labels: Lambdoidal suture, Coronal suture, Sphenoidal fontanel, Maxilla, Mandible, Mastoid fontanel, Squamosal suture	While the two main fontanels having obstetric significance in the fetal head are anterior fontanel (bregma) and posterior fontanel (lambda), there are smaller fontanels present at each side of the head. Present anteriorly is sphenoidal fontanel and posteriorly is the mastoid fontanel. These fontanels are visible if the fetal skull is seen from the side as shown in the Figure 2.2.2B.	Both anterior and posterior fontanels may be felt readily during labor, and their recognition gives important information concerning the presentation and position of the fetus.
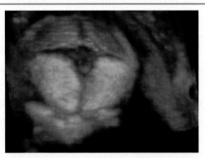 **Fig. 2.2.2C:** Anterior fontanel (bregma)	Anterior fontanel is formed by joining of four sutures: frontal suture (anteriorly); sagittal suture (posteriorly) and coronal sutures on the two sides (laterally). It measures about 3 cm in each of the dimensions (AP and transverse).	The palpation of anterior fontanel on vaginal examination is of great obstetric significance. Palpation of anterior fontanel indicates degree of flexion of fetal head. Presence of this fontanel facilitates molding of fetal head. The membranous nature of anterior fontanel helps in accommodating the rapid growth of brain during neonatal period. Floor of the anterior fontanel reflects the intracranial status. The floor may be depressed in case of dehydration and elevated in case of hydrocephalus or other conditions with raised intracranial tension.
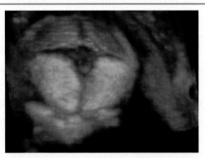 **Fig. 2.2.2D:** Three-dimensional ultrasound view of the fetus showing anterior fontanel (bregma)	Figure 2.2.2D shows a three-dimensional ultrasound view of the fetus demonstrating an anterior fontanel. Sutures and fontanels of fetal head can be visualized with three-dimensional ultrasound later during the first trimester.	The size of anterior fontanel can normally be observed to be increasing in size throughout the gestation. However, its size in relation to the volume of fetal head reduces due to the development of brain and growth of cranial bones. Measurement of size of the anterior fontanel on ultrasound proves to be useful because abnormal dimensions of the fontanel may be associated with underlying fetal anomalies. Studies have shown the anterior fontanel to be enlarged during the second trimester ultrasound in cases of Down's syndrome.

Picture	Clinical Description	Management/Clinical Features
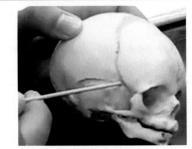 Fig. 2.2.2E: Posterior fontanel	Figure 2.2.2E shows the posterior fontanel which is triangular in shape (measuring about half inch in each dimension) and is present on the posterior aspect of skull. It has a membranous floor which becomes bony by term.	Posterior fontanel is formed by the joining of three sutures: sagittal suture (anteriorly) and lambdoid sutures on the two sides. The clinical significance of posterior fontanel is that it indicates the position of fetal head in relation to the maternal pelvis.
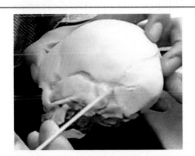 Fig. 2.2.2F: Sphenoid fontanel	Sphenoid fontanel is present between the coronal sutures (which connects the frontal and parietal bones) and squamosal sutures (which connect the temporal squama with lower border of parietal bone).	Sphenoid fontanel is present between the frontal bone and anterior lip of the parietal bone, and the temperal bone and the greater wing of sphenoid.
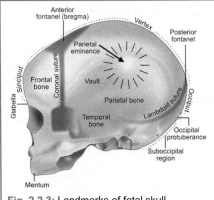 Fig. 2.2.2G: Mastoid fontanel	Mastoid fontanel is present between the lambdoidal sutures (which connect the parietal and temporal bone with the occipital bone) and squamosal sutures.	Mastoid fontanel is present between the temporal, occipital and parietal bones.

2.2.3: Landmarks of Fetal Skull

Picture	Clinical Description	Management/Clinical Features
Fig. 2.2.3: Landmarks of fetal skull	Figure 2.2.3 shows important landmarks of fetal skull, which include the sinciput, occiput, and anterior and posterior fontanel.	Palpation of occiput is important because it gives an idea about the flexion of fetal head. In a completely flexed head, the occiput and posterior fontanel can be palpated. However, the anterior fontanel cannot be palpated. The more deflexed the fetal head, the more likely is the anterior fontanel to be palpated.

Picture	Clinical Description	Management/Clinical Features

2.2.4: Sutures of Fetal Skull

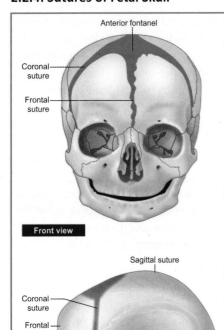

Front view

Side view

Fig. 2.2.4: Sutures of fetal skull

Figure 2.2.4 shows all the important sutures of fetal skull. Sutures can be defined as narrow ridges of connective tissue joining the flat bones of the skull.

The fetal skull has four main sutures and are as follows:

- *Sagittal or longitudinal suture*: Lies longitudinally across the vault of the skull in midline between the two parietal bones.
- *Coronal sutures*: These sutures are present between the parietal and frontal bones and extend transversely on either side from the anterior fontanels.
- *Lambdoid sutures*: This suture separates the occipital bone from the two parietal bones and extends transversely both on the right and left side from the posterior fontanel.
- *Frontal suture*: This suture is present between the two halves of the frontal bone in the skull of infants and children and usually disappears by the age of 6 years.

2.2.5: Diameters of Fetal Skull

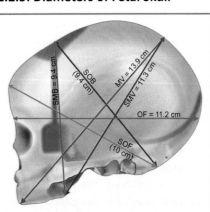

Fig. 2.2.5: Diameters of fetal skull (SOB, suboccipilobregmatic; MV, mentovertical; SMV, submentovertical; OF, occipitofrontal; SOP, suboccipitofrontal)

The important AP diameters of the fetal skull are shown in the adjacent Figure. Suboccipitobregmatic diameter extends from the nape of the neck to the center of bregma. Suboccipitofrontal extends from the nape of the neck to the anterior end of anterior fontanel or center of sinciput. Occipitofrontal diameter extends from the occipital eminence to the root of nose (glabella). Mentovertical diameter extends from midpoint of the chin to the highest point on sagittal suture. Submentovertical diameter extends from the junction of the floor of the mouth and neck to the highest point on sagittal suture. Submentobregmatic diameter extends from the junction of the floor of the mouth and neck to the center of bregma.

Important transverse diameters of the fetal skull are as follows:

Biparietal diameter (9.5 cm): It extents between the two parietal eminences. This diameter nearly always engages.

Supersubparietal diameter (8.5 cm): It extends from a point placed below one parietal eminence to a point placed above the other parietal eminence of the opposite side.

Bitemporal diameter (8 cm): Distance between the anteroinferior ends of the coronal sutures.

Bimastoid diameter (7.5 cm): Distance between the tips of the mastoid process. This diameter is nearly incompressible.

Picture	Clinical Description	Management/Clinical Features

2.3: OBSTETRIC EXAMINATION

2.3.1: General Physical Examination

2.3.1.1: Measurement of Weight and Body Mass Index

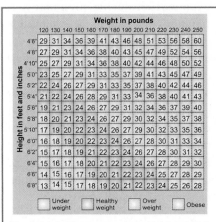

Fig. 2.3.1.1: Measurement of weight and body mass index

Body mass index (BMI), which is also known as the Quetelet index, is calculated by dividing the woman's weight in kilograms by height in meters square.

$BMI = Wt/ht^2 = kg/m^2$

Suggested weight gain during pregnancy is based on the woman's BMI as follows:

- In case of an underweight woman (BMI < 18.5), recommended weight gain during pregnancy is 12.5–18 Kg.
- In a woman with normal weight (BMI of 18.5–24.9), recommended weight gain is 11.5–16 Kg.
- In an overweight woman (BMI of 25.0–29.9), recommended weight gain is 7–11.5 Kg.
- In a woman with twin gestation, recommended weight gain is about 15.5–20.4 kg.

2.3.1.2: Distribution of Weight Gain During Pregnancy

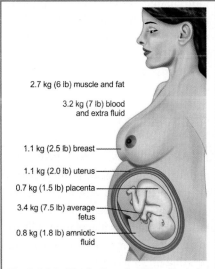

2.7 kg (6 lb) muscle and fat
3.2 kg (7 lb) blood and extra fluid
1.1 kg (2.5 lb) breast
1.1 kg (2.0 lb) uterus
0.7 kg (1.5 lb) placenta
3.4 kg (7.5 lb) average fetus
0.8 kg (1.8 lb) amniotic fluid

Fig. 2.3.1.2: Distribution of weight gain during pregnancy

Gestational weight gain amounts to about 28–29 pounds. Distribution of weight gain during pregnancy is described in Figure 2.3.1.2.

Out of 12.5 kg of average weight gain during pregnancy, approximately 3.5 kg is fat. The components of gestational weight gain are summarized below:

- *Products of conception*: Fetus (7.5–8.5 pounds), placenta and umbilical cord (1.5 lbs), and amniotic fluid (1.8 lbs).
- *Fluids in the extra-fetal tissues, gained by the mother in order to support pregnancy*: This amounts to about 6.7-7.0 lbs. The increase in intravascular blood volume, a normal physiological change occurring during pregnancy, amounts to about 4.0 lbs, whereas increase in tissue fluids amounts to about 2.7–3 lbs.
- *Maternal reserves*: There is about 1.0 lbs deposits of fat in breast and 7.5 lbs deposits in form of proteins and fat over rest of the body, particularly, uterus (amounting to about 1.5–2 lbs) and abdominal tissues, muscles of the back and upper thighs (6 lbs), which serve as an energy reservoir during time of labor and lactation. Altogether, the maternal reserves are responsible for about 8.5 lbs of weight gain during pregnancy.

Picture	Clinical Description	Management/Clinical Features

2.3.1.3: Head-to-toe Examination (A to I)

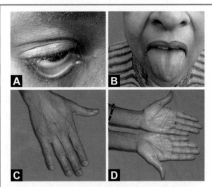

Figs 2.3.1.3 (A to D): Pallor is observed in: (A) lower palpebral conjunctiva; (B) tongue; (C) nailbed and (D) palm of hands

Figures 2.3.1.3 (A to D) demonstrate the areas in the human body, which the clinician must examine in order to diagnose pallor, which is commonly related to anemia during pregnancy. Reduced supply of oxyhemoglobin to the skin and mucous membranes is likely to result in their paleness, which can be detected on clinical examination. The areas in the body where pallor can be commonly observed include the lower palpebral conjunctiva, dorsal surface of tongue, palms of hand and nail beds.

General physical examination forms an important component of clinical examination during pregnancy. It comprises of a head-to-toe examination of the pregnant woman to look for clinical signs suggestive of any medical disorder. The important parameters, which must be assessed at the time of general physical examination during pregnancy, include measurement of maternal weight (for calculation of BMI), blood pressure measurement, and clinical assessment for edema, pallor, jaundice and thyroid enlargement.

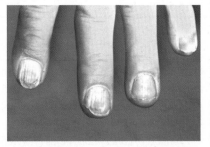

Fig. 2.3.1.3E: Nail changes suggestive of koilonychia

Figure 2.3.1.3E shows nail changes suggestive of koilonychia. This is a clinical finding where the nails lose their normal convexity and become depressed or flat or acquire a slight concavity. This results in production of spoon-shaped nails.

Presence of spoon-shaped nails is usually suggestive of hypochromic anemia, especially iron deficiency anemia. Other nail changes suggestive of systemic diseases, which can be observed include clubbing (inflammatory bowel disease); pitting (psoriasis); and onycholysis (connective tissue disorders, etc.)

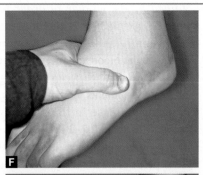

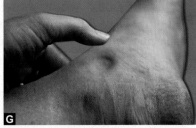

Figs 2.3.1.3 (F and G): (F) Testing for edema; (G) Presence of pitting edema in the feet

Edema is an observable swelling, which occurs due to accumulation of fluid in the body tissues. Pitting edema can be demonstrated as shown in Figures 2.3.1.3 (F and G). Pitting edema is usually demonstrated in the dependent parts of the body such as feet/ankles or the sacral region.

Pitting edema can be shown by application of pressure to the swollen area by pressing the skin with a finger. This results in an indentation in cases of pitting edema. This indentation is likely to persist for some time even after the pressing finger has been released.

Picture	Clinical Description	Management/Clinical Features
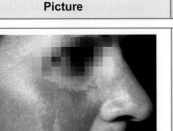 **Fig. 2.3.1.3H:** Melasma: skin change during pregnancy:	Figure 2.3.1.3H shows melasma, a frequently encountered skin change during pregnancy. It is usually produced under the effect of hormones such as estrogen and progesterone.	While it does not cause any other clinical symptom, it may be of cosmetic concern. It may disappear on its own following delivery of the baby. However, some cases may require treatment, which may comprise of one of the following: • Creams containing tretinoin, azelaic acid, topical corticosteroids, etc. • Chemical peels, microdermabrasion • Laser treatment (in extreme cases) • Topical depigmentary agents • Galvanic or ultrasonic facials
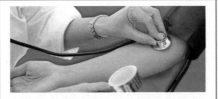 **Fig. 2.3.1.3I:** Measurement of blood pressure during pregnancy	Correct method for measurement of blood pressure during pregnancy has been illustrated in Figure 2.3.1.3I and has been described in details in Section 5 (5.2.4).	Blood pressure should be taken routinely during each antenatal visit in every pregnant woman. This is especially important to rule out preeclampsia which may present with devastating consequences both for the mother and the baby during pregnancy.

2.3.1.4: Breast Examination (A and B)

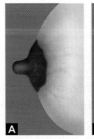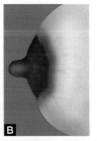 **Figs 2.3.1.4 (A and B):** (A) Breasts of a nonpregnant woman; (B) Breasts of a pregnant woman	Figures 2.3.1.4 (A and B) illustrate the changes in breasts occurring during pregnancy. There is pronounced pigmentation of the areola and nipples. There is also appearance of secondary areola, Montgomery's tubercles and presence of increased vascularity. For details regarding the changes in breasts occurring during pregnancy, kindly refer to Section 1.	Routine breast examination during antenatal examination is not recommended for the promotion of postnatal breastfeeding. Changes in the breasts are best evident in the primigravida in comparison to multigravida. Presence of secretions from the breasts of a primigravida who has never lactated is an important sign of pregnancy.

2.3.2: Abdominal Examination

2.3.2.1: Inspection of the Abdomen (A to D)

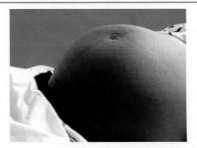 **Fig. 2.3.2.1A:** Abdominal distension	Figure 2.3.2.1A shows abdominal distension in a pregnant woman at term. Abdominal distension makes the abdomen look spherical in shape at 40 weeks of gestation.	Upon inspection of abdomen in case of a pregnant woman, the distension usually becomes visible after 16 weeks of gestation, when the uterus becomes an abdominal organ. With increasing abdominal distension as the period of gestation progresses the umbilicus becomes everted.

Picture	Clinical Description	Management/Clinical Features
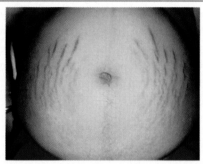 Fig. 2.3.2.1B: Linea nigra	Figure 2.3.2.1B shows the presence of linea nigra over the abdomen of a pregnant woman.	This is a blackish-brown line about 1 cm in width which runs in the midline from the xiphisternum to the pubic symphysis. This pigmentary change is probably related to the secretion of melanocyte stimulating hormone from anterior pituitary. Production of estrogen and progesterone in the body may also be responsible for producing this line. It usually disappears following delivery of the baby.
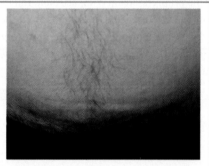 Fig. 2.3.2.1C: Stria gravidarum	Figure 2.3.2.1C shows presence of stria gravidarum over the abdomen of a pregnant woman. Stria gravidarum are linear, slightly depressed marks varying in length and width. They are found over lower anterior abdominal wall, usually below the umbilicus. Occurrence of stria gravidarum is probably related to mechanical stretching of skin and production of aldosterone during pregnancy.	The production of stria gravidarum can be minimized by controlling the weight gain during pregnancy and massaging the skin with lubricants such as olive oil. Application of creams containing glycolic acid, zinc sulfate and tyrosine as well as laser treatment (pulsed dye laser, 585 nm) is likely to produce an improvement and reduction in skin discoloration.
Fig. 2.3.2.1D: Presence of previous cesarean scar over the abdomen	Figure 2.3.2.1 shows a scar mark related to a cesarean section performed in this patient at the time of previous pregnancy. During that time, a Pfannenstiel incision was given.	At the time of abdominal inspection, it is important to observe the abdomen for presence of pregnancy related skin changes (linea nigra, stria gravidarum, etc.), presence of any varicosities, previous scar marks, etc. Presence of a previous scar mark could be related to an abdominal operative surgery done in past. Presence of scar mark related to cesarean delivery makes the patient at high risk due to a definite risk associated with uterine rupture in case of vaginal delivery in the present and future pregnancies. Moreover, the abdominal incision in future operative deliveries should be given in such a way that it also includes the scar mark of previously performed surgery.

Picture	Clinical Description	Management/Clinical Features

2.3.2.2: Abdominal Palpation (A to E)

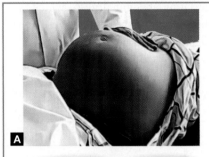

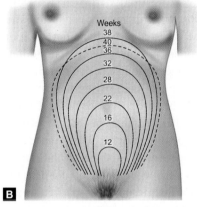

Weeks
38
40
36
32
28
22
16
12

Figs 2.3.2.2 (A and B): (A) Measurement of fundal height; (B) Correlation of fundal height with period of gestation

In order to measure the fundal height, firstly the dextrorotated uterus is centralized, following which the ulnar border of clinician's left hand is placed at the upper level of the fundus. The uterine height corresponds to the period of gestation. With increasing period of gestation, the height of the uterus increases. The rough estimation of fundal height with increasing period of gestation is shown in Figures 2.3.2.2 (A and B).

A rough estimation of the gestational age based on the fundal height is as follows:
- Midpoint between umbilicus and pubic symphysis: 16 weeks
- Lower level of umbilicus: 20 weeks
- Middle of umbilicus: 22 weeks
- Upper level of umbilicus: 24 weeks
- One-third of the distance between umbilicus and xiphisternum: 28 weeks
- Two-thirds of the distance between umbilicus and xiphisternum: 32 weeks
- Xiphisternum: 36 weeks
- One-third (of the distance between umbilicus and xiphisternum) below the xiphisternum: 40 weeks. The slight reduction in fundal height at 40 weeks is related to the engagement of fetal presenting part at term.

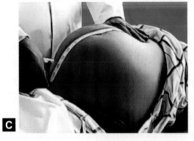

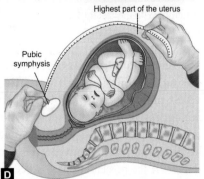

Highest part of the uterus

Pubic symphysis

Figs 2.3.2.2 (C and D): (C) Measurement of symphysis-fundal height; (D) Diagrammatic representation of symphysis fundal height

Fundal height is determined by measuring the distance from the pubic symphysis to the highest part of the uterus and comprises of the following steps:

After centralizing the dextrorotated uterus, the upper border of the fundus is located by the ulnar border of left hand and this point is marked by placing one finger there. The distance between the upper border of the symphysis and the marked point is measured in centimeters with the help of a measuring tape.

After 24 weeks, the symphysis-fundal height measured in centimeters corresponds to the period of gestation up to 36 weeks. Though a variation of 2 cm (more or less) is regarded as normal, there are numerous conditions where the symphysis-fundal height may not correspond with the period of gestation (e.g. polyhydramnios, oligohydramnios, intrauterine growth retardation, etc.)

Picture	Clinical Description	Management/Clinical Features
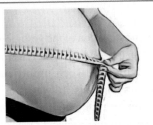 **Fig. 2.3.2.2E:** Measurement of abdominal girth	Figure 2.3.2.2E shows the method for measurement of abdominal girth in a pregnant woman. The abdominal girth is usually measured at the level of umbilicus.	In normal pregnancy after 32 weeks of gestation abdominal girth, which is 2 inches less than the period of gestation is regarded as normal. Abdominal girth of ≤ 31 inches at 36–40 weeks of gestation is indicative of IUGR. In nonpregnant woman, measurement of abdominal girth is an indicator of obesity.

2.3.2.3: Leopold's Maneuvers (A to D)

Picture	Clinical Description	Management/Clinical Features
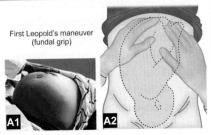 **Figs 2.3.2.3 (A1 and A2):** Fundal grip (Leopold's first maneuver)	Fundal grip (Leopold's first maneuver) is conducted while facing the patient's face. This helps the obstetrician to identify which of the fetal poles (head or breech) is present at the fundus. The fundal area is palpated by placing both the hands over the fundal area. Palpation of broad, soft, irregular mass at the fundus is suggestive of fetal legs and/or buttocks, thereby pointing toward cephalic presentation. Palpation of a smooth, hard, globular, ballotable mass at the fundus is suggestive of fetal head and points toward breech presentation.	Obstetric grips must be conducted when the uterus is relaxed and not when the woman is experiencing contractions. The mother should be comfortable lying in supine position and her abdomen is to be bared. She should be asked to semiflex her thighs in order to relax the abdominal muscles. These maneuvers can be used by experienced clinicians as an effective screening tool for detecting fetal malpresentation, particularly in settings where ultrasound may not be readily available.
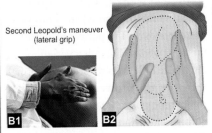 **Figs 2.3.2.3 (B1 and B2):** Lateral grip (Leopold's second maneuver)	Lateral grip (Leopold's second maneuver) is also conducted while facing the patient's face. The clinician's hands are placed flat over the abdomen on the either side of the umbilicus. Lateral grip helps the clinician in identifying the position of fetal back, limbs and shoulder in case of vertex or breech presentation.	The orientation of the fetus can be determined by noting whether the back is directed vertically (anteriorly, posteriorly) or transversely. In case of transverse lie, hard round globular mass suggestive of fetal head can be identified horizontally across the maternal abdomen. The fetal back can be identified as a smooth curved structure with a resistant feel.
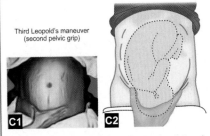 **Figs 2.3.2.3 (C1 and C2):** Second pelvic grip (Pawlik's grip) or third Leopold's maneuver	Second pelvic grip is performed while facing the patient's face. The clinician places the outstretched thumb and index finger of the right hand keeping the ulnar border of the palm on the upper border of the patient's pubic symphysis. Further details would be revealed by the next maneuver.	If a hard globular mass is gripped during this maneuver, it implies vertex presentation. A soft broad part is suggestive of fetal breech. If the presenting part is not engaged, it would be freely ballotable between the two fingers. If the presenting part is deeply engaged, the findings of this maneuver simply indicate that the lower fetal pole is in the pelvis. In case of transverse presentation, the pelvic grip is empty.

Picture	Clinical Description	Management/Clinical Features
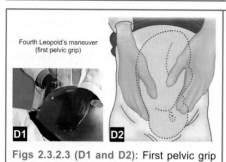 Fourth Leopold's maneuver (first pelvic grip) **D1** **D2** **Figs 2.3.2.3 (D1 and D2):** First pelvic grip (fourth Leopold's maneuver)	The objective of the first pelvic grip is to determine the amount of head palpable above the pelvic brim in case of a cephalic presentation. First pelvic grip is performed while facing the patient's feet. While performing this maneuver, tips of three fingers of each hand are placed on the either side of the midline in downward and backward direction in order to deeply palpate the fetal parts present in the lower pole of the uterus.	In case of vertex presentation, a hard smooth globular mass suggestive of fetal head can be palpated on pelvic grip. In case of breech presentation, broad soft, irregular mass is palpated.

2.3.2.4: Evaluation of Engagement of Fetal Head (A to E)

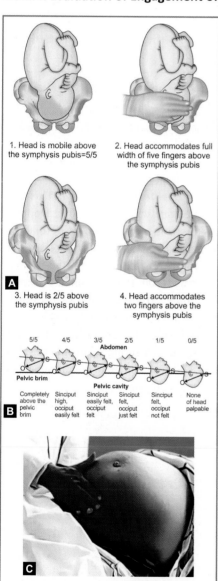 1. Head is mobile above the symphysis pubis=5/5 2. Head accommodates full width of five fingers above the symphysis pubis **A** 3. Head is 2/5 above the symphysis pubis 4. Head accommodates two fingers above the symphysis pubis **B** **C** **Figs 2.3.2.4 (A to C):** Abdominal examination for fetal descent	As shown in Figures 2.3.2.4 (A and B), the assessment of fetal descent through the abdominal examination is done by using the fifth's formula. In this method, number of fifths of fetal head above the pelvic brim is estimated. The amount of fetal head that can be palpated per abdominally is estimated in terms of finger breadth which is assessed by placing the radial margin of the index finger above the symphysis pubis successively. Depending upon the amount of fetal head palpated per abdominally, other fingers of the hand can be placed in succession, until all the five fingers cover the fetal head.	A free-floating head would be completely palpable per abdomen. This head accommodates full width of all the five fingers above the pubic symphysis and can be described as 5/5. A head which is fixing but not yet engaged may be three fifths palpable per abdominally and is known as 3/5. A recently engaged fetal head may be two-fifths palpable per abdominally and is known as 2/5, while a deeply engaged fetal head may not be palpable at all per abdominally and may be described as 0/5.

Picture	Clinical Description	Management/Clinical Features

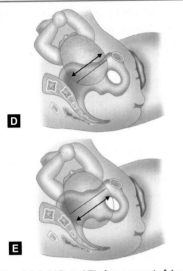

D

E

Figs 2.3.2.4 (D and E): Assessment of descent of fetal heat through the pelvic cavity

With the engagement of fetal head, the lower pole of the head (unmolded) can be felt on vaginal examination at or below the ischial spines. Figure 2.3.2.4D shows that the biparietal diameter of the unengaged head has yet not negotiated through the pelvic brim. On the other hand, in case of engaged head, the biparietal diameter of the head is at the level of ischial spines, or lower (2.3.2.4E). Even after the engagement has occurred, the head has to negotiate a distance of few centimeters as the distance between pelvic inlet and ischial spines is 5 cm, whereas that between the biparietal plane of head and vertex is about 3 cm.

With the progress of second stage of labor, there is progressive downward movement of the fetal head in relation to the pelvic cavity. Engagement is said to have occurred when largest diameter of presenting part passes through pelvic inlet.

Engagement of the fetal presenting part is of great importance as it helps in ruling out fetopelvic disproportion. Engagement of fetal presenting part is evident from abdominal and vaginal examination.

2.3.2.5: Fetal Heart Auscultation (A to H)

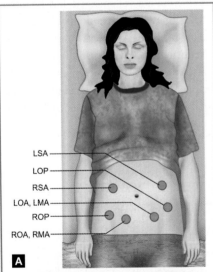

LSA
LOP
RSA
LOA, LMA
ROP
ROA, RMA

A

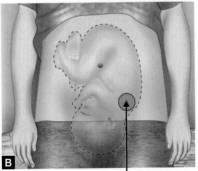

B

Location of FHR in LOA position

Figs 2.3.2.5 (A and B): (A) Location of fetal heart rate; (B) Location of fetal heart rate in left occiput anterior position

The fetal well-being is usually assessed by listening to the fetal heart. The region of maternal abdomen where the heart sounds are most clearly heard would vary with the presentation and extent of descent of the presenting part.

The abbreviations in the adjacent Figure are as follows:
LSA, left sacroanterior;
LOP, left occopitoposterior;
RSA, right sacroanterior;
LOA, left occipitoanterior;
LMA, left mentoanterior;
ROP, right occipitoposterior;
RMA, right mentoanterior

The fetal heart rate can be monitored in the following ways:
- *Electronic fetal monitoring*: Using an external fetal monitor
- *Intermittent auscultation*: This can be done with the help of a Doppler instrument or Pinard's fetoscope or even an ordinary stethoscope. If the heart rate is within the normal range (100–160 beats/minute), shows good variability, shows presence of accelerations and provides no evidence of decelerations, it is said to be "reassuring". This implies that the baby is in good condition and is tolerating labor well.

Picture	Clinical Description	Management/Clinical Features
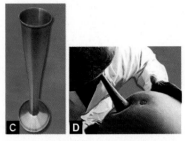 Figs 2.3.2.5 (C and D): (C) Fetoscope; (D) Using a fetoscope to measure the fetal heart rate	As previously described, monitoring of the fetal heart rate can be performed using intermittent auscultation using a fetoscope [Figures 2.3.2.5 (C and D)].	If the woman has no associated risk factor (postmaturity, IUGR fetus, history of preeclampsia, gestational diabetes, etc.) and her previous cardiotocograph trace is normal, the heart rate of the fetus can be monitored intermittently at regular intervals using a fetoscope. A stethoscope or a hand-held Doppler device can also be used instead of fetoscope.
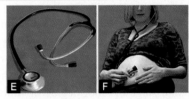 Figs 2.3.2.5 (E and F): (E) Stethoscope; (F) The woman listening to the fetal heart sounds using the stethoscope	Figures 2.3.2.5 (E and F) illustrate the measurement of fetal heart rate using the stethoscope by the pregnant woman herself.	Whatever method for monitoring of fetal heart is used, the main aim of the obstetrician is to assess the fetal heart rate and to assess its relationship with the uterine contractions.
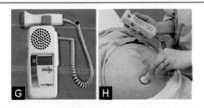 Figs 2.3.2.5 (G and H): Hand-held Doppler device	Figures 2.3.2.5 (G and H) demonstrate the measurement of fetal heart rate using hand-held Doppler device.	Evaluation of fetal heart rate using intermittent auscultation with hand-held Doppler device can be used throughout the antenatal period as well as during the progress of labor. However, as the labor progresses, it may become difficult to interpret the fetal heart rate properly.

2.3.3: Vaginal Examination

2.3.3.1: Changes in Cervix During Pregnancy and Labor

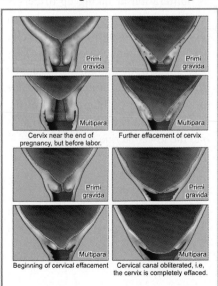 Fig. 2.3.3.1: Changes in cervix during pregnancy and labor	Figure 2.3.3.1 illustrates changes occurring in the cervical canal during pregnancy and labor both in multigravida and primigravida. These mainly comprise of cervical dilatation and effacement.	In primigravida, the effacement starts occurring before the dilatation. In these cases, dilatation only occurs once the cervix has completely effaced or has been completely taken up. On the other hand, in multigravida both cervical dilatation and effacement occur simultaneously.

| Picture | Clinical Description | Management/Clinical Features |

2.3.3.2: Cervical Dilatation

See Figures 2.4.1.1 (A to D).

2.3.3.3: Cervical Effacement

See Figures 2.4.1.2 (A and B).

2.4: NORMAL LABOR

2.4.1: Changes in Pelvic Organs at the Time of Labor

2.4.1.1: Cervical Dilatation (A to D)

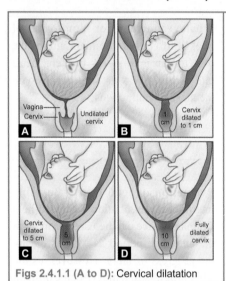

Figs 2.4.1.1 (A to D): Cervical dilatation

Cervical dilatation can be defined as the gradual opening up of cervix from 0 cm to 10 cm. [The cervical dilatation is usually described in terms of centimeters (1–10 cm)]. The cervix is said to be fully dilated when it measures about 10 cm.

The force of uterine contractions exerts a centrifugal pull over the cervix resulting in its distension. This process is known as cervical dilatation. After the cervix is completely dilated (10 cm), the second stage of labor begins in which there is progressive descent of the fetal presenting part, which is used to assess the progress of labor.

2.4.1.2: Cervical Effacement (A to C)

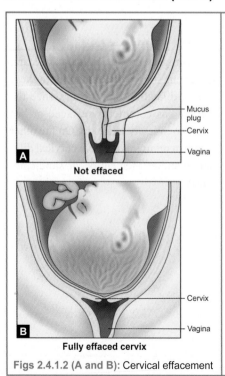

Not effaced

Fully effaced cervix

Figs 2.4.1.2 (A and B): Cervical effacement

As shown in Figures 2.4.1.2 (A and B) cervical effacement can be defined as the gradual thinning, shortening or drawing up of the cervix. It is usually measured in terms of percentage from 0% to 100%.

Cervical effacement can be defined as obliteration or taking up of cervix resulting in conversion of cervical canal (about 2 cm in length) into a circular orifice with paper thin edges. This takes place from above downward. The cervical effacement primarily results due to taking up or pulling upward of the muscular fibers at the level of internal os into the lower uterine segment.

Picture	Clinical Description	Management/Clinical Features
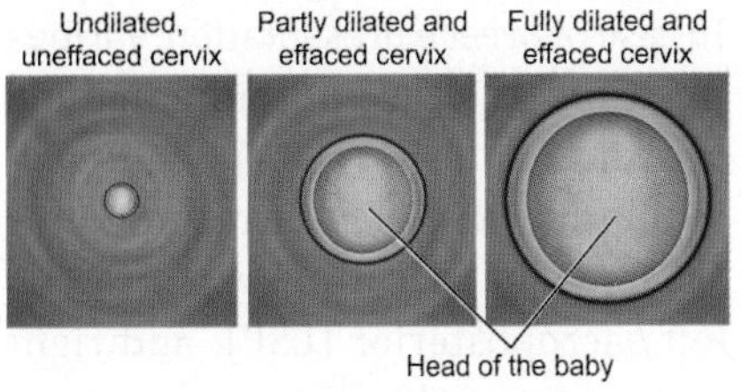 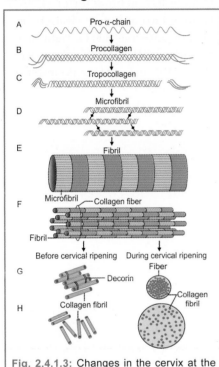 Fig. 2.4.1.2C: Cervical effacement	Figure 2.4.1.2C shows changes in cervical canal in relation to fetal head with progressive dilatation and effacement. When the cervix becomes as thin as the corresponding lower uterine segment, it is known as 100% or completely effaced.	During cervical effacement the edges of internal os are drawn upward several centimeters to become part of the lower uterine segment. When the cervix is reduced to one half of its original length, it is 50% effaced.

Fig. 2.4.1.2C: Cervical effacement

2.4.1.3: Changes in the Cervix at the Molecular Level

Picture	Clinical Description	Management/Clinical Features
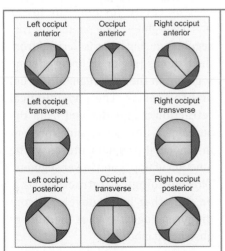 Fig. 2.4.1.3: Changes in the cervix at the molecular level	Figure 2.4.1.3 illustrates changes occurring in the cervix at molecular level at the time of cervical effacement and dilatation. During labor, the cervix retains its structural integrity, but at the same time becomes ripened (more distensible). The human cervix is composed of extracellular connective tissues. The main components of the extracellular matrix are type 1 and type 3 collagen. Various other substances such as glycosaminoglycans, proteoglycans (dermatan sulfate, hyaluronic acid, etc.), fibronectin, elastin, etc. may also be present.	At the time of cervical ripening, there is an increase in the percentage of soluble collagen and changes in the microstructure of collagen fibers, which promotes cervical softening. There occurs cross-linking between the collagen fibers. There is an increase in the content of hyaluronic acid which causes water to intercalate between the collagen fibers resulting in their segregation.

Fig. 2.4.1.3: Changes in the cervix at the molecular level

2.4.1.4: Fetal Position (A and B)

Picture	Clinical Description	Management/Clinical Features
Fig. 2.4.1.4A: Various positions possible in case of vertex presentation	Fetal position can be defined as the relationship between the denominator of the presenting part with the maternal pelvis. Figure 2.4.1.4A illustrates the six positions possible with vertex position. These include: left occiput anterior (LOA), right occiput anterior (ROA), left occiput transverse; (LOT), right occiput transverse (ROT), left occiput posterior; (LOP) and right occiput posterior (ROP).	The fetal position gives an idea regarding whether the presenting part is directed towards the front, back, left or right of the birth passage.

Fig. 2.4.1.4A: Various positions possible in case of vertex presentation

Picture	Clinical Description	Management/Clinical Features
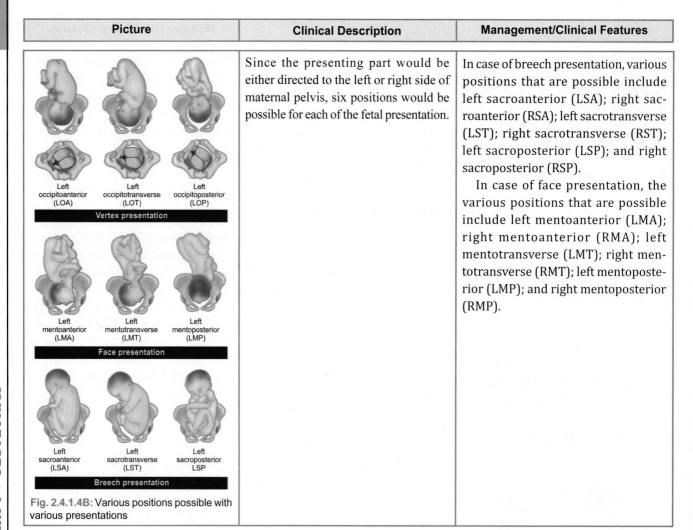**Fig. 2.4.1.4B:** Various positions possible with various presentations	Since the presenting part would be either directed to the left or right side of maternal pelvis, six positions would be possible for each of the fetal presentation.	In case of breech presentation, various positions that are possible include left sacroanterior (LSA); right sacroanterior (RSA); left sacrotransverse (LST); right sacrotransverse (RST); left sacroposterior (LSP); and right sacroposterior (RSP). In case of face presentation, the various positions that are possible include left mentoanterior (LMA); right mentoanterior (RMA); left mentotransverse (LMT); right mentotransverse (RMT); left mentoposterior (LMP); and right mentoposterior (RMP).

2.4.1.5: Changes in Uterus at Term

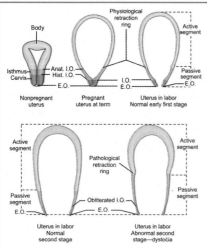**Fig. 2.4.1.5:** Progressive development of uterine segments at term (IO, internal os; EO, external os; Anat, anatomical; Hist, histological)	The adjacent figure shows comparison between the nonpregnant uterus, uterus at term and the uterus at the time of labor. During pregnancy, there occurs enlargement of the uterus due to hypertrophy and hyperplasia of the individual muscle fibers under the influence of hormones such as estrogen and progestogens. During early labor, there occurs hypertrophy and elongation of cervical isthmus by nearly three times its original size.	With the increasing period of gestation, the isthmus starts unfolding from above in downward direction until it gets incorporated into the uterine cavity, forming the lower uterine segment. The passive uterine segment during labor is derived from the isthmus (region of lower uterine segment in the nonpregnant uterus) and the cervix. The physiological retraction ring is derived from the anatomical internal os, and is present in a normal pregnant uterus at the junction of upper and lower segment. The pathological retraction ring, on the other hand, develops from the physiological ring at the time of obstructed labor.

Picture	Clinical Description	Management/Clinical Features

2.4.1.6: Stages of Labor (A to C)

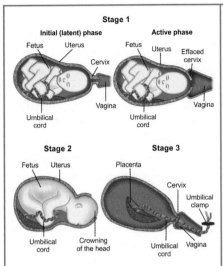

Fig. 2.4.1.6A: Stages of normal labor

Figure 2.4.1.6A describes the various stages of labor, which are as follows:

- *Stage I*: Starts from the onset of true labor pains and ends with complete dilatation of cervix.
- *Stage II*: This starts from full dilatation of cervix and ends with expulsion of the fetus from birth canal. This phase lasts for approximately 50 minutes in primigravida and 20 minutes in multigravida.
- *Stage III*: It begins after expulsion of the fetus and is associated with expulsion of placenta and membranes. This stage lasts for 15 minutes in both primigravida and multigravida
- *Stage IV*: This is the stage of observation, which lasts for at least 1 hour after the expulsion of afterbirths.

Since the true labor pains begin from the first stage of labor, the woman must be advised to relax and not to exhaust herself. Breathing exercises may prove to be useful. She should be advised to eat a light diet and drink lot of fluids in order to prevent dehydration. Since the uterine contractions further increase in frequency and intensity during the second stage, breathing and relaxation exercises are even more useful. If the pain is unbearable, the patient may be prescribed analgesic medicines. Sitting on a birthing ball may also be of some help to the woman.

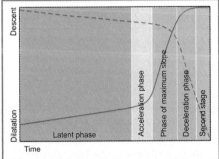

Fig. 2.4.1.6B: Graphical representation of normal labor

Friedman's (1978) graphical representation of normal progress of labor using parameters, such as cervical dilatation and descent of fetal head, has been described in Figure 2.4.1.6B While the cervical dilatation follows a sigmoid curve, descent of the fetal head through the birth canal follows a hyperbolic-shaped curve.

The graph in the adjacent figure illustrates that stage I can be divided into the following phases:

- *Latent phase*: This phase is associated with slow and gradual cervical effacement and dilatation (up to 3 cm).
- *Active phase*: This phase is associated with active cervical dilatation (3–10 cm) and fetal descent. It comprises of the following: acceleration phase, phase of maximum slope and deceleration phase.

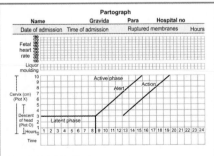

Fig. 2.4.1.6C: Partogram

Normal labor should be plotted graphically on a partogram as shown in Figure 2.4.1.6C. Partogram is the graphical record of the progress of labor. Dilatation of cervix and descent of fetal presenting part is plotted, which gives an estimate about the progress of first stage of labor. The partograph clearly identifies women showing abnormal progress of labor who are likely to benefit from early intervention (medical or surgical induction of labor). The partograph is divided into a latent phase and an active phase.

The latent phase ends while the active phase begins when the cervix is 3 cm dilated. Cervical dilation and descent of the presenting part are plotted in relation to an alert line and an action line. Alert line starts at the end of latent phase and ends with the full dilation of the cervix (10 cm) within 7 hours (at the rate of 1 cm/hour). The action line is drawn 4 hours to the right of the alert line. Labor is considered to be abnormal when the cervicograph crosses the alert line and intervention is required when it crosses the action line.

Picture	Clinical Description	Management/Clinical Features

2.4.1.7: Mechanism of Uterine Contractions During Labor

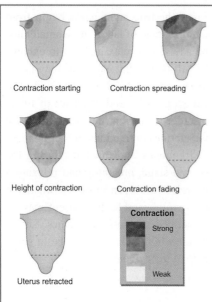

Fig. 2.4.1.7: Mechanism of uterine contractions during labor

As shown in the adjacent figure, uterine contractions normally start from the fundal region and spread downwards. They are mild-moderate in intensity during the first stage and become moderate-severe during the second stage. Uterine contractions usually follow a rhythmic pattern, with periods of contractions followed by periods of relaxation in between, which would allow the woman to rest. Contractions can vary in intensity from mild, moderate to strong. Contractions lasting less than 20 seconds are mild; those lasting for 20–40 seconds are moderate; and strong contractions are those lasting for more than 40 seconds.

Uterine contractions occur as a consequence of underlying electrical activity of myometrial cells. This is probably due to the stretch of the uterine musculature related to an increase in the uterine volume and the effect of hormones (particularly estrogen). The upper uterine segment actively contracts to push the fetus into the lower uterine segment. Since the lower uterine segment largely remains inert, it allows the fetus to descend against the cervix. In the early stages of labor, the frequency of the uterine contractions may be after every 10–15 minutes, lasting for about 30–60 seconds. However as the labor progresses, the frequency and duration of uterine contractions greatly increases with contractions occurring after every 1–2 minutes and lasting for about 60–120 seconds.

2.4.2: Examination of Baby at the Time of Labor

2.4.2.1: Lie of Fetus

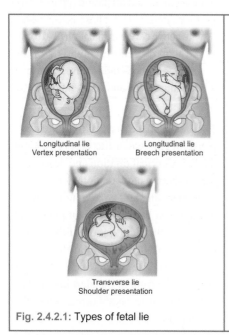

Fig. 2.4.2.1: Types of fetal lie

As shown in Figure 2.4.2.1 fetal lie refers to the relation of long axis of the fetus to long axis of uterus or maternal spine. Lie can be longitudinal, oblique or transverse. About 99% of the fetuses at term present with longitudinal lie.

Fetal lie refers to the relationship of cephalocaudal axis or long axis (spinal column) of fetus to the long axis of the centralized uterus or maternal spine. Various types of fetal lie are as follows:

Longitudinal lie: The maternal and fetal long axes are parallel to each other.

Transverse: The maternal and fetal long axes are perpendicular to each other.

Oblique lie: The maternal and fetal long axes cross each other obliquely or at an angle of 45°. The oblique lie is usually unstable and becomes longitudinal or transverse during the course of labor.

| Picture | Clinical Description | Management/Clinical Features |

2.4.2.2: Fetal Presentation

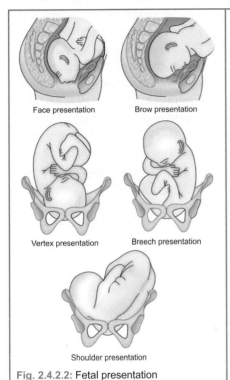

Face presentation   Brow presentation

Vertex presentation   Breech presentation

Shoulder presentation

Fig. 2.4.2.2: Fetal presentation

Fetal presentation can be described as the fetal body part, which occupies the lower pole of the uterus and thereby first enters the pelvic passage. Fetal presentation is determined by fetal lie and may be of three types: cephalic, podalic (breech) or shoulder and is shown in Figure 2.4.2.2.

Portion of the fetal presenting part, which is in close proximity to internal os and is felt by the examining fingers through the dilated cervix is called the presenting part. In case of cephalic presentation, commonest fetal presenting part is the vertex.

Cephalic or the head presentation is the commonest and occurs in about 97% of fetuses. Breech and shoulder presentations are less common and may pose difficulty for normal vaginal delivery. Thus, these two presentations are also known as malpresentations. The presenting part may be brow or face depending upon the degree of flexion of the fetal head.

2.4.2.3: Fetal Attitude or Posture (A and B)

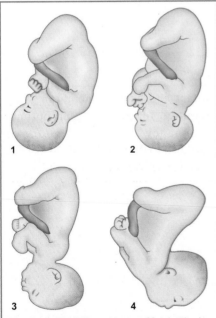

1   2

3   4

Fig. 2.4.2.3A: Different types of fetal attitudes
1: Complete flexion; 2: Moderate flexion. 3: Poor flexion; 4: Hyperextension

During the later months of pregnancy, the fetus adopts a characteristic posture called attitude. Usually, this posture is associated with flexion at all the fetal joints.

Exceptions to normal attitude of flexion include extension of the head in cephalic position or legs in breech position. The clinical significance of fetal attitude is that with the increasing degree of deflexion, the engaging diameter of fetal head progressively increases. In these cases, normal vaginal delivery may become difficult.

On the other hand, the engaging diameter is smallest in case of completely flexed head or completely extended head. In these cases, the fetal head can negotiate through the maternal pelvis and normal vaginal delivery is possible.

Picture	Clinical Description	Management/Clinical Features
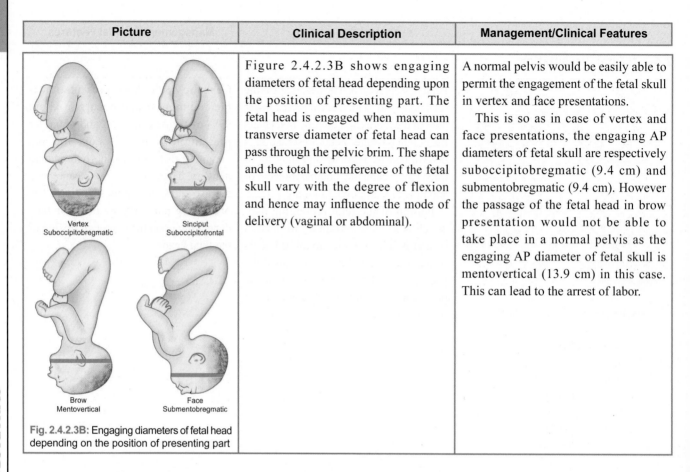 **Fig. 2.4.2.3B:** Engaging diameters of fetal head depending on the position of presenting part	Figure 2.4.2.3B shows engaging diameters of fetal head depending upon the position of presenting part. The fetal head is engaged when maximum transverse diameter of fetal head can pass through the pelvic brim. The shape and the total circumference of the fetal skull vary with the degree of flexion and hence may influence the mode of delivery (vaginal or abdominal).	A normal pelvis would be easily able to permit the engagement of the fetal skull in vertex and face presentations. This is so as in case of vertex and face presentations, the engaging AP diameters of fetal skull are respectively suboccipitobregmatic (9.4 cm) and submentobregmatic (9.4 cm). However the passage of the fetal head in brow presentation would not be able to take place in a normal pelvis as the engaging AP diameter of fetal skull is mentovertical (13.9 cm) in this case. This can lead to the arrest of labor.

2.4.2.4: Fetal Position (A to C)

Kindly refer to 2.4.1.4 for details related to fetal position.

2.4.2.5: Fetal Membranes

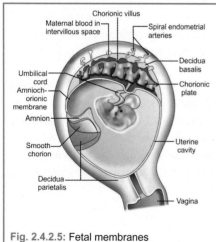 **Fig. 2.4.2.5:** Fetal membranes	Fetal membranes or chorioamniotic membranes include amnion (inner layer) and chorion (outer layer). These surround and protect the developing fetus. The amnion is a translucent layer adjacent to amniotic fluid. Chorion on the other hand is an opaque membrane attached to the uterine decidua. Extracelomic cavity is present between the amnion and chorion until 3 months of gestation. After 3 months, the membranes fuse with one another.	Intact and healthy membranes are required for achieving an optimal pregnancy outcome. Rupture of membrane (ROM) is usually associated with the delivery of baby.

Picture	Clinical Description	Management/Clinical Features

2.4.2.6: Artificial Rupture of Membranes

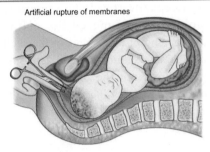

Artificial rupture of membranes

Fig. 2.4.2.6: The procedure of surgical rupture of membranes

The surgical process of artificial ROM is demonstrated in Figure 2.4.2.6 and comprises of the following steps:
- After placing the woman in lithotomy position, under all aseptic precautions, two fingers smeared with antiseptic ointment are introduced inside the vagina.
- Using the index and the middle fingers, the fetal membranes are swept free from the lower uterine segment as far as can be reached with fingers.
- While the fingers are still in the cervical canal, with the palmar surface upward, a long Kocher's forceps with closed blades is introduced along the palmer aspect of the fingers up to the membranes.
- The blades of the Kocher's forceps are opened to grasp the membranes and tear it using twisting movements.

Surgical methods such as low ROM and stripping of membranes are often used for induction of labor. At the time of surgical induction, when the membranes rupture, there is a visible gush of amniotic fluid. If the head is not engaged, an assistant must push the head to fix it to the brim prior to the procedure in order to prevent cord prolapse.

2.4.2.7: Station of Fetal Head

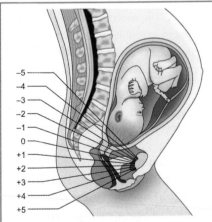

Fig. 2.4.2.7: Descent of fetal head in relation to the station on vaginal examination

The level of the fetal presenting part is usually described in relation to the ischial spines, which is halfway between the pelvic inlet and pelvic outlet. When the lowermost portion of the fetal presenting part is at the level of ischial spines, it is designated as "zero" station. The ACOG has devised a classification system that divides the pelvis above and below the spines into fifths. This division represents the distance in centimeters above and below the ischial spine. Thus, as the presenting fetal part descends from the inlet toward the ischial spine, the designation is −5, −4, −3, −2, −1, and then 0 station.

Below the ischial spines, the fetal head passes through +1, +2, +3, +4 and +5 stations till delivery (Fig. 2.4.2.7).

The engagement of the fetal head is assessed on abdominal and not on vaginal examination. However the vaginal examination does help in assessing the descent of fetal presenting part. Plus 5 (+5) station represents that the fetal head is visible at the introitus.

If the leading part of the fetal head is at the zero station or below, the fetal head is engaged. This implies that the biparietal plane of the fetal head has passed through the pelvic inlet. However in the presence of excessive molding or caput formation, engagement may not have taken place even if the head appears to be at zero station.

2.4.2.8: Molding in Different Types of Cephalic Presentations

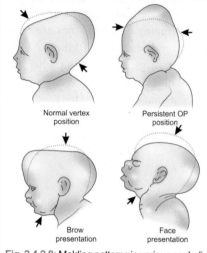

Fig. 2.4.2.8: Molding patterns in various cephalic presentations

Molding is the overlapping of the fetal skull bones at the regions of the sutures, which may occur during labor due to the head being compressed as it passes through the maternal pelvis. Molding results in the compression of the engaging diameter of the fetal head with the corresponding elongation of the diameter at right angles to it. For example, if the fully flexed fetal head engages in the suboccipitobregmatic diameter, this diameter gets compressed. At the same time, the mentovertical diameter (which is at right angles to the suboccipitobregmatic diameter) gets elongated.

In a cephalic (head) presentation, molding is diagnosed by feeling overlapping of the sutures of the skull on vaginal examination and assessing whether or not the overlap can be corrected by pressing gently with the examining finger.

2.4.2.9: Grade I Molding of Fetal Scalp Bones

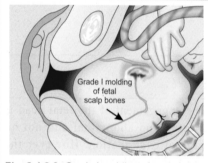

Fig. 2.4.2.9: Grade I molding of scalp bones

Figure 2.4.2.9 shows grade I molding of the fetal head. For grading the degree of molding of fetal head, the occipitoparietal and the sagittal sutures are palpated, and the relationship of the two adjacent bones is assessed.

Grading of the molding can be described as follows:
Grade 0: Normal separation of the bones with open sutures.
Grade 1 (mild molding): Bones touching each other.
Grade 2 (moderate molding): Bones overlapping, but can be separated.
Grade 3 (severe molding): Bones overlapping, but cannot be separated.

2.4.3: Induction of Labor (A to C)

Regime	Starting dose	Incre-mental dose (mU/min)	Dosage interval (min)	Maximum dose (mU/min)
Low dose	5–1	1	30	20
	1–2	2	40	40
O'Driscoll (high dose)	6	6	15	42

(Reduced to 3 mU/min with first episode of hyperstimulation and to 1 mU/min with subsequent bouts)

A

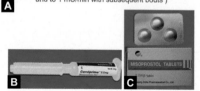

B **C**

Figs 2.4.3 (A to C): (A) Dosage protocol of oxytocin; (B) Induction using ceviprime gel; (C) Induction with misoprostol

Induction of labor can be defined as commencement of uterine contractions before the spontaneous onset of labor with or without ruptured membranes. Induction of labor comprises of cervical ripening and labor augmentation. Oxytocin is an uterotonic agent which stimulates uterine contractions and is used for both induction and augmentation of labor. It can be started in low dosage regimens of 0.5–1.5 mU/minute or the high dosage regimen of 4.5–6.0 mU/minute, with incremental increases of 1.0–2.0 mU/minute at every 15–40 minutes.

Pharmacological methods for cervical ripening commonly comprise of prostaglandins [dinoprostone (PGE2), or misoprostol (PGE1)]. PGE2 helps in cervical ripening and is available in the form of gel (prepidil or cerviprime) or a vaginal insert (cervidil). Prepidil comprises of 0.5 mg of dinoprostone in a 2.5 mL syringe. The gel is injected intracervically every 6 hours for up to three doses in a 24-hour period. Use of misoprostol for cervical ripening as recommended by the ACOG is a dose of 25 mg placed transvaginally at every 3 hourly intervals for a maximum of four doses.

Picture	Clinical Description	Management/Clinical Features

2.5: ABNORMAL LABOR

2.5.1: Obstructed Labor

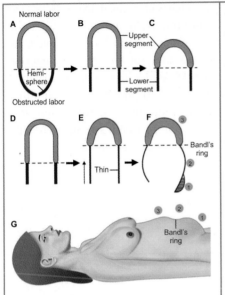

Fig. 2.5.1: Obstructed labor

Obstructed labor can be defined as a condition in which the progressive descent of the presenting part through the maternal genital tract is arrested despite of strong uterine contractions.

In primigravidas as a result of obstructed labor, features of maternal exhaustion and sepsis are apparent. However, the uterus becomes inert. On the other hand, in multigravidae, the uterus responds vigorously at the time of obstruction, which may eventually lead to the rupture of uterus. Tonic contractions in the face of uterine obstruction result in formation of a circular groove between the upper and lower uterine segment, known as the pathological retraction ring or Bandl's ring. Eventually, there is rupture of uterus as the lower segment gives way due to marked thinning of the uterine wall.

Management of obstructed labor comprises of the following steps:
- Most important step in the prevention of obstructed labor is early recognition of prolonged labor or abnormal progress of labor by plotting the progress of labor on a partograph.
- Taking steps for relieving the obstruction as soon as possible
- Checking against dehydration and ketoacidosis
- Controlling sepsis
- Correction of fluid and electrolyte balance
- Antibiotics: Usually a combination of third generation cephalosporin (e.g. ceftriaxone) and metronidazole is administered.
- A timely cesarean section gives the best results.

2.5.2: Prolonged Labor

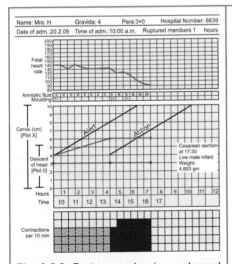

Fig. 2.5.2: Partogram showing prolonged labor in a fourth gravida patient (with no previous live baby). A cesarean delivery was eventually performed in this patient when the cervicograph crossed the action line

Prolonged labor or dystocia of labor (dysfunctional labor) is defined as difficult labor or abnormally slow progress of labor.

Abnormal progress of labor defined as lack of change or minimal change in cervical dilatation or effacement during a 2-hour period (for each of the phase: latent and active phase) in a woman having regular uterine contractions before the beginning of active phase of labor or as a descent of less than or equal to 1.0 cm/hour in nullipara and less than or equal to 2.0 cm/hour in multipara during the second stage of labor (from complete cervical dilatation to delivery). Assisted vaginal delivery in the form of vacuum or forceps application can serve as a good option in cases of delayed second stage. Cesarean section may be required when vaginal delivery appears to be unsafe.

Patients with prolonged latent phase can be managed in the following ways:
- *Therapeutic rest*: This involves administration of an intramuscular dose of 15 mg of morphine, following which the majority of patients would go to sleep within an hour.
- *Stimulation with oxytocin*: In cases of uterine hypocontractility, oxytocin (30 units diluted in 500 mL of saline) must be started at a rate of 0.5–1.0 mU/minute and gradually increased by 1–2 mU/minute at every 20–30 minutes, until an adequate pattern of contractions is achieved. If there is no response even after 3 hours of augmentation with oxytocin, cesarean section may be required due to the possibility of an underlying cephalopelvic disproportion.
- *Discontinuation of regional anesthesia*
- *Assisted vaginal delivery*

2.5.3: Hand Prolapse

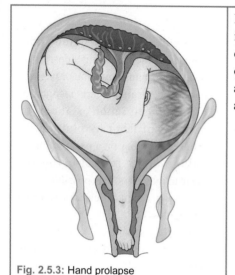

Fig. 2.5.3: Hand prolapse

In cases of transverse lie due to the ill-fitting fetal part, the sudden ROMs can result in the escape of large amount of liquor and the prolapse of fetal arm. Prolapse of fetal arm is often accompanied by a loop of cord.

Arm prolapse must be managed by an emergency cesarean delivery. Neglected arm prolapse in case of primigravida may result in uterine inertia. Though the uterus does not rupture, the condition is associated with significant maternal morbidity. In multigravida, on other hand, there may be formation of a retraction or Bandl's ring, eventually resulting in uterine rupture.

2.5.4: Pathological Retraction Ring

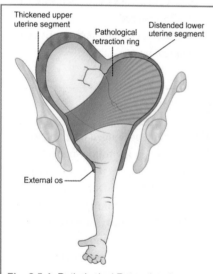

Fig. 2.5.4: Pathological Retraction ring

If the transverse lie with or without a prolapsed arm is left neglected, a series of complications including obstructed labor can occur. In primigravidas as a result of obstructed labor, features of maternal exhaustion and sepsis are apparent. However the uterus becomes inert. On the other hand, in multigravidae, the uterus responds vigorously at the time of obstruction. In order to push out the fetus, the upper uterine segment thickens whereas the lower uterine segment distends. A pathological retraction ring forms at the junction of upper and lower uterine segments (Fig. 2.5.4).

If the uterine obstruction is not immediately relieved, the intensity of uterine contractions increases. As the frequency of uterine contraction increases, there is a progressive reduction in the relaxation phase. This results in setting up of a phase of tonic contractions. Retraction of upper uterine segment continues, this causes the lower uterine segment to elongate, become progressively thinner in order to accommodate the fetus which is being pushed down from the upper segment.

This results in formation of a circular groove between the upper and lower uterine segment. This is known as the pathological retraction ring or Bandl's ring. As the degree of obstruction increases, the retraction ring becomes more prominent. Eventually, there is rupture of uterus as the lower segment gives way due to marked thinning of the uterine wall. There is an increased incidence of dehydration, ketoacidosis, septicemia, rupture uterus, postpartum hemorrhage, shock, peritonitis, injury to the genital tract, etc. All these factors result in increased rate of both maternal and fetal morbidity, and mortality.

Picture	Clinical Description	Management/Clinical Features

2.6: NORMAL VAGINAL DELIVERY

2.6.1: Delivery of Fetal Head (A to C)

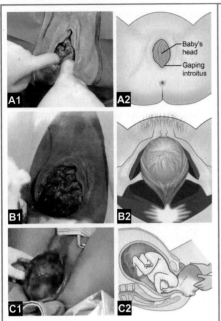

Figs 2.6.1 (A to C): Delivery of fetal head: (A1 and A2) Baby's head visible through the vaginal introitus; (B1 and B2) Crowning of the fetal head; (C1 and C2) Delivery of the fetal head (*Courtesy*: Rekha Khandelwal)

Delivery of fetal head: With the increasing descent of the head, the perineum bulges and thins out considerably. As the largest diameter of the fetal head distends the vaginal introitus, the crowning is said to occur [Figs 2.6.1 (A and B)].

- As the head distends the perineum and it appears that tears may occur in the area of vaginal introitus, mediolateral surgical incision called episiotomy may be given (only if the obstetrician feels its requirement).
- As the fetal head progressively distends the vaginal introitus, the obstetrician in order to facilitate the controlled birth of the head must place the fingers of one hand against the baby's head to keep it flexed and apply perineal support with the other hand. Increasing flexion of the fetal head would facilitate delivery of the smallest diameter of fetal head.

The most commonly adopted position at the time of delivery is dorsal lithotomy position.

- Vulvar and perineal cleaning and draping with antiseptic solution must be done.
- The sterile drapes must be placed in such a way that only the area immediately around the vulva and perineum is exposed.
- Delivery of the fetal head can be achieved with help of Ritgen's maneuver. In this maneuver, one of the obstetrician's gloved hands is used for exerting downward and forward pressure on the chin through the perineum, just in front of the coccyx. The other hand exerts pressure superiorly against the occiput. This helps in providing controlled delivery of the head and favors extension at the time of actual delivery so that the head is delivered with its smallest diameter passing through the introitus and minimal injury occurs to the pelvic musculature.

2.6.2: Delivery of Fetal Shoulders (A to C)

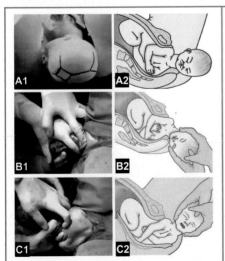

Figs 2.6.2 (A to C): Delivery of fetal shoulders: (A1 and A2) External rotation of head allowing delivery of shoulders; (B1 and B2) Delivery of anterior shoulder; (C1 and C2) Delivery of posterior shoulder (*Courtesy*: Rekha Khandelwal)

Delivery of the shoulders: Following the delivery of head, the fetal head falls posteriorly, while the face comes in contact with the maternal anus. As the restitution or external rotation of the fetal head occurs, the occiput turns toward one of the maternal thighs and the head assumes a transverse position. This movement implies that bisacromial diameter has rotated and has occupied the AP diameter of the pelvis. Soon the anterior shoulder appears at the vaginal introitus. Following the delivery of the anterior shoulder, the posterior shoulder is born. The obstetrician must move the baby's head posteriorly to deliver the shoulder that is anterior.

- Once the baby's head delivers, the woman must be encouraged not to push. The baby's mouth and nose must be suctioned.
- The obstetrician must then feel around the baby's neck in order to rule out the presence of cord around the neck. If the cord is around the neck but is loose, it should be slipped over the baby's head. However, if the cord is tight around the neck, it should be doubly clamped and cut before proceeding with the delivery of fetal shoulders.

2.6.3: Remaining Part of Delivery (A to C)

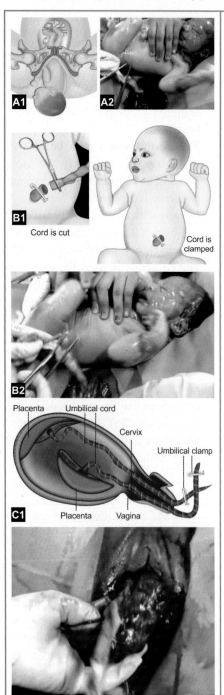

Cord is cut

Cord is clamped

Placenta   Umbilical cord

Cervix

Umbilical clamp

Placenta   Vagina

Figs 2.6.3 (A to C): Delivery of rest of the fetal body: (A1 and A2) Delivery of rest of the body; (B1 and B2) Clamping and cutting the umbilical cord; (C1 and C2) Delivery of the placenta (*Courtesy*: Rekha Khandelwal)

Delivery of the rest of the body: Delivery of the shoulders is followed by the delivery of the rest of the body. The rest of the baby's body must be supported with one hand as it slides out of the vaginal introitus.

Clamping the cord: Once the entire baby has delivered, the umbilical cord must be clamped and cut, if not done earlier.

- The baby must be placed over the mother's abdomen and then handed over to the assisting nurse or the pediatrician.

Delivery of placenta: Following the delivery of baby, the obstetrician must look for signs of placental separation (see Section 5).

- The third stage of labor must be actively managed.

Delayed clamping of the cord is a strategy sometimes employed, which would help in preventing the development of anemia by transferring about 80 ml of blood equivalent to 50 mg of iron) from the placenta to the neonate.

- Following the delivery, the baby's body must be thoroughly dried, the eyes be wiped and baby's breathing must be assessed.
- In order to minimize the chances of aspiration of amniotic fluid, soon after the delivery of the thorax, the face must be wiped, and the mouth and fetal nostrils must be aspirated.
- The baby must be covered with a soft, dry cloth and a blanket to ensure that the baby remains warm and no heat loss occurs.

Picture	Clinical Description	Management/Clinical Features

2.6.4: Mechanism of Delivery of Head in Occipitolateral Position (A to E)

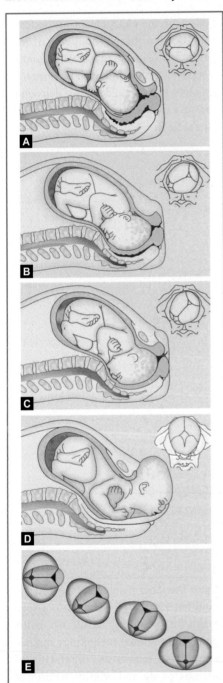

Figs 2.6.4 (A to E): Mechanism of delivery of fetal head: (A) Engagement, flexion and descent; (B) Further descent and internal rotation; (C) Complete rotation and beginning of extension; (D) Delivery of head by complete extension; (E) Diagram showing internal rotation of head to pass through pelvis

In normal labor, the fetal head enters the pelvic brim most commonly through the available transverse diameter of the pelvic inlet. This is so as the most common fetal position is occipitolateral (transverse) position. In some cases the fetal head may enter through one of the oblique diameters. The fetal head with left occipitoanterior position enters through right oblique diameter, whereas that with right occipitoanterior position enters through left oblique diameter of the pelvic inlet. Left occipitoanterior (LOA) position is slightly more common than the right occipitoanterior position as the left oblique diameter is encroached by the rectum. The engaging AP diameter of the fetal head is suboccipitobregmatic (9.4 cm) in position of complete flexion. The engaging transverse diameter of the fetal head is biparietal diameter (9.5 cm).

The cardinal fetal movements during the occipitolateral position comprise of the following: engagement, flexion, descent, internal rotation, crowning, extension, restitution, external rotation of the head and expulsion of the trunk. These movements are as follows:

Engagement: See 2.3.2.4

Descent: Descent of the fetal head is a continuous process which occurs throughout the second stage of labor.

Flexion: In normal cases, increased flexion of fetal chin against chest, help in presenting the smallest fetal diameter, i.e. the suboccipitobregmatic diameter.

Internal rotation: Fetal head rotates as it reaches the pelvic floor. In the occipitolateral position, there is anterior rotation of the fetal head by 2/8th of the circle in such a way that the occiput rotates anteriorly from the lateral position toward the pubic symphysis. The internal rotation of the fetal head by 2/8th of the circle is likely to cause the torsion of fetal neck by 2/8th of the circle. Since the neck would not be able to sustain this much amount of torsion, there would be simultaneous rotation of the fetal shoulders in the same direction by 1/8th of the circle. This would place the shoulders in an oblique diameter, i.e. right oblique with right occipitolateral and left oblique with left occipitolateral.

Crowning: During crowning, biparietal diameter of the fetal head stretches the vaginal introitus. Even as the uterine contractions cease, the head would not recede back during the stage of crowning.

Extension: Fetal head pivots under symphysis pubis and emerges out through extension, followed by occiput, then the face and finally the chin.

2.6.5: Mechanism of Delivery of Fetal Shoulders in Occipitoanterior Position (A to D)

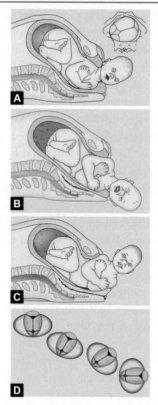

Figs 2.6.5 (A to D): Mechanism of delivery of fetal shoulders: (A) Restitution and external rotation; (B) Delivery of anterior shoulder; (C) Delivery of posterior shoulder; (D) Diagram showing external rotation of shoulders to pass through pelvis

Restitution: Following the delivery of fetal head, the neck which had undergone torsion previously, now untwists and aligns along with the long axis of the fetus.

External rotation of the head: As the undelivered shoulders rotate by 1/8th of the circle to occupy the AP diameter of the pelvis, this movement is visible outside in form of the external rotation of fetal head, causing the head to further turn to one side.

Following the engagement of the fetal shoulders in the AP diameter of the pelvis, anterior shoulder slips under symphysis pubis, followed by posterior shoulder. Once shoulders have delivered, the rest of the trunk is delivered by lateral flexion.

2.7: LABOR ANALGESIA

2.7.1: Normal Dermatome Distribution

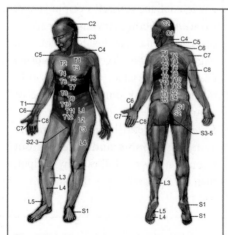

Fig. 2.7.1: Normal dermatome distribution

Dermatome refers to the area of skin supplied by a single nerve. Figure 2.7.1 shows normal dermatome distribution in human body. Knowledge regarding dermatomes supplying the pelvic and abdominal regions provides adequate information to the clinician regarding the nerves which need to be blocked so as to provide relief of pain during labor and delivery or at the time of operative procedures such as cesarean delivery, administration of episiotomy, etc.

Since the labor pain can be severe and debilitating, the clinicians often seek ways for providing relief from this pain. Nonregional techniques include supportive measures, inhalation of nitrous oxide and administration of parenteral opioids. Regional techniques are also commonly used for providing labor analgesia. Epidural analgesia is one such regional technique, which provides good pain relief during labor. This can be in form of caudal epidural analgesia or lumbar epidural analgesia.

Picture	Clinical Description	Management/Clinical Features

2.7.2: Normal Pain Pathway During Labor

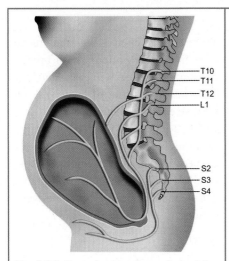

Fig. 2.7.2: Normal pain pathway during labor

The uterus including the cervix and lower uterine segment is supplied by afferents that pass from the uterus to the spinal cord by accompanying sympathetic nerves from T10 to L1. These nerves pass through the inferior hypogastric plexus, the hypogastric nerve, the superior hypogastric plexus, the lumbar and lower thoracic sympathetic chain and the nerves from T10 to L1 (as shown in the adjacent figure). The pain sensation is predominantly carried by the C fibers.

Pain of the first stage of labor is due to uterine contractions and stretching of the cervix which is most likely to cause stimulation of afferent fibers accompanying sympathetic pathway from T10 to L1. Fetus often exerts pressure over the periuterine tissues in lumbosacral region causing the stimulation of lumbosacral plexus (L5 to S1). Pressure by the presenting part over the bladder, urethra and rectum is likely to cause stimulation of S2 to S4. Distension and tearing of vagina is also likely to cause stimulation of somatic fibers of the following fibers:
- Pudendal nerve (S2 to S4)
- Genitofemoral nerve (L1 to L2)
- Ilioinguinal nerve (L1)
- Posterior cutaneous nerve of thigh (S2 to S3)

2.7.3: Pain Relief During Labor

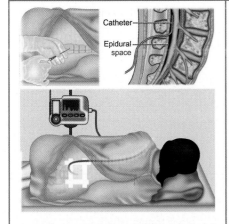

Fig. 2.7.3: Administration of epidural analgesia

Epidural analgesia has presently become a commonly employed technique for providing pain relief during labor. Epidural analgesia should be administered only once the diagnosis of labor has been established and the patient requests for pain relief. It should be provided by practitioners only in settings where facilities for resuscitation are immediately available. This technique involves injection of a local anesthetic agent into the epidural space (between the dura mater and the ligamentum flavum) in the space between the vertebra L3 and L4. An indwelling catheter is usually kept in place for repeat injections or continuous infusion. Following the loading dose, epidural analgesia may be maintained either with intermittent bolus injections or continuous epidural infusion. Patient controlled epidural analgesia may also be used.

Administration of epidural analgesia comprises of the following steps:
- Under all aseptic precautions, the epidural needle is inserted in the epidural space between the vertebra L3 and L4.
- An epidural catheter is threaded by 3–5 cm into the epidural space.
- A test dose of 3 mL of 1.5% lidocaine with 1:200,000 epinephrine or 3 mL of 0.25% bupivacaine with 1:200,000 epinephrine is injected.
- If the test dose is negative, loading dose comprising of approximately 10 mL of 0.25% bupivacaine (marcaine) or 0.25% of ropivacaine, with or without a small dose of a lipid-soluble opioid (e.g. fentanyl or sufentanil), are injected.

2.8: BREECH VAGINAL DELIVERY

2.8.1: Different Types of Breech Presentations

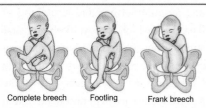

Complete breech   Footling   Frank breech

Fig. 2.8.1: Different types of breech presentations

In breech presentation, the fetus lies longitudinally with the buttocks presenting in the lower pole of the uterus. The different types of breech presentations are shown in the adjacent figure and are described below:

Frank breech: Buttocks present first with flexed hips and legs extended on the abdomen.

Complete breech: The buttocks present first with flexed hips and flexed knees. Feet are not below the buttocks.

Footling breech: One or both feet present as both hips and knees are in extended position.

There are two choices regarding mode of delivery for patients with breech presentation: breech vaginal delivery (also known as trial of breech) or an elective cesarean section.

There has been much controversy regarding choosing the best option for delivery. Parents must be informed about potential risks and benefits to the mother and neonate for each of the delivery options.

2.8.2: Different Positions of Breech

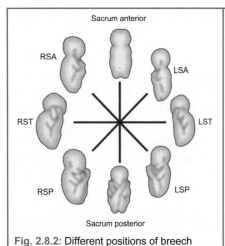

Sacrum anterior

RSA

LSA

RST

LST

RSP

LSP

Sacrum posterior

Fig. 2.8.2: Different positions of breech

The denominator of breech presentation is considered to be the sacrum. Depending on the relationship of the sacrum with the sacroiliac joint, the various positions of the breech, which are possible include:
- The left sacroanterior (LSA) position
- Right sacroanterior (RSA) position
- Right sacroposterior (RSP) position
- Left sacroposterior (LSP) position

Of the various possible positions of breech, LSA position is the most common position. In this position, the bitrochanteric diameter of the buttocks (9.5 cm) enters the pelvic inlet through the right oblique diameter of the pelvic brim.

2.8.3: Ultrasound Examination Showing Breech Gestation

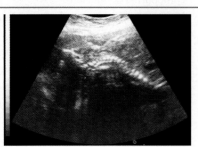

Fig. 2.8.3: Ultrasound examination showing breech presentation

As shown in the adjacent figure, ultrasound helps in establishing the diagnosis of abnormal presentation and confirming breech presentation.

The other things which can be seen on the ultrasound include the following:
- Presence of uterine and/or fetal anomalies
- Extension of fetal head: "Star gazing sign" can be observed if the degree of extension of fetal head is more than 90°.
- Fetal maturity and adequacy of liquor
- Placental location and grading
- Ruling out multiple gestation

Picture	Clinical Description	Management/Clinical Features

2.8.4: Mechanism of Breech Vaginal Birth till Delivery of Hips (A to C)

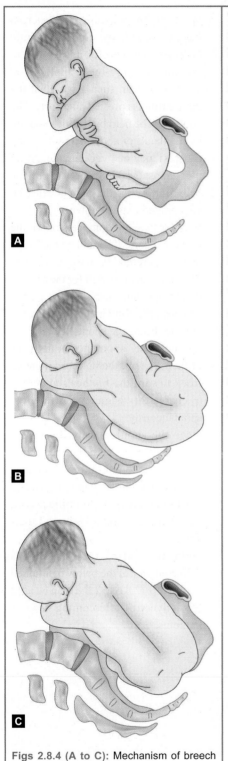

A

B

C

Figs 2.8.4 (A to C): Mechanism of breech vaginal birth until the delivery of hips

The breech most commonly presents in LSA position, which causes the bitrochanteric diameter of the buttocks (9.5 cm) to enter through the pelvic inlet in the right oblique diameter of the pelvic brim (Fig. 2.8.4A). Once the bitrochanteric diameter has passed through the oblique diameter of pelvis, engagement is said to occur (Fig. 2.8.4B). With full dilatation of the cervix, the buttocks descend deeply into the pelvis. When the buttocks reach the pelvic floor, the anterior hip which reaches the pelvic floor first, internally rotates through 45° so that the bitrochanteric diameter lies in the AP diameter of the pelvic outlet. With continuing fetal descend, the anterior buttock appears at the vulva. With further uterine contractions there is delivery of anterior hip followed by that of posterior hip by lateral flexion (Fig. 2.8.4C). The anterior hip slips out under the pubic symphysis followed by the lower limbs and feet.

The following steps must be taken at the time of breech vaginal delivery:
- Once the buttocks have entered the vagina and the cervix is fully dilated, the woman must be advised to bear down with the contractions.
- Episiotomy may be performed, if the perineum appears very tight.
- A "no touch policy" by the clinician must be adopted until the buttocks and lower back deliver till the level of umbilicus. At this point the baby's shoulder blades can be seen.
- Sometimes the clinician may have to make use of maneuvers like Pinard's maneuver and groin traction (will be described later), if the legs have not delivered spontaneously.

2.8.5: Mechanism of Breech Vaginal Birth till Delivery of Entire Body besides the Head (A to C)

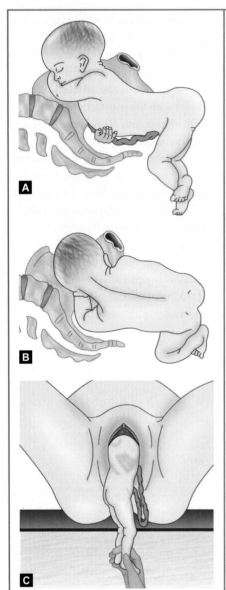

Figs 2.8.5 (A to C): Mechanism of breech vaginal birth till the delivery of entire body except the fetal head

Following the delivery of buttocks and legs, sacrum rotates by 45° in the direction opposite to the internal rotation, resulting in the external rotation of the breech. This causes the back to turn anteriorly. With continuing descend, the bisacromial diameter (12 cm) of the shoulders engages in right oblique diameter of the pelvis and descent continues. On touching the pelvic floor, the anterior shoulders undergo internal rotation by 45° so that the bisacromial diameter lies in the AP diameter of the outlet (Fig. 2.8.5A). Simultaneously, the buttocks and sacrum externally rotate anteriorly through 45°. As the anterior shoulder impinges under the pubic symphysis, the posterior shoulders and arm are born over the perineum followed by the delivery of anterior shoulder (Fig. 2.8.5B). Following the delivery, anterior shoulders undergo restitution through 45° and assume a right oblique position. At the same time the neck undergoes torsion of 45°. As a result, the engaging diameter of the head (suboccipitofrontal diameter 10.5 cm) or suboccipitobregmatic diameter engages in the left oblique diameter of the pelvis (Fig. 2.8.5C). Descent into the pelvis occurs with flexion of the fetal head. The flexion of fetal head is often maintained by uterine contractions aided by suprapubic pressure applied by the delivery assistant at the time of delivery. When the head reaches the pelvic floor, it undergoes internal rotation by 45° so that the sagittal sutures lie in the AP diameter of the pelvis, with the occiput present anteriorly and brow in the hollow of the sacrum. As the nape of the neck impinges against the pubic symphysis, the chin, mouth, nose, forehead, bregma and occiput are born over the perineum by flexion.

- Once the buttocks, hips and sacrum have delivered, the clinician should be extremely careful and gentle in holding the baby by wrapping it in a clean cloth in such a way that the baby's trunk is present anteriorly. The baby must be held by the hips and not by the flanks or abdomen as this may cause kidney or liver damage. At no point, must the clinician try to pull the baby out; rather the patient must be encouraged to push down.
- In order to avoid compression on the umbilical cord, it should be moved to one side, preferably in the sacral bay. The clinician must wait for the arms to deliver spontaneously. If arms are felt on chest, the clinician must allow the arms to disengage spontaneously one by one. After spontaneous delivery of the first arm, the buttocks must be lifted toward the mother's abdomen to enable the second arm to deliver spontaneously.
- Once the shoulders are delivered, the baby's body with the face down must be supported on the clinician's forearm. The clinician must be careful not to compress the umbilical cord between the infant's body and their arm.
- Once the entire fetal body has delivered, one of the below mentioned maneuvers (2.8.6 to 2.8.8) can be used for delivery of aftercoming head of the fetus.

2.8.6: Burns Marshall Technique for Delivery of Fetal Head (A and B)

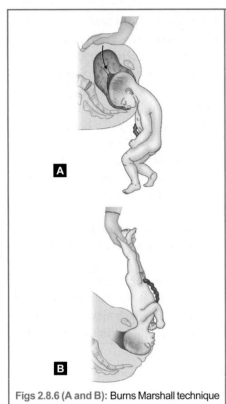

A

B

Figs 2.8.6 (A and B): Burns Marshall technique

Burns Marshall technique: Following the delivery of shoulders and both the arms, the baby must be let to hang unsupported from the mother's vulva. This would help in encouraging flexion of fetal head (Fig. 2.8.6A). The nursing staff must be further advised to apply suprapubic pressure in downward and backward direction, in order to encourage flexion of the baby's head. As the nape of baby's neck appears, efforts must be made by the clinician to deliver the baby's head by grasping the fetal ankles with the finger of right hand between the two. Then the trunk is swung up forming a wide arc of the circle, while maintaining continuous traction when doing this (Fig. 2.8.6B). The left hand is used to provide pelvic support and to clear the perineum off successively from the baby's face and brow as the baby's head emerges out.

Intrapartum care for patients undergoing breech vaginal delivery:
- Informed consent must be taken from the patient after explaining that the trial of breech can fail in 20% cases, thereby requiring a cesarean section.
- Increased maternal and fetal surveillance is required.
- Maternal intravenous line must be set up as the mother may require emergency induction of anesthesia at any time.
- Women should be advised to remain in bed to avoid the risk of premature rupture of membrane and risk of cord prolapse.
- Active management of labor preferably using a partogram needs to be done.
- Following the rupture of membranes, a vaginal examination needs to be performed to rule out cord prolapse.
- Breech presentation should be confirmed by an ultrasound examination in the labor ward.

2.8.7: Mauriceau Smellie Veit Maneuver

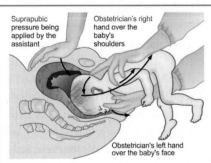

Suprapubic pressure being applied by the assistant

Obstetrician's right hand over the baby's shoulders

Obstetrician's left hand over the baby's face

Fig. 2.8.7: Mauriceau Smellie Veit maneuver

This is another commonly used maneuver for the delivery of aftercoming fetal head and is named after the three clinicians who had described the method of using this grip. This maneuver comprises of the following steps:
- The baby is placed face down with the length of its body over the supinated left forearm and hand of the clinician.
- The clinician must then place the first (index) and second finger (middle finger) of this hand on the baby's cheekbones and the thumb over the baby's chin. This helps in facilitating flexion of the fetal head. The next steps to be followed are described in the adjacent column.

- An assistant may provide suprapubic pressure to help the baby's head remain flexed. The right hand of the clinician is used for grasping the baby's shoulders. The little finger and the ring finger of the clinician's right hand is placed over the baby's right shoulder, the index finger over the baby's left shoulder and the middle finger over the baby's suboccipital region. With the fingers of right hand in this position, the baby's head is flexed toward the chest. At the same time, left hand is used for applying downward pressure on the jaw to bring the baby's head down until the hairline is visible.
- Thereafter the baby's trunk is carried in upward and forward direction toward the maternal abdomen, till the baby's mouth, nose and brow and lastly the vertex and occiput have been released.

Picture	Clinical Description	Management/Clinical Features

2.8.8: Delivery of Aftercoming Head Using Forceps

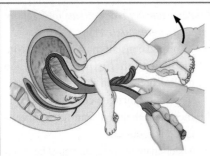

Fig. 2.8.8: Delivery of aftercoming head using forceps

Nowadays forceps are commonly used to deliver the aftercoming head of the breech (Fig. 2.8.8). Use of forceps helps in better maintenance of flexion of fetal head and helps in transmitting the force to the fetal head rather than the neck. This helps in reducing the risk of fetal injuries.

For delivery of fetal head using forceps, the following steps are required:
- Ordinary forceps or Piper's forceps (specially designed forceps with absent pelvic curve) can be used.
- While the clinician is applying forceps, the baby's body must be wrapped in a cloth or towel and held on one side by the assistant. Left blade of the forceps is applied first followed by the right blade and the handles are locked.
- The forceps are used for both flexing and delivering the baby's head.
- The head must be delivered slowly over 1 minute in order to avoid sudden compression or decompression of fetal head, which may be a cause for intracranial hemorrhage.

2.8.9: Lovset's Maneuver for Extended Arms (A to C)

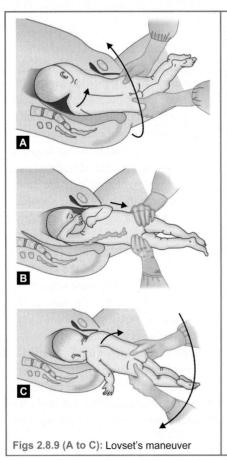

Figs 2.8.9 (A to C): Lovset's maneuver

If the baby's arms are stretched above the head or folded behind the neck (nuchal displacement), the maneuver called Lovset's maneuver is used for delivery of fetal arms. This maneuver is based on the principle that due to the curved shape of the birth canal when the anterior shoulder is above the pubis symphysis, the posterior shoulder would be below the level of pubic symphysis. The maneuver should be initiated only when the fetal scapula becomes visible underneath the pubic arch and includes the steps shown in Figures 2.8.9 (A to C).

The Lovset's maneuver comprises of the following steps:
- First the baby is lifted slightly to cause lateral flexion of the trunk.
- Then the baby which is held by pelvifemoral grip is turned by half a circle, keeping the back uppermost. Simultaneously downward traction is applied, so that the arm that was initially posterior and below the level of pubic symphysis now becomes anterior and can be delivered under the pubic arch.
- Delivery of the arm can be assisted by placing one or two fingers on the upper part of the arm. Then the arm is gradually drawn down over the chest as the elbow is flexed, with the hand sweeping over the face.
- In order to deliver the second arm, the baby is again turned by 180° in the reverse direction, keeping the back uppermost and applying downward traction and then delivering the second arm in the same way under the pubic arch as the first arm was delivered.

Picture	Clinical Description	Management/Clinical Features

2.8.10: Delivery of Shoulder, which is Posterior

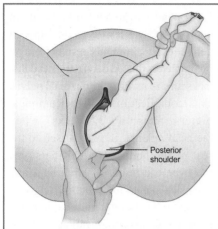

Fig. 2.8.10: Delivery of shoulder, which is posterior

If the clinician is unable to turn the baby's body to deliver the arm that is anterior first, through Lovset's maneuver, then the clinician can deliver the shoulder that is posterior, first (as shown in Figure 2.8.10).

Delivery of the posterior shoulder involves the following steps:

- The clinician must hold and lift the baby up by the ankles. At the same time the baby's chest must be moved toward the woman's inner thighs. The clinician must then hook the baby shoulder with fingers of his/her hand. This would help in delivering the shoulder that is posterior, followed by the delivery of arm and hand.
- Then the baby's back should be lowered down, still holding it by ankles. This helps in the delivery of anterior shoulder followed by the arm and hand.

2.8.11: Groin Traction

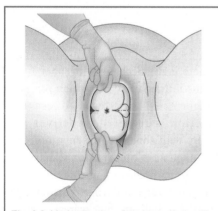

Fig. 2.8.11: Application of double groin traction

If the buttocks and hip do not deliver by themselves, the clinician can make use of simple maneuvers including groin traction (described in adjacent figure) or Pinard's maneuver (2.8.12) to deliver the legs. Groin traction could be of two types: single or double groin traction.

In single groin traction, the index finger of one hand is hooked in the groin fold and traction is exerted toward the fetal trunk rather than toward the fetal femur, in accordance with the uterine contractions. In double groin traction (Fig. 2.8.11), the index fingers of both the hands are hooked in the groin folds and then traction is applied.

2.8.12: Pinard's Maneuver (A to C)

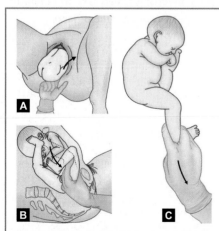

Figs 2.8.12 (A to C): Steps for performing Pinard's maneuver

Pinard's maneuver is a method commonly used at the time of breech extraction. This maneuver aims at bringing down the foot in cases where the fetal leg is extended, e.g. frank breech.

In this maneuver pressure is exerted against the inner aspect of the knee (popliteal fossa), with help of the middle and index fingers of the clinician. As the pressure is applied, the knee gets flexed and abducted. This causes the lower leg to move downward, which is then swept medially and gently pulled out of the vagina.

Picture	Clinical Description	Management/Clinical Features

2.8.13: Dührssen's Incision

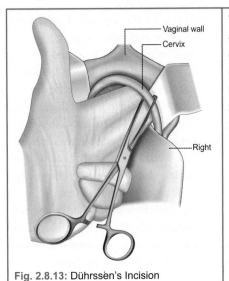

Fig. 2.8.13: Dührssen's Incision

This is the incision, which is about 1–3 cm deep made through several portions of the cervical canal (commonly at 2', 6', or 10'O clock positions). Administration of this incision may be necessary to relieve cervical entrapment and to facilitate the delivery of fetal head.

Fetal head entrapment may occur in approximately 8.5% of vaginal breech deliveries. It commonly results from an incompletely dilated cervix and head that lacks time to mold to the maternal pelvis. This complication is higher amongst preterm fetuses (< 32 weeks), when the head is larger in comparison to the rest of the body. Cervical incisions, however, can result in hemorrhage and extension into the lower uterine segment. Therefore the operator must be equipped to deal with this complication.

2.9: TRANSVERSE LIE

2.9.1: Different Positions of Transverse Lie (A and B)

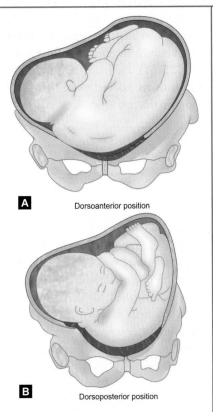

A Dorsoanterior position

B Dorsoposterior position

Figs 2.9.1 (A and B): (A) Dorsoanterior position; (B) Dorsoposterior position

Transverse lie is an abnormal fetal presentation in which the fetus lies transversely with the shoulders presenting in the lower pole of the uterus. In this presentation, long axis of the fetus is perpendicular to the maternal spine. As a result, the presenting part becomes the fetal shoulder.

The denominator is the fetal back. Depending on whether the position of the fetal back is anterior, posterior, superior or inferior, the following positions are possible:

- *Dorso-anterior*: The most common position where the fetal back is anterior.
- *Dorso-posterior*: Fetal back is posterior.
- *Dorso-superior*: Fetal back is directed superiorly.
- *Dorso-inferior*: Fetal back is directed inferiorly.

Depending on the position of the fetal head, the fetal position can be described as right or left.

There is no mechanism of labor for a fetus in transverse lie, which remains uncorrected until term. A cesarean section is required to deliver the baby with shoulder presentation. The management options for transverse lie during pregnancy include external cephalic version during the antenatal period or delivery by cesarean section (elective or an emergency). At some centers, stabilizing induction is used for converting transverse to cephalic presentation at the time of labor.

Picture	Clinical Description	Management/Clinical Features

2.9.2: Vaginal Touch Picture of Shoulder Presentation (A and B)

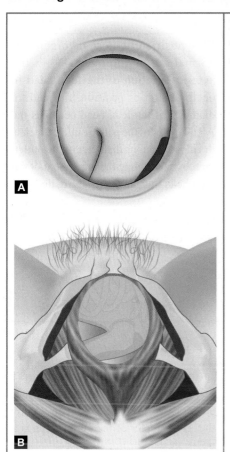

A

B

Figs 2.9.2 (A and B): (A) Vaginal touch picture in case of shoulder presentation; (B) Fetal shoulder as identified on vaginal examination

Figures 2.9.2 (A and B) show the findings observed on vaginal examination in cases of transverse lie.

On vaginal examination during the antenatal period, the pelvis appears to be empty. Even if something is felt on vaginal examination, no definite fetal part may be identified.

At the time of labor, on vaginal examination, fetal shoulder including scapula, clavicle and humerus, and grid iron feel of fetal ribs can be palpated. Due to ill-fitting fetal part, an elongated bag of membranes may be felt on vaginal examination. If the membranes have ruptured, the fetal shoulder can be identified by feeling the acromion process, the scapula, clavicle, axilla, ribs and intercostal spaces.

Ribs and intercostal spaces upon palpation give feeling of grid iron. If the arm prolapse has occurred, the fetal arm might be observed lying outside the vagina.

2.9.3: Ultrasound Examination in Case of Transverse Lie

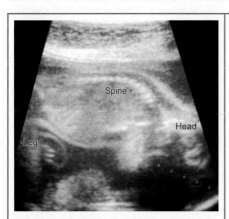

Spine

Head

Leg

Fig. 2.9.3: Ultrasound examination at 24 weeks gestation showing transverse lie

Ultrasound helps in confirming the presence of transverse lie as shown in the adjacent figure.

The other things which can be observed on the ultrasound include the following:
- Presence of uterine and/or fetal anomalies
- Fetal maturity
- Placental location and grading
- Adequacy of liquor
- Ruling out multiple gestation

Picture	Clinical Description	Management/Clinical Features

2.10: ABNORMAL POSITIONS

2.10.1: Occipitoanterior Position

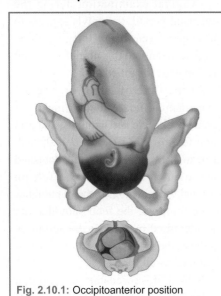

Fig. 2.10.1: Occipitoanterior position

In cases of occipitoanterior position on vaginal examination, the sagittal sutures lie in one of the oblique diameters (right or left) of the pelvic inlet. In LOA position, the sagittal diameter lies in the right oblique diameter of the pelvic inlet.

This position is most favorable for normal vaginal delivery. With the anterior rotation of the fetal head in occipitoanterior position, the sagittal diameter of the fetal head occupies the AP diameter of the pelvic outlet, which is the most spacious diameter of the outlet, thereby facilitating the movement of the fetal head outside the pelvic outlet.

2.10.2: Occipitotransverse Position

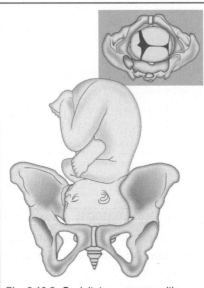

Fig. 2.10.2: Occipitotransverse position

Figure 2.10.2 illustrates the fetal head in occipitotransverse position. In cases of occipitotransverse position on vaginal examination, the sagittal sutures lie in the transverse diameter of the pelvis and both the fontanels are palpable. This position occurs due to anterior rotation by one-eight of the circle in case of oblique occipitoposterior position or it may occur due to nonrotation in case of primary occipitotransverse position.

In most cases of occipitotransverse position, the sagittal sutures rotate anteriorly by 2/8th of a circle to occupy the AP diameter of the outlet. This is a position, which is the most favorable for normal vaginal delivery. Sometimes the occipitotransverse position can lead to deep transverse arrest. In cases of deep transverse arrest, the fetal head gets captured in this position and the sagittal suture fails to move anteriorly, the position which favors normal vaginal delivery. Neither sinciput nor occiput leads the fetal head as a result of which further labor gets arrested and there is no advancement of fetal head. The head lies deep in the pelvic cavity at the level of ischial spines and there is no progress in the descent of fetal head even after half an hour to one hour following complete cervical dilatation. In these cases, the mother must not be encouraged to push down because it may not resolve the problem. Operative cesarean delivery appears to be the safest option for delivery in cases of deep transverse arrest.

Picture	Clinical Description	Management/Clinical Features

2.10.3: Occipitoposterior Position

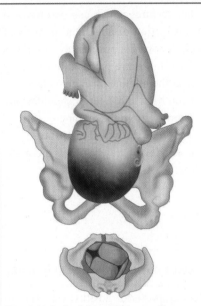

Fig. 2.10.3: Occipitoposterior position

This is a type of abnormal position of the vertex where the occiput is placed over the left sacroiliac joint [left occipitoposterior (LOP) or fourth vertex] or right sacroiliac joint [right occipitoposterior (ROP) or third vertex] or directly over the sacrum (direct occipitoposterior position). ROP position is more common than the LOP.

Manual rotation of fetal head or rotation using Kielland's forceps, both of which were previously performed, are no longer done nowadays.

In majority of cases, long anterior rotation of head occurs. Delivery, therefore, in majority of cases occurs spontaneously or with low forceps or ventouse. Management in the cases of occipitoposterior position at the time of labor comprises of following steps:

- Watchful expectancy hoping for fetal descent and anterior rotation of the occiput
- Intravenous infusion of ringer lactate must be started in anticipation of prolonged labor.
- Bed rest must be advised to avoid early ROM.
- Pelvis must be assessed for adequacy.
- Liberal episiotomy should be given to prevent perineal tears.
- Though in cases of occipitoposterior positions, ventouse application can be sometimes done, nowadays, cesarean section is the most commonly used mode of delivery in cases where there is failure of instrumental delivery or there is presence of an obstetric indication for cesarean delivery.

2.10.4: Causes of Occipitoposterior Position (A to D)

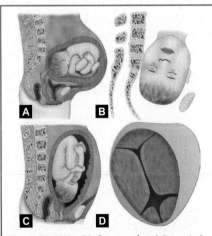

Figs 2.10.4 (A to D): Causes of occipitoposterior position: (A) Pendulous abdomen found in multipara; (B) Flat sacrum with deflexed head leads to further deflexion and occipitoposterior position; (C) Placenta placed on the anterior abdominal wall; (D) Android pelvis

Some common causes of occipitoposterior position are demonstrated in the adjacent figure and are as follows:

- Presence of an anthropoid or android pelvis
- Maternal kyphosis
- Marked deflexion of fetal head
- High pelvic inclination
- Attachment of placenta on the anterior uterine wall
- Brachycephaly of fetal head
- Abnormal uterine contractions
- Other conditions favoring occipitoposterior position include placenta previa, pelvic tumors, pendulous abdomen, polyhydramnios, multiple pregnancy, etc.

Diagnosis of occipitoposterior position is usually made on clinical examination. Findings on vaginal examination are as follows:

- Presence of an elongated bag of membranes
- Sagittal sutures occupy any of the oblique diameters of the pelvis
- Posterior fontanel is felt near the sacroiliac joint
- Anterior fontanel can be felt more easily due to the deflexed head.

Picture	Clinical Description	Management/Clinical Features

2.10.5: Inspection of Abdomen (Comparison between Occiput Anterior and Occiput Posterior Position) (A and B)

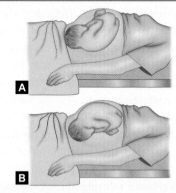

Figs 2.10.5 (A and B): Comparison between occiput anterior and occiput posterior position on abdominal examination

Figure 2.10.5 shows comparison between the appearances of abdomen in cases of occipitoposterior and occipitoanterior positions. On abdominal inspection there is flattening of the abdomen below the umbilicus in cases of occipitoposterior position. On the other hand, there is fullness of the abdomen below the umbilicus in occipitoanterior position. In occipitoposterior position, the fetal back is directed posteriorly, whereas the limbs are directed anteriorly. The abdomen looks flattened due to the absence of round contour of the fetal back.

Other features which can be observed on inspection of abdomen in cases of occipitoposterior position are as follows
- Fetal limbs are palpated more easily near the midline on either side
- Fetal back and anterior shoulders are far away from the midline
- The fetal heart sound (FHS) is difficult to locate and may be best heard in the region of flanks.

2.10.6: Palpation of Fetal Head (Comparison between Occiput Anterior and Occiput Posterior Position) (A and B)

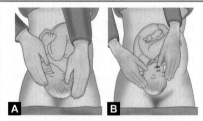

Figs 2.10.6 (A and B): Palpation of fetal head: (A) Occiput anterior position; (B) Occiput posterior position

Figure 2.10.6 shows comparison between the palpation of fetal head in cases of occipitoposterior and occipitoanterior positions. On pelvic grip in cases with occipitoposterior position, the head is not engaged. Also, the cephalic prominence is not felt as prominently as felt in occipitoanterior position due to deflexed head.

Occipitoposterior position can be considered as an abnormal position of the vertex rather than an abnormal presentation. Cesarean section is not indicated per se in the cases of occipitoposterior position.

2.10.7: Consequences Related to Occipitoposterior Position

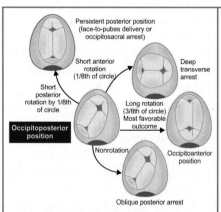

Fig. 2.10.7: Consequences related to occipitoposterior position

In majority of cases of occipitoposterior position, good uterine contractions result in the flexion of fetal head. Descent occurs and the occiput undergoes rotation by 3/8th of the circle to lie behind the pubic symphysis, resulting in an occipitoanterior position. In a small number of cases, the outcome may be favorable, resulting in short anterior rotation, nonrotation and short posterior rotation. In case of short anterior rotation, the occiput rotates through 1/8th of the circle anteriorly so that the sagittal sutures lie in the bispinous diameter. This position is known as the "deep transverse arrest".

In case of nonrotation of the occiput, sagittal sutures lie in the oblique diameter. Further progress of labor is unlikely and this is known as oblique posterior arrest.

Various complications related to occipitoposterior position are as follows:
- Prolonged duration of both first and second stages of labor (due to labor dystocia; delayed engagement of the fetal head and abnormal uterine contractions with slow dilatation of cervix).
- Early ROM
- Extreme degree of molding of fetal skull can result in tentorial tears.
- Increased tendency for postpartum hemorrhage.
- High chances of perineal injuries and trauma including complete perineal tears.
- Increased maternal and perinatal morbidity.

Picture	Clinical Description	Management/Clinical Features

2.10.8: Persistent Occipitoposterior Position

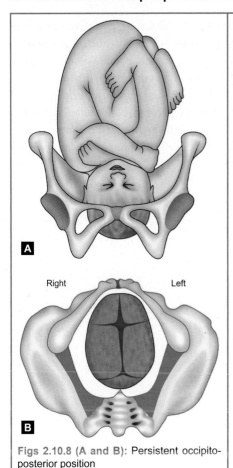

A

Right   Left

B

Figs 2.10.8 (A and B): Persistent occipito-posterior position

In cases of persistent occipitoposterior position, due to deflexed head, the occiput fails to rotate forward. Instead the sinciput reaches the pelvic floor first and rotates forward. As a result, the baby is born facing the pubic bone (face-to-pubis delivery). Due to deflexed head, the occipitofrontal diameter (11.5 cm) enters the pelvis leading to delayed engagement.

In case of short posterior rotation, posterior rotation of the sinciput occurs by 1/8th of the circle, putting the occiput in the sacral hollow.

This position is known as persistent occipitoposterior position. Under favorable conditions with an average-sized baby, spacious pelvis and good uterine contractions, spontaneous face-to-pubis delivery can occur. If conditions are not favorable, delivery may not occur, resulting in an occipitosacral arrest. In these cases cesarean delivery may be required.

2.10.9: Molding of Fetal Head Following Persistent Occipitoposterior Position

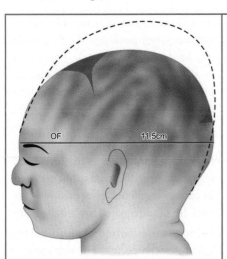

OF   11.5cm

Fig. 2.10.9: Molding of fetal head following persistent occipitoposterior position (OF, Occipitofrontal)

In cases of fetal head in persistent occipitoposterior position, characteristic molding of head is observed with the caput succedaneum present on the anterior part of the parietal bone.

On vaginal examination, anterior fontanel is felt behind the pubic symphysis and a large caput succedaneum may be seen masking this. If the pinna of the ear is observed to be pointing toward the mother's sacrum, it indicates an occipitoposterior position.

2.10.10: Mechanism of Vaginal Delivery in Case of Occipitoposterior Position (A to D)

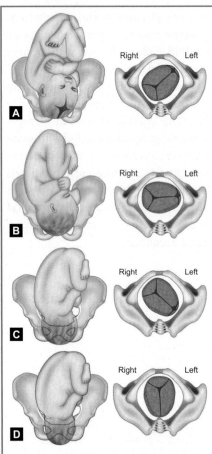

Figs 2.10.10 (A to D): Mechanism of vaginal delivery in case of occipitoposterior position

Figures 2.10.10 (A to D) demonstrate the mechanism of normal vaginal delivery in cases of right occipitoposterior position. Descent of the head occurs with increased flexion. As the fetal head enters the maternal pelvis, sagittal sutures are in right oblique diameter of the pelvis. With the increasing descent, occiput and shoulders rotate by 1/8th of the circle forward due to which the sagittal sutures of fetal head occupy the transverse diameter of pelvis. With increasing descent, occiput and shoulders have rotated further 1/8th of circle (total of 2/8th of a circle) forward due to which the sagittal sutures occupy left oblique diameter of the pelvis. The position therefore becomes right occipitoanterior. As further rotation of fetal occiput occurs, sagittal sutures now lie in the AP diameter of the pelvis. This way occiput has undergone rotation by a total 3/8th of the circle forward.

In 90% cases of occipitoposterior position, delivery occurs normally through vaginal route as long anterior rotation occurs by 3/8th of circle, bringing the occiput anteriorly. This kind of favorable outcome occurs in cases with good uterine contractions, well-flexed fetal head and roomy pelvis.

2.10.11: Face Presentation

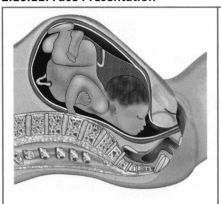

Fig. 2.10.11: Face presentation

This is an abnormal fetal position characterized by an extreme extension of the fetal head so that the fetal face rather than the fetal head becomes the presenting part and the fetal occiput comes in direct contact with the back. Ultrasonography must be performed in order to assess fetal size and to rule out the presence of any bony congenital malformations.

Abdominal examination: In case of mentoanterior positions, the fetal limbs can be palpated anteriorly. Fetal chest is also present anteriorly against the uterine wall. The FHS is thus clearly audible. On abdominal palpation, the groove between the head and neck is not prominent and cephalic prominence lies on the same side as the fetal back. On pelvic grip, the head is not engaged. In case of mentoposterior positions, the back is better palpated toward the front.

Vaginal examination: The following structures can be felt: alveolar margins of the mouth, nose, malar eminences, supraorbital ridges and the mentum. Also, there is absence of meconium staining on examining fingers.

2.10.12: Different Positions in Case of Face Presentation

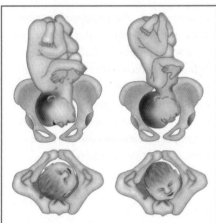

Fig. 2.10.12: Different positions in case of face presentation

Denominator in the cases of face presentation is mentum or chin.

Four positions are possible depending on the position of the chin with left or right sacroiliac joints:

- Right mentoposterior position (deflexed LOA)
- Left mentoposterior position [deflexed right occipitoanterior (ROA)]
- Left mentoanterior position (deflexed ROP)
- Right mentoanterior position (deflexed LOP).

Most common type of face presentation is left mentoanterior position.

Delivery occurs spontaneously in most of cases of face presentation. In presence of normal cervical dilatation and descent, there is no need for the obstetrician to intervene. Labor will be longer, but if the pelvis is adequate and the head rotates to a mentoanterior position, a vaginal delivery can be expected. The mechanism of delivery and corresponding body movements in case of anterior face presentations are similar to that of the corresponding occipitoanterior position. The only difference being that delivery of head occurs by flexion rather than extension. The engaging diameter is submentobregmatic in case of a fully extended head. If the head rotates backward to a mentoposterior position, a cesarean section may be required. In case of posterior face presentations, the mechanism of delivery is same as that of occipitoposterior position except that the anterior rotation of the mentum occurs in only 20–30% of the cases.

In the remaining 70–80% cases, there may be incomplete anterior rotation, no rotation or short posterior rotation of mentum. There is no possibility of spontaneous vaginal delivery in case of persistent mentoposterior positions. Cesarean section may be required in these cases.

2.10.13: Brow Presentation

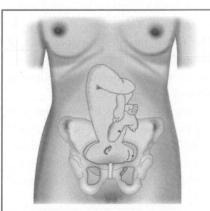

Fig. 2.10.13: Brow presentation

This is a type of cephalic presentation where the fetal head is incompletely flexed as shown in the adjacent figure. The head is short of complete extension, which could have resulted in a face presentation. As a result, presenting part becomes the brow. On vaginal examination, the occiput and sinciput are palpated at the same level.

Since the engaging diameter of the head is mentovertical (14 cm), there would be no mechanism of labor with an average-sized baby and a normal pelvis. Vaginal delivery may be the possible option only in cases where there is spontaneous conversion to face or vertex presentation. Therefore, after ruling out the cephalopelvic disproportion and fetal congenital anomalies, the obstetrician must await for spontaneous vaginal delivery. In cases where this does not occur, cesarean section is the best method for delivery.

2.10.14: Compound Presentation

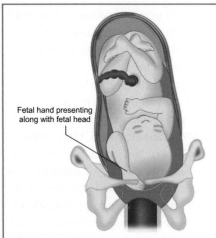

Fetal hand presenting along with fetal head

Fig. 2.10.14: Compound presentation

In compound presentation, one or two of the fetal extremities enter the pelvis simultaneously with the presenting part. The most common combinations are head-hand; breech-hand and head-arm-foot. The predisposing factors for the development of compound presentation include factors such as prematurity; multiparity; twin/multiple gestation; pelvic tumors; cephalopelvic disproportion; macerated fetus, etc.

In most cases, the prolapsed extremity does not cause any interference with the normal progress of labor and vaginal delivery. Moreover, the prolapsed limbs spontaneously rise up with the descent of the presenting part in most of the cases. In presence of cephalopelvic disproportion and/or cord prolapse, cesarean section is required.

2.10.15: Cord Presentation

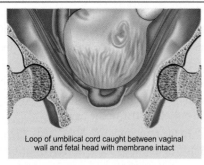

Loop of umbilical cord caught between vaginal wall and fetal head with membrane intact

Fig. 2.10.15: Cord presentation

Cord presentation is the presence of one or more loops of umbilical cord between the fetal presenting part and the cervix, with the membranes being intact. It usually occurs due to ill-fitting fetal presenting part in the lower uterine segment. This could be related to various causes, such as prematurity, contracted pelvis, polyhydramnios, pelvic tumors, etc. The condition is related with high mortality rate due to fetal asphyxia, resulting from the following causes:

- Mechanical compression of the umbilical cord between fetal presenting part and bony pelvis
- Spasm of the blood vessels within the umbilical cord when exposed to the external environment.

Cord prolapse is associated with higher mortality than cord presentation.

Prevention and first aid:

- Artificial ROM should be avoided whenever possible if the presenting part has yet not engaged or is mobile.
- In cases where ROM becomes necessary even in such circumstances, this should be performed in an operation theater with facilities available for an immediate cesarean birth.
- In cases of cord presentation where immediate vaginal delivery is not possible, consent should be taken and immediate preparations be made for an urgent cesarean delivery.
- To prevent cord compression, it is recommended that the presenting part be elevated either manually or by filling the urinary bladder with normal saline.

Definitive Management

Definitive management comprises of immediate delivery. In cases where cervix is fully dilated, the following options can be considered:

- *Vertex presentation*: In cases where head has engaged, mode of delivery should be ROM, followed by forceps delivery.
- *Breech presentation*: The delivery option in these cases is ROM followed by breech extraction.

Picture	Clinical Description	Management/Clinical Features

2.10.16: Cord Prolapse

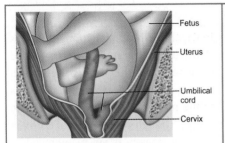

Fig. 2.10.16: Cord prolapse

Cord prolapse has been defined as descent of the umbilical cord through the cervix alongside the presenting part (occult presentation) or past it (overt presentation) in the presence of ruptured membranes. In occult prolapse, the cord cannot be felt by the examiner's fingers at the time of vaginal examination. In overt cord prolapse, the cord is found lying inside the vagina or outside the vulva following the ROM.

In cases of cord prolapse where immediate vaginal delivery is not possible, assistance should be called immediately; venous access should be obtained, consent taken and immediate preparations be made for an urgent cesarean delivery. The following steps can be followed until facilities for cesarean section are made available:

- To prevent vasospasm, there should be minimal handling of loops of cord lying outside the vagina, which can be covered with surgical packs soaked in warm saline.
- To prevent cord compression, it is recommended that the presenting part should be elevated either manually or by filling the urinary bladder with normal saline.
- Cord compression can be further reduced by advising the mother to adopt knee-chest position or head-down tilt (preferably in left lateral position).

Spontaneous vaginal delivery may be allowed in cases of dead fetus.

2.10.17: Ultrasound Examination in Case of Cord Prolapse/Presentation

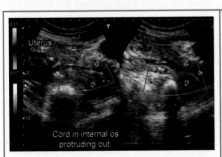

Fig. 2.10.17: Color Doppler ultrasound showing cord prolapse

Figure 2.10.17 describes the findings of ultrasound examination in case of cord prolapse/presentation. In this case, the internal os appears dilated with umbilical cord within the cervix; this finding is diagnostic of cord prolapse.

Clinical examination helps in detecting this condition in most of the cases. In cases where a clinical diagnosis of cord prolapse is made, it is necessary to establish whether the fetus is living or not. Various investigations, which could help in the diagnosis of cord prolapse or presentation include the following:

- *Cardiotocography*: There may be variable decelerations of heart rate pattern on continuous electronic fetal monitoring.
- *Ultrasound examination*: Ultrasound may help in identification of umbilical cord within the cervix.

2.11: FETAL MONITORING USING CARDIOTOCOGRAPHY

2.11.1: Electronic External Fetal Heart Rate Monitoring

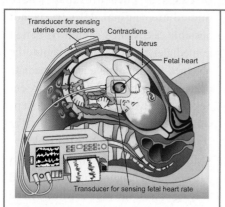

Fig. 2.11.1: Electronic external fetal heart rate monitoring

Electronic fetal monitoring has been defined by both ACOG and RCOG as monitoring the baby's heart rate for indicators of stress, usually during labor and birth using electronic fetal heart-rate monitoring device. Electronic fetal monitoring can be of two types: external and internal cardiac monitoring. Figure 2.11.1 shows the process of electronic external fetal cardiac monitoring.

External fetal heart monitoring (EFM) as shown in the adjacent figure is performed by attaching the cardiotocograph machine through external transducers to the mother's abdomen with elastic straps. Though routine use of EFM in every pregnancy is not recommended, it is widely used in the assessment of fetal health, particularly in high-risk pregnancies and unbooked patients with low-risk pregnancy, presenting for the first time late in labor.

2.11.2: Cardiotocograph Machine

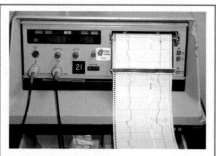

Fig. 2.11.2: Cardiotocograph machine

Cardiotocometer ("cardio"—heart; "toco"—labor; "meter"—measure) machine comprises of an ultrasound to monitor the fetal heart rate and a tocodynamometer which monitors contraction patterns. The transducers use Doppler ultrasound to detect fetal heart motion, and the information is sent to the fetal heart monitor, which calculates and records the fetal heart rate on a continuous strip of paper. Modern cardiotocographic machines comprise of microprocessors and make use of mathematical procedures, which helps in improving the fetal heart-rate signal and the accuracy of fetal heart recording.

Electronic fetal heart monitoring is commonly used for assessing the fetal well-being within the contracting uterus and for detecting signs of fetal distress. ACOG recommends that the speed of the cardiotocography (CTG) paper within the cardiotocographic machine should be set at 1 cm/minute, and fetal heart rate (FHR) range display must be set at 50–210 BPM. Correct date and time of recording should be noted by the obstetrician upon commencement of CTG, and it should be labeled with the mother's name, date, time commenced and hospital record number. The CTG should be interpreted in combination with the woman's complete history. As far as possible the clinician should be present throughout the time period when the fetal heart tracing is being taken. Continuous CTG monitoring is not recommended in all cases. However, it may be required whenever there is an evidence of fetal compromise.

Picture	Clinical Description	Management/Clinical Features

2.11.3: An Obstetrician Taking a Cardiotocographic Trace of a Patient in Labor

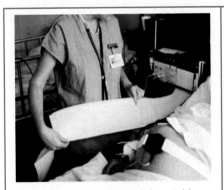

Fig. 2.11.3: An obstetrician taking a cardiotocographic trace of a patient in labor

Figure 2.11.3 shows an obstetrician taking cardiotocographic trace of a pregnant patient. At the time of cardiotocography, electronic fetal monitors are used to detect and trace the fetal heart rate and uterine contractions. Fetal heart-rate monitoring is performed using an external transducer, which is placed on the maternal abdomen with help of ultrasound gel and held in place by a lightweight stretchable band or an elastic belt. The external transducer comprises of piezoelectrical crystal, which can emit and receive ultrasound waves. The fetal heart rate is calculated from echo signal by the application of the Doppler principle.

The typical fetal monitor strip consists of two rows of graphs; the upper graph charting the fetal heart rate (in beats per minute) and the lower graph charting the mother's contractions (in mm Hg). The normal fetal heart rate range is between 120 BPM to 160 BPM. Each small square of the charts represents a span of 10 seconds, equaling 1 minute for every 6 small squares across.

2.11.4: Characteristics of the Fetal Heart Rate that Need to be Assessed

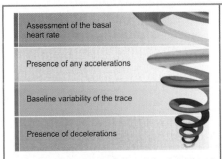

Fig. 2.11.4: Characteristics of the fetal heart rate that need to be assessed

The assessment of the fetal heart trace requires the clinician to look for the characteristics enumerated in Figure 2.11.4. Based on the assessment of these four characteristics of the fetal heart-rate pattern, the fetal trace can be classified as normal, suspicious (non reassuring) or abnormal (pathological or ominous). A cardiotocograph is considered to be normal when all the four features fall into the reassuring category. This implies that baseline heart rate varies from 120 BPM to 160 BPM, shows baseline variability of $\geq$ 5 BPM, there is absence of decelerations and presence of accelerations. It is considered to be suspicious when one of the features falls into the non reassuring category, whereas the remainder of the features are reassuring. However, when two or more cardiotocographic features fall under the non reassuring category, it is considered as pathological.

While reassuring patterns are associated with good fetal outcome, non reassuring patterns are not. Non reassuring patterns, such as severe fetal tachycardia, bradycardia and late decelerations with good short-term variability require interventions to rule out fetal acidosis. Ominous patterns require emergency intrauterine fetal resuscitation and immediate delivery. The characteristics of uterine contractions that need to be assessed include the rate, intensity, duration, regularity and baseline tone between contractions.

Picture	Clinical Description	Management/Clinical Features

2.11.5: Reassuring Fetal Heart-Rate Patterns

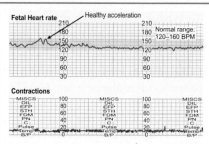

Fig. 2.11.5: Reassuring fetal heart-rate patterns

Figure 2.11.5 illustrates reassuring heart rate pattern on fetal heart-rate trace.

Reassuring fetal heart-rate pattern can be defined as follows:
- Baseline fetal heart rate of 120–160 BPM, having preserved beat-to-beat variability.
- There may be accelerated lasting for 15 seconds or more above the baseline, peaking to 15 or more BPM.

Fetal heart tracing should be interpreted using a systematic approach, which involves evaluation of four main parameters, such as baseline heart rate, variability, absence of decelerations and presence of accelerations.

2.11.6: A Heart-Rate Tracing Showing Fetal Bradycardia

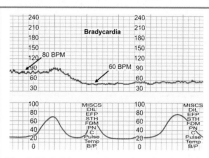

Fig. 2.11.6: A heart-rate tracing showing fetal bradycardia

Fetal bradycardia is defined when fetal heart rate is less than 120 BPM and lasts 10–15 minutes or longer. A borderline fetal bradycardia (FHR of 110–119 BPM) in the absence of other fetal heart changes does not signify fetal compromise. Moderate bradycardia is a FHR of 80–100 BPM, and severe bradycardia is 80 BPM or less lasting for 3 minutes or longer. Bradycardia is a late sign of fetal hypoxia (a continued lack of oxygen supply to fetus). One of the most important causes of baseline fetal bradycardia is fetal hypoxemia and metabolic acidosis. Mild bradycardia can also sometimes results from compression of the umbilical cord.

Since fetal bradycardia is an emergency, seeking immediate assistance becomes mandatory.

Bradycardia resulting from cord compression usually gets corrected on its own as the fetus moves. Discontinuing the drug use or neutralizing its action by using an antidote can rectify bradycardia resulting from the drug use.

2.11.7: A Tracing Showing Tachycardia

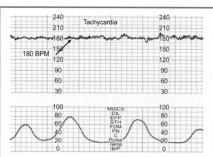

Fig. 2.11.7: A fetal heart tracing showing tachycardia

Fetal tachycardia is said to be present when the fetal heart rate exceeds 160 BPM. Fetal tachycardia is identified, when this increase in heart rate lasts for 10 minutes or longer. While mild tachycardia may be a physiological finding, tachycardia of 200 BPM or more may be ominous.

Baseline tachycardia may be an early clinical sign of fetal hypoxia. However, complicated baseline tachycardia, i.e. associated with loss of baseline variability and/or deceleration of any type or heart rate of more than or equal to 200 BPM is extremely ominous and may be associated with fetal acidosis and high-risk of fetal decompensation.

Tachycardia in absence of other ominous findings usually settles on giving adequate analgesia. Since fever is another important cause of tachycardia, maternal temperature should be taken every 2 hours in labor. Often fetal tachycardia returns to normal when steps for reducing maternal fever or infection are taken. Treatment of the underlying cause of tachycardia (e.g. stopping the use of drug causing tachycardia) usually helps in taking care. Teachycardia greater than 200 BPM requires urgent fetal blood sampling and pH estimation, followed by immediate delivery.

PART I ❖ OBSTETRICS

Picture	Clinical Description	Management/Clinical Features

2.11.8: Short-term Variability

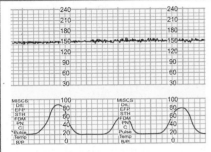

Fig. 2.11.8: Short-term variability

Baseline variability implies that the FHR is under constant variation from the baseline. A normal, healthy fetus should exhibit average to moderate variability varying between 5 BPM to 15 BPM every 10–20 seconds, i.e. at the frequency of three to six cycles per minute. Normal beat-to-beat variability indicates the ability of the fetal heart to respond to external stimuli through a well-balanced sympathetic and parasympathetic nervous system. Variability can normally be both short term and long term. The adjacent figure illustrates short-term variability.

Beat-to-beat or short-term variability is the oscillation of the FHR around the baseline in amplitude of 5–10 BPM. The minute irregularity that occurs from one beat to the other on the CTG trace line, responsible for giving it a saw-toothed appearance, represents the real beat-to-beat or short-term variability of FHR. This signifies the variation in the interval between two R-waves on the fetal ECG. Short-term variability being so minute may be difficult to assess visually.

2.11.9: Long-term Variability

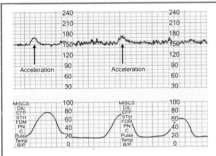

Fig. 2.11.9: Long-term variability

Long-term variability denotes the fluctuations or oscillatory changes that occur during the course of 1 minute in the fetal heart tracing relative to its baseline rate. Though by definition long-term variability is to be judged on 1 minute tracing; for proper interpretation, it must be analyzed for several minutes (about 3–5 minutes). Long-term variability is mostly controlled by the autonomic nervous system. The magnitude of long-term baseline variability can be found out by drawing a line along the highest and lowest projection of FHR trace during 1 minute.

Chronic hypoxia and fetal acidosis invariability results in reduced variability of less than 5 BPM. Persistently minimal or absent FHR variability appears to be the most significant intrapartum sign of fetal compromise. On the other hand, the presence of good FHR variability may not always be predictive of a good outcome. Other causes of reduced variability include fetal prematurity, fetal sleep; administration of drugs including central nervous system depressant drugs (diazepam, pethidine), $MgSO_4$ and local anesthetic drugs (drugs with "caine" group) to the mother, and baseline tachycardia (especially severe tachycardia of greater than 180 BPM).

2.11.10: Reduced Baseline Variability of Less than 5–10 BPM over a Period of Time

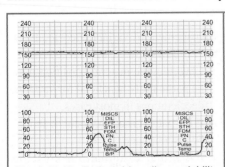

Fig. 2.11.10: Reduced baseline variability of less than 5–10 BPM over a period of time

Beat-to-beat or short-term variability normally varies between 5 BPM and 15 BPM. The adjacent figure illustrates a cardiotocographic tracing showing baseline variability of less than 5–10 BPM over a period of time.

Chronic hypoxia typically affects the parasympathetic control resulting in the loss of baseline variability of FHR. Fetal acidosis invariability results in reduced variability of less than 5 BPM. Persistently minimal or absent FHR variability appears to be the most significant intrapartum sign of fetal compromise.

2.11.11: Early Deceleration

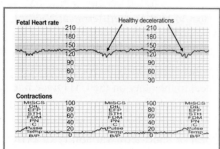

Fig. 2.11.11: Early deceleration

A sudden decrease in FHR by more than 15 BPM lasting for more than 15 seconds, but less than 2 minutes from the baseline is considered as a deceleration and can be either periodic or episodic. Periodic decelerations can be further subclassified into following three types based on their relation to the specific period of uterine contraction: early, late and variable decelerations. Figure 2.11.11 shows the pattern of early deceleration. The onset and return of the deceleration typically coincides with the start and end of the contraction respectively.

The obstetrician should always remember that presence of decelerations during labor is not always ominous, as during labor it is possible for some nonpathological type of early decelerations to occur as well (e.g. due to compression of head in the first or second stage of labor). However, their occurrence during the antenatal period should always be considered to be pathological. Typically, early decelerations during labor do not require any treatment other than continued observation and reassessment. Uncomplicated early deceleration does not signify hypoxia or acidosis, hence immediate intervention is usually not necessary.

2.11.12: Early Deceleration (Magnified View)

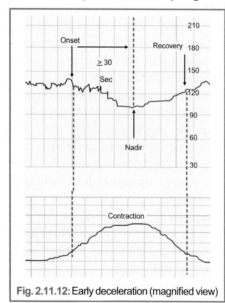

Fig. 2.11.12: Early deceleration (magnified view)

An early deceleration is a deceleration pattern in which the decrease in the fetal heart rate starts at about the same time as the onset of the contraction and the nadir of deceleration coincides with the peak of contraction. Since the decelerations start very shortly after the beginning of contractions, they are known as early. These decelerations recover fully by the end of the uterine contraction.

Though most of the times early decelerations are nonpathological, if early decelerations appear on the CTG trace, the obstetrician must perform a prompt vaginal examination in order to assess the progress of labor, adequacy of pelvic passage and to exclude cord prolapse. Also, it is possible that there is coexistant hypoxia. The obstetrician, therefore, needs to keep a close watch on such tracing to assess if other ominous features (absence of variability) are making their appearance or not.

2.11.13: Variable Decelerations

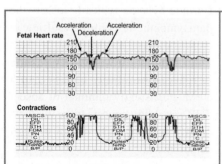

Fig. 2.11.13: Variable decelerations

Variable decelerations are named so as they can occur at any time during a contraction. These decelerations are often variable in duration, intensity and timing. Cord compression is usually responsible for variable decelerations. However, severe atypical (associated with loss of variability) variable decelerations are commonly associated with fetal acidosis and low APGAR scores.

Management of variable decelerations is as follows:
- Changing the maternal position may be particularly beneficial for variable decelerations in most cases.
- If the patient is on oxytocin, it should be discontinued.
- A vaginal examination must be performed to rule out cord prolapse.

Picture	Clinical Description	Management/Clinical Features

2.11.14: Variable Decelerations (Magnified View)

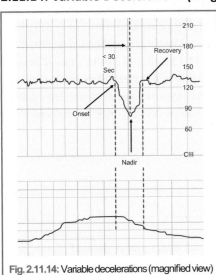

Fig. 2.11.14: Variable decelerations (magnified view)

Variable decelerations are characterized by a frequently short acceleration pattern followed by a rapid deceleration for some seconds, then a rapid rise and a short acceleration before returning to baseline. This results in accelerations "shoulders" before and after a deceleration and is responsible for their V or W-shape.

Besides the steps mentioned in 2.11.13, other steps which may be taken are:
- Amnioinfusion to be considered in cases of oligohydramnios.
- Administration of 100% O_2 by a tight face mask.

2.11.15: Late Deceleration (Magnified View)

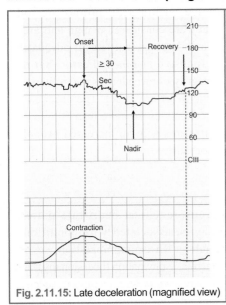

Fig. 2.11.15: Late deceleration (magnified view)

Onset of late decelerations occurs after the beginning of the contraction, and the nadir of the deceleration occurs after the peak of the contraction. Since deceleration starts late in the contraction, hence it is known as late deceleration. There must be presence of consecutive three or more late decelerations following normal fetal heart trace, for the diagnosis of late deceleration to be made.

Immediate steps for management are as follows:
- The patient must be placed in left lateral position.
- O_2 must be administered to the mother with help of a tight face mask.
- Medications like oxytocin, etc. which by causing uterine contractions can further result in placental insufficiency must be discontinued.
- Maternal hypotension can be corrected by administration of IV fluids.
- In case of uterine hyperstimulation, uterine relaxants like terbutaline 0.25 mg can be administered subcutaneously.

2.11.16: Late Decelerations with Preserved Baseline Variability

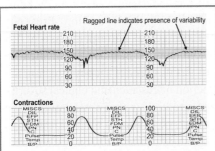

Fig. 2.11.16: Late decelerations with preserved baseline variability

Late decelerations are the most ominous fetal heart-rate pattern. Late decelerations are associated with reduced placental perfusion resulting in uteroplacental insufficiency, which can result in development of hypoxia and metabolic abnormalities. Figure 2.11.15 shows late decelerations with preserved baseline variability. Persistent late decelerations with decreased or absent variability is associated with an even worse prognosis.

If despite the above mentioned steps (2.11.15), maternal decelerations persist for more than 30 minutes, measurement of fetal scalp pH is indicated. Scalp pH of greater than or equal to 7.25 is considered to be reassuring. However, pH between 7.2–7.25 is considered equivocal and must be repeated within 30 minutes. If scalp pH is less than 7.2 or there is continued presence of late decelerations with absent variability, the obstetrician must try to deliver the baby as soon as possible.

Picture	Clinical Description	Management/Clinical Features

2.11.17: Mild and Severe Variable Decelerations

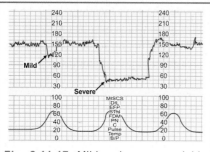 Fig. 2.11.17: Mild and severe variable decelerations	As previously described, variable decelerations are frequently V-shaped or W-shaped due to their variable intensity. The severity of variable decelerations is determined by how low the FHR drops, and how long the episode lasts. These decelerations are classified as severe if they last more than 60 seconds or if the fetal heart rate drops to less than 90 BPM.	Management of mild variable decelerations has been described in 2.11.13 and 2.11.14. In case of severe variable decelerations indicative of fetal hypoxia and acidosis, emergency cesarean delivery may be required.

2.11.18: Acceleration of Fetal Heart

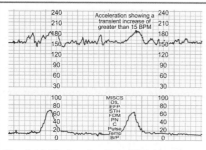 Fig. 2.11.18: Acceleration of fetal heart	Accelerations are transient increases in the fetal heart rate caused by fetal movement. The 15 × 15 rule (increase in FHR by more than 15 BPM for more than 15 seconds) is a good indicator of fetal well-being and adequate oxygen reserve. In the normal mature fetus, accelerations can be triggered by fetal body movements, sounds, and other stimuli.	Fetal heart rate is defined as reactive if there are fetal heart accelerations resulting in an increase of 15 BPM above baseline for at least 15 seconds duration, twice within a 20-minute period. They are considered benign and are a reassuring sign that fetus is adequately responsive and an indicator that the integrity of mechanisms controlling the fetal heart are intact. The absence of accelerations for more than 80 minutes correlates with an increased neonatal morbidity.

2.11.19: True Sinusoidal Pattern

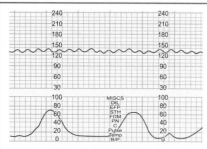 Fig. 2.11.19: True sinusoidal pattern	A sinusoidal pattern is one in which the amplitude of oscillations and period of short-term (beat-to-beat variability) remains more or less constant. This gives the fetal heart trace a smooth, undulating, regular wavy appearance. The fetal heart pattern is labeled as sinusoidal, if this pattern lasts for at least 10 minutes. In this pattern, the amplitude of oscillations usually varies between 5 BPM to 15 BPM with a fixed period of three to five cycles per minute. Fetal activity may be minimal or absent, and FHR accelerations are usually lacking. A true sinusoidal pattern is rare, but ominous and is associated with high rate of fetal morbidity and mortality.	Sinusoidal fetal heart-rate pattern may be associated with conditions, such as Rh isoimmunization, severe anemia, asphyxiation (occasionally), and maternal administration of some sedative and analgesic drugs like mepridine, pethidine, butorphanol, etc. Treatment of the underlying cause usually helps in treating this condition. Presence of sinusoidal pattern in case of Rh isoimmunized pregnancies is indicative of fetal anemia. Depending on the period of gestation and clinical severity of situation, either fetal intrauterine transfusion (prior to birth) or exchange transfusion (after birth) may be required. Sinusoidal pattern due to pethidine can be treated by administration of naloxone.

Picture	Clinical Description	Management/Clinical Features

2.11.20: Pseudosinusoidal Pattern

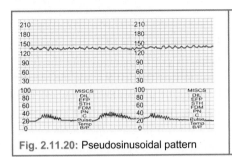

Fig. 2.11.20: Pseudosinusoidal pattern

Sinusoidal pattern is known as the pseudosinusoidal pattern, when in the in-between period, the baseline variability is preserved. It is not flattened as in the true sinusoidal pattern.

This type of sinusoidal pattern, which alternates with normal fetal heart pattern does not carry ominous significance and usually does not require any treatment.

2.11.21: Saltatory Pattern

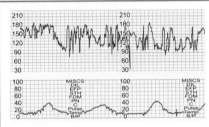

Fig. 2.11.21: Saltatory pattern

Saltatory fetal heart pattern comprises of rapidly occurring couples of acceleration and deceleration causing relatively large oscillations of the baseline fetal heart rate.

This pattern is usually caused by acute hypoxia or mechanical compression of the umbilical cord. It is considered a non reassuring pattern, but it is not usually an indication for immediate delivery and responds with conservative therapy such as:
- Changing the maternal position
- Administration of oxygen by mask to the mother
- Discontinuation of sedatives or oxytocics.

2.11.22: Set of Telemetry System (A and B)

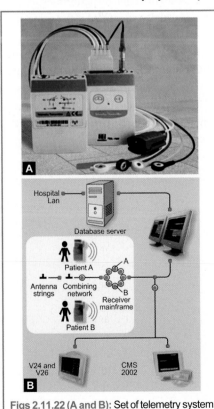

Figs 2.11.22 (A and B): Set of telemetry system

Since the conventional CTG monitoring largely restricts the maternal mobility, a new type of monitoring, namely the telemetry, which is a lot like the regular electronic fetal monitoring, was introduced to help the mother maintain her mobility. Through this technique, the fetal heart tones are transmitted to the nurses' station through the use of radiowaves.

A channel is assigned to each telemetry transmitter. Each transmitter is linked to a particular receiver in the main frame. The raw data from each transmitter after being relayed is processed by the main frame. This information is sent to the central station through a direct wired connection.

Telemetry has yet not been shown to improve the false positive rate associated with external monitoring. However, it does eliminate many of the problems associated with maternal immobility and positioning, by allowing the mother to maintain mobility. At present telemetry is not available in all hospitals.

2.12: OBSTETRIC MANEUVERS

2.12.1: External Cephalic Version through Forward Roll (A to D)

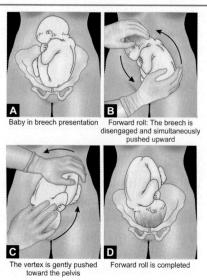

Figs 2.12.1 (A to D): External cephalic version through forward roll

External cephalic version (ECV) is a procedure in which the clinician externally rotates the fetus from a breech presentation into cephalic presentation. The procedure of ECV can be performed by two methods: forward roll or through back flip. The procedure of forward role has been described in the adjacent figure, while the procedure of back flip has been described in 2.12.2 (A to C)

While performing ECV, the clinician helps in gently manipulating the fetal head toward the pelvis while the breech is brought up cephalad toward the fundus. The clinician must attempt a forward roll first and then a backward roll, if the initial attempt is unsuccessful. The fetal head is manipulated to move it in the forward direction. This method is usually helpful if the spine and head are on opposite sides of the maternal midline. If the forward roll is unsuccessful, a second attempt is usually made in the opposite direction.

2.12.2: External Cephalic Version through Back Flip (A to C)

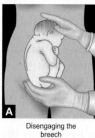

Disengaging the breech

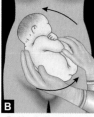

Pushing the breech upward and gently guiding the vertex toward the pelvis

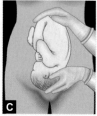

Completing the back flip

Figs 2.12.2 (A to C): External cephalic version through back flip

The procedure of ECV initially became popular in the 1960s and 1970s, following which its use reduced due to the reports of fetal deaths related to the procedure. It was reintroduced in 1980s and became increasingly popular in the 1990s, with increased advancement in the field of fetal monitoring. Routine use of external version has been observed to reduce the rate of cesarean delivery by about two-thirds.

The manipulation of fetal head in the backward direction by performing a back flip is usually attempted if the spine and head of the fetus are on the same side of the maternal midline. While doing the ECV, the fetus should be moved gently rather than using forceful movements. The procedure should only be performed in a facility equipped for emergency cesarean section.

Picture	Clinical Description	Management/Clinical Features

2.12.3: External Cephalic Version in Case of Transverse Lie (A and B)

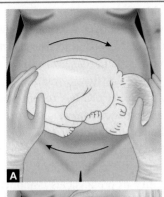

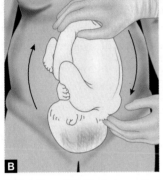

Figs 2.12.3 (A and B): Technique of external cephalic version in case of transverse lie

External cephalic version is a procedure in which the clinician externally rotates the fetus from a transverse lie into a cephalic presentation. The use of ECV helps in producing considerable cost savings in the management of the fetus in transverse lie by reducing the rate of cesarean section because the only available option in cases of uncorrected transverse lie is delivery by cesarean section.

Prior to the procedure of ECV, the following are done:
- The patient is placed in a supine or slight Trendelenburg position.
- Ultrasonic gel is applied liberally over the abdomen in order to decrease friction and to reduce the chances of an overvigorous manipulation. The procedure of ECV comprises of the following steps:
- External version can be performed by a clinician who is experienced in the procedure along with his/her assistant.
- Initially, the clinician grasps the fetus from its two poles.
- While performing the ECV, the clinician helps in gently manipulating the fetal head toward the pelvis while the podalic pole is brought up cephalad toward the fundus.
- While doing the ECV, the fetus should be moved gently rather than using forceful movements.

2.12.4: Internal Version

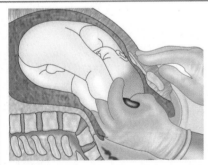

Fig. 2.12.4: Technique of internal podalic version

The technique of internal podalic version is shown in the adjacent figure. The procedure must be ideally performed under general anesthesia with the uterus sufficiently relaxed. Under all aseptic precautions the obstetrician introduces one of his/her hands into the uterine cavity in a cone-shaped manner. The hand is passed along the breech to ultimately grasp the fetal foot, which is identified by its heel. While the foot is gradually brought down, obstetrician's other hand present externally over the abdomen helps in gradually pushing the cephalic pole upward. Rest of the delivery is completed by breech extraction. Following the delivery of the baby, routine exploration of the cervicovaginal canal must be done to exclude out any injuries.

The only indication for internal version in modern obstetrics is the transverse lie of second twin. Besides this indication, the procedure of internal version has no place in modern obstetrics.

In case of vaginal delivery for twin gestation, following the delivery of the first twin in vertex presentation, the lie of second fetus is checked through abdominal examination. If the lie of second twin is transverse, external version must be attempted in order to correct the fetal lie. If the external version fails, internal version under general anesthesia can be attempted.

2.12.5: First Line Maneuvers for Shoulder Dystocia (A to C)

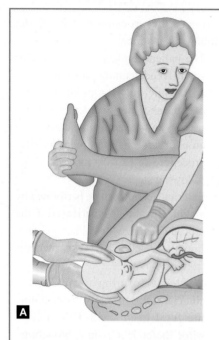

A

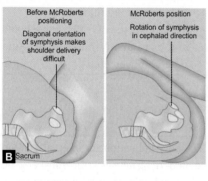

Before McRoberts positioning

Diagonal orientation of symphysis makes shoulder delivery difficult

McRoberts position

Rotation of symphysis in cephalad direction

B Sacrum

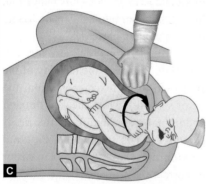

C

Figs 2.12.5 (A to C): (A and B) McRobert's maneuver; (C) Application of suprapubic pressure

McRobert's maneuver and application of suprapubic pressure are amongst few of the initial steps which must be employed in cases of shoulder dystocia. McRobert's maneuver is the single most effective intervention, which is associated with success rate as high as 90% and should be the first maneuver to be performed. The McRobert's maneuver involves sharp flexion and abduction of the maternal hips and positioning the maternal thighs on her abdomen. This maneuver helps in cephalad rotation of the symphysis pubis and the straightening of lumbosacral angle. This maneuver, by straightening the sacrum tends to free the impacted anterior shoulder. Suprapubic pressure (also known as Rubin I maneuver) in conjunction with McRobert's maneuver is often all that is required to resolve 50–60% cases of shoulder dystocias. By application of suprapubic pressure, the obstetrician makes an attempt to manually dislodge the anterior shoulder from behind the symphysis pubis.

Shoulder dystocia can be defined as the inability to deliver the fetal shoulders after the delivery of the fetal head without the aid of specific maneuvers (other than the gentle downward traction on the head). The ACOG has recommended that an estimated fetal weight of over 4.5 kg should be considered as an indication for delivery by cesarean section in order to reduce the potential morbidity and mortality in pregnancies complicated with maternal diabetes mellitus since this is an important risk factor for development of shoulder dystocia.

Picture	Clinical Description	Management/Clinical Features

2.12.6: Second Line Maneuvers for Shoulder Dystocia (A to C)

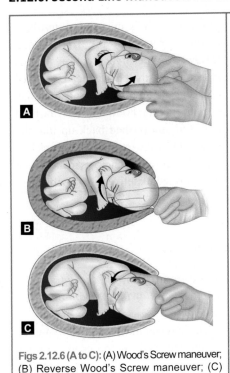

Figs 2.12.6 (A to C): (A) Wood's Screw maneuver; (B) Reverse Wood's Screw maneuver; (C) Rubin II maneuver

In case of the failure of first line maneuvers, such as Mc Robert's maneuver and suprapubic pressure, the second line maneuvers for resolution of shoulder dystocia must be employed. These include "enter the pelvis maneuvers" (internal rotation), such as Rubin II maneuver, Wood's Screw maneuver and reverse Wood's Screw maneuver

Rubin II maneuver: In this maneuver, the obstetrician inserts the fingers of his/her right hand into the vagina and applies digital pressure on to the posterior aspect of the anterior shoulder, making an attempt to push it toward the fetal chest. This rotates the shoulders forward into the more favorable oblique diameter.

Wood's Screw maneuver: In this maneuver, the obstetrician's hand is placed behind the posterior shoulder of the fetus. The shoulder is rotated progressively by 180° in a corkscrew manner so that the impacted anterior shoulder is released.

Reverse Wood's Screw maneuver: In this maneuver the obstetrician applies pressure to the posterior aspect of the posterior shoulder and attempts to rotate it through 180° in the direction opposite to that described in the Screw maneuver.

2.12.7: Delivery of Posterior Arm in Case of Shoulder Dystocia (A to C)

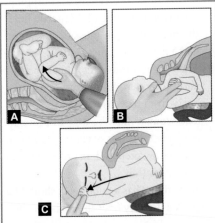

Figs 2.12.7 (A to C): Delivery of posterior arm: (A) The clinician's hand is introduced into the vagina along the posterior shoulder. Keeping the arm flexed at the elbow, it is swept across the fetal chest; (B) The fetal hand is grasped and the arm is extended out along the side of the face; (C) The posterior arm and shoulder are delivered from the vagina

Delivery of posterior arm is another effective maneuver for resolving shoulder dystocia. The steps for performance of this maneuver are described in Figures 2.12.7 (A to C).

In this maneuver, the obstetrician places his or her hand behind the posterior shoulder of the fetus and locates the arm. This arm is then swept across the fetal chest and delivered. With the posterior arm and shoulder now delivered, it is relatively easy to rotate the baby, dislodge the anterior shoulder and allow delivery of the remainder of the baby.

2.12.8: Third Line Maneuvers for Shoulder Dystocia (A and B)

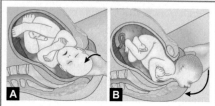

Figs 2.12.8 (A and B): Zavanelli's maneuver

Several third line methods have been described for cases of shoulder dystocia, which are resistant to all simple measures (including the first and second line maneuvers). Some of these maneuvers include cleidotomy, symphysiotomy and the Zavanelli's maneuver. These maneuvers are rarely employed in today's modern obstetric practice.

The Zavanelli's maneuver involves cephalic replacement of the head followed by cesarean section. In this maneuver, firstly the fetal head is rotated back into its prerestitution position, i.e. occiput anterior. Following this, the head is flexed and pushed back up into the vagina. Once the fetal head gets back into the pelvis, an emergency cesarean section is performed to deliver a live baby.

2.13: CESAREAN DELIVERY

2.13.1: Administration of Anesthesia and Cleaning and Draping the Abdomen (A to C)

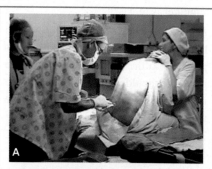

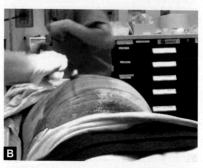

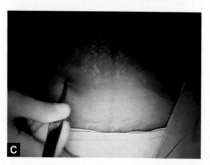

Figs 2.13.1 (A to C): (A) Administration of spinal anesthesia; (B) Cleaning the abdomen with betadine solution; (C) Checking the effect of anesthesia (*Courtesy*: Rekha Khandelwal)

Administration of anesthesia
Women who are having a cesarean delivery must preferably be offered regional anesthesia because it is safer and results in lower maternal and neonatal morbidity in comparison to general anesthesia.

Preparation of the skin
- The woman's pubic hair must not be shaved prior to surgery as this may increase the risk of wound infection. The hair may be trimmed, if necessary.
- Routine cleaning of the patient's skin at the proposed site of incision must be done with antiseptic solution (e.g. betadine) before surgery in order to reduce the risk of postoperative wound infections. The antiseptic solution must be applied three times on the incision site using a high-level disinfected ring forceps and cotton or gauze swab.

While application of the anesthetic agent, the following precautions need to be taken:
- The surgeon must begin applying the antiseptic at the proposed incision site and move outward in a circular motion away from the site of incision. In the end, the inner aspects of thighs and umbilicus must be swabbed.
- At the time of cleaning and draping, after reaching edge of the sterile field, the previous swab must be discarded and a new swab must be used.
- The surgeon must keep his/her arms and elbows high and surgical gown away from the surgical field.
- The woman must be draped immediately after the area of surgery has been adequately prepared, in order to avoid contamination.
- If the drape has a window, it should be placed directly over the incision site.

Picture	Clinical Description	Management/Clinical Features

2.13.2: Steps of Cesarean Section until the Visualization of Peritoneum (A to D)

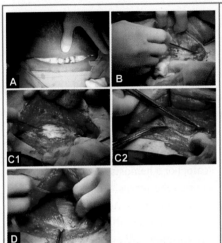

Figs 2.13.2 (A to D): (A) Giving a skin incision; (B) Dissection of the fat; (C1 and C2) Exposure and dissection of rectus sheath; (D) Separation of the rectus muscle to visualize the parietal peritoneum (*Courtesy*: Rekha Khandelwal)

Skin incision
A vertical or transverse incision can be given over the skin.

Dissecting the rectus sheath
After dissecting through the skin, subcutaneous fat and fascia, the anterior rectus sheath is reached. The rectus sheath is cut, following which the cut edges of the incised rectus sheath are carefully separated out from the underlying rectus muscle and pyramidalis with help of blunt and sharp dissection, to expose transversalis fascia and peritoneum.

Skin incision
The most commonly used type of transverse incision in case of cesarean delivery is a sharp (Pfannenstiel) type of incision. Pfannenstiel incision is slightly curved, transverse skin incision made at the level of pubic hairline, about an inch above the pubic symphysis and is extended somewhat beyond the lateral borders of rectus abdominis muscle.

Dissecting the rectus sheath
Rectus sheath can be cut using sharp dissection by using a scalpel to incise the rectus sheath throughout the length of the incision.

2.13.3: Steps of Cesarean Section until the Separation of Visceral Peritoneum (A to D)

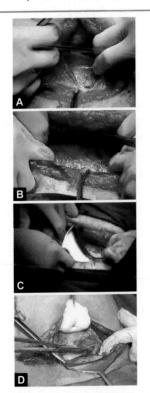

Figs 2.13.3 (A to D): (A) Opening the parietal peritoneum; (B) Visualization of uterus; (C) Insertion of Doyen's retractor; (D) Separating and cutting the visceral layer of peritoneum (*Courtesy*: Rekha Khandelwal)

Opening the peritoneum: The transversalis fascia and peritoneal fat are dissected carefully, to reach the underlying peritoneum. After placing two hemostats about 2 cm apart to hold the peritoneum, it is carefully opened. The peritoneum is superiorly incised up to the level of incision and inferiorly to a point just above the peritoneal reflection over the bladder. Once the parietal peritoneum has been opened, the uterus becomes visible.

Insertion of the Doyen's retractor: Following the dissection of parietal peritoneun, the Doyen's retractor is inserted to expose the lower uterine segment. The loose fold of the uterovesical peritoneum over the lower uterine segment is then grasped with the help of forceps and incised transversely with help of scissors. The underlying bladder is then separated by blunt dissection. Finally, the lower flap of peritoneum and the adjacent areolar tissue is also retracted by the Doyen's retractor to clear the lower uterine segment.

Opening the peritoneum: Before opening the peritoneum, the layers of peritoneum must be carefully examined to be sure that omentum, bowel or bladder is not lying adjacent to it and they do not get injured while cutting the peritoneum.

Insertion of the Doyen's retractor: Following the dissection of parietal peritoneum and insertion of Doyen's retractor, the surgeon must then check, if the uterus is dextrorotated, by identifying the round ligaments. If found to be dextrorotated, its position must be corrected prior to administration of the uterine incision.

2.13.4: Steps of Cesarean Section until Delivery of the Baby and Placenta (A to D)

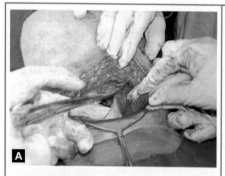

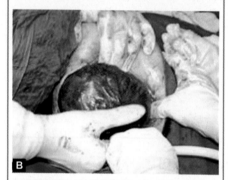

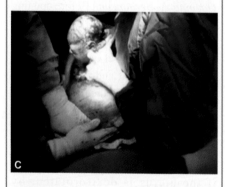

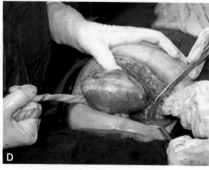

Figs 2.13.4 (A to D): (A) Giving a uterine incision; (B) Delivery of fetal head; (C) Delivery of the rest of baby; (D) Delivery of the placenta (*Courtesy*: Rekha Khandelwal)

Uterine incision: An incision is made in the lower uterine segment about 1 cm below the upper margin of peritoneal reflection and about 2–3 cm above the bladder base. While making an incision in the uterus, a curvilinear mark of about 10 cm length is made by the scalpel, cutting partially through the myometrium. Following this, a small cut (about 3 cm in size) is made using the scalpel in the middle of this incision mark, reaching up to, but not through the membranes. The rest of the incision can be completed either by stretching the incision, using the tips of two index fingers along both the sides of the incision mark or using bandage scissors, to extend the incision on two sides. As the fetal membranes bulge out through the uterine incision, they are ruptured. The amniotic fluid, which is released following the rupture of membranes, is sucked with help of a suction machine.

Delivery of the infant: In case of cephalic presentation, once the fetal presenting part becomes visible through the uterine incision, the surgeon places his/her right hand below the fetal presenting part and grasps it. In case of cephalic presentation the fetal head is then elevated gently, using the palms and fingers of the hand. Delivery is completed in the manner similar to normal vaginal delivery. Once the baby's shoulders have delivered, an IV infusion containing 20 U of oxytocin per liter of crystalloids is infused at a rate of 10 mL/minute, until effective uterine contractions are obtained. Following the delivery of the baby, the cord is clamped and cut, and the baby is handed over to the pediatrician.

Placental removal: At the time of cesarean section, the placenta should be removed using controlled cord traction.

Uterine incision

While giving the uterine incision, use of bandage scissors may be especially required in cases where the lower uterine segment is thickened and the uterine incision cannot be extended using the fingers. If the lower uterine segment is very thin, injury to the fetus can be avoided, by using the handle of the scalpel or a hemostat (an artery forceps) to open the uterus. In case the surgeon feels that lateral extension of the uterine incision is a possibility, he/she can use several alternatives, such as making a J-shaped, U-shaped or T-shaped incision.

Delivery of the infant

Delivery of the fetal head should be in the same way as during the normal vaginal delivery. There is no need for routine use of forceps in order to deliver the fetal head. Forceps should be used for the delivery of fetal head at the time of cesarean delivery, only if there is difficulty while delivering the baby's head.

Placental removal

Following the delivery of the placenta, the remnant bits of membranes and decidua are removed using a sponge-holding forceps.

Picture	Clinical Description	Management/Clinical Features

2.13.5: Steps of Cesarean Section Involving Closure of the Uterine Cavity and Rectus Sheath (A to D)

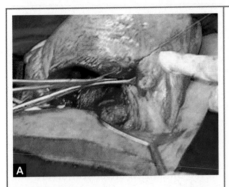

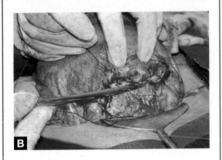

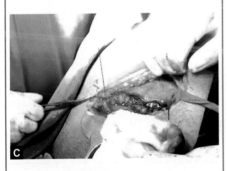

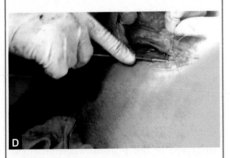

Closure of the uterine incision: The cut edges of the uterine incision are then identified and grasped with the help of Green Armytage clamps. The uterine angles are usually grasped with Allis forceps. The main controversy related to the closure of the uterine incision is whether the closure should be in form of a single-layered or a double-layered closure. The current recommendation by National Collaborating Center for Women's and Children's Health (2004) is to close the uterus in two layers as the safety and efficacy of closing uterus in a single layer is presently uncertain. Following the uterine closure, swab and instrument count is done. Once the count is found to be correct, the abdominal incision is closed in layers.

Peritoneal closure: In our setup, the edges of visceral peritoneum overlying the uterus and bladder are approximated using 2-0 chromic catgut. We routinely do not perform the closure of the parietal peritoneum.

Closure of the rectus sheath: Rectus sheath closure is performed after identifying the angles and holding them with Allis forceps. The angles must be secured using 1-0 vicryl sutures.

Closure of the uterine incision: Both single-layered and double-layered closure of uterine incision are being currently practiced. Though single layered closure is associated with reduced operative time and reduced blood loss in the short term, the risk of the uterine rupture during subsequent pregnancies is increased. Prior to the closure of uterine incision, it is a good practice to inspect the adnexa (both the tubes and ovaries). Individual bleeding sites can be approximated with the help of figure-of-eight sutures.

Peritoneal closure: The current recommendation by RCOG is that neither the visceral nor the parietal peritoneum should be sutured at the time of cesarean section, as this reduces the operative time and the requirement for the postoperative analgesia.

Closure of the rectus sheath: The rectus layer is closed with help of continuous locked sutures placed no more than 1 cm apart. Hemostasis must be checked at all levels.

Figs 2.13.5 (A to D): (A) Holding the uterine angles using allies forceps; (B) Stitching the uterine incision; (C) Uterine incision has been completely stitched; (D) Stitching the rectus sheath (*Courtesy*: Rekha Khandelwal)

2.13.6: Steps of Cesarean Section Involving Closure of the Subcutaneous Fat and Skin (A to C)

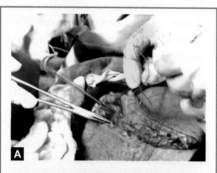
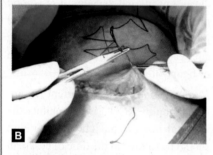
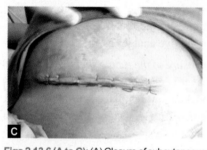

Figs 2.13.6 (A to C): (A) Closure of subcutaneous fat; (B) Closure of skin; (C) Skin incision following complete closure (*Courtesy*: Rekha Khandelwal)

Closure of subcutaneous space: There is no need for the routine closure of the subcutaneous tissue space, unless there is more than 2 cm of subcutaneous fat.

Skin closure: Skin closure can be either performed, using subcutaneous, continuous repair absorbable or nonabsorbable stitches or using interrupted stitches with nonabsorbable sutures or staples. In our setup skin is closed with vertical mattress sutures of 3-0 or 4-0 silk. Following the skin closure, the vagina is swabbed dried and dressing is applied to the wound.

Closure of subcutaneous space: Routine closure of the subcutaneous space (< 2 cm) has not been shown to reduce the incidence of wound infection or wound dehiscence.

Skin closure: Obstetricians should be aware that presently the differences between the use of different suture materials and methods of skin closure at the time of cesarean section are not certain.

2.14: INSTRUMENTAL DELIVERY

2.14.1: Forceps

2.14.1.1: Classification of Forceps Delivery

Procedure	Criteria
Outlet forceps	The fetal scalp is visible at the introitus, without separating the labia; the sagittal suture is in AP diameter or LOA or LOP position and the rotation does not exceed 45°
Low forceps	Leading point of fetal skull is at station +2. The degree of rotation does not matter.
Midpelvic	Station is above +2 cm, but the head is engaged

Fig. 2.14.1.1: Classification of forceps delivery

The ACOG (2007) criteria for classification of instrumental delivery (both forceps and vacuum) according to the station and rotation of fetal head are described in the adjacent figure. The revised classification uses the level of the leading bony point of the fetal head in centimeters, measured from the level of the maternal ischial spines to define station ($\pm$ 5 cm) of the fetal presenting part.

High forceps deliveries, used in previous classification systems, which defined them as procedures performed when the head was not engaged, are no longer included in the present classification system. According to ACOG (1994) and Society of Obstetricians and Gynaecologists of Canada (2005), "high forceps deliveries are not recommended in modern obstetric practice".

Picture	Clinical Description	Management/Clinical Features

2.14.1.2: Types of Forceps (A to D)

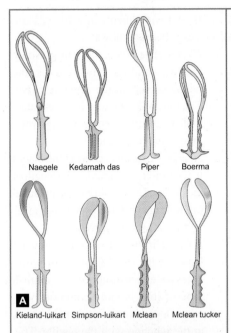

Naegele   Kedarnath das   Piper   Boerma

A

Kieland-luikart   Simpson-luikart   Mclean   Mclean tucker

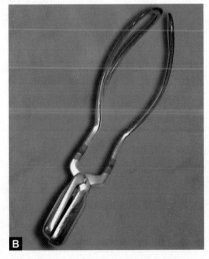

B

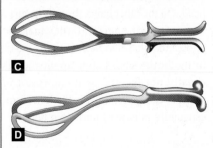

C

D

Figs 2.14.1.2 (A to D): Types of forceps: (A) Different types of forceps used in clinical practice; (B) Wrigley's forceps; (C) Kielland's forceps; (D) Piper's forceps

Figure 2.14.1.2 illustrates different types of forceps employed in the clinical practice. Wrigley's forceps (Fig. 2.14.1.2B) is the most commonly used outlet forceps. Kielland's forceps (Fig. 2.14.1.2C) is used for the rotation of fetal head. Piper's forceps (Fig. 2.14.1.2D) is used for the delivery of the aftercoming head of the breech.

Different types of forceps commonly used in the clinical setup are described below:

Wrigley's forceps: This is designed for use when the head is on the perineum and local anesthesia is being used. It is a short, light instrument having pelvic and cephalic curves and an English lock.

Kielland's forceps: Dr Christian Kielland introduced The Kielland's forceps in 1915. This forceps was originally designed to facilitate rotation and extraction of the fetal head, arrested in the deep transverse or occipitoposterior position.

The blades of Kielland's forceps have only a slight pelvic curve to enable the operator to safely rotate the forceps blade inside the vaginal canal. The shanks of the forceps blades are overlapping and joined by a sliding lock in comparison to the English lock, which is present in most classical forceps.

Piper forceps: Pipers forceps was introduced by Dr Edmund B. Piper in 1924. This forceps was designed to facilitate delivery of the aftercoming fetal head in breech deliveries. Piper forceps have long shanks with a backward curve. This causes the handles to fall below the level of blades, which helps the surgeon to directly apply the forceps blades to the baby's aftercoming head, without the necessity of elevating the baby's body above the horizontal.

2.14.1.3: Different Components of Forceps

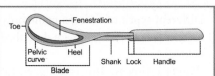

Fig. 2.14.1.3: Different components of forceps

Forceps are composed of two branches, each of which has four major components, blade, shank, lock and handle.

Different components of a forceps can be described as follows:

- *Blades*: The blades help in grasping the fetus and have two curves, the pelvic curve and the cephalic curve. The forceps blades may be fenestrated, with the fenestrations providing firmer grip of the fetal head.
- *Shanks*: The shanks connect the blades to the handles and provide the length of the device. They could be either parallel (as in Wrigley's forceps) or crossing (as in Tucker McLane forceps).
- *Lock*: The lock is the articulation between the shanks. Many different types have been designed. The English type of lock is more common type, where a socket is located on the shank at the junction with the handle. This fits into a socket located similarly over the opposite shank.
- *Handles*: The handles are where the operator holds the device and applies traction to the fetal head. The handles may be fenestrated at times to allow a firmer hold over the fetal head.

2.14.1.4: Different Curves of Forceps

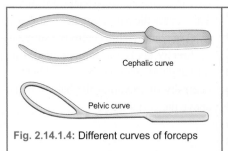

Fig. 2.14.1.4: Different curves of forceps

The forceps blades have two curves, i.e. the cephalic curve and the pelvic curve. In cephalic application, the forceps blades are applied along the sides of the head, grasping the biparietal diameter in between the widest part of the blades. The long axis of the blades corresponds more or less to the occipitomental plane of the fetal head. Since this method of application results in negligible compression effect on the cranium, it is favored over pelvic method of application. Pelvic application consists of application of forceps blades along the sides of lateral pelvic wall, ignoring the position of fetal head.

The pelvic curve corresponds to the axis of birth canal, whereas the cephalic curve conforms to the shape of fetal head. The cephalic curve is adapted to provide a good application to the fetal head. On the other hand, the pelvic curve conforms to the axis of birth canal and allows the blades to fit in with the curve of the birth canal. Pelvic application is usually not favored as it can result in serious compression on the cranium, especially in case of unrotated head.

2.14.1.5: Assembly of the Blades of Forceps Prior to Application

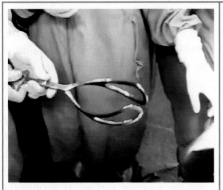

Fig. 2.14.1.5: Assembly of the blades of forceps prior to application

Prior to the application, the blades are assembled together and locked. This is known as ghost application and helps in identification of the left and right blade of forceps. Following the identification of two blades, the left blade is applied first followed by the right one. Figures 2.14.1.6 to 2.14.1.8 represent a demonstration of a simple outlet-forceps delivery for an occipitoanterior position and are described next in details.

The success of instrumental vaginal delivery, using forceps largely depends upon the technique of forceps application. Knowledge regarding the exact position of the fetal head is of utmost importance before the application of forceps. The "cephalic application", which involves application of blades of forceps on the two sides of fetal head, is largely preferred over the pelvic application.

2.14.1.6: Application of Both the Blades of Forceps (A to D)

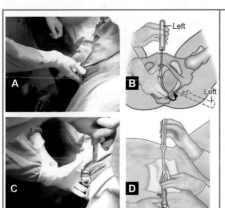

Figs 2.14.1.6 (A to D): (A) Application of left blade of forceps; (B) Diagram showing the introduction of left blade of forceps on the left side of the pelvis; (C) Application of right blade of forceps; (D) Diagram showing the introduction of right blade of forceps by the right hand, while the left blade is held by an assistant

The blades of the forceps are usually applied when the uterus is relaxed and not when the woman is experiencing uterine contractions. However once properly applied, the blades may be left in place, if a contraction occurs at the time of placement.

Application of the left blade of forceps: Before the application of forceps blades, the surgeon holds the left handle of the left branch of forceps between the fingers of left hand, as if holding a pencil. The shank is held perpendicular to the floor and under the guidance of the fingers of the right hand, the left blade is inserted into the posterior half of the left side of the pelvis along the left vaginal wall. The left hand guides the handle in a wide arc until the blade is in place. As the blade is introduced into the vagina, it is brought to a horizontal position. This blade may be either left in place to stand freely on its own or is held in place without pressure by an assistant.

Application of the right blade of forceps: The right blade of the forceps is held in the right hand and introduced into the right side of the pelvis in the similar manner.

After ensuring proper anesthesia, an empty bladder and other prerequisites for forceps application, the fetal position and fetal heart rate are checked again.

The left and right blades of forceps are identified by assembling the blades prior to application.

| Picture | Clinical Description | Management/Clinical Features |

2.14.1.7: Locking the Blades of Forceps (A to D)

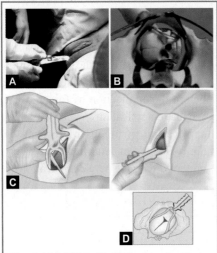

Figs 2.14.1.7 (A to D): (A) Locking the blades of the forceps; (B) Demonstration of correct application of the forceps blades over the fetal skull; (C) Performing and episiotomy. A left mediolateral episiotomy is shown here; (D) The forceps have been locked. The inset shows a left occipitoanterior fetal position, where appropriately applied blades are equidistant from the sagittal sutures

Locking the blades of the forceps: With insertion of the right blade, the forceps should be locked without pressure.

Checking the proper application of forceps: The forceps blades must be applied directly to the sides of fetal head along the occipitomental diameter. In case of occiput anterior position, appropriately applied blades are equidistant from the sagittal sutures. In a proper cephalic application, the long axis of the blades corresponds to the occipitomental diameter, with the ends of the blades lying over the posterior cheeks. An episiotomy may be given if the blades of the forceps have been correctly applied, the blades have been locked and head is observed to be distending the perineum. If not given at this point, an episiotomy may be given later at the time of application of traction.

Checking the proper application of forceps: In case of occiput anterior position, the shanks of the blades must be perpendicular to the sagittal suture and there must be only a fingertip or less space between the heel of the blade and sagittal suture. When the forceps have been correctly applied, the blades lie over the parietal eminence, the shank should be in contact with the perineum and the superior surface of the handle should be directed upward. In this position, the forceps should lock easily without any force and stand parallel to the plane of the floor.

Locking the blades of the forceps: In case there is trouble locking the blades of forceps, it implies that they have not been properly applied. Even if the blades do get locked up, they might just slip off when the traction is applied.

2.14.1.8: Application of Traction (A to D)

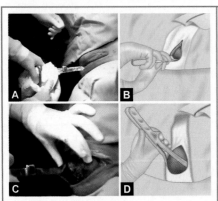

Figs 2.14.1.8 (A to D): (A) Application of horizontal traction with the operator seated; (B) Diagram showing application of traction in horizontal direction until the perineum begins to bulge; (C) As the fetal occiput bulges out, the traction is applied in the upward direction; (D) Diagram showing application of traction in the upward direction with the bulging of occiput

Application of traction: When the operator is sure that the blades have been placed appropriately, traction can be applied. The traction is usually applied in the direction of pelvic axis and at all times must be gentle and intermittent. The operator should be seated in front of the patient, with elbows kept pressed against the sides of the body. Initially, the traction is applied in a horizontal direction until the perineum begins to bulge.

Episiotomy: With the application of traction, as the vulva starts getting distended by the fetal occiput, an episiotomy may be performed, if the operator feels that it would facilitate the delivery process. As the fetal occiput emerges out, the handles of forceps are gradually elevated, eventually pointing almost directly upward as the parietal bones emerge. This facilitates the delivery of head by extension.

Traction: At all times, the surgeon should be careful toward avoiding the use of undue force. To avoid excessive force during traction, the force should be exerted only through the wrist and forearms. Traction should be applied intermittently, synchronous with the uterine contractions and the fetal head should be allowed to recede inside during the periods of uterine relaxation. The safe limit for the amount of traction to be applied, in order to accomplish safe fetal head descent has been considered to be about 45 pounds in primiparas and 30 pounds in multiparas.

Episiotomy: Though the administration of an episiotomy is not deemed essential in all cases, in our setup, an episiotomy is usually performed in all cases of forceps deliveries.

Picture	Clinical Description	Management/Clinical Features

2.14.1.9: Application of Forceps in Occipitoposterior Position

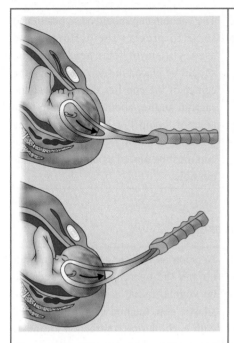

Fig. 2.14.1.9: Application of forceps in occipitoposterior position

Delay in the second stage of labor due to persistent occipitoposterior position or deep transverse arrest is an indication for application of forceps. Method of application of forceps is shown in Figure 2.14.1.9. In case of direct occiput posterior position, long-axis traction forceps are used.

The blades are applied in such a way that they correctly grip the fetal head and are equidistant from the midline of the face and brow. The toes of the blade curve toward the mouth rather than facing toward the ears. Traction is first applied in downward/backward direction until the forehead emerges under the symphysis pubis. The handles are then gradually elevated so that the occiput is flexed and it emerges over the perineum. With the emergence of occiput, the handles are depressed to deliver the face and forehead, thereby completing face-to-pubis delivery.

2.14.2: Vacuum Application

2.14.2.1: Vacuum Equipment (A to E)

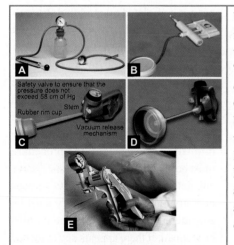

Figs 2.14.2.1 (A to E): Vacuum equipment: (A) Vacuum device, having a rigid metal cup, as invented by Malmström; (B) Hand-held vacuum device with soft silastic cup; (C) Mitysoft Bell cup; (D) M-style mushroom cup; (E) Hand operated suction control device for vacuum extractor system

Ventouse is an instrument, which assists in delivery of the fetus by creating a vacuum between it and the fetal scalp. The pulling force in case of vacuum extraction helps in dragging the cranium. Originally, vacuum devices, as invented by Malmström, had a rigid metal cup with a separate suction catheter attached laterally and connected to a foot-or hand-operated pedal. The newer devices available nowadays have a lax cup, are intended for single use and are disposable.

The instrument as devised by Malmström comprises of three parts: (1) suction cup, (2) vacuum generator and (3) traction tubing device.

The newer vacuum devices available nowadays have soft or semi-rigid cups available in different shapes and sizes. Most of these devices use hand-pump suction, which requires an assistant or can be used by the obstetrician (herself or himself).

2.14.2.2: Application of Vacuum Cup over the Fetal Head

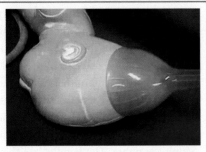

Fig. 2.14.2.2: Application of vacuum cup over the fetal head

The adjacent figure demonstrates the method of application of vacuum cup over the fetal head.

The vacuum cup should be so positioned so as to prevent the deflexion and asyncylitism of fetal head. The cup should be placed in such a way that the center of the cup lies directly over the sagittal suture, about 6 cm behind the anterior fontanel or 3 cm in front of the posterior fontanel. As a general rule, the cup must be placed as far posteriorly as possible.

2.14.2.3: Procedure of Vacuum Application in Occipitoanterior Position (A and B)

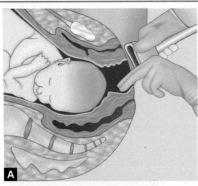

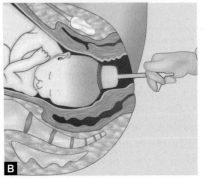

Figs 2.14.2.3 (A and B): Procedure of vacuum application in occipitoanterior position

The actual steps of vacuum extraction in case of occiput anterior position are shown in Figures 2.14.2.3 (A and B) and comprise of the following steps:

- Under all aseptic precautions, the patient's perineum and external genitalia are cleaned and draped.
- The patient's labia are separated, following which the vacuum (soft) cup, which has been compressed and folded, prior to insertion, is applied.
- The cup is inserted gently by pressing it in inward and downward direction, so that the inferior edge of the cup lies close to the posterior fourchette.
- Once the cup has been properly placed, vacuum must be created.
- The obstetrician must place the fingers of one hand against the suction cup and grasp the handle of the instrument with the other hand, following which the vacuum is applied.
- In order to achieve effective traction, a pressure of at least 0.6–0.8 kg per cm^2 must be created.
- The pressure must be gradually created by increasing suction by 0.2 kg per cm^2 every 2 minutes.

Prior to the application of traction, an episiotomy may be performed. For this a pudendal nerve block serves as an optimal form of anesthesia.

As soon as the vacuum has been built up and the operator has checked that no vaginal tissue is trapped inside the silastic cup, traction should be applied with each uterine contraction in line of pelvic axis. The direction of traction should be at right angles to the plane of the cup. The patient is encouraged to push at the same time, so that a minimum amount of traction is required to complete the delivery. As the head clears the pubic symphysis, delivery of the head is completed by modified Ritgen's maneuver. Vacuum extraction should not be attempted for more than 20 minutes. It usually becomes obvious within six to eight pulls, whether delivery would be successful or not. The procedure should be abandoned, if delivery is not achieved or the labor does not progress. Under ordinary circumstances, the procedure must be abandoned after three successive cup detachments. In these cases forceps delivery or abdominal delivery must be considered. The procedure should also be stopped, if there appears any evidence of maternal or fetal trauma.

Picture	Clinical Description	Management/Clinical Features

2.14.2.4: Procedure of Vacuum Application in Occipitoposterior Position (A and B)

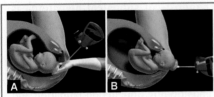

Figs 2.14.2.4 (A and B): Vacuum application in occipitoposterior position

Correct placement of the vacuum cup over the fetal head helps in creating proper flexion in case of deflexed head. Figure 2.14.2.4 shows the procedure of application of the vacuum cup over the fetal head.

The vacuum cup must be placed over the leading point of fetal head. In case of occipitoposterior position the cup must be located 2–3 cm above the posterior fontanel. At the time of cup placement, in order to prevent the entrapment of maternal tissues within the vacuum cup, the full circumference of the cup must be palpated, both before and after the vacuum has been created, as well as prior to the application of traction.

2.14.2.5: Correct Placement of Vacuum Cup over the Fetal Head

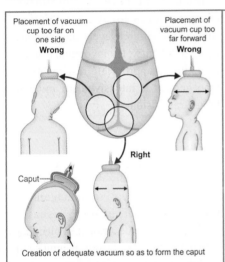

Fig. 2.14.2.5: Correct placement of vacuum cup over the fetal head

In case of an occipitoanterior position, the cup should be placed in such a way that the edge of the cup is located approximately over the posterior fontanel as most of the cups have a diameter of 5–7 cm. This positioning helps in maintaining flexion of the fetal head and avoids traction over the anterior fontanel.

If the cup is placed anteriorly on the fetal cranium near the anterior fontanel rather than over the occiput, this may result in undue extension of the cervical spine. Similarly, if the cup is asymmetrically placed in relation to the sagittal suture, it is likely to worsen asynclitism.

While positioning the cup, the obstetrician must be careful that no maternal soft tissues get trapped between the vacuum cup and fetal head.

2.14.2.6: Fetal Head Injuries due to Vacuum Application

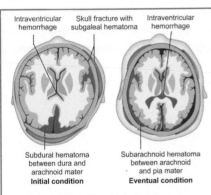

Fig. 2.14.2.6: Fetal head injuries due to vacuum application

Use of vacuum can result in development of various head injuries (as shown in Figure 2.14.2.6), such as scalp lacerations, bruising, subgaleal hematomas, cephalohematomas, intracranial hemorrhage, subdural hematoma, subarachnoid hematoma, intraventricular hemorrhage, etc. Other types of fetal injuries include neonatal jaundice, subconjunctival hemorrhage, clavicular fracture, shoulder dystocia, injury of VI and VII cranial nerves, Erb's palsy, retinal hemorrhage, fetal death, etc.

Signs and symptoms of serious intracranial injury in a neonate include apnea, bradycardia, bulging fontanels, convulsions, irritability, lethargy and poor feeding.

2.14.2.7: Subgaleal Hematoma (A and B)

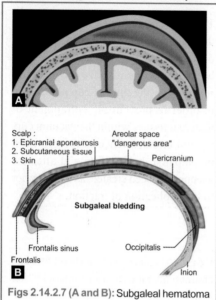

Scalp:
1. Epicranial aponeurosis
2. Subcutaneous tissue
3. Skin

Areolar space "dangerous area"

Pericranium

Subgaleal bledding

Frontalis sinus

Occipitalis

Frontalis

Inion

Figs 2.14.2.7 (A and B): Subgaleal hematoma

Subgaleal or subaponeurotic hematomas occur as a result of bleeding in the potential space between the skull periosteum and epicranial aponeurosis. Since the collection occurs above the periosteum, it can cross the sutures lines. Subgaleal hematoma must be suspected in case of boggy scalp swelling, swelling crossing the suture lines and an expanding head circumference.

Diagnosis of subgaleal hematoma is established on the basis of history and physical examination. The diffuse, progressive, fluctuant, head swelling related to subgaleal hematoma shifts with repositioning, indents on palpation and is not limited by suture lines. Optimal clinical diagnosis is made through CT or MRI scan.

Subgaleal hematoma at times can result in severe hypovolemia. In suspected cases, hemoglobin levels must be immediately measured. Even if found to be normal, monitoring of hemoglobin levels, coagulation studies and bilirubin levels must be done every 6–8 hourly. Hypovolemia usually responds to appropriate resuscitation, management in intensive care unit and blood transfusion.

2.14.2.8: Cephalohematoma (A and B)

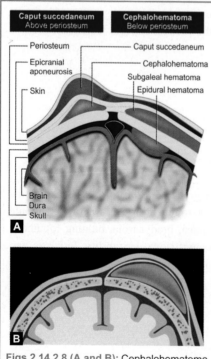

Caput succedaneum
Above periosteum

Cephalohematoma
Below periosteum

Periosteum

Caput succedaneum

Epicranial aponeurosis

Cephalohematoma

Subgaleal hematoma

Skin

Epidural hematoma

Brain

Dura

Skull

Figs 2.14.2.8 (A and B): Cephalohematoma

Vacuum deliveries are associated with higher chances of development of neonatal cephalohematoma, in comparison with forceps delivery. The resolution of cephalohematomas can result in the development of hyperbilirubinemia over long term. In case of cephalohematoma, bleeding occurs beneath the periosteum, between the skull and the periosteum. As a result, the boggy swelling associated with cephalohematoma is limited by the suture lines in contrast to the subgaleal hematomas, which are not limited by the suture lines.

Cephalhematoma also needs to be differentiated from caput succedaneum, which is a swelling of the scalp occurring as a result of pressure from the uterus or vaginal wall at the time of delivery in case of vertex presentation. It heals on its own within 2–3 days after delivery and is present above the periosteum in contrast to cephalohematoma, which is present below the periosteum.

The swelling usually disappears on its own and conservative management including observation is usually sufficient. Since the amount of bleeding is usually not very heavy, hemoglobin studies are not required in most cases. Coagulation studies may be required in cases where underlying bleeding disorders are suspected and bilirubin levels may be required in cases where there is appearance of jaundice. CT scan may be required in cases where there is appearance of neurological symptoms.

2.15: OBSTETRIC HYSTERECTOMY

2.15.1: Steps of Obstetric Hysterectomy until Clamping of Uterine Vessels (A to D)

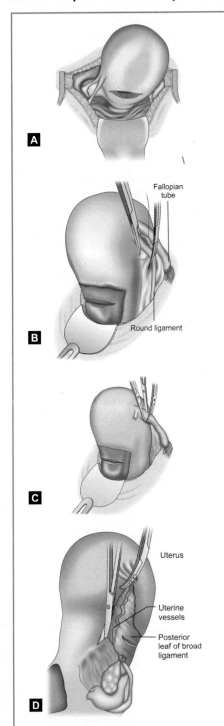

Figs 2.15.1 (A to D): (A) Incision in the uterus as a result of cesarean section; (B) Camping, cutting and ligating the round ligaments; (C) The utero-ovarian ligaments and fallopian tubes are clamped and cut bilaterally; (D) Tracing the path of the uterine vessels

The steps of obstetric hysterectomy until clamping of uterine vessels are as follows:

- After giving a vertical fascial incision (about 2–3 cm in length) and dissection of various layers of abdomen (rectus fascia and peritoneum), the uterus is reached.
- The round ligaments are clamped, cut and double ligated with Kocher's clamps.
- From the cut edge of the round ligament, the anterior leaf of the broad ligament is opened. The broad ligament is incised up to the point where the bladder peritoneum is reflected on to the lower uterine surface in the midline.
- The surgeon must use his/her two fingers in order to push the posterior leaf of the broad ligament forward, just under the tube and ovary, near the uterine edge. A hole of the size of a finger must be made in the broad ligament, using scissors.
- Through this hole, the right fallopian tube and utero-ovarian ligaments are doubly clamped with a Kocher's clamp. The medial round ligament clamp is replaced to encompass the adnexal structures. The adnexal pedicle is then divided between the medial clamp and the two lateral clamps.
- The surgeon must dissect the bladder downward off the lower uterine segment using finger or scissors. The pressure must be directed downward, but inward toward the cervix and the lower uterine segment.
- The surgeon must also feel for the joint between the uterus and cervix to identify the uterine blood vessels.

The uterine vessels are then doubly clamped at an angle of 90° on each side of the cervix and then ligated doubly with a No. 0 chromic catgut suture.

A vertical skin incision and dissection of various abdominal layers is not required if a cesarean section had been performed prior to the hysterectomy.

In these women, following the delivery of the baby and the placenta, the uterine incision may be stitched in cases where appreciable amount of bleeding is occurring. Instead of stitching the uterine incision, sponge holding forceps or Green Armytage forceps can be applied at the margin of uterine incision for achieving hemostasis. If bleeding is minimal, neither of the above maneuvers is required and the uterine incision can be left as such. Once the uterine vessels have been correctly ligated, the bleeding usually stops and the uterus starts looking pale.

Picture	Clinical Description	Management/Clinical Features

2.15.2: Steps of Obstetric Hysterectomy from Clamping Cardinal Ligaments until the Vault Closure (A to D)

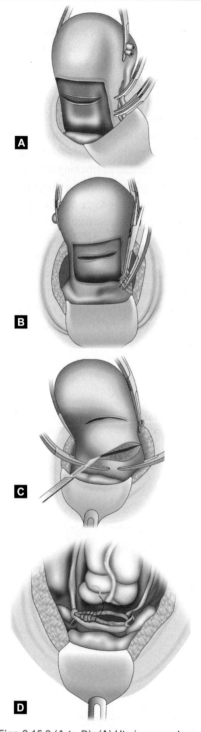

A

B

C

D

Figs 2.15.2 (A to D): (A) Uterine vessels are clamped, cut and ligated bilaterally; (B) Cardinal and uterosacral ligaments are clamped, cut and ligated bilaterally; (C) Separating the uterus from the vaginal vault; (D) Closure of the vaginal vault

In case of a total hysterectomy following the clamping of uterine vessels, the additional steps required are as follows:

- The posterior leaf of broad ligament is divided inferiorly toward the uterosacral ligament.
- The bladder and the attached peritoneal flap are again deflected and dissected from the lower uterine segment and retracted out of the operative field. If the bladder flap is unusually adherent, a careful sharp dissection may be necessary.
- The uterosacral and the cardinal ligaments are then clamped, cut and ligated.
- As the upper 2 cm of the vagina gets free of the attachments, the vagina must be circumcised as close to the cervix as possible, clamping any bleeding points as they appear.

In case of a subtotal hysterectomy the uterus must be amputated, above the level where the uterine arteries are ligated, using scissors.

- The cervical stump must be closed with interrupted 2-0 or 3-0 chromic catgut or polyglycolic sutures.

Some surgeons prefer to close the vaginal cuff, while the others prefer to leave it open.

Before closing the abdomen in either case, total or subtotal hysterectomy, the surgeon must carefully check various structures such as the cervical stump, leaves of broad ligament and other pelvic floor structures for any signs of bleeding. Bladder must also be checked for any signs of injury. Any injury, if identified, must be repaired before closing the abdomen.

- There is no need to close the bladder or abdominal peritoneum. Fascia must be closed using continuous No. 0 chromic catgut or polyglycolic sutures.
- If there are no signs of infection, the skin can be closed using vertical mattress sutures of 3-0 nylon or silk, and a sterile dressing may be applied.

2.16: INTRAUTERINE FETAL DEATH

2.16.1: Spalding Sign

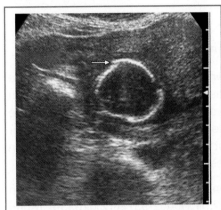

Fig. 2.16.1: Spalding sign: showning overlapping of the fetal skull bones (indicated by arrow)

Intrauterine fetal death can be defined as the diagnosis of the stillborn infant (with the period of gestation being > 28 weeks and fetal weight > 500 g).

Fetal deaths may be divided into two: (1) antepartum intrauterine death (IUD) (fetal deaths occurring in the antenatal period) and (2) intrapartum IUD (fetal deaths occurring during labor). Definitive diagnosis is made by observing the lack of fetal cardiac motion during a 10-minute period of careful examination with real-time ultrasound. There may be presence of Spalding sign (irregular overlapping of the cranial bones) on sonographic examination, which is a feature diagnostic of intrauterine fetal demise (Fig. 2.16.1). Other signs of fetal death may include hyperflexion of the spine; crowding of ribs, and appearance of gas shadows in the heart and great vessels (Robert's sign).

Management in these cases comprises of the following steps:

- Reassurance to be provided to the bereaving parents.
- Diagnosis and treatment of abnormality, if possible.
- In most of the cases, spontaneous expulsion occurs within 2 weeks of birth.
- In cases where spontaneous expulsion does not occur, induction by oxytocin infusion or prostaglandins (PGE2 gel or 25–50 mg of misoprostol) may be required.
- Fibrinogen levels to be estimated on a weekly basis. Falling fibrinogen levels to be arrested by controlled infusion of heparin.
- Postmortem examination: Examination of the dead baby and placenta needs to be done in order to detect the cause of death.
- Autopsy and chromosomal analysis for detection of fetal anomalies and dysmorphic features need to be done.

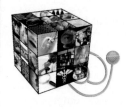

1. BLUNT VERSUS SHARP EXPANSION OF THE UTERINE INCISION DURING CESAREAN DELIVERY

Meta-analyses involving four randomized trials (1731 patients) have shown that blunt expansion of the uterine incision in comparison to the sharp one at the time of cesarean delivery is associated with a significant reduction in the amount of blood loss. Moreover, this has been found to be associated with an insignificant increase in the number of unintended extensions in the blunt group and no difference in the incidence of endometritis. However in this review, data from one recently completed trial (535 patients) is yet not available. Therefore, this conclusion may change, once data from a new unpublished large clinical trial becomes available.

Source: Xu LL, Chau AM, Zuschmann A. Blunt vs sharp uterine expansion at lower segment cesarean section delivery: a systematic review with metaanalysis. Am J Obstet Gynecol. 2012;pii: S0002-9378(12)02033-9. [Epub ahead of print]

2. USE OF INHALED ANALGESICS FOR PAIN RELIEF DURING LABOR

Use of inhaled nitrous oxide and flurane derivatives helps in effectively reducing the intensity of labor pains. Presently, however, the use of inhaled analgesic drugs is not an option in the US and most other countries except UK and Canada.

Source: Klomp T, van Poppel M, Jones L, et al. Inhaled analgesia for pain management in labour. Cochrane Database System Rev. 2012;9:DOI:10.1002/14651858.CD009351.pub2.

3. TRANEXAMIC ACID FOR CESAREAN SECTION

Use of tranexamic acid effectively helps in reducing intrapartum and postpartum bleeding amongst patients giving birth by cesarean section. Moreover, the use of tranexamic acid has not been found to be associated with any significant complications such as venous thromboembolism, gastrointestinal problems, hypersensitivity, etc.

Source: Sentürk MB, Cakmak Y, Yildiz G, et al. Tranexamic acid for cesarean section: a double-blind, placebo-controlled, randomized clinical trial. Arch Gynecol Obstet. 2012. [Epub ahead of print]

4. SURGICAL STAPLES COMPARED WITH SUBCUTICULAR SUTURE FOR SKIN CLOSURE AFTER CESAREAN DELIVERY

Closure of the skin incision at the time of cesarean delivery with staples in comparison with subcuticular stitches is associated with significantly increased rate of composite wound morbidity. This was primarily related to an increased rate of wound disruption amongst those patients in whom staples were used.

Source: Dana F, Chapman VJ, Jeff S, et al. Surgical staples compared with subcuticular suture for skin closure after cesarean delivery: a randomized controlled trial. Obstetrics & Gynecology. 2013(January);121(1): pp. 33-8..

Obstetrics

Section 3

Early Pregnancy Complications

SECTION OUTLINE

3.1: ECTOPIC PREGNANCY

3.1.1: Definition of Ectopic Pregnancy (A and B)

Picture	Medical/Surgical Description	Management/Clinical Highlights
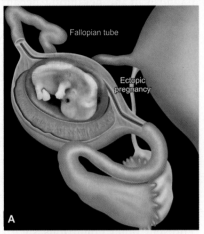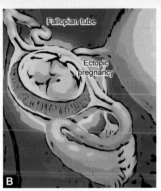**Figs 3.1.1 (A and B):** Ectopic pregnancy: (A) Diagrammatic representation of ectopic pregnancy; (B) Computerized generation of the image showing an artist's interpretation of ectopic pregnancy	Ectopic means "out of place". In an ectopic pregnancy, the fertilized ovum gets implanted outside the uterus as a result of which the pregnancy occurs outside the uterine cavity. Ectopic pregnancy usually occurs as a result of delay or prevention in passage of the blastocyst to the uterine cavity.	Ectopic pregnancies constitute nearly 2% of total pregnancies and are associated with premature implantation of blastocyst in the extrauterine tissues. Risk factors for ectopic pregnancy include previous history of tubal ligation, use of intrauterine devices, history of pelvic inflammatory diseases, use of fertility drugs, etc.

3.1.2: Occurrence of Ectopic Pregnancy at Various Locations

Picture	Medical/Surgical Description	Management/Clinical Highlights

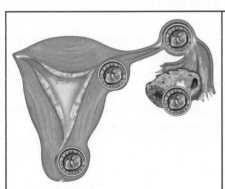**Fig. 3.1.2:** Occurrence of ectopic pregnancy at various locations	Average incidence for occurrence of ectopic pregnancy at various locations is as follows:
	• Fallopian tube: 97%
	  – Ampulla: 80%
	  – Isthmus: 11%
	  – Fimbria: 4%
	  – Cornua: 2%
	  – Interstitium: 3%
	• Abdominal cavity, ovary and cervix: 3%
		Most commonly, i.e. in nearly 95% of cases, the fertilized ovum gets implanted inside the fallopian tube. The ovum buries into the tube and induces a decidual reaction in the cells of the endosalpinx. However, this reaction is feeble. Also, there occurs invasion of the trophoblastic cells into the wall of the fallopian tube. As a result, there is a high risk of choriodecidual hemorrhage and of erosion or rupture of the tubal wall.

3.1.3: Types of Ectopic Pregnancy (A to D)

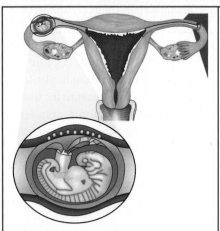

Fig. 3.1.3A: Section through the fallopian tube showing detailed view of ectopic pregnancy

Though ectopic pregnancy can develop at several locations, fallopian tubes are the most common site of ectopic pregnancy. In the fallopian tube itself, the ectopic can be present at several locations such as ampulla, isthmus, fimbria, interstitium, etc. Ampulla being the most spacious part of fallopian tube is the most common site for the location of tubal ectopic. Tubal ectopic pregnancy is associated with factors such as pelvic inflammatory disease or tubal surgery.

Ectopic pregnancy can be difficult to diagnose in the beginning because symptoms are often very much similar to those of a normal early pregnancy. These can include missed periods, breast tenderness, nausea, vomiting or frequent urination.

The typical triad on history for ectopic pregnancy includes bleeding, abdominal pain and a positive pregnancy test result. However, while these symptoms are typical for an ectopic pregnancy, they do not imply that an ectopic pregnancy is necessarily present and could also represent other conditions such as threatened abortion.

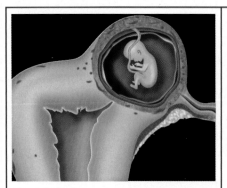

Fig. 3.1.3B: Cornual ectopic pregnancy

Also known as interstitial pregnancy, cornual pregnancy is located in the cornual (interstitial) part of fallopian tube. Some predisposing factors for cornual ectopic pregnancy include factors such as presence of rudimentary horn, previous salpingectomy and proximal intratubal adhesions. Since the interstitial portion of the tube is surrounded by uterine myometrium, it can expand significantly when it hosts a pregnancy. The cornu of the uterus usually ruptures between 12 to 16 weeks of pregnancy.

Early diagnosis is important and is enabled by the use of transvaginal sonography (TVS). The treatment is primarily surgical, and involves removal of the products of conception (POC) and surgical repair of the uterus. The dearth of myometrium around the gestational sac (< 5 mm); an empty uterine cavity; gestational sac separate from the uterine cavity; and presence of an echogenic line, extending from the endometrial cavity to the corner next to the gestational mass (interstitial line sign) on ultrasound examination are diagnostic of cornual pregnancy. A ruptured interstitial pregnancy is a medical emergency, requiring immediate surgical intervention, either in form of laparoscopy or laparotomy for controlling the bleeding and removing the ectopic pregnancy.

Picture	Medical/Surgical Description	Management/Clinical Highlights
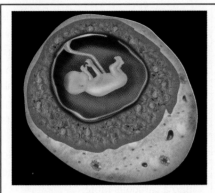 **Fig. 3.1.3C:** Ovarian ectopic pregnancy	Ovarian ectopic pregnancies are located inside the ovaries and occur rarely. It usually results because the ovum released during ovulation is not picked up by the fimbriated end of the tube. Instead it fertilizes within the ovary and gets implanted there. Since ovarian tissue is not able to support the growth of gestational sac for long, it eventually bursts open, resulting in an intra-abdominal bleeding, which must be treated like a medical emergency.	Once the ovarian ectopic pregnancy is identified, oophorectomy or salpingo-oophorectomy may be performed either by laparoscopy or laparotomy depending on the patient's condition and extent of destruction that has occurred. In case of limited damage to the ovaries, ovarian wedge resection may be performed or treatment may be initiated with help of methotrexate.
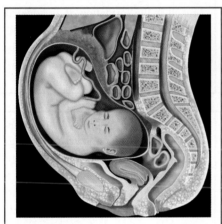 **Fig. 3.1.3D:** Abdominal ectopic pregnancy	In abdominal pregnancy, the pregnancy gets implanted in the peritoneal cavity, outside the fallopian tubes and ovary. These pregnancies can rarely result in the delivery of a viable infant, though the outcome can be equally fatal as compared to ectopic pregnancy at other locations. Abdominal pregnancies comprise about 1% of cases of ectopic pregnancy. Various locations where ectopic pregnancy can get implanted include Pouch of Douglas (POD), omentum, bowel mesentery, etc.	On clinical examination, fetal parts of the baby can be easily palpated. The diagnosis of this condition is established on sonography or magnetic resonance imaging (MRI). Rupture of abdominal ectopic pregnancy can result in severe intraperitoneal bleeding, which must be treated as a medical emergency. Treatment is primarily surgical involving the removal of fetus either through laparoscopy or laparotomy. Methotrexate or embolization can also be used for termination of pregnancy.

3.1.4: Course of Ectopic Pregnancy with Increasing Gestation (A to C)

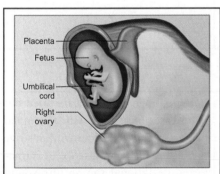 **Fig. 3.1.4A:** Ectopic pregnancy at 8 weeks of gestation	A classical ectopic pregnancy normally does not develop into a live birth. The extrauterine locations may be able to sustain the gestational sac up to 6–8 weeks of gestation at the most. Figure 3.1.4A shows ectopic pregnancy at 8 weeks of gestation.	The extrauterine locations do not have sufficient space or nurturing tissues to support a growing pregnancy. Since none of these areas have been equipped by nature to support a growing pregnancy, with the continuing growth of the fetus, the gestational sac and the organ containing it eventually burst open, resulting in rupture.

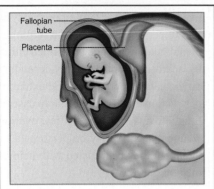

Fig. 3.1.4B: Ectopic pregnancy at 12 weeks of gestation

Figure 3.1.4B shows ectopic pregnancy in the fallopian tubes at 12 weeks of gestation. The gestation reached up to 12 weeks of gestation, considering the fact that it was present in the spacious ampullary part of the tube.

Though the pregnancy at ectopic locations rarely reaches term, it can sometimes grow up to 8–12 weeks of gestation, before rupturing eventually. The other courses, which the implanted tubal pregnancy can take are as follows:
- *Tubal abortion*: The pregnancy gets aborted out through the tube.
- *Tubal mole*: The embryo dies due to faulty environment and gets converted into a carneous mole.
- *Chronic ectopic adnexal mass*: After a slight or moderate bleeding, the hemorrhage may get arrested and result in the formation of an adnexal mass involving the tube and ovaries.
- *Fetal survival to term*: This usually does not occur as the fetus is commonly unable to develop.

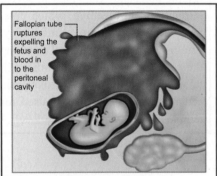

Fig. 3.1.4C: Ruptured ectopic pregnancy with increasing gestational age

Although spontaneous resolution of ectopic pregnancy can sometimes occur, patients are at a risk of tubal rupture and catastrophic hemorrhage. The fallopian tube may rupture due to its thin lumen at the isthmus. The lumen is incapable of distension due to burrowing in and erosion by the blastocyst. Tubal rupture is usually intraperitoneal and may result in severe bleeding and partial or complete extrusion of chorionic villi resulting in hemodynamic instability and shock like features.

Rupture of gestational sac at an ectopic location can result in severe bleeding, sometimes even endangering the woman's life. As a result, it remains a major cause of maternal morbidity and mortality when misdiagnosed or left untreated.

3.1.5: Ultrasound for Diagnosis of Ectopic Pregnancy (A to G)

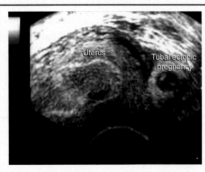

Fig. 3.1.5A: Ectopic pregnancy in left tube

Ectopic pregnancy can have multiple presentations on ultrasonography. Most common type of presentation is empty uterus with or without presence of free fluid in the POD and a complex tubal adnexal mass.

Ectopic pregnancy must be ruled out in all cases presenting with abdominal pain or vaginal bleeding with positive pregnancy test and absence of intrauterine gestational sac on ultrasound examination.

PART I ❖ OBSTETRICS

Picture	Medical/Surgical Description	Management/Clinical Highlights
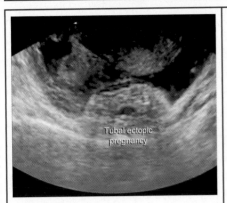 **Fig. 3.1.5B:** Bagel's sign	Presence of "Bagel's sign" on TVS can be defined as thickened fallopian tube due to the presence of gestational sac inside it. There is a thick, bright echogenic, ring-like structure, which is located outside the uterus, having a gestational sac containing an obvious fetal pole, yolk sac or both. This usually appears as an intact, well defined tubal ring (Doughnut or Bagel's sign). Though this finding confirms the diagnosis of ectopic pregnancy, it may not always be present.	Ultrasonography, especially TVS should be the initial investigation of choice for women in their first trimester, who are suspected to be having an ectopic pregnancy. TVS has been reported to have sensitivity of 90%, specificity of 99.8%, with positive and negative predictive values of 93% and 99.8% respectively.
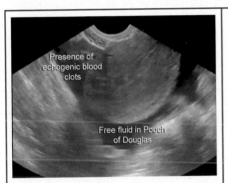 **Fig. 3.1.5C:** Free fluid in the Pouch of Douglas	Figure 3.1.5C shows presence of free fluid in the POD, which is suggestive of a tubal ectopic. This forms the basis of the diagnostic test "culdocentesis" in which aspiration of blood/blood clots from the POD is indicative of ectopic pregnancy.	The free fluid in this case comprises of blood and blood clots, resulting from rupture of ectopic pregnancy, which accumulate in the most dependent part of pelvis, i.e. the rectouterine pouch or cul-de-sac or POD or in the intraperitoneal gutters (Morrison pouch).
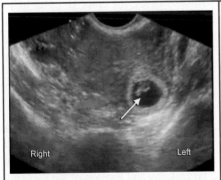 **Fig. 3.1.5D:** Cornual ectopic pregnancy (indicated by arrow)	Figure 3.1.5D shows presence of a gestational sac in the left horn of the bicornuate uterus. A gestational sac with a sonolucent center can be identified. It is surrounded by a thick, concentric, echogenic ring located within one of the horns of bicornuate uterus and contains a fetal pole.	A normal gestational sac, a sign of normal intrauterine pregnancy, comprises of an ovoid collection of fluid adjacent to the endometrial stripe. It can be visualized by means of the transvaginal probe at a gestational age of about 5 weeks. It can often be seen when it is 2 or 3 mm in diameter and should be consistently seen at 5 mm. The earliest embryonic landmark, the yolk sac, appears when the sac is 8 mm or more in diameter, usually during the 5th week of gestation. Cardiac activity can be seen with endovaginal scanning when the embryo reaches 4–5 mm in diameter, at a gestational age of 6–6.5 weeks.

Picture	Medical/Surgical Description	Management/Clinical Highlights

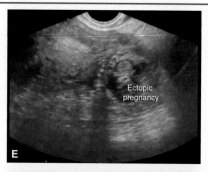

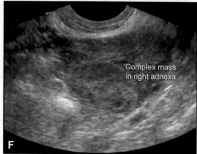

Figs 3.1.5 (E and F): (E) Left sided ectopic pregnancy; (F) Complex right adnexal mass

Figure 3.1.5E represents a tubal gestational sac, which was about 10–12 weeks in size and fetal heart rate could be observed on ultrasound examination. Severe adnexal tenderness with probe palpation was also observed, which is also suggestive of ectopic pregnancy. In Figure 3.1.5F, no definite gestational sac could be identified. Hematosalpinx (presence of free fluid or blood in the fallopian tubes) probably resulted in an echogenic complex mass in this case.

Signs of a definite ectopic pregnancy on ultrasound include presence of a thick, bright echogenic, ring-like structure, which is located outside the uterus, having a gestational sac containing an obvious fetal pole or yolk sac or both. This usually appears as an intact, well-defined tubal ring (Doughnut or Bagel's sign). Though this finding confirms the diagnosis of ectopic pregnancy, it may not always be present.

An empty uterus or a pseudogestational sac on TVS images in patients with a serum β hCG level greater than the discriminatory cut-off value is also considered to be an ectopic pregnancy until proven otherwise.

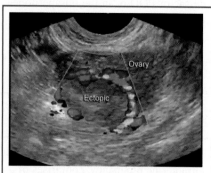

Fig. 3.1.5G: Doppler ultrasound in the same case as shown in Figure 3.1.5F

In case of presence of a complex adnexal mass on transvaginal ultrasound (Fig. 3.1.5F), a Doppler ultrasound was performed. It showed "ring of fire" appearance on Doppler ultrasound due to increased vascularity. In cases of suspicious adnexal masses, presence of gestational sac at any location (intrauterine or extrauterine) is associated with increased vascularity, which may result in a "ring of fire" appearance on Doppler ultrasound.

Commonly, ectopic pregnancy may appear as a complex inhomogeneous adnexal mass on an ultrasound. Unfortunately, it may not be possible to identify a gestational sac every time. In these cases, it may become difficult to reach the correct diagnosis. In such cases, the color Doppler helps in confirming the diagnosis. In the cases like these, it is important to separate the mass from ovary by applying pressure with a transducer.

3.1.6: Diagnostic Laparoscopy for Diagnosis of Ectopic Pregnancy (A to D)

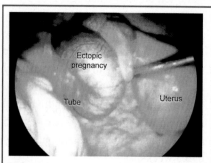

Fig. 3.1.6A: Ectopic pregnancy in the right tube

Sometimes in case of doubt, laparoscopic examination may be performed to diagnose an ectopic pregnancy. In case, the diagnosis of ectopic pregnancy is confirmed on laparoscopic examination, definitive treatment (salpingectomy or salpingostomy) may be carried out at the same time.

By the early 20th century, the standard treatment for ectopic pregnancy included laparotomy and ligation of the bleeding vessels with removal of the affected tube (salpingectomy).

Now in the 21st century, the treatment modality has shifted toward minimal invasive surgery (operative laparoscopy) and salpingostomy, which have largely replaced laparotomy and salpingectomy.

Picture	Medical/Surgical Description	Management/Clinical Highlights
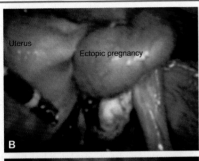 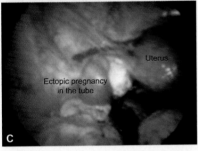 **Figs 3.1.6 (B and C):** Tubal ectopic pregnancy	Figures 3.1.6 (B and C) demonstrate the laparoscopic appearance of tubal ectopic pregnancy on the left and right side respectively.	Whenever the tubal ectopic pregnancy is diagnosed or suspected, the patient should be admitted immediately to the hospital. If the patient is in a state of shock, it needs to be treated first. Transfusion with blood, plasma or substitutes needs to be arranged as soon as possible. If in shock, resuscitation and surgery at the same time can be lifesaving. Immediate laparotomy and clamping of the bleeding vessels may be the only way of saving the life of a moribund patient.
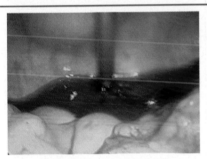 **Fig. 3.1.6D:** Presence of clotted blood in the Pouch of Douglas	Figure 3.1.6D demonstrates the presence of echogenic or sonolucent fluid in the cul-de-sac.	The process of culdocentesis can help diagnose the presence of blood in the cul-de-sac.

3.1.7: Culdocentesis for the Diagnosis of Ectopic Pregnancy

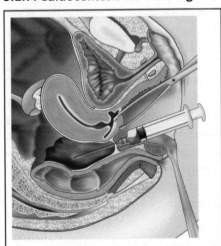 **Fig. 3.1.7:** Culdocentesis for the diagnosis of ectopic pregnancy	Figure 3.1.7 demonstrates the process of culdocentesis for the diagnosis of ectopic pregnancy. After inserting a bivalve Cusco's speculum inside the vagina, the posterior lip of cervix is held with a tenaculum and pulled to straighten out the uterus. Local anesthetic agent is then infiltrated into the vaginal mucosa of posterior fornix, following which an 18 gauge spinal needle, attached to a 20 mL syringe is introduced through the posterior vaginal wall into the peritoneal space of rectouterine pouch in order to aspirate the fluid from the Cul-de-sac. The test is said to be positive when more than 2 mL of nonclotting blood is obtained.	Culdocentesis can be performed to help diagnose blood in the cul-de-sac. Presence of nonclotted blood in the POD is diagnostic of chronic hemorrhage in the peritoneal cavity and is suggestive of a ruptured ectopic pregnancy. Before the widespread use of ultrasound, culdocentesis was commonly used as a diagnostic test for ectopic pregnancy. Even today, this method can be used in unstable patients where ultrasonography is not immediately available.

3.1.8: Salpingectomy for Treatment of Ectopic Pregnancy (A to E)

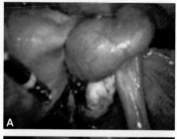

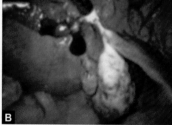

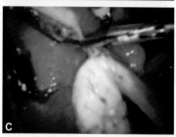

Figs 3.1.8 (A to C): (A) Laparoscopic appearance showing presence of ectopic pregnancy in the left tube; (B and C) Bipolar dissection and cutting along the mesenteric border of the tube after applying traction on the fimbrial end of the tube

Salpingectomy involves removal of the ectopic pregnancy along with the fallopian tube of affected side. Regardless of the route of approach (whether laparotomy and laparoscopy), decision for salpingectomy is taken after considering the factors such as condition of the patient, desire for future child-bearing, condition of the other fallopian tube and ovary, etc. Steps of salpingectomy have been demonstrated in Figures 3.1.8 (A to E). The mesosalpinx must be continued to be clamped, cut and ligated until the tube is free and can be removed.

Salpingectomy is indicated in the following situations:
- The tube is severely damaged.
- There is uncontrolled bleeding.
- There is a large tubal pregnancy of size > 5 cm.
- The ectopic pregnancy has ruptured.
- The woman has completed her family and future fertility is not desired.
- Ectopic pregnancy has resulted due to sterilization failure.
- Ectopic pregnancy has occurred in a previously reconstructed tube.
- Patient requests sterilization.
- Hemorrhage continues to occur even after salpingotomy.
- Cases of chronic tubal pregnancy.

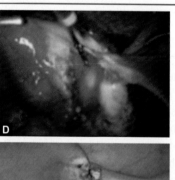

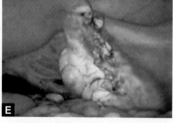

Figs 3.1.8 (D and E): (D) The bipolar dissection and cutting is continued as close to the uterine cornu as possible; (E) Appearance of uterus and tubes following left salpingectomy

As shown in Figures 3.1.8 (D and E) the dissection is continued up to the right uterine cornu and a small portion of the tube is left attached to the uterine cornu.

Surgical treatment in form of open surgery (laparotomy) or minimal invasive surgery (laparoscopy) is the most commonly used treatment option. The procedures, which can be performed at the time of both laparotomy and laparoscopy, include salpingectomy or salpingotomy. In a hemodynamically stable patient, a laparoscopic approach is preferable to laparotomy. If the woman is not hemodynamically stable, the most expedient method of surgical management should be chosen, i.e. laparotomy.

Picture	Medical/Surgical Description	Management/Clinical Highlights

3.1.9: Salpingotomy for Treatment of Ectopic Pregnancy (A to D)

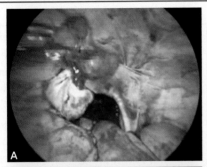

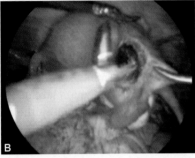

Figs 3.1.9 (A and B): (A) Laparoscopic view showing how the tube containing ectopic pregnancy is grasped, before giving the incision; (B) A small 1 cm incision is given over the tubal ectopic

Tube-sparing salpingostomy or salpingotomy is a procedure in which the gestational sac is removed, without the removal of tube, through a 1-cm-long incision on the tubal wall. The procedure of salpingotomy is illustrated in Figures 3.1.9 (A to D). After infiltrating the mesosalpinx with vasopressin (20 IU in 50 mL normal saline), 1–2 cm incision is made on the antimesenteric side of the tube. The next steps are discussed below in Figures 3.1.9 (C and D).

Salpingotomy is preferred over salpingectomy because not only is it less invasive, but it is also associated with comparable rates of subsequent fertility and ectopic pregnancy. Laparoscopic salpingotomy should especially be considered as the primary modality of treatment if the woman has contralateral tube disease and desires future fertility. When salpingotomy is used for the management of tubal pregnancy, follow-up protocols (weekly serum β hCG levels) are necessary for the identification and treatment of women with persistent disease.

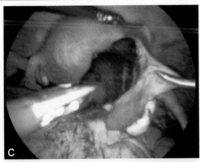

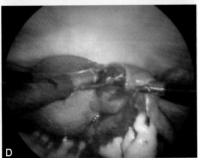

Figs 3.1.9 (C and D): (C) Tubal contents protruding from the incision are removed out from the tube; (D) After the complete removal of tubal contents, the entire salpingotomy incision is left unstitched and only the bleeding vessels on the incision site are coagulated

A syringe filled with saline is inserted deep into the incision and the fluid is injected forcefully in such a way so as to dislodge the ectopic pregnancy and clots. The contents of ectopic pregnancy and clots are aspirated out. Following this, the bed of the ectopic pregnancy must be irrigated well. The tubal incision is left unstitched. Applying pressure with blunt tissue forceps for 5 minutes may help control bleeding. If the bleeding still continues, the vessels on the incision site must be coagulated.

Postoperative follow-up in these cases comprises of the following steps:
• Regular follow-up must be done following surgery in order to ensure that the patient's hCG levels have returned to zero. This may take several weeks. Elevated hCG levels could mean that some ectopic trophoblastic tissue, which was missed at the time of removal, is still remaining inside.
• This tissue may have to be removed using methotrexate or additional surgery.

3.2: HYDATIDIFORM MOLE

3.2.1: Definition (A and B)

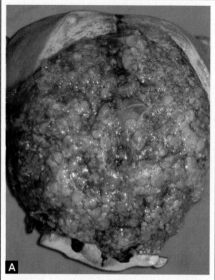

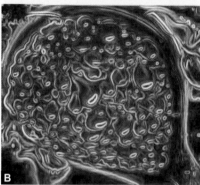

Figs 3.2.1 (A and B): Hydatidiform mole (H. mole): (A) Clinical specimen of complete hydatidiform mole; (B) Computerized generation of the image showing an artist's interpretation of H. mole

Hydatidiform mole (H. mole) belongs to a spectrum of disease known as gestational trophoblastic disease (GTD), resulting from overproduction of the chorionic tissue, which is normally supposed to develop into the placenta. H. mole can be considered as a neoplasm of trophoblastic tissue and involves both syncytiotrophoblast and cytotrophoblast.

H. moles are nonviable and genetically abnormal conceptions, showing excessive expression of paternal genes.

In this condition, the placental tissues develop into an abnormal mass. Often, there is no fetal mass at all. However sometimes, partial moles may show presence of fetal tissue.

GTD can be classified as follows: benign forms (90%) and malignant forms (10%). The benign form includes complete hydatidiform mole (CHM) and partial hydatidiform mole (PHM).

Malignant forms, collectively also known as gestational trophoblastic tumors, include entities such as invasive mole, choriocarcinoma, placental site trophoblastic tumor and epithelioid trophoblastic tumor.

3.2.2: Structure of Molar Vesicles

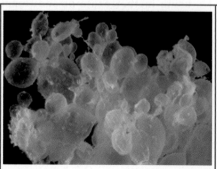

Fig. 3.2.2: Magnified view showing the vesicular structures

Figure 3.2.2 illustrates a magnified view showing vesicular grape-like structures. In this condition, the entire embryonic chorionic tissue gets converted into grape-like structures, in which each vesicle is connected to each other with help of fine stalk-like structures.

H. mole is an abnormal pregnancy in which placental villi become edematous (hydropic) and start proliferating. During the formation of H. mole, firstly there is an edema of the whole central core, causing the villus to develop into a rounded cyst-like structure filled with watery fluid.

Picture	Medical/Surgical Description	Management/Clinical Highlights

3.2.3: Histological Appearance of Complete Hydatidiform Mole

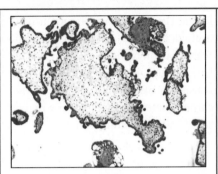

Fig. 3.2.3: Histological appearance of complete hydatidiform mole

The diagnosis of H. mole is confirmed by histological examination. Therefore all POC from nonviable pregnancies must be submitted for routine pathological evaluation. On pathologic evaluation, there is hydropic swelling of the villi and hyperplasia of both syncytiotrophoblasts and cytotrophoblasts. Complete mole does not contain any fetal tissue.

Management of benign GTD comprises of evacuation of the uterine contents with the help of suction evacuation, irrespective of the uterine size. Due to the lack of fetal parts, a suction catheter, up to a maximum size of 12 mm is usually sufficient for evacuating all complete molar pregnancies. Prior to evacuation, an intravenous line must be set up. Blood should be crossmatched and kept available. Cervical dilatation is usually not required prior to dilatation. Serum hCG levels must be measured at every follow-up visit for first 6 months (until 2 years) to see if they are regressing, plateauing or declining.

3.2.4: Histological Appearance of Partial Hydatidiform Mole

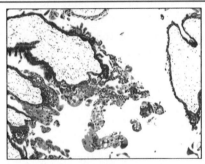

Fig. 3.2.4: Histological appearance of partial hydatidiform mole

There is hydropic swelling of the villi and hyperplasia of syncytiotrophoblasts only. Fetal tissue may sometimes be present in PHM. However this fetal tissue is usually nonviable. Even if fetal tissue is viable, fetus is often severely growth restricted or may have multiple anomalies.

Management in these cases is similar as discussed in 3.2.3.

3.2.5: Pathogenesis of Complete Hydatidiform Mole (A and B)

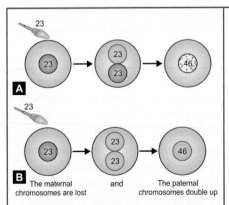

Figs 3.2.5 (A and B): Pathogenesis of complete H. mole: (A) Normal process of fertilization; (B) Formation of a complete H. mole

In the normal process of fertilization, a sperm fertilizes an ovum resulting in formation of a diploid zygote (containing 46 chromosomes). In a CHM mole, all chromosomes are derived from the father by means of either monospermic or dispermic fertilization.

Monospermic fertilization results from fertilization of a sperm with an anucleate oocyte. The genetic material is duplicated, resulting in a 46XX karyotype. Rarely, CHM can also be produced due to dispermic fertilization in which there is fertilization of two different sperms with an anucleate oocyte.

Both complete and partial H. moles overexpress paternal genes. CHMs are usually diploid, with all chromosomes being derived from the father. 46XX karyotype is found in 90% of CHMs. A few cases may also have a 46XY karyotype.

3.2.6: Pathogenesis of Partial Hydatidiform Mole (A and B)

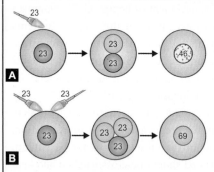

Figs 3.2.6 (A and B): Pathogenesis of partial H. mole: (A) Normal process of fertilization; (B) Formation of a partial hydatidiform mole

Figure 3.2.6A shows normal process of fertilization. Figure 3.2.6B shows the pathogenesis of PHM. In this case, two different sperms fertilize with an ovum, resulting in the formation of a triploid karyotype having two sets of paternal chromosomes and one set of maternal chromosomes (69XXX, 69XXY or 69XYY).

Partial Hydatidiform moles are usually triploid, formed as a result of dispermic fertilization. About 10% of PHMs have tetraploid or higher karyotypes consisting of multiple sets of paternal chromosomes in combination with one set of maternal chromosomes.

3.2.7: Ultrasound for the Diagnosis of Hydatidiform Mole

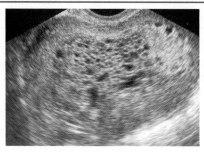

Fig. 3.2.7: Ultrasound showing hydatidiform mole

Figure 3.2.7 shows an ultrasound picture in case of a molar pregnancy in which there is presence of numerous anechoic cysts with intervening hyperechoic material giving a "snow storm appearance". In a typical sonographic appearance of CHM in the second and third trimesters, there may be presence of an enlarged uterine endometrial cavity containing homogeneously hyperechoic endometrial mass with innumerable anechoic cysts sized 1–30 mm. Ultrasound may also show presence of theca lutein cysts in the ovaries.

Sonography is the imaging investigation of choice to confirm the diagnosis of H. mole. Sonographic examination is not only helpful in establishing the initial diagnosis, it also helps in assessing the response to treatment regimes; determining the degree of invasion in malignant forms of gestational trophoblastic neoplasia (GTN); determining the disease recurrence in malignant forms of GTN and evaluation of liver metastasis.

While sometimes the sonographic picture of both H. mole and missed abortion may appear similar, a complete mole is usually associated with higher serum levels of β hCG in comparison with the cases of missed abortion.

3.2.8: Magnetic Resonance Imaging

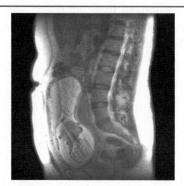

Fig. 3.2.8: Magnetic resonance imaging showing hydatidiform mole

Figure 3.2.8 shows MRI examination in a 25-years-old woman who presented at 10 weeks of gestation with elevated levels of β hCG and no visible gestational sac on ultrasound examination. On sagittal T2 weighted magnetic resonance images, there was presence of high-signal-intensity heterogeneous material filling the uterine cavity. Histopathological examination of the evacuated materials confirmed the presence of complete molar pregnancy.

At present, MRI plays no role in the diagnosis of H. mole. Presently, it is not an essential investigation for management of nonmetastatic molar gestation. However it is beneficial in diagnosing the metastatic disease. MRI is also used for characterizing the degree of myometrial and/or parametrial invasion and for assessing the response to chemotherapy.

3.2.9: Theca Lutein Cyst (A to C)

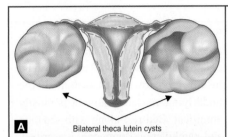

A

Bilateral theca lutein cysts

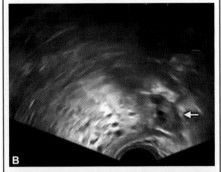

B

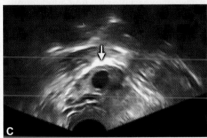

C

Figs 3.2.9 (A to C): Theca lutein cyst: (A) Diagrammatic representation; (B) Normal left sided ovary; (C) Right sided ovary with theca lutein cyst

Ultrasound in cases of molar gestation may also show the presence of theca lutein cysts in the ovaries. The presence of bilateral and/or large theca lutein cysts usually occurs in association with high serum β hCG levels of greater than 100,000 mIU/mL. High circulating levels of β hCG associated with H. mole usually causes ovarian hyperstimulation, resulting in formation of these cysts. In rare cases, theca lutein cysts may rupture, hemorrhage or may even cause ovarian torsion. On sonograms, theca lutein cysts appear as large, septate, cystic ovarian lesions. They may be unilateral or bilateral and at times may be extremely large.

If the theca lutein cysts are large, transvaginal scanning may be of little value in arriving at the correct diagnosis. In these cases, transabdominal scanning may be required for complete visualization of enlarged ovaries. However, before making the diagnosis of theca lutein cysts, the radiologist must exclude the possibility of a preexisting or concomitant cystic ovarian neoplasm.

A repeat sonographic evaluation must be done following suction evacuation after serum β hCG levels have normalized.

In most patients, no treatment is required because theca lutein cysts regress within 8–12 weeks after the evacuation of H. mole.

3.2.10: Pulmonary Metastasis in Case of Hydatidiform Mole

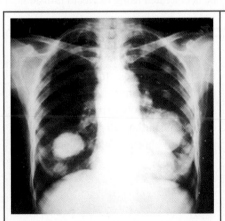

Fig. 3.2.10: X-ray showing cannon ball appearance of pulmonary metastasis

The lungs are the most common site for metastasis in case of malignant GTD and may show the presence of distinct nodules or cannon ball appearance as shown in Figure 3.2.10. Other radiographic patterns, which can be observed on the X-ray include an alveolar or snow storm pattern, pleural effusion and an embolic pattern caused by pulmonary arterial occlusion.

A suspicion of pulmonary metastasis on chest X-ray must be followed by a CT or MRI examination of both head and abdomen. If abdominal CT or MRI examination shows any evidence of metastatic disease, an ultrasound examination of the liver must be done in order to confirm the presence of hepatic metastatic disease.

Determination of cerebrospinal fluid or serum β hCG levels helps in detecting cerebral metastasis. Titers of greater than 1:60 are diagnostic of cerebral metastases.

3.3: MISCARRIAGE

3.3.1: Types of Miscarriage (A to D)

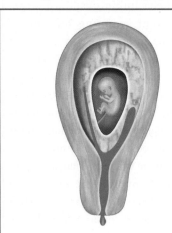

Fig. 3.3.1A: Threatened abortion

Threatened abortion is a type of abortion where the process of abortion has begun, but has yet not progressed to a stage from where the recovery would be impossible. In case of threatened abortion, despite of occurrence of bleeding or cervical discharge, the cervical os is closed. The fetal heart rate may be present and there may be normal intrauterine growth. The bleeding may sometimes stop on its own and pregnancy may continue normally. If the pregnancy continues, there may be increased chances of preterm labor, intrauterine growth retardation, placenta previa, etc.

Sonography can help differentiate between a viable or nonviable intrauterine pregnancy or an inevitable abortion. Therapy should be directed toward treatment of the underlying cause. Treatment is mostly empirical. Bed rest along with sedation and painkillers is commonly prescribed. Administration of progestogens and hCG may prove to be useful in some cases. Anti-Rh immune globulins must be administered to Rh negative nonsensitized women with symptoms of threatened abortion, at or after 12 weeks of gestation. However, no treatment is available, which can stop the process of abortion.

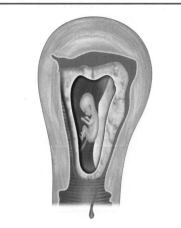

Fig. 3.3.1B: Inevitable abortion

Inevitable abortion is a type of abortion where the process of abortion has progressed to such an extent that the continuation of pregnancy is not possible. It is often associated with pain in abdomen and bleeding. The cervical os is open in these cases. This type of miscarriage may progress into either complete or incomplete miscarriage.

In case of excessive bleeding, intravenous drip should be started with 5% dextrose in water or 5% dextrose in saline. Blood should be arranged and crossmatched, following which it may be transfused. In these cases, an intravenous injection of oxytocin 5–10 units or ergometrine 0.5 mg could be given.

Arrangements should be made to evacuate the uterus as soon as possible. Suction evacuation can be used in case the period of gestation is less than 12 weeks. If the period of gestation is more than 12 weeks, the process of abortion can be accelerated using oxytocin infusion.

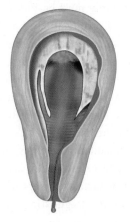

Fig. 3.3.1C: Incomplete abortion

When the process of inevitable abortion has progressed to such an extent that part of fetal products has been expelled out and part of it is still within the uterine cavity, it is known as incomplete abortion. This type of abortion is associated with pain and bleeding. Cervical os is open and some of the fetal tissues may have been passed out.

Treatment in cases of incomplete abortion is same as that discussed in cases of inevitable abortion. In case the size of uterus is more than 12 weeks, using a single dose of 600 μg misoprostol orally or 400 μg sublingually can facilitate the process of abortion to completion.

Picture	Medical/Surgical Description	Management/Clinical Highlights
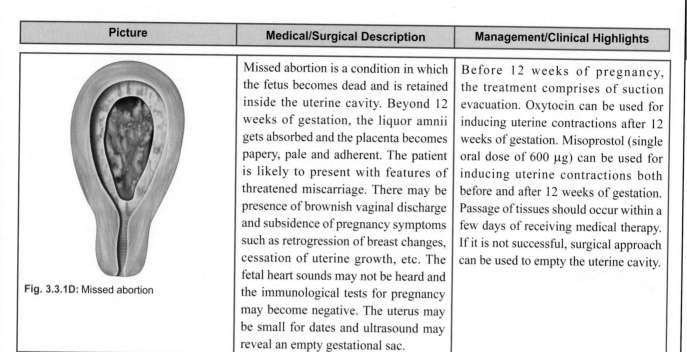 **Fig. 3.3.1D:** Missed abortion	Missed abortion is a condition in which the fetus becomes dead and is retained inside the uterine cavity. Beyond 12 weeks of gestation, the liquor amnii gets absorbed and the placenta becomes papery, pale and adherent. The patient is likely to present with features of threatened miscarriage. There may be presence of brownish vaginal discharge and subsidence of pregnancy symptoms such as retrogression of breast changes, cessation of uterine growth, etc. The fetal heart sounds may not be heard and the immunological tests for pregnancy may become negative. The uterus may be small for dates and ultrasound may reveal an empty gestational sac.	Before 12 weeks of pregnancy, the treatment comprises of suction evacuation. Oxytocin can be used for inducing uterine contractions after 12 weeks of gestation. Misoprostol (single oral dose of 600 µg) can be used for inducing uterine contractions both before and after 12 weeks of gestation. Passage of tissues should occur within a few days of receiving medical therapy. If it is not successful, surgical approach can be used to empty the uterine cavity.

3.3.2: Causes of Miscarriage

Picture	Medical/Surgical Description	Management/Clinical Highlights
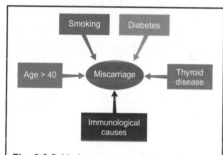 **Fig. 3.3.2:** Various causes of miscarriage	According to WHO and CDC, abortion can be defined as the termination of pregnancy prior to 20 weeks of gestation or birth of a fetus weighing less than 500 grams. Various causes of miscarriage are as follows: • *Genetic causes*: Changes in the number of chromosomes, e.g. trisomy, polyploidy, etc. or structural abnormalities of chromosomes, e.g. translocations, deletions, etc. • *Endocrinological causes*: These include causes such as luteal phase defects; thyroid disorders including both hypothyroidism and hyperthyroidism; diabetes mellitus; etc. • *Infections*: These include viral causes such as Rubella, Cytomegalovirus, HIV, etc.; parasitic causes such as toxoplasma, malaria, etc.; and bacterial causes such as Ureaplasma, Chlamydia, Brucella, etc.) • *Immunological causes*: These include autoimmune diseases, alloimmune diseases, thrombophilias, etc. • *Anatomical causes*: This can include abnormalities like bicornuate uterus, cervical incompetence, presence of uterine fibroids, etc.	Treatment is usually directed toward the management of underlying cause. Treatment of each type of abortion has been individually discussed.

3.3.3: APLA Syndrome as a Cause of Miscarriage

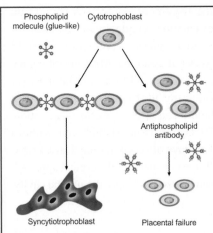

Fig. 3.3.3: APLA syndrome as a cause of miscarriage

Antiphospholipid antibody syndrome (APAS) is an autoimmune condition that has emerged as the most important treatable cause of recurrent miscarriage, early onset preeclampsia, preterm labor, low birthweight babies and intrauterine growth restriction. There are three primary classes of antibodies associated with the APAS:

- Anticardiolipin antibodies (directed against membrane anionic phospholipids)
- The lupus anticoagulant
- Antibodies directed against specific molecules including a molecule known as beta-2 glycoprotein I.

This disease causes miscarriage by forming antibodies against the body's own tissues and placenta, resulting in thrombosis of vessels, placental infraction, fetal hypoxia and ultimately fetal death.

Patients with recurrent pregnancy loss must be administered a prophylactic dose of subcutaneous heparin (preferably low-molecular-weight heparin) and low-dose aspirin. Since long-term use of heparin can cause osteoporosis, patients who require heparin administration throughout pregnancy should also receive calcium and vitamin D supplementation. Therapy is usually withheld at the time of delivery and is restarted after delivery, continuing for 6–12 weeks postpartum. Most obstetricians prefer to avoid the use of warfarin (coumadin) during pregnancy as it can cross the placental barrier and produce teratogenic changes in the fetus.

- Breast-feeding women may be administered the combination of heparin and warfarin. Some researchers have examined the use of combination comprising of aspirin and prednisone during pregnancy. Most of the studies suggest that complications associated with prednisone use usually outweigh the benefits associated.
- In patients for whom the treatment with aspirin and heparin is not successful, use of intravenous immunoglobulins can be used.

3.3.4: Absence of Blocking Antibodies as a Cause of Miscarriage

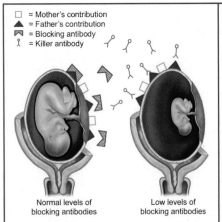

Fig. 3.3.4: Absence of blocking antibodies as a cause of miscarriage

Allotypic antigens in the trophoblast may elicit the production of antibodies, which are cytotoxic to peripheral leukocytes in blood. These antigens are called TLX (trophoblast lymphocyte cross-reactive antigens). If the embryo contains paternal TLX antigens which do not exist in the mother, it may mount a protective reaction, resulting in abortion. If the mother produces antipaternal blocking antibodies, these are able to produce a protective response, which helps in avoiding pregnancy rejection.

Immunotherapy with paternal pool leukocytes can be considered as an optimal solution for this problem. However, this therapy is presently in purely experimental stage and can be considered dangerous before further research is conducted.

Picture	Medical/Surgical Description	Management/Clinical Highlights

3.3.5: Asherman's Syndrome as a Cause of Recurrent Miscarriage

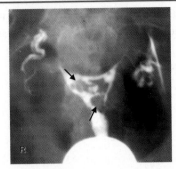

Fig. 3.3.5: Asherman's syndrome as a cause of recurrent miscarriage (arrows representing the presence of synechiae)

Diagnosis of Asherman's syndrome can be reached by doing tests like hysteroscopy, transvaginal ultrasound examination, hysterosalpingography, etc. Hysterosalpingogram (HSG) revealing irregular filling defects in the endometrium is suggestive of endometrial adhesions (arrows represent adhesions). The patient was diagnosed to be suffering from Asherman's syndrome on hysteroscopy on which resection of the intrauterine adhesions was done.

Asherman's syndrome is characterized by presence of intrauterine adhesions and synechiae within the uterine cavity. The most accurate method of diagnosis of Asherman's syndrome is direct visualization via hysteroscopic resection. These adhesions can also be removed on hysteroscopy. In order to prevent reformation of adhesions following surgery, prescription of estrogen supplementation or placement of a splint, balloon or copper device may prove useful.

3.3.6: Bicornuate Uterus as a Cause of Recurrent Miscarriage

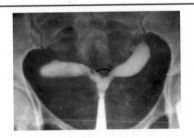

Fig. 3.3.6: Bicornuate uterus as a cause of recurrent miscarriage

Figure 3.3.6 shows an HSG demonstrating a single cervical canal and a possible duplication of the uterine horns. In this case, it was difficult to differentiate between bicornuate uterus and septate uterus on ultrasound alone. Since an angle of greater than 105° was found to be separating the two uterine horns on HSG, the diagnosis of bicornuate uterus was made.

Müllerian anomaly such as bicornuate uterus could be responsible for producing an abnormal or irregularly shaped uterus, which could result in improper implantation and/or growth of the embryo, thereby resulting in recurrent miscarriages. Management of cases of bicornuate uterus has been discussed in Section 12.

3.3.7: Presence of Uterine Septum as a Cause of Recurrent Miscarriage (A and B)

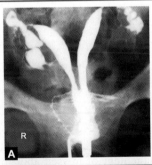
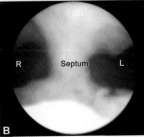

Figs 3.3.7(A and B): Presence of uterine septum as a cause of recurrent miscarriage: (A) View on hysterosalpingogram; (B) View on hysteroscopy

Figure 3.3.7A demonstrates an HSG showing presence of a uterine septum, which was confirmed on hysteroscopy. Figure 3.3.7B illustrates hysteroscopic visualization of uterine septum.

Since uterine septum is a relatively avascular structure, implantation of the gestational sac over the uterine septum is likely to result in a recurrent miscarriage. Management of uterine septum has been discussed in Section 12.

Picture	Medical/Surgical Description	Management/Clinical Highlights

3.3.8: Various Uterine Anomalies as Cause of Recurrent Miscarriage (A to C)

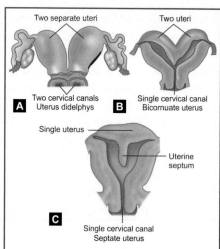

Figs 3.3.8 (A to C): Various uterine anomalies as cause of recurrent miscarriage: (A) Uterus didelphys; (B) Bicornuate uterus; (C) Septate uterus

Various anatomic abnormalities of the uterus are associated with 10–15% cases of recurrent second trimester miscarriages. Various Müllerian abnormalities such as septate uterus and bicornuate uterus are commonly associated with recurrent miscarriage due to poor blood supply to the conceptus as a result of the implantation of the gestational sac over relatively avascular septum. Uterus didelphys is commonly associated with preterm labor, but can also sometimes cause recurrent miscarriage.

Surgical correction of these various anomalies, which has been discussed in Section 12 helps in resolving the problem of recurrent miscarriage.

3.3.9: Diagnosis of Miscarriage Using Ultrasound (A to D)

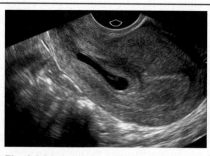

Fig. 3.3.9A: Inevitable abortion

The definition and clinical manifestations in case of inevitable abortion are discussed in Figure 3.3.1B. Figure 3.3.9A demonstrates the ultrasound findings in case of inevitable abortion. There is a loss of definition of gestational sac, resulting in a smaller diameter of gestational sac. There are no central echoes in the gestational sac which are normally indicative of a healthy pregnancy. Fetal cardiac activity is normally absent.

Management of inevitable abortion is discussed in 3.3.1B.

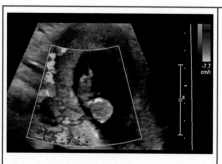

Fig. 3.3.9B: Missed abortion

The definition and clinical manifestations in case of missed abortion are discussed in Figure 3.3.1D. Figure 3.3.9B demonstrates the ultrasound findings in case of missed abortion. There was absence of the growth of the fetal pole over a 5 days observation period. The fetal heart rate was also absent.

Management of missed abortion has been discussed in 3.3.1D.

Picture	Medical/Surgical Description	Management/Clinical Highlights
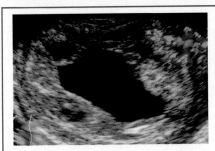 **Fig. 3.3.9C:** Anembryonic pregnancy as observed on color Doppler ultrasound	Figure 3.3.9C shows an anembryonic pregnancy where there is large gestational sac having a size 3 × 2 cm. The gestational sac was empty without having presence of yolk sac or fetal pole. The pregnancy may be deemed abnormal if no yolk sac appears at the gestational sac size of 10 mm or no fetal pole is seen at the gestational sac size of 18 mm. If the gestational sac has an irregular or scalloped appearance, that is also abnormal.	In a normal TVS, the yolk sac is normally visible by 5–5.5 weeks, fetal pole is visible by 5.5–6 weeks and fetal heart beat by 6 weeks. Gestational sac is the first to appear at 4.5–5 weeks. All these findings are likely to appear 1 week later on the transabdominal scan. Normally when a gestational sac is observed on TVS, levels of β hCG in the serum can vary between 1,500 IU and 2,000 IU.
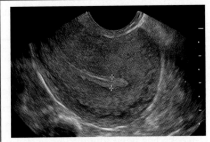 **Fig. 3.3.9D:** Complete abortion	Figure 3.3.9D shows an ultrasound image in case of a complete abortion, where the gestational sac and POC have been completely expelled out. As a result, the triple line uterine endometrium with an empty uterine cavity can be seen on TVS.	Since the gestational sac and POC have been completely expelled out, no treatment is usually required. Management is largely expectant, comprising of patient observation for presence of abnormal uterine bleeding or uterine hypotonia.

3.4: CERVICAL INCOMPETENCE

3.4.1: Definition (A to D)

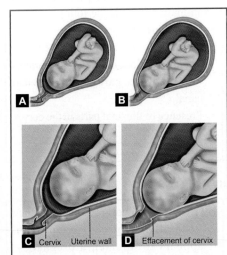 **Figs 3.4.1 (A to D):** Changes associated with cervical incompetence in comparison to normal pregnancy: (A) Normal pregnancy; (B) Incompetent cervix; (C) The fetus is within the uterus; (D) The cervix is thinned and dilated, allowing the fetus to drop down and protrude into the vaginal canal	Cervical incompetence is a common cause of recurrent second trimester miscarriages and was defined by Palmer and La Comme as a condition in which the pregnant woman's cervix starts dilating and effacing before her pregnancy has reached term, usually between 16 and 28 weeks of gestation. Therefore, the woman with cervical incompetence is unable to retain the fetus during her pregnancy.	If left untreated, cervical incompetence may cause rupture of fetal membranes, which may be accompanied by the expulsion of fetus. Cervical incompetence is probably responsible for causing 20–25% of miscarriages in the second trimester. Surgical treatment of cervical incompetence has been described next in the text (3.4.4 to 3.4.7).

Picture	Medical/Surgical Description	Management/Clinical Highlights

3.4.2: Anatomical Changes in the Endocervical Canal

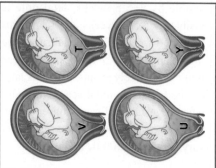

Fig. 3.4.2: Anatomical changes in the endocervical canal associated with cervical incompetence

Figure 3.4.2 illustrates anatomical changes occurring in the endocervical canal in a patient with cervical incompetence. With the progressive dilatation of internal cervical os and cervical shortening associated with cervical effacement, the cervical canal undergoes changes in shape from being T-shaped in nonpregnant state to Y-shaped in early pregnancy, then to V-shaped and ultimately into U-shaped. This ultimately results in bulging of fetal membranes, premature rupture of membranes and abortion.

The patient usually presents with a significant cervical dilatation of 2 cm or more in the early pregnancy. The cervical length is usually less than 25 mm.

In the second trimester, cervix may dilate up to 4 cm in association with active uterine contractions. This may be associated with rupture of the membranes resulting in the spontaneous expulsion of the fetus. On clinical examination, the cervical canal may be dilated and effaced. Fetal membranes may be visible bulging through the cervical os.

3.4.3: Ultrasound Changes in the Endocervical Canal

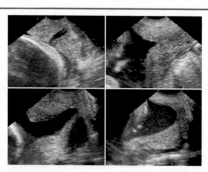

Fig. 3.4.3: Ultrasound changes in endocervical canal with cervical incompetence

Figure 3.4.3 illustrates various ultrasound changes in response to various anatomical changes occurring in the cervix as described in Figure 3.4.2. Cervical dilation and effacement produces changes in the cervix in form of T, Y, V, U (can be remembered using the mnemonic "Trust Your Vaginal Ultrasound"). T-shaped cervix on ultrasound examination points toward a normal cervix. As the internal cervical os opens and the membranes start herniating into the upper part of endocervical canal, the cervical shape on ultrasound changes into a Y. With the further progression of above mentioned cervical changes, Y shape changes into V and then eventually into U.

Serial sonographic evaluation of the cervix for funneling and shortening in response to transfundal pressure, every 2 weeks has been found to be useful in the evaluation of incompetent cervix. Besides changes in cervical shape observed on transvaginal ultrasound, other findings observed on ultrasound examination include the following:
- Cervical length < 25 mm
- Funneling of cervix: Funneling implies herniation of fetal membranes into the upper part of endocervical canal.
- Presence of the fetal parts in the cervix or vagina.

3.4.4: McDonald's Procedure for Surgical Correction of Cervical Incompetence

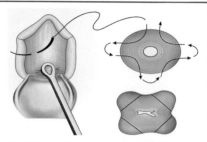

Fig. 3.4.4: McDonald's procedure for surgical correction of cervical incompetence

Figure 3.4.4 presents a diagrammatic representation of McDonald's procedure. This procedure, which is performed vaginally, involves placement of a purse string suture around the ectocervix at the level of internal cervical os. This suture on approximation is likely to tighten the internal cervical os.

No treatment for cervical incompetence is generally required, except when it appears to threaten a pregnancy. Cervical incompetence can be treated using surgery involving placement of a cervical cerclage suture, which reinforces the cervical muscle. Surgical repair of the cervix can be done using a vaginal or abdominal approach.

Picture	Medical/Surgical Description	Management/Clinical Highlights

3.4.5: Steps of McDonald's Procedure (A to G)

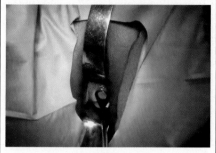

Fig. 3.4.5A: Exposing the cervix

In order to expose the cervix as shown in Figure 3.4.5A, the posterior vaginal wall is retracted with Sim's speculum, whereas the anterior lip of cervix is held with a sponge holding forceps.

The McDonald's procedure is a simple procedure not involving bladder dissection or complete burial of the sutures. The McDonald's suture can be easily removed at the time of delivery. The stitch can also be applied when the cervix is effaced or the fetal membranes are bulging.

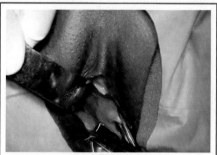

Fig. 3.4.5B: Taking the first stitch

The first stitch is taken between 6 O'clock and 7 O'clock positions.

The stiches must be taken through the substance of cervix. Care must however be taken not to enter the cervical canal.

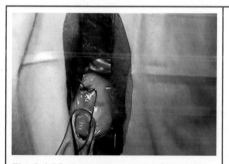

Fig. 3.4.5C: Taking the second stitch

The second stitch is taken anteriorly between 12 O'clock and 1 O'clock positions.

In McDonald's procedure, no bladder dissection is required as in Shirodkar's procedure.

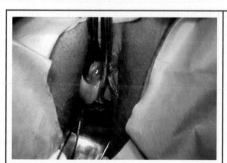

Fig. 3.4.5D: Taking the last stitch

The last stitch is taken between 6 O'clock and 7 O'clock positions.

In the original McDonald's procedure, the suture begins at 12 O'clock position and ended also at 12 O'clock position. Therefore, the knot was tied anteriorly. Anterior knot may be associated with bladder irritation or cystitis. In the modified McDonald's procedure, commonly performed nowadays, the suture begins at about 6 O'clock position and also ends here. As a result, the knot is tied posteriorly.

Picture	Medical/Surgical Description	Management/Clinical Highlights
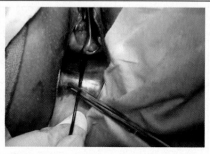 **Fig. 3.4.5E:** Tying the knot posteriorly	A knot is tied posteriorly by taking the long ends of first and last stitch.	The purse string suture, which is placed, is usually removed at 37 weeks, unless there is a reason (e.g. infection, preterm labor, preterm rupture of membrane, etc.) requiring an earlier removal.
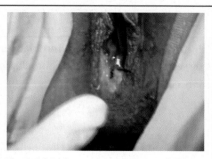 **Fig. 3.4.5F:** Cutting the excessive length of thread from the knot	Excessive length of the thread is cut about 2 cm from the knot.	The disadvantage of the procedure is the occurrence of excessive vaginal discharge with the exposed suture material.
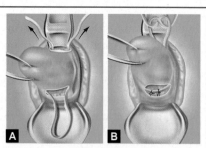 **Fig. 3.4.5G:** Appearance of cervix following surgery	The ends of the knot can be visualized, protruding slightly from the introitus from where it can be easily grasped to cut the knot at the time of removal.	The knot must be removed at 37 weeks of gestation or earlier if the patient goes into labor.

3.4.6: Shirodkar's Procedure for Surgical Correction of Cervical Incompetence (A and B)

Figs 3.4.6 (A and B): Application of Shirodkar's stitch: (A) Following the incision of vaginal mucosa and reflection of bladder anteriorly and rectum posteriorly, a 5 mm mersilene band is passed below the vaginal mucosa laterally on both sides; (B) Following the application of this band, it is secured in its position	In this procedure, suture is placed submucosally as close to the internal os as possible by giving incisions over the mucosa both on the anterior and posterior aspects of the cervix. This is followed by dissection and separation of the bladder and the rectum from both anterior and posterior surface of the cervix respectively.	In Shirodkar's procedure, a permanent purse string suture which would remain intact for life is applied. Therefore the patient has to be delivered by a cesarean section. This procedure is usually performed under spinal or epidural anesthesia.

Picture	Medical/Surgical Description	Management/Clinical Highlights

3.4.7: Wurm's Procedure

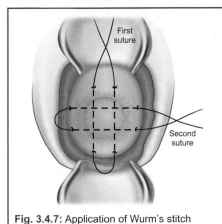

Fig. 3.4.7: Application of Wurm's stitch

| | Also known as Hefner's cerclage, Wurm's stitch is performed by application of U or mattress sutures. | This stitch appears to be most useful when minimal length of cervical canal has been left as a result of premature cervical effacement. |

3.5: MEDICAL TERMINATION OF PREGNANCY USING VACUUM ASPIRATION

3.5.1: Instruments Used for Vacuum Aspiration (A to E)

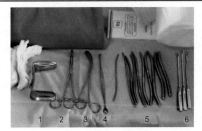

Fig. 3.5.1A: Tray containing various equipment used for suction evacuation: (1) Sim's speculum; (2) Sponge holder; (3) Vulsellum; (4) Anterior vaginal wall retractor; (5) Hegar's dilators of increasing sizes; (6) Uterine curettes of varying sizes

| | Figures 3.5.1 (A to E) show various instruments which are used at the time of vacuum aspiration for medical termination of pregnancy (MTP). Figure 3.5.1A demonstrates a tray containing various equipment used for suction evacuation. Each of the individual instruments has been dealt with individually in details below. | Surgical techniques for MTP in the first trimester of pregnancy practically comprise entirely of vacuum or suction techniques. The terms "vacuum curettage" or "uterine aspiration" or "vacuum aspiration" are often used interchangeably. They all refer to evacuation of the uterus by suction, regardless of the source of the suction. |

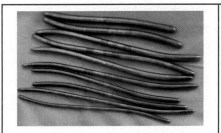

Fig. 3.5.1B: Hegar's dilators in different sizes

| | Mechanical dilation using physical dilators is currently the most frequently used method of dilating the cervix, which is commonly performed prior to surgical evacuation. Though a variety of dilators are available, Hegar's dilators (as shown in Figure 3.5.1B) are most commonly used. They are available in various sizes varying from 4 mm to 12 mm. Dilation is usually done up to 10 mm. | These are blunt-ended instruments, graduated on both the ends. They are available in different sizes, of which different sizes vary by 1 mm. The dilatation is initially started using smaller dilators and then generally large dilators are used, one after the other. |

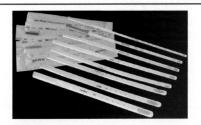

Fig. 3.5.1C: Karman's cannulas in various sizes

| | Figure 3.5.1C shows plastic cannulas of various sizes (from the smallest to the largest). These are named as Karman's cannulas. | Karman's cannulas are connected to the suction machine at one end and are inserted into the uterine cavity through the cervix after appropriate cervical dilatation. Insertion of Karman's cannula helps in the suction of uterine contents, which are then aspirated out into the suction machine. |

Picture	Medical/Surgical Description	Management/Clinical Highlights
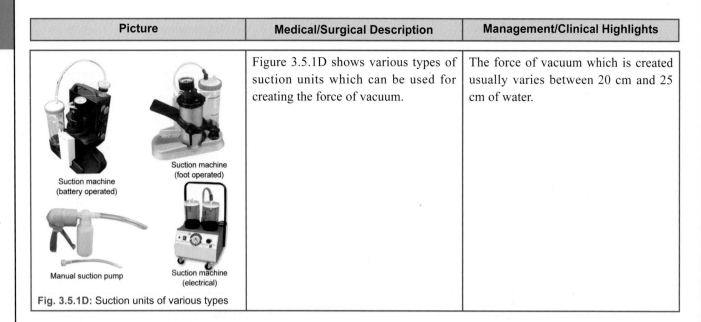 **Fig. 3.5.1D:** Suction units of various types	Figure 3.5.1D shows various types of suction units which can be used for creating the force of vacuum.	The force of vacuum which is created usually varies between 20 cm and 25 cm of water.
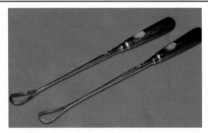 **Fig. 3.5.1E:** Uterine curettes of varying sizes	Figure 3.51E shows uterine curettes. They are available in different sizes varying from smallest to largest.	A sharp curettage is performed by some surgeons at the end of the procedure, just to confirm that the procedure has been completely performed. This step is considered as controversial and not performed by everyone, because the use of sharp curettage may slightly increase the amount of blood loss.

3.5.2: Steps of the Procedure of Vacuum Aspiration (A to F)

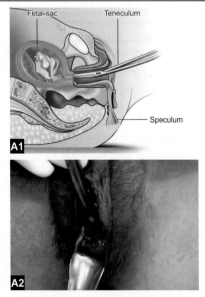 **Figs 3.5.2 (A1 and A2):** Retracting the posterior wall of the vagina with Sim's speculum and grasping the anterior lip with vulsellum	The cervix is exposed after retracting the posterior vaginal wall using Sim's vaginal speculum. The anterior lip of the cervix is held using a vulsellum or tenaculum.	Once the cervix has been properly visualized, paracervical block is given. Though suction evacuation is commonly performed under local anesthesia (paracervical block and sedation), general anesthesia may be required at times. This, however, may be associated with a greater blood loss in comparison to local anesthesia.

Picture	Medical/Surgical Description	Management/Clinical Highlights

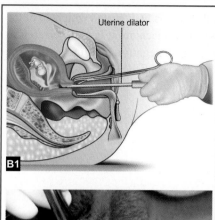

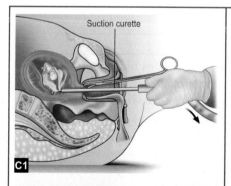

Figs 3.5.2 (B1 and B2): Dilating the external cervical os with Hegar's dilator

The cervix is then serially dilated, using a series of metallic or plastic dilators. While dilating the cervix, the dilators must be held in a pen holding fashion and an undue force must not be applied over the cervix. The dilators must be inserted slowly and gently. This practice is both safe and less painful. If resistance is experienced, the operator should return to the previous dilator, reinsert it and allow it to remain in place for a minute or so before attempting to insert the next large dilator.

Safe dilation depends on the operator's proper determination of the direction of the endocervical canal at the time of bimanual examination. Failure to appreciate that the uterus is retroverted may result in an anterior perforation.

The rule normally followed is that "the size of the suction cannula to be used for the procedure must be equivalent to the size of the uterus". The dilation of the cervix must be approximately 0.5–1 mm more than the size of suction cannula to be used.

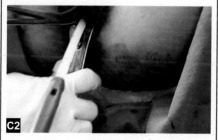

Figs 3.5.2 (C1 and C2): Insertion of Karman's cannula for producing suction

A plastic Karman's cannula is then inserted inside the uterine cavity. Once the cannula has been inserted, the clinician must connect the cannula to a suction machine. The cannula is rotated at an angle of 360° and moved by 1–2 cm, back and forth, till the entire uterine cavity has been evacuated. The cannula can be gently rotated several times. When one round of suction is complete, the cannula tip is pulled back to the region just above the internal os, but not out of it. Care should be taken not to rotate the cannula inside the cervix.

Evacuation is said to be complete, when no more contents are observed to be coming out of the uterine cavity; instead of the uterine contents, air bubbles start appearing in the cannula and/or the uterine cavity appears to be firm and gritty. Once the surgeon is sure that the procedure is complete, the cannula is removed after disconnecting the suction.

Picture	Medical/Surgical Description	Management/Clinical Highlights
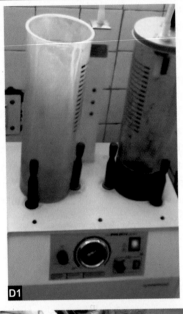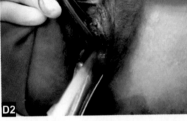**Figs 3.5.2 (D1 and D2):** (D1) Suction being generated through suction machine; (D2) Suction generated through the suction machine helps in aspiration of the products of conception	Karman's cannula is connected to the suction machine, which generates pressure equivalent to 60–70 mm Hg or 20–25 cm of water.	Pressure is first created with help of the suction machine. It is then released to create a negative pressure within the uterine cavity to help suck out the uterine contents.
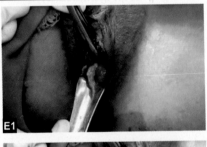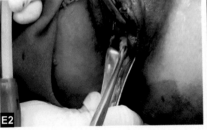**Figs 3.5.2 (E1 and E2):** Removal of protruding products of conception using an ovum's forceps	Figures 3.5.2 (E1 and E2) show the removal of protruding POC using an ovum's forceps.	The aspirated tissue must be sent for histopathological examination to confirm for the presence of chorionic villi in the aspirated tissues.

Picture	Medical/Surgical Description	Management/Clinical Highlights
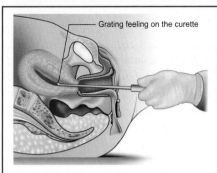 Fig. 3.5.2F: The evacuation of the uterine contents is almost complete resulting in a grating feeling	When the procedure of evacuation is complete, a grating feeling may be observed at the time of suctioning or curettage. Methergine 0.25 mg IM may be administered after the procedure in order to facilitate uterine contractions, thereby reducing the amount of bleeding.	The patient must be observed in the recovery room for 2–3 hours before discharge. • In case of pain, analgesic drugs may be prescribed. • If the procedure is performed under general anesthesia, the patient can be discharged after a few hours, once she has stabilized. • Women who are rhesus-negative can be given Rh immune globulins immediately following the procedure. • A woman who has undergone MTP must be counseled regarding the use of contraception in future, in order to prevent the reoccurrence of unwanted pregnancies. Immediate contraception in form of IUCD insertion or placement of a subdermal rod, intramuscular depot medroxyprogesterone acetate injections, etc. may be provided after the procedure depending on the patient's wishes. • The patients are scheduled for a follow-up visit, 1–2 weeks after abortion.

3.5.3: Use of Laminaria Tents for Cervical Dilatation (A and B)

Picture	Medical/Surgical Description	Management/Clinical Highlights
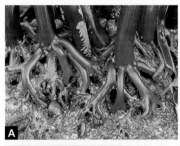 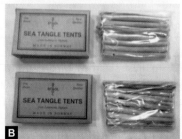 Figs 3.5.3 (A and B): Use of laminaria tents for cervical dilatation: (A) Sea weed laminaria; (B) Laminaria tents	Laminaria tents are natural cervical ripening agents, which are made from dried seaweed stems.	Besides Hegar's dilators, other methods of cervical dilatation include osmotic dilatation using laminaria tents or use of pharmacological dilatation using medications such as misoprostol. Laminaria tents can also be used for cervical dilation to induce labor and delivery. Recently, there has been a decline in the use of laminaria tents due to an increased rate of infection as a result of ineffective sterilization techniques used on the plants prior to drying.

3.6: MEDICAL TERMINATION OF PREGNANCY

3.6.1: Instruments Used for Manual Vacuum Aspiration (A to E)

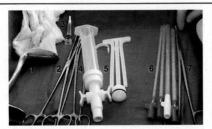

Fig. 3.6.1A: Equipment tray with unassembled vacuum aspiration syringe: (1) Sim's speculum; (2) Vulsellum; (3) Silicone gel; (4) Syringe; (5) Plunger; (6) Suction cannula; (7) Sponge holder

The most important component in this equipment tray is manual vacuum aspiration (MVA) syringe, which is kept unassembled.

Manual vacuum aspiration is a simple and safe method for MTP in a small uterus (preferably before 10 weeks of gestation) and can be performed as an outpatient procedure.

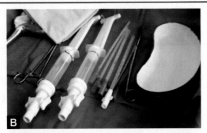

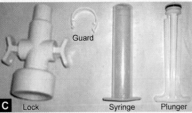

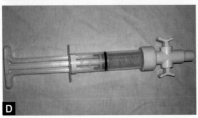

Figs 3.6.1 (B to D): Manual vacuum aspiration syringe: (B): Equipment tray with assembled vacuum aspiration syringe; (C) Different parts of a vacuum aspirator syringe; (D) An assembled vacuum aspirator syringe

The MVA syringe comprises of the following components:
- A syringe with a valve/lock, which can be used for locking the syringe.
- Plunger
- Guard

Since there is no requirement of performing cervical dilation prior to the procedure of MVA, it is associated with minimal rate of complications, particularly uterine perforations.

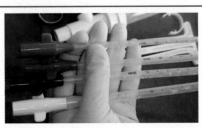

Fig. 3.6.1E: Different sized cannulae used for manual vacuum aspiration

The suction cannulas for MVA are available in different sizes, which can be identified by the color of the cannula.

The smallest sized cannula is green in color and 5 mm in size. The next one is blue in color, which is 6 mm in size. The brown-colored cannula is 7 mm in size. The largest cannula is white in color and 8 mm in size.

Picture	Medical/Surgical Description	Management/Clinical Highlights

3.6.2: Procedure of Manual Vacuum Aspiration (A to F)

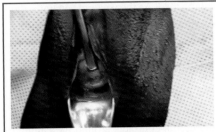

Fig. 3.6.2A: The posterior vaginal wall is retracted using Sim's speculum and the anterior lip is held with a vulsellum

The cervix is exposed by retracting the posterior vaginal wall with Sim's speculum and anterior lip of vagina with a vulsellum.

Manual vacuum aspiration is more cost effective than suction evacuation and is the only surgical procedure which can be used in a uterus less than 6 weeks in size.

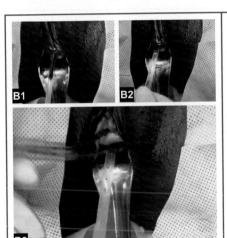

Figs 3.6.2 (B1 to B3): Using suction cannula of different sizes to serially dilate the cervix

Suction cannulas of progressively increasing sizes are used for serially dilating the cervix. The suction cannula of appropriate size (equal to the period of gestation) is then slowly pushed into the uterine cavity until it touches the fundus, but it is usually not advanced for more than 10 cm.

Prior dilation with Hegar's dilators is usually not required in these cases. Introduction of suction cannulas of progressively increasing size helps in dilating the cervix.

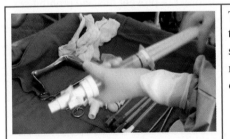

Fig. 3.6.2C: Charging the vacuum aspiration syringe

The process of creating vacuum inside the syringe is known as charging the syringe. The syringe is charged and kept ready before attaching it to the suction cannula.

The syringe is charged by first inserting the plunger inside the syringe, placing the guard and locking the syringe. The plunger is then pulled out to create the vacuum.

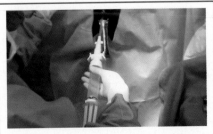

Fig. 3.6.2D: Attaching the manual vacuum aspiration syringe to the suction cannula

The charged MVA syringe is then attached to the suction cannula.

The pinch valve on the syringe is released to transfer the vacuum through the cannula to the uterine cavity.

The vacuum of the charged syringe helps in separating the POCs from uterine wall, following which they are sucked inside the syringe. To avoid losing the vacuum, the cannula must not be withdrawn past the cervical os.

Picture	Medical/Surgical Description	Management/Clinical Highlights
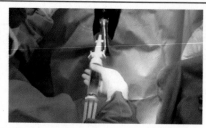 **Fig. 3.6.2E:** The products of conception fill the syringe due to the force exerted by vaccum	The remainder of uterine contents is evacuated by gently rotating the syringe from side to side (10 to 12 O'clock) and then moving the cannula gently and slowly back and forth within the uterine cavity. When the process of evacuation is complete, the cannula must be withdrawn, the syringe be detached and cannula be placed in decontamination solution.	If the vacuum is lost, it must be re-established. As the vacuum separates the uterine contents, they slowly start filling the syringe. In case, the syringe is more than half full, it should be emptied and the vacuum be re-established. As the process of evacuation gets completed, no more tissue is seen in the cannula and the uterus contracts around the cannula producing a grating sensation.
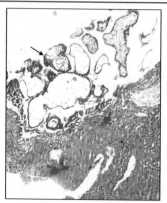 **Fig. 3.6.2F:** The histopathological appearance of the evacuated products	The evacuated uterine products must be sent for histopathological examination to confirm the diagnosis. Histological appearance in case of the evacuated POC can be observed in the adjacent figure, where cut section of various placental villi can be observed (indicated by arrows).	Histopathological examination helps in ruling out presence of other pathologies such as hydatidiform mole.

3.6.3: PNDT Act

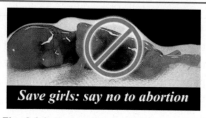 **Fig. 3.6.3:** Performing abortion in cases of female fetuses is illegal in India	Prenatal sex determination is a crime in India because this practice is likely to promote female feticide and abortion.	In order to prevent this and prohibit sex selection before and after conception, the PC & PNDT (Preconception and Prenatal Diagnostic Test: Prohibition of Sex Selection) act, 1994 was implemented.

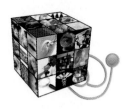

EVIDENCE-BASED BREAKTHROUGH FACTS

1. CHEMOTHERAPY AND HUMAN CHORIONIC GONADOTROPIN CONCENTRATIONS SIX MONTHS AFTER UTERINE EVACUATION OF MOLAR PREGNANCY

Chemotherapy may not be started in every patient with raised hCG concentrations after 6 months of evacuation of H. mole. It is important to see if these values have been increasing or falling over the period of time. While increasing or persistently high values are an indication for starting chemotherapy, surveillance policy (without starting chemotherapy) appears to be an acceptable option in patients with low and declining concentration of hCG, even 6 months after the evacuation of H. mole.

Source: Agarwal R, Teoh S, Short D, et al. Chemotherapy and human chorionic gonadotropin concentrations 6 months after uterine evacuation of molar pregnancy: a retrospective cohort study. Lancet. 2012;379:130.

2. PRECONCEPTIONAL LAPAROSCOPIC ABDOMINAL CERCLAGE

Preconception laparoscopic transabdominal cerclage serves as an effective option for preventing repeated pregnancy loss in certain patients. Women with a shortened or absent cervix or those in whom previous transvaginal cerclage surgery had been unsuccessful serve as the best candidates for transabdominal laparoscopic cerclage.

Source: Burger NB, Einarsson JI, Brolmann HA, et al. Preconceptional laparoscopic abdominal cerclage: a multicenter cohort study. Am J Obstet Gynecol. 2012;207(4):273.e1-273.e12.

Obstetrics

Section 4

Complications of Pregnancy

SECTION OUTLINE

4.1: MULTIFETAL GESTATION

4.1.1: Definition (A and B)

Picture	Medical/Surgical Description	Management/Clinical Highlights
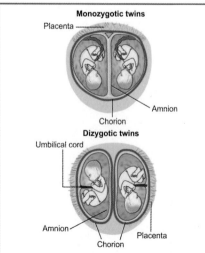 **Figs 4.1.1 (A and B):** Multifetal gestation: (A) Twin gestation; (B) Ten-years-old live quadruplet siblings from China with their mother (*Source*: Mail Today, 2012)	Development of two or more embryos simultaneously in a pregnant uterus is termed as multifetal gestation. Development of two fetuses simultaneously is known as twin gestation; development of three fetuses simultaneously as triplets; four fetuses as quadruplets; five fetuses as quintuplets and so on.	In case of multifetal gestation, following findings may be observed on abdominal examination: • On inspection, there may be abdominal overdistension (barrel-shaped abdomen). • The uterus may be palpable abdominally earlier than 12 weeks of gestation. • In the second half of pregnancy, the women may present with a uterine size more than the period of gestation and/or higher than expected weight gain in comparison to singleton pregnancies. • Height of the uterus is greater than period of amenorrhea (fundal height is typically 5 cm greater than the period of amenorrhea in the second trimester). • Abdominal girth at the level of umbilicus is greater than the normal abdominal girth at term. • On palpation, there may be presence of multiple fetal parts (e.g. palpation of two fetal heads). • There may be presence of hydramnios. • Two fetal heart sounds (FHS) can be auscultated over the abdomen, located at two separate spots separated by a silent area in between.

4.1.2: Difference Between Monozygotic and Dizygotic Twins

Monozygotic twins — Placenta, Amnion, Chorion; **Dizygotic twins** — Umbilical cord, Amnion, Placenta, Chorion. **Fig. 4.1.2:** Difference between monozygotic and dizygotic twins	Monozygotic or identical twins are formed due to division of a fertilized ovum into two. As a result, the two fetuses are of the same sex, they share the same placenta, same genetic features (DNA finger printing) and same blood group. The intervening membrane is composed of three layers: a fused chorion in the middle surrounded by amnion on two sides. Abnormal fetal growth and congenital malformations are more common amongst the monozygotic twins, and these twins comprise one-third of total cases of twins.	Dizygotic or nonidentical twins are formed as a result of fertilization of two or more ova by sperms. As a result, the two fetuses have different sexes; they have a separate placenta each; different genetic features (DNA finger printing) and can have different blood groups. The intervening membrane is composed of four layers, two chorions in the middle surrounded by amnion on two sides. Abnormal fetal growth and congenital malformations are less common amongst the dizygotic twins, and these twins comprise nearly two-thirds of total cases of twins.

Picture	Medical/Surgical Description	Management/Clinical Highlights

4.1.3: Formation of Twins (A to C)

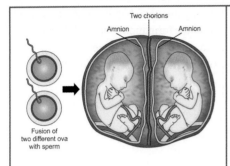

Fig. 4.1.3A: Formation of dizygotic twins

When two or more ova are fertilized by sperms, the result is development of dizygotic twins or nonidentical twins or fraternal twins.

Since each ovum is fertilized by two separate sperms, the two embryos can be of different sexes. Furthermore, in dizygotic twins the two embryos have separate placentae and there is no communication between the fetal vessels of the two embryos.

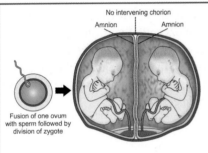

Fig. 4.1.3B: Formation of monozygotic twins

Monozygotic twins are formed due to the division of a single fertilized egg into two distinct fetuses after a variable number of divisions.

Different types of monozygotic twins which can be formed include diamniotic dichorionic monozygotic twins, diamniotic monochorionic monozygotic twins, monoamniotic monochorionic monozygotic twins and conjoined or Siamese monozygotic twins.

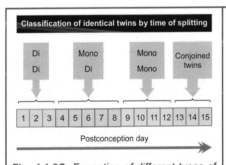

Fig. 4.1.3C: Formation of different types of monozygotic twins (DiDi: Diamniotic dichorionic; Mono Di: Monochorionic diamniolic; Mono Mono: Monoamniotic, Monochorionic)

Different types of monozygotic twins can result depending on the timing of the division of the fertilized ovum.

If the division of fertilized ovum occurs between days 1 and 3, diamniotic dichorionic monozygotic twins are formed; if division occurs between days 4 and 7, diamniotic monochorionic monozygotic twins are formed; if division occurs between the days 8 and 12, monoamniotic monochorionic monozygotic twins are formed and division between the days 13 and 15 results in the formation of conjoined or Siamese monozygotic twins.

4.1.4: Different Types of Monozygotic Twins (A to C)

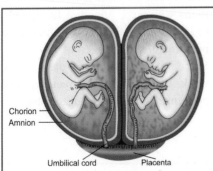

Fig. 4.1.4A: Diamniotic dichorionic monozygotic twin pregnancy

Formation of diamniotic dichorionic monozygotic twin pregnancy is associated with development of two chorions and two amnions. Moreover, there is development of two distinct placentae or a single fused placenta.

In case of diamniotic dichorionic monozygotic twins, the embryo splits at or before 3 days of gestation. This type of monozygotic twin accounts for nearly 8% of all twin gestations.

Picture	Medical/Surgical Description	Management/Clinical Highlights
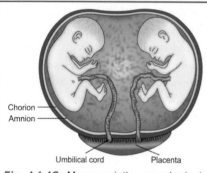 **Fig. 4.1.4B:** Diamniotic monochorionic monozygotic twin pregnancy	Formation of diamniotic monochorionic twin pregnancy is associated with development of a single chorion and two amnions. Usually there is a single fused placenta.	In case of diamniotic monochorionic twins, the cleavage division is delayed until the formation of inner cell mass and the embryo splits between 4 and 7 days of gestation. Nearly 20% of all twins are of this type.
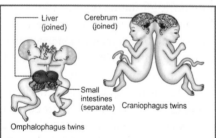 **Fig. 4.1.4C:** Monoamniotic monochorionic monozygotic twin pregnancy	Formation of monoamniotic monochorionic monozygotic twins is associated with development of a single chorion and a single amnion. Usually there is a single fused placenta.	In monoamniotic monochorionic monozygotic twins, the embryo splits between 8 and 12 days of gestation. Such types of monozygotic twins are rare, accounting for less than 1% of all twin gestations.

4.1.5: Conjoined or Siamese Monozygotic Twins (A to F)

Picture	Medical/Surgical Description	Management/Clinical Highlights
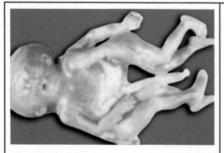 **Fig. 4.1.5A:** Different types of conjoined twins	In case of conjoined or Siamese twins, the embryo splits at or after 13 days of gestation, resulting in development of conjoined twins, which share a particular body part with each other.	Different types of conjoined twins, which can result, are: thoracophagus twins (joined at the chest); omphalophagus twins (joined at the anterior abdominal wall); craniophagus twins (joined at the head); pyophagus (joined at the buttocks) and ischiophagus twins (joined at the ischium). Development of such type of monozygotic twins is extremely rare.
Fig. 4.1.5B: Autopsy specimen of craniophagus twins	Figure 4.1.5B shows the autopsy specimen of craniophagus twins.	In this case, the diagnosis of conjoined twins who were joined at the region of head was established by ultrasound performed at 12 weeks of gestation. Since the fetuses died in utero at 24 weeks of gestation, hysterectomy was performed to deliver the dead babies.

Picture	Medical/Surgical Description	Management/Clinical Highlights
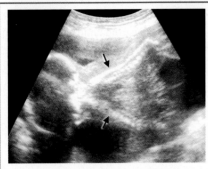 **Fig. 4.1.5C:** Ultrasound appearance of thoracophagus twins	Figure 4.1.5C shows ultrasound appearance of twins fused in the region of anterior chest wall. Both the twins appear to be facing one another, with their heads being at the same plane and level. Moreover, the thoracic cages of both the twins appear unusually close to one another.	Other ultrasonographic features which can help in the diagnosis of conjoined twins are as follows: • Repeat ultrasound examination done at an interval of few days or even few weeks is unable to show any change in the relative positions of the fetuses. • The fetal heads may appear to be unusually hyperextended.
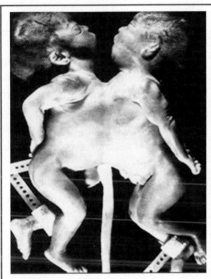 **Fig. 4.1.5D:** Autopsy specimen of thoracophagus twins	In this case the diagnosis of thoracophagus twins was established accidently during the second trimester ultrasound performed at 16 weeks. The patients decided to continue with the pregnancy.	If the pregnancy is allowed to continue, delivery by Cesarean section is the only option followed by surgical separation of the babies after birth. In this case an elective caesarean delivery was performed at term. The two twins died immediately after birth.
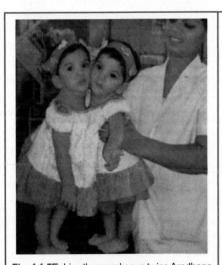 **Fig. 4.1.5E:** Live thoracophagus twins Aradhana and Stuti who have been separated after birth (*Source*: Navbharat times, June 2012)	Two live thoracophagus twins, belonging to the Betul district in Madhya Pradesh (India) had a fused liver and separate hearts with a single fused pericardium.	A surgery lasting for nearly 12 hours was successfully performed on June 20, 2012 on these twins by a team of doctors from both India and abroad. Firstly the pericardium was separated followed by the liver. Unfortunately, one of the twins, Aradhana died after 1 month following surgery as a result of two heart attacks which she suffered from during this time.

Picture	Medical/Surgical Description	Management/Clinical Highlights

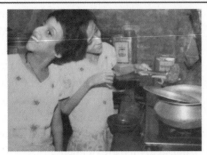

Fig. 4.1.5F: Live craniophagus 16-years-old twins Saba and Farah Shakeel (*Source*: Mail Today, July 20, 2012)

The Figure 4.1.5F shows live craniophagus twins, belonging to Patna region, India, joined in the head region, sharing a common brain.

They have yet not undergone any surgery because the family has not given permission for performance of surgery, which is too risky to be performed.

4.1.6: Different Types of Twin Presentations (A to E)

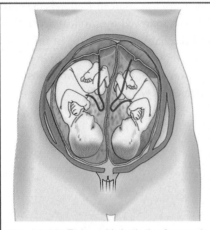

Fig. 4.1.6A: Twins with both the fetuses in vertex presentation

Twins with both the fetuses in vertex presentation is the commonest type of twin presentation and is present in about 40% cases. If the first twin is in vertex position, a vaginal delivery must be conducted to deliver this twin, provided there are no fetal or obstetric indications for cesarean delivery.

Delivery of the first twin in vertex position is conducted in a manner similar to that of a singleton pregnancy. Special precautions, which need to be taken include the following:
- IM methergine is not to be given at the birth of anterior shoulders of the first twin.
- Cord of the first baby is clamped and cut, and the baby is handed over to the pediatrician.
- After the delivery of first baby, a vaginal examination is performed to confirm the position of second baby. If the second baby is in vertex position, a vaginal delivery is performed.

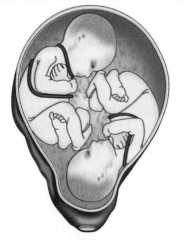

Fig. 4.1.6B: Twins with first fetus as vertex and second as breech

Twins with first fetus in vertex and second in breech position are present in about 25% cases.

If the second twin is in breech presentation, expected fetal weight is between 2 kg and 3 kg, fetal head is well flexed and the size of second twin is smaller than that of the first twin, a spontaneous or assisted breech delivery can be considered in case of complete/frank breech. Footling breech can be delivered by breech extraction. In case the second twin in breech presentation has a weight greater than 3 kg or less than 2 kg or the size of second twin is larger than that of first twin, a cesarean delivery is usually preferred.

Picture	Medical/Surgical Description	Management/Clinical Highlights
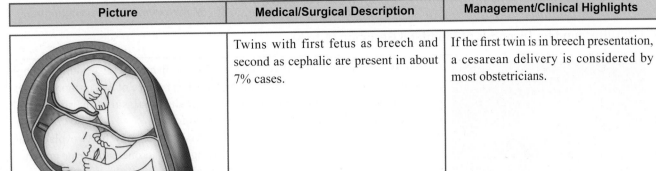 **Fig. 4.1.6C:** Twins with first fetus as breech and second as cephalic	Twins with first fetus as breech and second as cephalic are present in about 7% cases.	If the first twin is in breech presentation, a cesarean delivery is considered by most obstetricians.
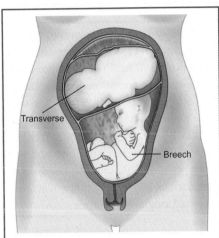 **Fig. 4.1.6D:** Twins with first fetus as breech and second as transverse	Twins with the first as breech and second as transverse are present in about 3% cases.	In these cases, delivery by cesarean section appears to be most useful.
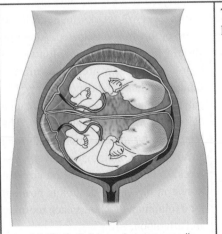 **Fig. 4.1.6E:** Both fetuses in transverse lie	Twins with both the fetuses in transverse lie are present in about 3% cases.	Presence of both the fetuses in transverse lie is the most definitive indication for cesarean delivery.

4.1.7: Ultrasound for Diagnosis of Multifetal Gestation (A to K)

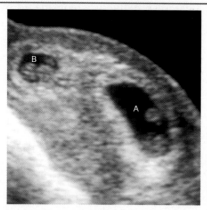

Fig. 4.1.7A: Presence of two gestational sacs with A = 7.6 weeks and B = 5.7 weeks

Presence of multiple fetuses and/ or multiple placentas on ultrasound examination is the most diagnostic feature of multifetal gestation.

In case of multifetal gestation, there may be presence of two or more fetuses or gestational sacs on ultrasound examination.

Also, there may be two placentas lying close to one another or presence of a single large placenta with a thick dividing membrane. This dividing layer could be composed of maximum up to four membranes (two layers of chorion fused in the middle, surrounded by amnion). Twin peak sign is another feature suggestive of multifetal gestation on ultrasound examination (Fig. 4.1.7K).

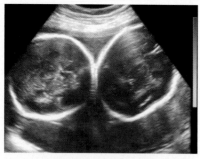

Fig. 4.1.7B: Ultrasound of the same patient at 30 weeks, showing two fetal heads

In the same patient as shown in Figure 4.1.7A when an ultrasound examination was performed at 30 weeks of gestation, two fetal heads were identified suggestive of twin gestation. Since both the fetuses were in vertex presentation, a vaginal delivery was planned for this patient.

In case of multifetal gestation, there is an additional calorie requirement to the extent of 300 kcal per day above that required for a normal singleton gestation or 600 kcal more in comparison with the nonpregnant state. Iron requirement must be increased to the extent of 60–100 mg per day and folic acid to 1 mg per day. Calcium also needs to be prescribed above the requirements for a normal singleton gestation.

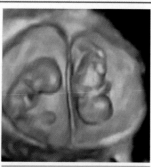

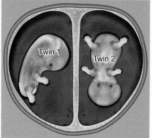

Twin 1 Twin 2

Fig. 4.1.7C: Three-dimensional ultrasound showing diamniotic dichorionic twins at 9 weeks

Figure 4.1.7C demonstrates three-dimensional ultrasound showing twin pregnancy at 9 weeks of gestation. There are two embryos with two distinctive placentas. The intervening membrane between the twins is composed of four layers: two chorions in the middle surrounded by a layer of amnion on either side.

In case of multifetal gestation, there is a requirement for increased frequency of antenatal visits. The patient should be advised to visit the antenatal care clinic every 2 weeks, especially if some problem is anticipated. Attention should be focused on evaluation of blood pressure, proteinuria, uterine fundus height and fetal movements. The patient should be advised to maintain a daily fetal movement count chart. The fetal growth should be monitored using an ultrasound examination every 3–4 weeks. The patient should be advised to rest in the lateral decubitus position for a minimum of 2 hours each morning and afternoon.

Picture	Medical/Surgical Description	Management/Clinical Highlights
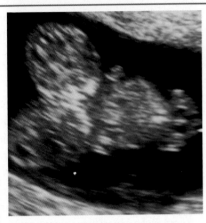 **Fig. 4.1.7D:** Conjoined twins fused in the region of thorax and abdomen	Figure 4.1.7D shows conjoined twins fused in the region of thorax and abdomen at 12 weeks of gestation. Other ultrasound features of conjoint twins have been discussed in 4.1.5.	In case the parents decide to continue with the pregnancy, delivery by cesarean section and surgical separation of the two twins after birth is the preferred option.
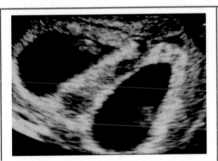 **Fig. 4.1.7E:** Diamniotic dichorionic twins at 7 weeks of gestation	Figure 4.1.7E shows diamniotic dichorionic twins at 7 weeks of gestation. There are two separate chorionic sacs surrounding each of the two amniotic sacs, with each sac containing an embryo. The intervening membrane between the twins is composed of four layers: two layers of chorion in the middle surrounded by a layer of amnion on either side.	Since multifetal gestation is associated with increased perinatal and maternal mortality, efforts must be taken to prevent the occurrence of multifetal gestation in the first place. Methods for primary prevention of multifetal gestation include limiting the number of embryos transferred in IVF and close counseling/monitoring of women using ovulation induction therapies. Since 2001, the Human Fertilization and Embryology Authority (UK) has recommended that the maximum number of embryos to be transferred per cycle of IVF must be limited to two.
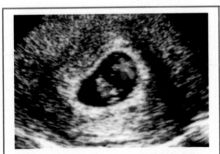 **Fig. 4.1.7F:** Monoamniotic monochorionic twins at 7 weeks of gestation	Figure 4.1.7F show monoamniotic monozygotic twins at 7 weeks of gestation. The two embryos are surrounded by a single amnion and a single chorion. As a result, there is no intervening membrane between the two fetuses.	Secondary prevention methods are commonly employed to help reduce the occurrence of twin gestation and other higher order pregnancies through the procedure of multifetal pregnancy reduction. In this procedure, potassium chloride is injected into the selected fetuses under either transabdominal or transvaginal ultrasound guidance, usually between 9 and 12 weeks of gestation.

Picture	Medical/Surgical Description	Management/Clinical Highlights
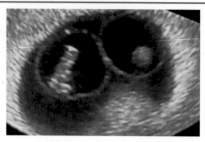 **Fig. 4.1.7G:** Monochorionic diamniotic twins	Figure 4.1.7G shows monochorionic diamniotic twins. Each embryo is surrounded by a separate amniotic sac. However there is common chorionic sac which surrounds the two amniotic sacs. As a result the intervening membrane between the two twins comprises of two layers of amnion.	Some of the steps which can be taken to prevent preterm labor in cases of twin gestation are as follows: • Bed rest • Administration of tocolytic agents • Regular monitoring of uterine activity, if possible, using external cardiotocography in which uterine contractions along with the fetal heart rate are continuously monitored. • The women should be advised to contact her midwife/obstetrician as soon as she experiences a contraction.
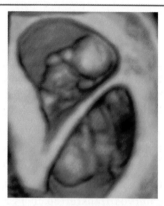 **Fig. 4.1.7H:** Three-dimensional view of diamniotic dichorionic twins at 10 weeks of gestation	Figure 4.1.7H demonstrates a three-dimensional ultrasound showing diamniotic dichorionic twins at 10 weeks of gestation. The intervening membrane between the two twins is composed of four layers: two intervening layers of chorion surrounded by a layer of amnion on either side.	Increased fetal surveillance is required in the cases of multifetal gestation. Since presence of multifetal gestation can produce numerous complications for the fetuses, which can result in significant neonatal morbidity and mortality, stringent fetal surveillance during the antenatal and intrapartum period becomes mandatory. Fetal monitoring can be done with the help of serial ultrasound examination, biophysical profile (BPP), nonstress test (NST), amniotic fluid index (AFI) and Doppler ultrasound examinations.
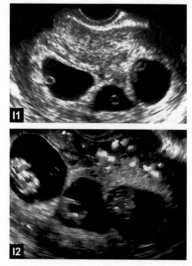 **Figs 4.1.7 (I1 and I2):** Triplets at 7 weeks of gestation: (I1) Transvaginal ultrasound; (I2) Color Doppler ultrasound	Figures 4.1.7 (I1 and I2) shows triplets at 7 weeks of gestation. Three separate gestational sacs, each having an embryo can be observed. The three fetuses share a common placenta as observed on Doppler ultrasound examination.	In cases of multifetal gestation, the following precautions need to be observed in the intrapartum period: • Blood to be arranged and kept cross-matched. • Pediatrician/anesthesiologist needs to be informed. • Patient should be advised to stay in bed as far as possible in order to prevent premature rupture of membranes. • Prophylactic administration of corticosteroids for attaining pulmonary maturity in cases of anticipated preterm deliveries. • IV access in the mother must be established.

Picture	Medical/Surgical Description	Management/Clinical Highlights
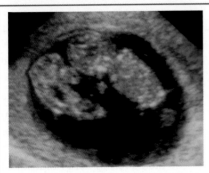 **Fig. 4.1.7J:** Monochorionic monoamniotic twins	Figure 4.1.7J illustrates the ultrasound appearance of monochorionic mono-amniotic twins. Due to the absence of any intervening membrane between the two twins, such twins are likely to have increased risk of complications such as cord entanglement, twin-to-twin transfusion syndrome (TTTS), vascular anastomosis, etc.	Other steps which must be observed in intrapartum period include the following: • Epidural analgesia for relief from pain is preferred as it can be rapidly extended in caudal direction in case a procedure like internal podalic version or cesarean section is required. • Vaginal examination must be performed soon after the rupture of membranes to exclude cord prolapse and to confirm the presentation of first twin. • Two healthcare professionals (one obstetrician and one pediatrician) should be available for each anticipated fetus. At least one of these persons should be well-versed in neonatal resuscitation. • Method for intrapartum fetal monitoring has been described in 4.1.8.
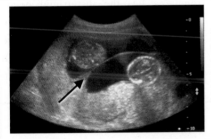 **Fig. 4.1.7K:** Lambda sign (indicated by arrow)	The lambda sign, also known as twin peak refers to the triangular projection of placental tissue extending from placental surface upward to a variable distance into the intertwin membrane, where it appears to be gradually tapering, resulting in the formation of triangular projection.	This sign is indicative of dichorionic diamniotic twin pregnancy. It is also indicative of extension of placental villi into the potential space formed as a result of reflection of apposed layers of amniotic and chorionic membranes from each fetus in case of dichorionic diamniotic twins.

4.1.8: Monitoring of Multifetal Pregnancy During Labor

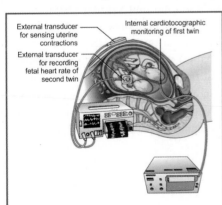 **Fig. 4.1.8:** Monitoring of multifetal pregnancy during labor	If the membranes have ruptured, the first twin can be monitored with help of internal cardiotocography, whereas the second twin can be monitored with help of external cardiotocography as shown in the adjacent figure.	In case of multifetal gestation, labor should be monitored with help of a partogram and the heart rate of both the fetuses must be monitored preferably using a cardiotocogram.

4.1.9: Antepartum Management of Twins

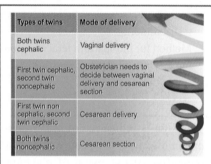

Steps in management	Strategy
Prevention of anemia	Supplementation with iron and folic acid
Early detection of preeclampsia	Regular blood pressure monitoring
Prevention of preterm delivery	Patient education, and counseling regarding preterm delivery and labor
Early detection of complications	Serial ultrasonograms

Fig. 4.1.9: Antepartum management of twins

Principles for antepartum management of multifetal gestation are as follows:
- Steps to be taken for prevention of preterm labor
- Increased daily requirement for dietary calories, proteins and mineral supplements
- Increased frequency of antenatal visits
- Increased fetal surveillance

Development of anemia in cases of multifetal gestation can be prevented by supplementation with iron and folic acid. Early detection of preeclampsia can be done by regular monitoring of blood pressure and urine examination for proteinuria. Fetal growth and well-being can be monitored by serial ultrasound examinations. Patient must be educated regarding the signs of development of preterm labor.

4.1.10: Mode of Delivery of Twins

Types of twins	Mode of delivery
Both twins cephalic	Vaginal delivery
First twin cephalic, second twin noncephalic	Obstetrician needs to decide between vaginal delivery and cesarean section
First twin non cephalic, second twin cephalic	Cesarean delivery
Both twins noncephalic	Cesarean section

Fig. 4.1.10: Mode of delivery of twins

In case the first twin is delivered by vaginal route, delivery of the first baby should be conducted according to guidelines for normal pregnancy. Ergometrine is not to be given at the birth of first baby. Cord of the first baby should be clamped and cut to prevent exsanguination of the second twin in case communicating blood vessels between the two twins exist.

If both the twins are in cephalic presentation, the mode of delivery is usually vaginal unless there is an indication for cesarean delivery. In case of first twin in cephalic presentation and second twin in noncephalic presentation (breech/transverse lie), the obstetrician needs to decide between vaginal or cesarean delivery. If the first twin is in noncephalic presentation or both the twins are in noncephalic presentation, cesarean delivery is invariably performed.

4.1.11: Designation of Twins In Utero

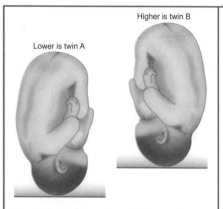

Higher is twin B

Lower is twin A

Fig. 4.1.11: Designation of twins in utero

In case of twin gestation, the twin which presents first (whose presenting part is palpated first on vaginal examination), is designated as twin A. On the other hand, the twin which presents next (whose presenting part can be palpated on vaginal examination, following the delivery of first twin) is designated as twin B.

Following the delivery of twin A and before the delivery of twin B, an abdominal and vaginal examination should be performed to confirm the lie, presentation and FHS of the second baby. External version can be attempted at the time of abdominal examination, in case the lie of twin B is transverse. Vaginal examination also helps in diagnosing cord prolapse, if present.

4.1.12: Complications of Twin Gestation

4.1.12.1: Twin-to-Twin Transfusion Syndrome (A to E)

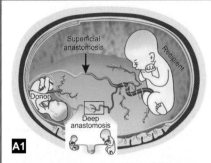

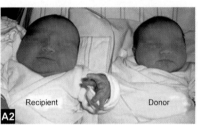

Figs 4.1.12.1 (A1 and A2): Twin-to-twin transfusion syndrome

Twin-to-twin transfusion syndrome is a rare complication that can occur in monozygotic monochorionic twins, which causes the blood to pass from one twin to the other.

As a result of the vascular communications, one of the twins, which donates blood (donor twin) becomes thin and undernourished, while the other twin who receives blood (recipient twin) grows at the expense of donor twin.

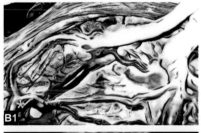

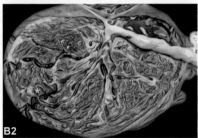

Figs 4.1.12.1 (B1 and B2): Placental specimen in a patient with TTTS (area of anastomosis is indicated by an asterisk)
(*Source*: Computerized generation of the image)

Twin-to-twin transfusion syndrome usually occurs due to the presence of placental vascular communications, which can be seen in this figure.

Since more advanced stages of TTTS have a worse prognosis in comparison to the earlier stages, when severe TTTS occurs at a very early gestational age (prior to 16 weeks), the option of termination of the pregnancy can be considered. The various therapies that are presently available, either involve balancing the fluid volumes between the two sacs or interrupting the communication of blood vessels between the twins. The treatment options that are currently available include options such as reduction amniocentesis, septostomy (microseptostomy), selective laser ablation of the placental anastomotic vessels, selective cord coagulation, etc. Complete bed rest along with nutritional supplementation (massive intake of proteins) has been recommended by some researchers as a therapy for this syndrome.

Picture	Medical/Surgical Description	Management/Clinical Highlights
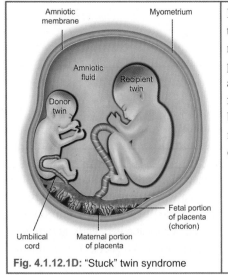 **Fig. 4.1.12.1C:** Diagrammatic representation of placenta showing arteriovenous anastomosis	The placental vascular anastomoses responsible for the development of TTTS could be from artery-to-artery (A-A); artery-to-vein (A-V) or from vein-to-vein (V-V).	Management of TTTS has been discussed in 4.1.12.1B.
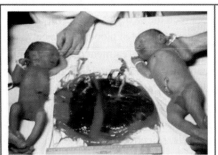 **Fig. 4.1.12.1D:** "Stuck" twin syndrome	In extreme cases of TTTS, the donor twin may donate so much blood to the recipient twin that it may not be able to produce any urine, thereby resulting in almost complete absence of amniotic fluid. As a result, the donor twin may become wrapped by its amniotic membrane, resulting in the formation of a "stuck" twin.	Management of TTTS has been discussed in 4.1.12.1B
Fig. 4.1.12.1E: Delivered specimen of dead donor/recipient twins	Figure 4.1.12.1E shows delivered specimen of dead donor/recipient twins. The donor twin (right) shows poor growth and appears pale, whereas the recipient is larger in size and plethoric (left).	The donor twin in TTTS usually shows poor growth, oliguria, anemia and hyperproteinemia, low or absent liquor, resulting in development of oligohydramnios, etc. On the other hand, the recipient twin shows polyuria, polyhydramnios and an enlarged urinary bladder. In the long run, this twin frequently develops polycythemia, biventricular cardiac hypertrophy and diastolic dysfunction with tricuspid regurgitation. The death of this twin eventually occurs due to congestive heart failure.

4.1.12.2: Twin Reversed Arterial Perfusion Syndrome (A to C)

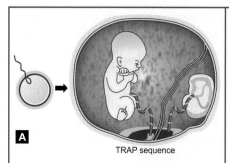

A

TRAP sequence

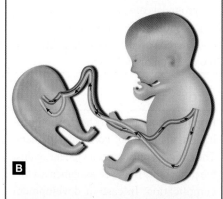

B

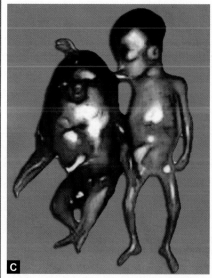

C

Figs 4.1.12.2 (A to C): Twin reversed arterial perfusion syndrome: (A) Diagram showing the twin reversed arterial perfusion syndrome; (B) Perfusion of the acardiac twin in a retrograde manner with poorly oxygenated blood which should have been delivered to the placenta; (C) Computerized generation of image showing a normal twin and an acardiac twin with poorly developed cephalic end

Acardiac twin or twin reversed arterial perfusion (TRAP) syndrome is an unusual form of TTTS. In these monochorionic twins, one twin develops normally while the other twin, known as an acardiac twin fails to develop a heart as well as other body structures. This twin acts as a recipient and depends on the normal donor (pump) twin for obtaining its blood supply via transplacental anastomoses and retrograde perfusion of the acardiac umbilical cord. Perfusion of the malformed (acardiac) fetus occurs via A-A and V-V anastomoses between the fetuses. Deoxygenated umbilical arterial blood from the donor flows into the umbilical artery of the recipient, with its direction reversed. In these pregnancies, the umbilical cord from the acardiac twin branches directly from the umbilical cord of the normal twin. This blood flow is reversed from the normal direction leading to the name for this condition—"twin reversed arterial perfusion syndrome". As a result, there is better perfusion of the lower part of the deformed body. On the other hand, the upper part of the body, showing lack of head, heart and upper extremities remains poorly perfused.

Normal twin (donor) eventually develops high output failure because it is responsible for maintaining the circulation of both the twins. Thus the circulatory load of the donor twin may become extremely large resulting in heart failure.

Doppler verification of reversed flow in the umbilical cord of the acardiac fetus helps in confirming the diagnosis. In some cases, the blood flow from the pump twin to the acardiac twin stops on its own and the acardiac twin stops growing. In other cases, the flow continues and the acardiac twin continues to increase in size. This eventually leads to heart failure and polyhydramnios in the pump twin. Radiofrequency ablation of a major blood vessel in the acardiac fetus often serves as the therapeutic strategy of choice. This procedure helps in stopping the blood flow and as a result the pump twin (normal twin) has to no longer send the blood to the acardiac twin.

4.1.12.3: Twin Embolization Syndrome

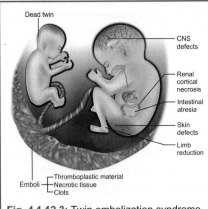

Fig. 4.1.12.3: Twin embolization syndrome

Twin embolization syndrome is a rare complication of monozygotic twins where in utero death of one of the twins has occurred. This may be associated with the passage of thromboplastic material from the dead twin into the circulatory system of surviving twin. This is likely to result in the ischemic structural defects of central nervous system, gastrointestinal and genitourinary tract of the surviving twin.

In instance of death of one of the babies in case of monozygotic twin gestation, the clinician must remain vigilant regarding the development of this syndrome in the surviving twin. In case of sonographic evidence of any defect in the central nervous system, gastrointestinal or genitourinary tract of the surviving twin, the parents must be counseled regarding the prognosis of surviving twin. Medical termination of the surviving twin can be considered based on the risk to fetus and the decision of parents.

4.1.12.4: Cord Entanglement

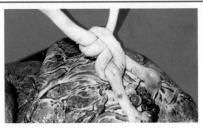

Fig. 4.1.12.4: Cord entanglement

Cord entanglement is a rare complication of monochorionic monoamniotic monozygotic twin pregnancy. Due to the absence of any intervening membrane between the two twins, the umbilical cords of these twins are likely to get entangled with each other.

Doppler ultrasound may help in confirming the diagnosis of cord entanglement. The clinician must remain vigilant against the probability of the development of this complication. In case of development of cord entanglement, the clinician may have to resort to immediate cesarean delivery, to save the twins.

4.2: ANTEPARTUM HEMORRHAGE

4.2.1: Placenta Previa

4.2.1.1: Definition

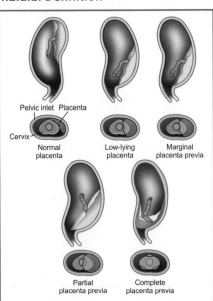

Fig. 4.2.1.1: Relationship of various types of placenta previa with the cervix

Placenta previa is one of the important placental causes of antepartum hemorrhage (APH) and can be defined as abnormal implantation of the placenta in the lower uterine segment. Depending on the location of placenta in the relation to cervical os, there can be four types of placenta previa: total placenta previa, partial, marginal and low-lying placenta previa.

Antepartum hemorrhage can be defined as hemorrhage from the genital tract occurring after the 28th week of pregnancy, but before the delivery of baby. True APH (due to placental causes) may mainly occur due to two conditions: placenta previa and abruption placenta. The cause of bleeding in these cases is related to mechanical separation of the placenta from the site of implantation. This usually occurs at the time of formation of the lower uterine segment, during third trimester, or during effacement and dilatation of the cervix at the time of labor.

Picture	Medical/Surgical Description	Management/Clinical Highlights

4.2.1.2: Types of Placenta Previa (A to D)

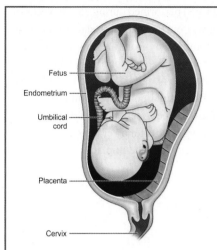

Fig. 4.2.1.2A: Total placenta previa

Total or central placenta previa is also known as type IV placenta previa. In this condition, the placenta completely covers the cervix.

Cesarean delivery is necessary for type IV placenta previa. In cases of severe bleeding, the most important step in management is firstly to stabilize the patient. The clinician must immediately arrange and crossmatch at least four units of blood and start blood transfusion, if required. All efforts must be made to shift her to the operating theater as soon as possible for an emergency cesarean delivery.

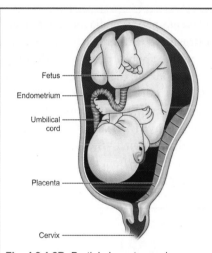

Fig. 4.2.1.2B: Partial placenta previa

Partial placenta previa is also known as type III placenta previa. In this condition, the placenta partly covers the cervical os.

Cesarean delivery is necessary for most cases of type III placenta previa.

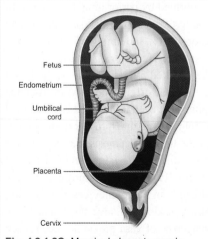

Fig. 4.2.1.2C: Marginal placenta previa

Marginal placenta previa is also known as type II placenta previa. In this condition, the placenta does not in any way cover the cervical os, but it approaches the edge of the cervix.

Cesarean delivery is necessary for most cases of posterior type II placenta previa. Patients with anterior type II placenta previa can be offered trial of labor by vaginal delivery, with arrangements for an urgent caesarean delivery in place in case of an emergency.

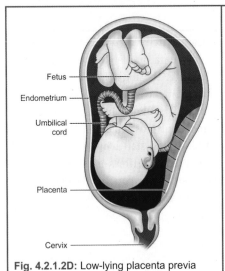

Fig. 4.2.1.2D: Low-lying placenta previa

Low-lying placenta previa is also known as type I placenta previa. Low-lying placenta is a term used to describe a placenta which is implanted in the lower uterine segment, but is not quite close enough to the cervix to qualify as marginal placenta previa.

If at the time of transvaginal sonography (TVS) performed during 35–36 weeks of gestation, the placental edge is more than 20 mm away from the cervical os, there are high chances for a vaginal delivery. The patient can be offered trial of labor with vaginal delivery in anticipation of high success rates. Nevertheless, the arrangements for an emergency cesarean delivery must be in place.

4.2.1.3: Placental Localization on Transabdominal Imaging

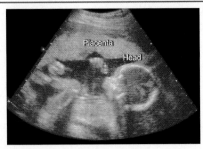

Fig. 4.2.1.3: Placental localization on transabdominal imaging

Vaginal examination must never be performed in suspected cases of placenta previa. The main way of confirming the diagnosis of placenta previa is by imaging studies, especially ultrasonography. Besides determining the placental position, ultrasound also helps in the assessment of fetal maturity, fetal well-being, fetal presentation and presence of congenital anomalies.

Placenta previa is diagnosed through ultrasound, either during a routine prenatal appointment or following an episode of vaginal bleeding. TVS is considered to be significantly more accurate than transabdominal sonography (TAS) and its safety is well established. On TVS examination, the actual distance from the placental edge to the margin of internal cervical os must be determined in millimeters.

4.2.2: Vasa Previa

4.2.2.1: Definition of Vasa Previa

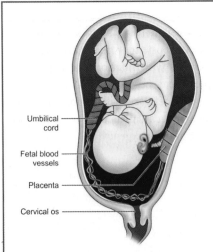

Fig. 4.2.2.1: Definition of vasa previa

Vasa previa is an uncommon obstetrical complication, which may be associated with a high risk of fetal demise, if it is not recognized before rupture of membranes. In vasa previa, umbilical vessels traverse the membranes in the lower uterine segment in front of the fetal presenting part. During uterine contractions, fetal vessels can get compressed resulting in fetal hypoxia and death. Patient with vasa previa presents with painless vaginal bleeding at the time of spontaneous rupture of membranes or amniotomy. Since the bleeding occurs from fetal vessels, fetal shock or demise can occur rapidly.

The presence of fetal blood can be confirmed by performing the Apt test. In this test, one drop of blood is added to nine drops of 1% sodium hydroxide in a glass test tube. The color of the test tube must be checked after 1 minute. If the blood is of fetal origin, the mixture remains pink. However, if the blood is of maternal origin, the mixture turns brown in color. If at the time of diagnosis, cervix is almost fully dilated, the fetus can be delivered vaginally. If cervix is not completely dilated, an emergency cesarean section must be done to save the fetus. If the diagnosis of vasa previa has been made in the antenatal period, the patient can be posted for an elective cesarean delivery.

4.2.2.2: Diagnosis of Vasa Previa

Picture	Medical/Surgical Description	Management/Clinical Highlights
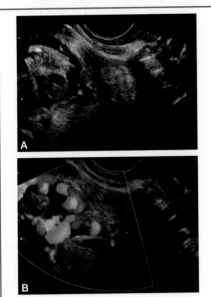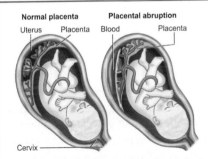**Figs 4.2.2.2 (A and B):** Diagnosis of vasa previa: (A) Transvaginal ultrasound; (B) Doppler ultrasound	Figure 4.2.2.2B illustrates a Doppler ultrasound photograph showing the presence of fetal vessels in front of the fetal presenting part. The diagnosis of vasa previa was established in this case.	When the diagnosis of vasa previa has been made during the antenatal period, the patient must be posted for an elective cesarean section at 37–38 weeks of gestation or when fetal lung maturation has been confirmed.

4.2.3: Abruptio Placenta

4.2.3.1: Placental Abruption and its Comparison with Normal Placenta

Picture	Medical/Surgical Description	Management/Clinical Highlights
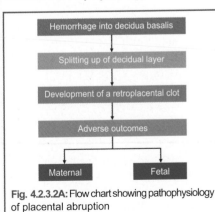**Fig. 4.2.3.1:** Placental abruption and its comparison with normal placenta	Placental abruption, also known as accidental hemorrhage can be defined as an abnormal, pathological separation of the normally situated placenta from its uterine attachment. As result, bleeding occurs from the opened sinuses present in the uterine myometrium.	In cases of abruption placenta, separation of the normally situated placenta results in hemorrhage into the decidua basalis. This causes the development of a retroplacental clot between the placenta and the decidua basalis.

4.2.3.2: Pathophysiology of Placental Abruption (A and B)

Picture	Medical/Surgical Description	Management/Clinical Highlights
Hemorrhage into decidua basalis → Splitting up of decidual layer → Development of a retroplacental clot → Adverse outcomes → Maternal / Fetal **Fig. 4.2.3.2A:** Flow chart showing pathophysiology of placental abruption	Figures 4.2.3.2 (A and B) illustrate the pathophysiology of placental abruption.	As a result of abnormal separation of a normally situated placenta, a retroplacental clot develops between the placenta and the decidua basalis, which interferes with the supply of oxygen to the fetus. This can lead to fetal distress, which can eventually cause fetal death.

Picture	Medical/Surgical Description	Management/Clinical Highlights
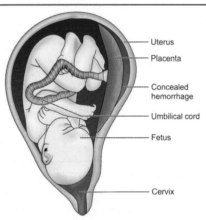 **Fig. 4.2.3.2B:** Pathophysiology of placental abruption	Figure 4.2.3.2B diagrammatically illustrates the pathophysiology of placental abruption.	In cases of abruption placenta, separation of the normally situated placenta results in hemorrhage into the decidua basalis. This causes internal bleeding, which can be either revealed or concealed.

4.2.3.3: Classification of Placental Abruption (A and B)

Picture	Medical/Surgical Description	Management/Clinical Highlights
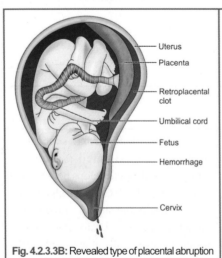 **Fig. 4.2.3.3A:** Concealed type of placental abruption	Based on the type of clinical presentation, there can be three types of placental abruption: revealed type, concealed type and mixed type.	In the concealed type of placental abruption, no actual bleeding is visible. The blood collects between the fetal membranes and decidua in form of the retroplacental clot. Though this type of placental abruption is usually rarer than the revealed type, it carries a higher risk of maternal and fetal hazards in comparison to the revealed type.
Fig. 4.2.3.3B: Revealed type of placental abruption	In the revealed type of placental abruption, following the placental separation, the blood does not collect between the fetal membranes and decidua, but moves out of the cervical canal and is visible externally.	Revealed type of placental abruption is commoner than the concealed variety. It is associated with a comparatively lower risk of maternal and fetal hazards in comparison to the concealed type.

4.2.3.4: Diagnosis of Placental Abruption

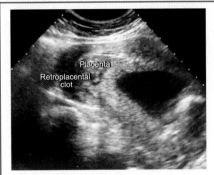

Fig. 4.2.3.4: Diagnosis of retroplacental clot on ultrasound examination

Ultrasound examination may help in showing the location of the placenta and thus would help in making or excluding the diagnosis of placenta previa. Ultrasound examination also helps in visualization of retroplacental clot (as shown in the adjacent figure), thereby confirming the diagnosis of placental abruption. Besides confirming the diagnosis, ultrasound examination also helps in checking the fetal viability and presentation.

Once the placental detachment has occurred in the cases of abruption placenta, presently there is no treatment to replace the placenta back to its original position. However, some of the steps can be taken to help reduce its occurrence:

- Early detection and treatment of preeclampsia
- Avoidance of smoking, drinking alcohol or using illicit drugs during pregnancy
- Avoidance of trauma
- Avoidance of sudden uterine decompression

4.2.3.5: Complications of Placental Abruption (A and B)

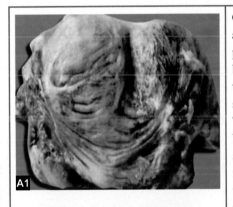

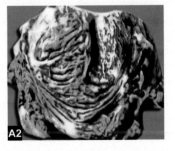

Figs 4.2.3.5 (A1 and A2): Couvelaire uterus: (A1) Photograph; (A2) Computerized generation of the image

Couvelaire uterus has been found to be associated with severe form of concealed placental abruption and is characterized by massive intravasation of blood into the uterine musculature up to the level of serosa (as shown in the adjacent figure). The blood gets infiltrated between the bundles of individual muscle fibers. As a result, the uterus becomes port wine in color. This is likely to interfere with uterine contractions and may predispose to the development of severe postpartum hemorrhage. There can be effusions of blood beneath the tubal serosa, connective tissues of broad ligaments, substance of the ovaries as well as presence of free blood in the peritoneal cavity.

The mother's hemodynamic status must be closely monitored. Intravenous access must be established with preferably two wide-bore intravenous lines. The patient should be kept warm and oxygen saturation maintained at > 95%. Blood should be crossmatched and kept arranged. Coagulation studies must also be performed. In case of atonic uterus, uterine contractions can be stimulated with help of intravenous oxytocin. In case of presence of any clots inside the uterus, they can be evacuated out. Couvelaire uterus per se is not an indication for cesarean hysterectomy. However in cases of uncontrollable postpartum hemorrhage, hysterectomy may be sometimes required.

Picture	Medical/Surgical Description	Management/Clinical Highlights
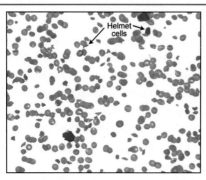 Fig. 4.2.3.5B: Peripheral smear in patient with disseminated intravascular coagulation, suggestive of hemolytic anemia. The black arrows point toward the helmet cells	In DIC, initially there is activation of the coagulation pathways, both intrinsic and extrinsic due to thromboplastin released from the decidual fragments and placental separation. As the process of coagulation continues, it results in consumption of various clotting factors and widespread deposition of fibrin. This can result in development of hypoxia, ischemia and necrosis, which ultimately results in end stage organ damage, especially renal and hepatic failure. The findings on peripheral smear in patients with DIC are suggestive of microangiopathic hemolytic anemia. The peripheral smear shows presence of multiple helmet cells, fragmented RBCs, microspherocytes and schistocytes, and paucity of platelet cells.	In the cases of DIC, fibrinogen levels are reduced; prothrombin time, APTT and thrombin time are prolonged; platelet levels are reduced, and levels of D-dimer and fibrinogen degradation products are increased. Treatment of DIC mainly involves the treatment of the underlying cause. Platelets can be transfused in patients at high risk of bleeding. Replacement therapy with fresh frozen plasma (FFP) in the dosage of 10–15 mg/kg body weight to maintain fibrinogen levels above 150 mg/dL may be administered. FFP usually contains the clotting factors V, VIII, XIII and antithrombin III. Transfusion of platelets, fibrinogen concentrates and cryoprecipitate (combination of fibrinogen and factor VIII) is also sometimes given.

4.3: RH NEGATIVE PREGNANCY

4.3.1: Pathophysiology of Rh Negative Isoimmunization (A to C)

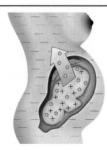 Fig. 4.3.1A: Rh positive antigens move into the maternal blood through placental circulation	Rh incompatibility may develop when a woman with Rh negative blood marries a man with Rh positive blood and conceives a fetus with Rh positive blood group (who has inherited the Rh factor gene from the father). Rh positive fetal red blood cells from the fetus leak across the placenta and enter the woman's circulation.	During the time of first Rh positive pregnancy, the production of maternal anti-Rh antibodies is relatively slow and usually does not affect that pregnancy. However, if the mother is exposed to the Rh D antigens during subsequent pregnancies, the immune response is quicker and much greater.
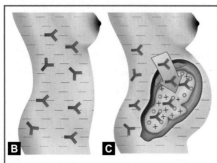 Figs 4.3.1 (B and C): These Rh positive antigens stimulate the formation of anti-Rh antibodies in the maternal circulation, which in subsequent pregnancies with Rh positive baby can destroy the fetal Rh positive cells	Throughout the pregnancy, small amounts of fetal blood can enter the maternal circulation (fetomaternal hemorrhage), with the greatest transfer occurring at the time of delivery or during the third trimester. This transfer stimulates maternal antibody production against the Rh factor, which is called isoimmunization. The process of sensitization has no adverse health effects on the mother.	The anti-D antibodies produced by the mother can cross the placenta and bind to Rh D antigen on the surface of fetal red blood cells, causing lysis of the fetal RBCs, resulting in development of hemolytic anemia. Severe anemia can lead to fetal heart failure, fluid retention and hydrops, and intrauterine death.

Picture	Medical/Surgical Description	Management/Clinical Highlights

4.3.2: Sinusoidal Fetal Heart Rate Pattern on Cardiotocography (Diagnostic of Rh Negative Isoimmunization)

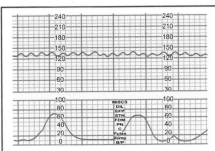

Fig. 4.3.2: Sinusoidal fetal heart rate pattern on cardiotocography (diagnostic of Rh negative isoimmunization)

Figure 4.3.2 shows sinusoidal heart rate pattern. A sinusoidal pattern is one in which the amplitude of oscillations and period of short-term (beat-to-beat variability) remains more or less constant. This gives the trace a smooth, undulating, regular wavy appearance. In this pattern, the amplitude of oscillations usually varies between 5 to 15 BPM with a fixed period of three to five cycles per minute. Fetal activity may be minimal or absent, and fetal heart rate accelerations are usually lacking.

The earliest warning of fetal anemia may be experienced by the mother in the form of reduced fetal body movements. External cardiotocography may show evidence of sinusoidal fetal heart rate patterns, and fetal BPP may also be affected. A true sinusoidal pattern is rare but ominous and is associated with high rates of fetal morbidity and mortality.

4.3.3: Liley's Chart

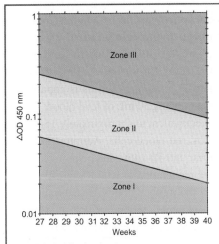

Fig. 4.3.3: Liley's chart

In cases of Rh isoimmunization, the fetus can be monitored for the development of anemia by performance of serial amniocentesis for calculating the ΔOD 450 values, which is then plotted over a standardized chart (Liley's chart or Queenan's chart). The only disadvantage of Liley's curve is that it is inaccurate before 26 weeks of gestation.

Zone III on the Liley's curve corresponds to severely affected infants, zone II to moderately affected infants and zone I to unaffected or mildly affected infants. If the amniotic fluid ΔOD 450 lies in zone I, the procedure should be repeated in 4 weeks. If the repeated ΔOD 450 values remain in the zone I, the infant should be delivered at the term.

If at any time, the ΔOD 450 value lies in the zone II, the procedure needs to be repeated at weekly intervals. If during the repeated test the ΔOD 450 values come to lie in the zone I, the test needs to be repeated again after 4 weeks. If during the repeated tests the ΔOD 450 values show a decreasing trend but still within the zone II, amniocentesis must be again repeated after 2 weeks. If the horizontal trend continues on successive repeated amniocentesis examinations, cordocentesis and evaluation of fetal hematocrit is required. If at any time, the Δ OD 450 values lies in the zone III or show a rising trend (moves from zone I or II to zone III), cordocentesis must be done and fetal hemoglobin values must be determined.

If fetal hematocrit values are less than 30%, intrauterine transfusion is indicated.

Picture	Medical/Surgical Description	Management/Clinical Highlights

4.3.4: Queenan's Chart

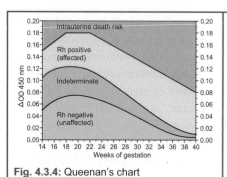

Fig. 4.3.4: Queenan's chart

Another chart called Queenan's chart (Fig. 4.3.4) is sometimes used instead of the Liley's chart. It has been found to be more accurate in comparison to the Liley's curve before 26 weeks of gestation. It can be used for the fetal assessment, starting from 14 weeks of gestation up to 40 weeks.

The Queenan's chart has been divided into four zones. The first zone in this curve corresponds to a nonaffected fetus. As the ΔOD 450 values move to higher zones, the chances of having an affected fetus also correspondingly increase. The values in the upper zone correspond to the higher risk of the fetal death.

4.3.5: Administration of Rh Anti-D Immunoglobulins

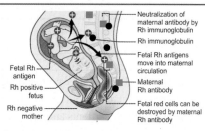

Fig. 4.3.5: Administration of Rh anti-D immunoglobulins

In cases where the father is Rh positive and the mother is Rh negative, it is important to detect the development of antibodies in the mother during antenatal period. The maternal antibody screen in order to detect presence of the antibodies needs to be carried out at 20, 24 and 28 weeks of gestation. The indirect Coomb's test is done to measure the presence of antibodies in the maternal blood. This test helps in detecting antibodies against fetal RBCs that are present unbound in the patient's serum.

Negative antibody titer on indirect Coomb's test can help identify the fetus that is not at risk.

In case, the antibody screen is negative, the patient should be administered 300 µg of immunoglobulins at 28 weeks of gestation in order to neutralize the fetal Rh antigens. This dose of anti-D immunoglobulins is capable of neutralizing 30 mL of fetal blood, which is equivalent to approximately 15 mL of fetal red blood cells. Administration of these anti-Rh antibodies helps in blocking the recognition of fetal Rh positive cells by the mother's body by neutralization of maternal antibodies before they can destroy the fetal Rh positive cells.

4.3.6: Process of Exchange Transfusion

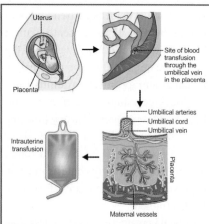

Fig. 4.3.6: Process of exchange transfusion

Exchange transfusion is a potentially lifesaving procedure that is done to counteract the effects of serious jaundice related to hemolytic anemia in a newborn child born to the mother with Rh incompatibility. It also helps in removing the circulatory antibodies. A unit of donor cells, which has freshly been donated and is devoid of Rh positive antigens is usually chosen. Crossmatching with maternal blood is performed, following which the blood is packed to a final hematocrit of 75–80% in order to allow the transfusion of minimal volume of blood.

The procedure of exchange transfusion comprises of the following steps:
- A plastic catheter is passed through the fetal umbilical vein into the inferior vena cava.
- In each cycle of exchange transfusion, about 5–20 mL of infant's blood is slowly withdrawn through a peripheral artery and at the same time an equal amount of fresh, prewarmed blood or plasma is injected into the infant's body through the umbilical vein.

This cycle is repeated until the required volume of blood has been replaced.

Picture	Medical/Surgical Description	Management/Clinical Highlights

4.3.7: Complications of Rh Negative Isoimmunization (A and B)

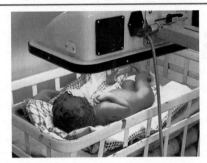 **Fig. 4.3.7A:** Baby with neonatal jaundice receiving phototherapy	Hemolysis due to Rh incompatibility may produce profound anemia, which may even result in fetal death in utero. As a compensatory mechanism to anemia, the fetal bone marrow starts producing immature erythroblasts into the fetal peripheral circulation. Excessive hemolysis results in excessive production of bilirubin, which is responsible for producing hyperbilirubinemia and jaundice.	Low levels of jaundice are not harmful but, if left untreated, higher levels may develop resulting in damage to specific areas of the neonatal brain, causing permanent brain damage (kernicterus). Postnatal jaundice can be treated with phototherapy (Fig. 4.3.7A) and exchange transfusion.
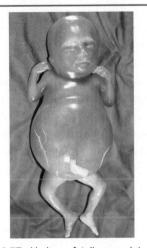 **Fig. 4.3.7B:** Hydrops fetalis associated with fetal ascites and skin edema	Hydrops fetalis is a condition, characterized by an accumulation of fluids within the baby's body, resulting in development of ascites, pleural effusion, pericardial effusion, skin edema, etc. In many cases, it may also cause polyhydramnios and placental edema. Pleural effusion may interfere with the normal process of breathing, whereas pericardial effusion may be associated with congestive heart failure. The fetus is particularly susceptible to interstitial fluid accumulation due to increased capillary permeability, hypoproteinemia and obstruction to lymphatic return.	Spontaneous remission of the condition has been reported in some cases. The following treatment strategies can be employed in cases of fetal hydrops: • Maternal antiarrhythmic agents (e.g. digoxin) for treatment of fetal arrhythmia • Fetal intrauterine transfusion for treatment of severe anemia • In utero fetal surgery (fetal thoracocentesis, paracentesis, etc.) The risks related to hydrops must be balanced against the benefits related to a particular treatment strategy. In case the fetal maturity has been attained, the affected fetus must be immediately delivered.

4.4: INTRAUTERINE GROWTH RETARDATION

4.4.1: Definition

4.4.1.1: Classification of Intrauterine Growth Retardation (IUGR)

Fig. 4.4.1.1: Classification of intrauterine growth retardation	IUGR refers to low birthweight infants whose birthweight is below the 10th percentile of the average for the particular gestational age. IUGR is also present when the birthweight is less than 2,500 g (5 pounds, 8 ounces) or when the abdominal circumference (AC) is less than 2.5th percentile. Some clinicians consider growth restriction when the fetal AC or the ratio of HC/AC or FL/AC is below the 10th percentile (or 2.5 standard deviation below the mean) of the average for that particular gestational age.	IUGR infants can be of two types, i.e. symmetric intrauterine growth retarded and asymmetric intrauterine growth retarded, depending on the stage of fetal growth at which the pathological insult occurred. If the pathological insult occurs at stage 1 of fetal growth, the process of cellular hyperplasia is mainly affected. This results in symmetrically growth restricted infants. If the pathological insult occurs at stage 3 of fetal growth, cellular hypertrophy is mainly affected. This results in asymmetrically affected growth restricted infants.

4.4.1.2: Causes of Intrauterine Growth Retardation

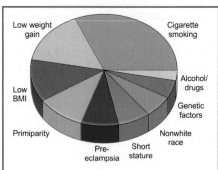

Fig. 4.4.1.2: Causes of intrauterine growth retardation (BMI, Body mass index)

Various causes of IUGR are as follows:

Maternal Factors
- Constitutionally small mothers
- Maternal malnutrition
- Tobacco smoking
- Excessive alcohol intake
- Strenuous physical work
- Poor socioeconomic conditions
- Preeclampsia and chronic hypertension
- Maternal anemia, especially sickle cell anemia

Fetal Factors
- Multiple pregnancy
- Chromosomal abnormalities
- Severe congenital malformations
- Chronic intrauterine infection

Placental Factors
- Poor placental function (placental insufficiency or inadequacy)
- Placental abnormalities including chorioangioma, circumvallate placenta, marginal or velamentous cord insertion, placenta previa, placenta abruption, etc.

Treatment of IUGR comprises of correction of primary abnormality [e.g. treatment of underlying maternal disease, stopping substance abuse, good nutrition, bed rest and maternal hyperoxygenation, use of steroids for fetal maturity (if gestational age is less than 32 weeks)], and fetal monitoring in form of serial sonograms, NST, contraction stress test, BPP and umbilical artery Doppler velocimetry. Immediate delivery may be required in cases of nonreassuring fetal status. If gestational age is more than or equal to 34 weeks and an abnormality is detected in the tests of fetal well-being, fetus must be delivered. In case of nonreassuring fetal response, low AFI and meconium stained liquor, amnioinfusion can be considered. Cesarean delivery must be conducted in case of deteriorating fetal status.

4.4.2: Diagnosis of Intrauterine Growth Retardation

4.4.2.1: Symphysis Fundus Growth Curves

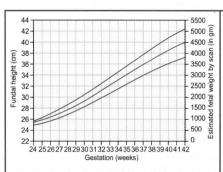

Fig. 4.4.2.1: Symphysis-fundal height chart

A customized fundal height chart, which is adjusted for various maternal variables including height, weight, parity, ethnicity, etc. helps in improving the accuracy of symphysis-fundus height (SFH) in predicting a small for gestational age fetus. SFH is measured in centimeters from the upper edge of the symphysis pubis to the top of the fundus of the uterus. After 24 weeks of gestation, SFH corresponds to the period of gestation. A lag of 4 cm or more is suggestive of fetal growth restriction. Ideally the SFH in centimeters should be plotted against the gestational age on the SFH chart.

The SFH curve compares the symphysis-fundus (S-F) height with the period of gestation. The middle line of the growth curve represents the 50th percentile, whereas the upper and lower lines represent the 95th and 5th percentiles, respectively. If intrauterine growth is normal, the S-F height will fall between the 5th and 95th percentiles. If IUGR is present, the S-F height would fall below the 5th percentile. Growth restriction is also suggested when three successive measurements of fetal weight "plateau" at approximately the same level, without necessarily crossing below the 5th percentile.

Picture	Medical/Surgical Description	Management/Clinical Highlights

4.4.2.2: Graphical Representation of Crown-rump Length Measurement

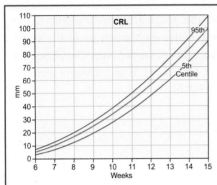

Fig. 4.4.2.2: Graphical representation of crown-rump length measurement

Crown-rump length (CRL) is an ultrasonic measurement which is made earliest in pregnancy, when the gestational age is between 7 weeks and 13 weeks. The graphical measurement of CRL according to the gestational age is shown in Figure 4.4.2.2. The upper and lower curves respectively represent the 95th and 5th percentiles for the CRL measurement according to the gestational age. Ultrasound measurement of CRL is described in Section 7.

The measurement of the CRL of the fetus gives most accurate measurement of the gestational age. Early in pregnancy, the accuracy of determining gestational age through CRL measurement is within ± 4 days, but later in pregnancy due to different growth rates of the fetus, the accuracy of determining gestational age with help of ultrasound is less. If the fetal growth is normal, the successive CRL measurements would fall between the 5th and 95th percentiles.

4.4.2.3: Graphical Representation of Biparietal Diameter Measurement

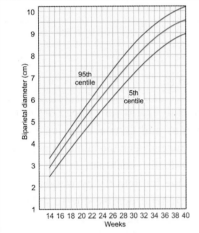

Fig. 4.4.2.3: Graphical representation of biparietal diameter measurement

Biparietal diameter (BPD) is the distance between the two sides of the head. BPD is usually measured after 13 weeks of pregnancy for dating of pregnancy. It increases from about 2.4 cm at 13 weeks to about 9.5 cm at term. The graphical measurement of BPD according to the gestational age is shown in Figure 4.4.2.3. Ultrasound measurement of BPD is described in Section 7.

The upper and lower curves respectively represent the 95th and 5th percentiles for the BPD measurement according to the gestational age. An obstetrician maintaining such a chart is able to efficiently monitor the fetal growth. The BPD remains the standard against which other parameters of gestational age assessment are compared. At 20 weeks of gestation, accuracy of BPD is within 1 week. If the fetal growth is normal, the successive BPD measurements would fall between the 5th and 95th precentiles.

4.4.2.4: Graphical Representation of Abdominal Circumference Measurement

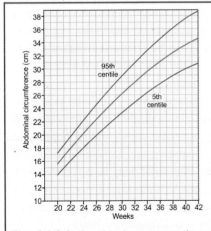

Fig. 4.4.2.4: Graphical representation of abdominal circumference measurement

Abdominal circumference is a measure of fetal abdominal girth. Figure 4.4.2.4 shows the graphical representation of AC measurement in relation to the gestational age. Ultrasound measurement of AC is described in Section 7.

If the AC measurement falls below the 5th percentile on the graph, a diagnosis of fetal growth restriction is made. If the fetal growth is normally occurring, the measurements of AC would fall between the two curves.

Picture	Medical/Surgical Description	Management/Clinical Highlights

4.4.2.5: Graphical Measurement of Femur Length

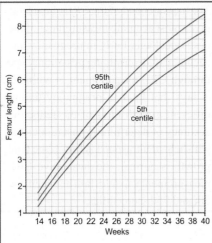

Fig. 4.4.2.5: Graphical measurement of femur length

Femur length is the length of femoral diaphysis, the longest bone in the body, and represents the longitudinal growth of the fetus. Its usefulness is similar to the BPD. It increases from about 1.5 cm at 14 weeks to about 7.8 cm at term. Ultrasound measurement of FL is described in Section 7.

If the fetal growth is normal, the successive measurements of FL would fall between the two lines. The ultrasound ratio of AC/FL is an important measure of IUGR.

4.4.3: Management of Cases of Intrauterine Growth Retardation

4.4.3.1: Deciding the Time of Delivery in Intrauterine Growth Retardation (A and B)

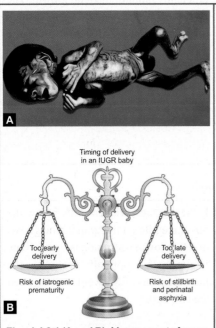

Figs 4.4.3.1 (A and B): Management of cases of intrauterine growth retardation: (A) IUGR baby (computerized graphic); (B) Deciding the time of delivery in IUGR babies

The most important goal of management in case of IUGR fetuses is to deliver the most mature fetus in the least compromised position and at the same time causing minimum harm to the mother.

Presently the Royal College of_Obstetricians and Gynaecologists (2002) recommends that the clinician needs to individualize each patient and decide the time for delivery by weighing the risk of fetal demise due to delayed intervention against the risk of long-term disabilities resulting from preterm delivery due to early intervention. The two main parameters for deciding the optimal time of delivery include results on various fetal surveillance techniques and gestational age. Also, the patient needs to be counseled regarding the potential risks associated with the two strategies.

Preterm delivery could be associated with future disabilities, intraventricular hemorrhage, sepsis and retinopathy of prematurity, etc. Delayed delivery on the other hand, may be associated with ischemic brain injury, periventricular leukomalacia, intraventricular hemorrhage and intrauterine death.

Picture	Medical/Surgical Description	Management/Clinical Highlights

4.5: AMNIOTIC FLUID AND ITS ABNORMALITIES

4.5.1: General Features Related to Amniotic Fluid

4.5.1.1: Amniotic Fluid Formation (A and B)

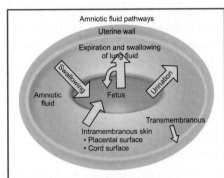

Fig. 4.5.1.1A: Amniotic fluid pathway

The amniotic fluid is the fluid which surrounds and protects the baby inside the intrauterine cavity.

Though the exact process of formation of amniotic fluid is yet not clear, it is believed to be formed by the following processes:
- Secretion from the amniotic cells
- Diffusion of maternal tissue fluid of decidua parietalis across the chorioamniotic membrane
- Diffusion from blood in intervillous space across the chorionic plate
- Respiratory tract secretions of the fetus
- Urine secreted by the fetal kidneys
- Water transport across the highly permeable skin of the fetus.

The amniotic fluid probably gets drained through the following processes:
- Diffusion into maternal tissue fluid of decidua parietalis across the chorioamniotic membrane.
- Fetal swallowing: Fetus begins swallowing at about 8−11 weeks of gestation.
- Reabsorption by the fetal intestines.

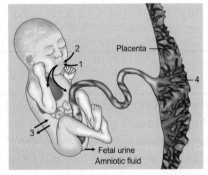

Fig. 4.5.1.1B: Formation of amniotic fluid
1. Fetal swallowing and reabsorption by intestine.
2. Exchange with respiratory tract reabsorption via lungs.
3. Exchange across fetal skin possible only for small lipid soluble gases.
4. Net water movement between mother and fetus across chorion frondosum.

The process of formation and absorption of amniotic fluid has been described in 4.5.1.1A. The process of production of amniotic fluid through fetal urine and fetal lung fluid production is balanced by removal of fluid through fetal swallowing and intramembranous absorption across the fetal surface of placenta.

Imbalance in the procedure of formation and removal, resulting in an increased production of fetal urine or lung fluids or reduced removal of fluid is responsible for development of hydramnios. Reduced fluid production and increased absorption, on the other hand, is responsible for oligohydramnios.

4.5.1.2: Classification of Amniotic Fluid Based on Four-Quadrant Index

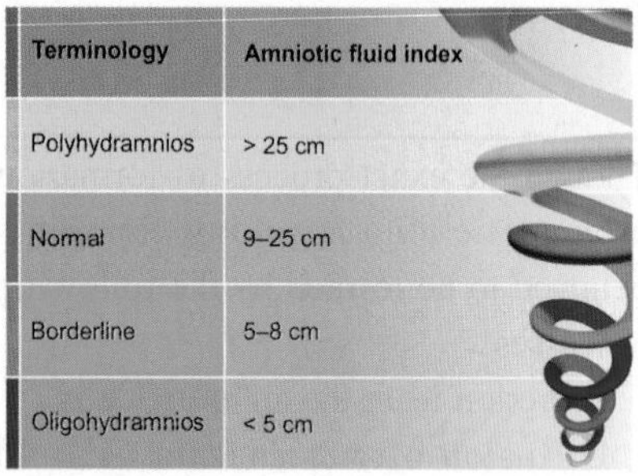

Terminology	Amniotic fluid index
Polyhydramnios	> 25 cm
Normal	9–25 cm
Borderline	5–8 cm
Oligohydramnios	< 5 cm

Fig. 4.5.1.2: Classification of amniotic fluid based on four-quadrant index

Amniotic fluid index (AFI) is obtained by measuring and adding together the vertical depth of the largest fluid pockets in each of the four abdominal quadrants. The AFI uses the 5th and 95th percentiles for gestational age to signify oligohydramnios and polyhydramnios respectively. If the amniotic fluid depth measures less than 5 cm (5th percentile), the woman is supposed to have oligohydramnios. If amniotic fluid levels add up to more than 25 cm (95th percentile), she is supposed to have polyhydramnios.

Classification system based on the volume of amniotic fluid:

Normal amniotic fluid: Adequate fluid, seen everywhere between the fetus and uterine wall varying in amount from 700 mL to 1 L at full term is considered as normal.

Oligohydramnios: Amniotic fluid volume is less than 200 mL. Maximum vertical pocket of fluid is between 1 to 2 cm. AFI is less than 5 cm.

Polyhydramnios: Amniotic fluid volume is 2,000 mL or greater at term. Maximum vertical pocket of fluid is greater than 8 cm. AFI is greater than 25 cm.

4.5.1.3: Classification of Amniotic Fluid Based on the Depth of Largest Pocket

Maximum vertical diameter	Interpretation
2–8 cm	Normal
1–2 cm	Marginal
< 1 cm	Oligohydramnios
> 8 cm	Polyhydramnios

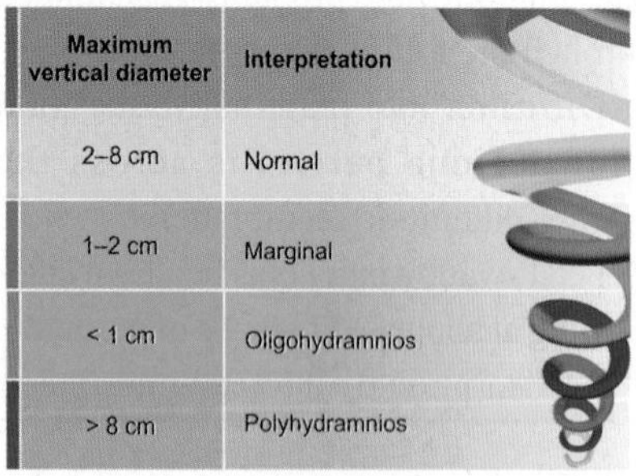

Fig. 4.5.1.3: Classification of amniotic fluid based on the depth of largest pocket

The two most commonly used techniques for ultrasound evaluation of amniotic fluid volume include the measurement of maximal vertical pocket depth of amniotic fluid and the measurement of AFI.

As the name suggests, the measurement of maximum vertical pocket depth involves the measurement of maximum vertical diameter of the deepest pocket of amniotic fluid identified upon ultrasound examination.

Presence of low amniotic fluid volumes may require additional fetal surveillance testing and use of potent glucocorticoids to accelerate fetal lung maturity in preterm pregnancies followed by their delivery.

4.5.1.4: Ultrasound of a Patient with Normal Amniotic Fluid Volume

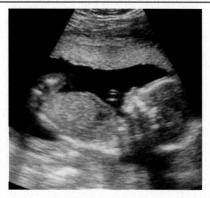

Fig. 4.5.1.4: Ultrasound of a patient with 32 completed weeks of gestation

The most commonly employed diagnostic methodology for evaluation of amniotic fluid is ultrasound. Figure 4.5.1.4 shows ultrasound of a patient with 32 completed weeks of gestation showing normal amniotic fluid volume. Adequate fluid can be seen everywhere between the fetus and uterine wall on this ultrasound.

Use of amniotic fluid volume evaluation during ultrasound examination has become important in the assessment of high-risk pregnancy because it forms basis for two important tests of fetal well-being, namely the BPP and the modified BPP both of which include ultrasound estimation of amniotic fluid volume.

4.5.1.5: Changes in Amniotic Fluid with Increasing Period of Gestation

Picture	Medical/Surgical Description	Management/Clinical Highlights
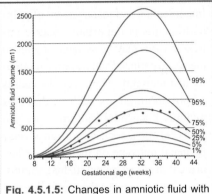 **Fig. 4.5.1.5:** Changes in amniotic fluid with increasing period of gestation	The amniotic sac that contains the fetus forms about 12 days after conception. Amniotic fluid immediately begins to fill the sac. In the early weeks of pregnancy, amniotic fluid mainly comprises of transudation of maternal serum. After about 20 weeks, when the fetal kidneys start functioning, fetal urine makes up most of the fluid.	As shown in the adjacent figure, with the fetal growth, the amount of amniotic fluid also goes on increasing in maximum number of normal pregnancies. It is about 30 mL at 10 weeks, 350 mL at 20 weeks and 700 mL to 1 L at full term. In normal fetuses, swallowing by the fetus, balanced by the production of fetal urine, helps in maintaining the amniotic fluid volume at a steady level.

4.5.2: Polyhydramnios

4.5.2.1: Ultrasound of a Fetus with Polyhydramnios

Picture	Medical/Surgical Description	Management/Clinical Highlights
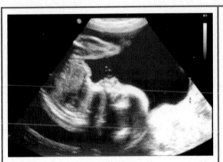 **Fig. 4.5.2.1:** Ultrasound of a fetus with polyhydramnios	Figure 4.5.2.1 shows ultrasound of a fetus with polyhydramnios. As discussed previously, the criteria for diagnosis of polyhydramnios is presence of AFI > 25 cm and the depth of maximum vertical pocket of amniotic fluid being greater than 8 cm.	Management of polyhydramnios comprises of the following: *Correction of the primary anomaly*: In cases of polyhydramnios, attempts must be made to correct the primary abnormality (e.g. correcting high blood sugar levels in women with gestational diabetes). *Decompression by amniocentesis*: For patients developing symptoms like respiratory embarrassment, excessive uterine activity, one of the available therapeutic options is decompression by amniocentesis, a procedure involving the removal of amniotic fluid. *Treatment with indomethacin*: Indmethacin is an antiprostaglandin, which acts by reversibly inhibiting the enzyme cyclooxygenase. This drug therefore helps in reducing amniotic fluid levels by reducing fetal urine production. It also helps in alleviating various complications (respiratory embarrassment, preterm labor, etc.) associated with polyhydramnios. Most clinicians recommend treatment with indomethacin (2.2–3.0 mg/kg body weight/day or 75 mg twice daily or 25 mg three times daily).

4.5.2.2: Causes of Polyhydramnios

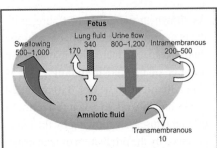

Fig. 4.5.2.2: Causes of polyhydramnios

In about two thirds of cases, the cause of polyhydramnios is unknown. Polyhydramnios is more likely to occur in the following maternal and fetal situations:

Fetal Causes
- *Congenital abnormalities*: Birth defects involving the gastrointestinal tract and central nervous system.
- *Twin-twin transfusion syndrome*
- *Parvovirus B19 infection*: Fetal infection, such as with Parvovirus B19, which in childhood may cause a mild illness called fifth disease, may sometimes result in polyhydramnios.

Maternal Causes
- Multiple gestation
- Maternal diabetes
- Rh blood incompatibilities between the mother and the fetus

Identification and management of polyhydramnios is important because untreated cases may be associated with an increased perinatal and maternal morbidity and mortality. Moreover, the causes of polyhydramnios such as diabetes mellitus, congenital malformations and twins are also associated with an adverse perinatal outcome on their own. When present in association with hydramnios, they further increase the morbidity.

4.5.2.3: Degrees of Polyhydramnios

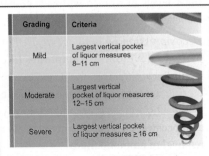

Grading	Criteria
Mild	Largest vertical pocket of liquor measures 8–11 cm
Moderate	Largest vertical pocket of liquor measures 12–15 cm
Severe	Largest vertical pocket of liquor measures ≥ 16 cm

Fig. 4.5.2.3: Degrees of polyhydramnios

Mild hydramnios can be defined as the presence of largest vertical pocket of liquor measuring between 8 cm and 11 cm. Moderate hydramnios can be defined as presence of largest vertical pocket of liquor measuring between 12 cm and 15 cm, whereas severe hydramnios is defined by the presence of largest vertical pocket of liquor greater than 16 cm.

Management of polyhydramnios is described in 4.5.2.1.

4.5.2.4: Fetus with Polyhydramnios

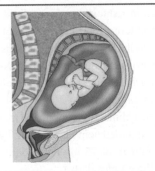

Fig. 4.5.2.4: Fetus with polyhydramnios

In case of polyhydramnios, the fetus is surrounded by excessive amount of amniotic fluid. The condition develops because the fetus is unable to swallow and/or absorb amniotic fluid in normal amounts. This could be related to the presence of some congenital abnormality such as duodenal atresia, esophageal atresia, anencephaly, etc.

Management of polyhydramnios is described in 4.5.2.1.

Picture	Medical/Surgical Description	Management/Clinical Highlights

4.5.3: Oligohydramnios

4.5.3.1: Ultrasound Scan of a Twenty-six Weeks Old Fetus Showing Oligohydramnios

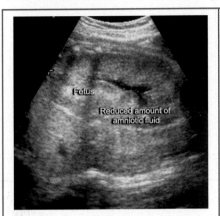 **Fig. 4.5.3.1:** Ultrasound scan of a 26-weeks-old fetus showing oligohydramnios	Figure 4.5.3 shows ultrasound appearance of a woman having oligohydramnios. This can be defined as presence of less than 200 mL of amniotic fluid at term or an AFI of less than 5 cm or presence of the largest pocket of fluid, which does not measure more than 1 cm at its largest diameter.	When a woman has too little amniotic fluid, it is termed as oligohydramnios. About 4% of women have been estimated to develop oligohydramnios at the time of their pregnancy. Though it commonly develops in the last trimester, it can also develop at any time during pregnancy.

4.5.3.2: Complications (A and B)

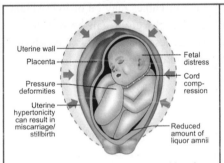 **Fig. 4.5.3.2A:** Complications resulting from oligohydramnios	Complications which can occur during early pregnancy due to presence of oligohydramnios include the following: • Amniotic adhesions causing deformities or constriction of the umbilical cord • Pressure deformities like clubfeet Complications which occur during late pregnancy include the following: • Fetal distress • Cord compression, resulting in fetal hypoxia • Intrauterine growth retardation • Prolonged rupture of membranes • Fetal malformations (renal agenesis, polycystic kidneys, urethral obstruction, etc.) • Postmaturity syndrome • Miscarriage • Stillbirth • Increased risk of meconium aspiration syndrome • Presence of oligohydramnios in late pregnancy is one of the signs of fetal distress and is often seen in association with IUGR. • Women with oligohydramnios are more likely to require a cesarean section in comparison to the normal women.	Women with otherwise normal pregnancies who develop oligohydramnios in near term probably need no treatment and their babies are likely to be born healthy. Nearly half the cases of oligohydramnios resolve themselves without treatment. However, obstetrician requires keeping close surveillance over such patients. If any one of the tests for fetal well-being shows abnormality, early delivery by fastest route may be required even if the fetus is preterm. The obstetrician may recommend weekly (or more frequent) ultrasound examinations to see if the level of amniotic fluid is decreasing to a dangerous point. If the level of amniotic fluid becomes inadequate, the clinician may recommend inducing labor early to help prevent complications during labor and delivery.

Picture	Medical/Surgical Description	Management/Clinical Highlights

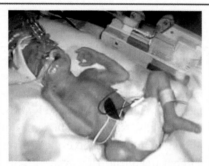

Uterus Decreased amniotic fluid Small lungs Enlarged kidneys Hydronephrosis Enlarged bladder Club feet **Fig. 4.5.3.2B:** Effects of oligohydramnios on various organ systems	Too little amniotic fluid early in pregnancy in cases of oligohydramnios can lead to compression of fetal organs, resulting in lung and limb defects, especially pressure deformities of feet such as clubfeet. The fetus is likely to have enlarged kidneys (hydronephrosis) and an enlarged bladder.	Management of cases of oligohydramnios has been described in 4.5.3.2A.

4.6: PRETERM BABY

4.6.1: Photograph of a Preterm Baby Born at Thirty Weeks of Gestation

Picture	Medical/Surgical Description	Management/Clinical Highlights
Fig. 4.6.1: Photograph of a preterm baby born at 30 weeks of gestation	Figure 4.6.1 shows photograph of a preterm baby born at 30 weeks of gestation weighing about 1 kg. The preterm baby is usually deficient in subcutaneous fat. As a result, the baby's skin appears pink in color, feels very thin and can easily wrinkle. The preterm baby's head circumference may exceed the waist circumference.	Birthweight of a normal term infant varies from 2,500 g to 3,999 g. Most preterm babies may be of low weight. Low birthweight can be defined as weight less than 2,500 g. Length of a preterm baby may be less than 47 cm.

4.6.2: Dubowitz (Ballard) Examination for Newborn

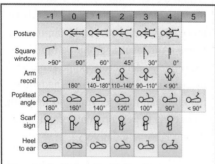

Picture	Medical/Surgical Description	Management/Clinical Highlights
Fig. 4.6.2: Dubowitz (Ballard) examination for newborn	Dubowitz (Ballard) examination is used for assessing fetal maturity based on the physical characteristics as well as the maturity of neuromuscular system. Points are given for each parameter, which is assessed. Low scores (–1 or 0) are given in case of extreme prematurity. High scores (4, 5) are given in case of postmaturity.	Physical characteristics, which are assessed, include parameters such as skin texture, lanugo hair, planter creases, breasts, eyes and ear, and appearance of the genitalia. Assessment of neuromuscular maturity includes evaluation of parameters such as posture, square window (flexion of baby's hand toward the wrist); arm recoil (angle of recoil following very brief extension of the upper extremity); heel to ear movement (passive resistance to extension of posterior hip flexor muscles); popliteal angle (resistance of baby's knee to extension) and scarf sign (how far the elbow can be moved across the baby's chest).

4.6.3: Clinical Features of a Newborn Preterm Baby in Comparison to a Term Baby (A to G)

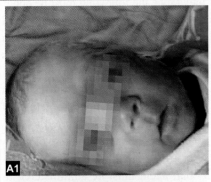

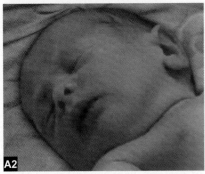

Figs 4.6.3 (A1 and A2): Facial appearance in a preterm newborn baby (upper) in comparison to a term baby (lower)

Figures 4.6.3 (A1 and A2) show facial appearance in a newborn preterm baby in comparison to a term baby. Premature/preterm birth refers to the birth of baby prior to 37 weeks of gestation. Since by that time many of the fetal organ systems may have not completely developed, the baby may have to face many physiological challenges while transition from intrauterine to extrauterine environment. In a preterm child the general activity is poor, and neonatal reflexes are poor and sluggish. There may be generalized hypotonia.

The individual features of a preterm baby in comparison to a normal one are described in separate sections below.

Skin of the preterm baby appeared thin, red and shiny with minimal amount of subcutaneous fat.

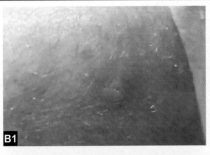

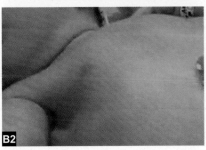

Figs 4.6.3 (B1 and B2): Breast nodule in a preterm newborn baby (upper) in comparison to a term baby (lower)
(*Courtesy*: Rajiv Khandelwal)

Breast nodule is small with size less than 5 mm in a preterm child. It may sometimes even be absent.

Steps for prevention of preterm birth are as follows:
- Identification and recognition of women at a high risk of preterm delivery
- Presence of infection such as urinary tract infection and lower genital tract infection must be treated.
- Administration of progestogens to reduce the incidence of preterm births must also be considered.

Picture	Medical/Surgical Description	Management/Clinical Highlights
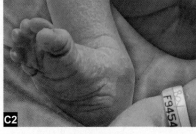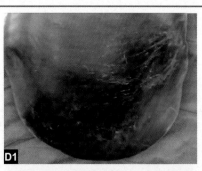**Figs 4.6.3 (C1 and C2):** Heel in a preterm baby (upper) in comparison to a term baby (lower) (*Courtesy*: Rajiv Khandelwal)	The entire sole is not covered with creases in case of a preterm child. Creases on the heel may be entirely absent or present only on the anterior one-third in the preterm babies. The entire sole is covered with creases in case of a term child.	In cases the preterm birth appears inevitable, the following must be done: • Glucocorticoids must be administered to enhance the fetal lung maturity in case of pregnancies less than 34 weeks gestation. • Administration of tocolytics must be considered until the effect of glucocorticoids has occurred. • In case of premature rupture of membranes, a broad-spectrum antimicrobial agent must be administered to prevent chorioamnionitis.
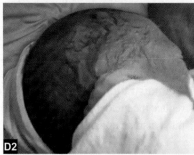**Figs 4.6.3 (D1 and D2):** Hair of a preterm baby (upper) in comparison to a term baby (lower) (*Courtesy*: Rajiv Khandelwal)	Scalp hair in a newborn preterm baby is fine, wooly and fuzzy whereas it is firmer in case of a term child.	Intrapartum management in cases of preterm babies comprises of the following steps: • Continuous electronic fetal heart rate monitoring • Broad-spectrum antibiotics such as ampicillin or penicillin G may be administered IV every 6 hourly until delivery. • Delivery should be preferably conducted in a tertiary care unit.

Picture	Medical/Surgical Description	Management/Clinical Highlights
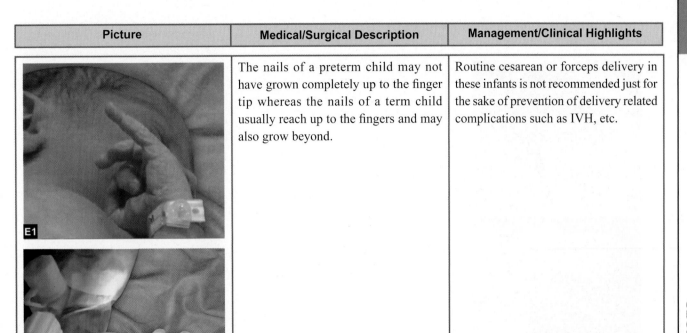 **Figs 4.6.3 (E1 and E2):** Nails of a preterm baby (upper) in comparison to a term baby (lower) (*Courtesy*: Rajiv Khandelwal)	The nails of a preterm child may not have grown completely up to the finger tip whereas the nails of a term child usually reach up to the fingers and may also grow beyond.	Routine cesarean or forceps delivery in these infants is not recommended just for the sake of prevention of delivery related complications such as IVH, etc.
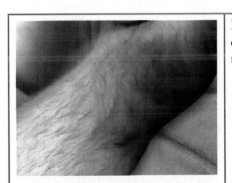 **Fig. 4.6.3F:** Presence of lanugo hair on the leg in a preterm baby (*Courtesy*: Rajiv Khandelwal)	In a preterm baby, the lanugo or fine downy hair are plentiful and may cover the entire body parts.	Following the delivery of the baby, the following steps must be taken: • Measures must be taken to clear the airways and initiate breathing. • Care of umbilical cord, eyes and administration of vitamin K should be done similar to the way done in a term baby. • Special consideration must be given toward the maintenance of body's thermal control, and monitoring of fetal heart rate and respiration. • Since such infants are at a risk of hypoglycemia, early feeding must be initiated.

Picture	Medical/Surgical Description	Management/Clinical Highlights
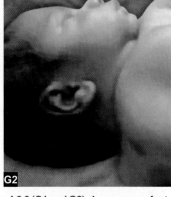 **Figs 4.6.3 (G1 and G2):** Appearance of external ear in a preterm baby (upper) in comparison to a term baby (lower) (*Courtesy*: Rajiv Khandelwal)	In a preterm child, the pinna of the ear is soft and pliable with no cartilage present. In case of a term infant, the ear cartilage is firm and well shaped.	All preterm infants having a period of gestation less than 35 weeks or birthweight less than 1,500 g must be admitted to the nursery. Infants with birth asphyxia and respiratory distress must also be admitted to the nursery. Oxygen therapy and/or mechanical ventilation may be considered in these babies.

4.6.4: Complications of Prematurity (A to D)

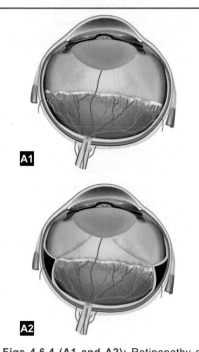 **Figs 4.6.4 (A1 and A2):** Retinopathy of prematurity: (A1) Stage 3; (A2) Stage 4	In the retinopathy of prematurity (ROP), there occurs neovascularization of blood vessels from the retina toward the center of eye. ROP is usually associated with low gestational age, low birthweight and/or prolonged exposure to oxygen. ROP can be divided into five stages. In stages 1 and 2, there is mild proliferation of blood vessels. With more advanced disease, there is enlargement and twisting of blood vessels. In the most advanced stage (stage 4 and 5), there occurs retinal detachment. Untreated advanced cases may at times result in blindness.	Retinopathy of prematurity is usually diagnosed by retinal examination with indirect ophthalmoscopy. Currently, no method is available which is likely to prevent the occurrence of ROP. Laser photocoagulation for destruction of avascular area of retina is the preferred treatment modality of choice for ROP. Cryotherapy is another mode of treatment, which can commonly be employed. Stage 1 and 2 ROP usually get better on their own. Scleral buckling and/or vitrectomy may be considered for advanced (stage 4 and 5) ROP. Intravitreal injection of bevacizumab has also been shown to be effective in the advanced cases of ROP.

Picture	Medical/Surgical Description	Management/Clinical Highlights
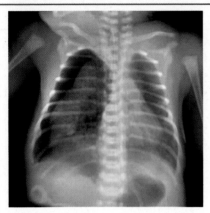 **Fig. 4.6.4B:** Respiratory distress syndrome	The adjacent X-ray image is of a newborn preterm baby, 2 days after birth. The image shows tension pneumothorax on right side with collapsed lung. As a result, the mediastinum is pushed toward the left side. Nasogastric tube, which has been inserted in the esophagus, can also be visualized. Based on the findings of clinical examination and various investigations, diagnosis of respiratory distress syndrome was made. Babies with respiratory distress syndrome lack a protein surfactant, which normally prevents the lung alveoli from collapsing. Administration of corticosteroids in cases of anticipated preterm delivery may help in promoting surfactant synthesis.	Treatment involves the following: • Baby should be admitted in neonatal intensive care unit and placed in a warm incubator with high humidity. • Treatment with a lung surfactant may be required. • Oxygen therapy with continuous positive airway pressure to deliver pressurized air to the baby's lungs • Mechanical breathing assistance • Intravenous administration of sodium bicarbonate for correction of acidosis • Correction of hypovolemia and electrolyte imbalance • Maintenance of nutrition through intragastric feeding.
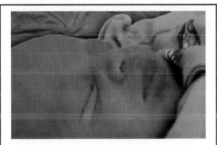 **Fig. 4.6.4C:** Physiological jaundice in the newborn baby (*Courtesy*: Rajiv Khandelwal)	Preterm babies are more likely to develop jaundice than the full-term babies because their livers are immature and may not be able to remove bilirubin efficiently from the blood. Presence of high levels of unconjugated bilirubin may result in the development of physiological jaundice, a type of nonhemolytic jaundice (usually with unconjugated bilirubin levels > 12 mg/dL). High levels of unconjugated bilirubin (> 20 mg/dL) may cause bilirubin staining of the basal ganglia and hippocampus, resulting in kernicterus.	Physiological jaundice usually appears by 2nd or 3rd day of life and disappears on its own by 7th−10th day of life. Therefore, no treatment is required in most cases. Careful observation is however required in preterm babies. If the unconjugated bilirubin levels rise beyond the critical levels (> 20 mg/dL), exchange transfusion may be required to prevent the development of kernicterus. Serum bilirubin levels must be measured at 24 hours of age with follow-up estimates done every 12−24 hours, till the levels stabilize. In case treatment is required, use of phototherapy and/or phenobarbitone is sufficient in most of the cases.
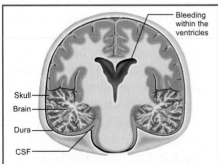 **Fig. 4.6.4D:** Intraventricular hemorrhage	Intraventricular hemorrhage usually develops within 72 hours of birth. Small hemorrhages in the germinal matrix usually resolve on their own without causing any impairment.	Severity of IVH can be assessed with the help of ultrasound and CT scan. Administration of corticosteroids, 24 hours prior to delivery can help to prevent or reduce the incidence of IVH. Avoiding significant hypoxia before and after delivery is of great importance in the prevention of IVH. Presently there is little evidence that routine cesarean delivery for preterm infants in cephalic presentation is likely to reduce the incidence of IVH.

Picture	Medical/Surgical Description	Management/Clinical Highlights

4.6.5: Management of Preterm Baby (A and B)

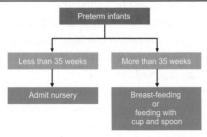

Fig. 4.6.5A: Algorithm for management of preterm baby

In early preterm babies (< 35 weeks) or with fetal weight less than 1,500 g, the baby must be admitted to the nursery. Infants with birth asphyxia and respiratory distress must also be admitted to the nursery. Wherever possible, early breast-feeding must be initiated. If breast milk is not available, consideration must be toward using appropriate preterm formula milk until the breast milk becomes available.

Considerations must be given to the following:
- Thermal regulation
- Monitoring of fetal heart rate and respiration
- Oxygen therapy
- Feeding the infant.

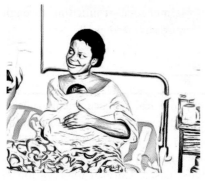

Fig. 4.6.5B: Kangaroo care
(*Source*: Computerized generation of image)

Kangaroo care or promoting skin-to-skin contact between the mother and the baby is a technique commonly used for taking care of preterm babies in settings with limited resources. In this method, the baby wearing only a diaper and with its head covered is placed in a flexed position, with direct skin-to-skin contact over the bare chest of an adult, mother (most commonly) or father or some other close relative. The baby is secured in position by wrapping it with the help of a stretchy cloth or wrap material.

Not only does this method promote physiological and psychological bonding between the parent and the child, it also promotes breast-feeding and lactation. It also helps in regulating the newborn's temperature, thereby preventing hypothermia.

4.7: POST-TERM PREGNANCY

4.7.1: Features of a Post-term Baby

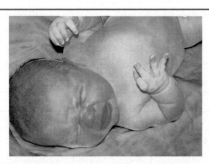

Fig. 4.7.1: Post-term macrosomic baby
(*Courtesy*: Rajiv Khandelwal)

Postdated pregnancy is the one, which has extended beyond the gestational age of 42 weeks starting from the day one of last menstrual period. Accurate dating of pregnancy is vital for the diagnosis of prolonged pregnancy.

Management of post-term pregnancy comprises of the following steps:
- Accurate assessment of gestational age in early pregnancy
- Antepartum fetal surveillance: This must be initiated between 41 weeks and 42 weeks of gestation, and can be initiated with the help of tests such as NST with AFI and/or BPP.
- Initiating delivery if the labor does not occur spontaneously: Delivery is recommended when the risks to the fetus due to continuation of pregnancy are greater than those which would be faced by the neonate after birth.

4.7.2: Management of Post-term Baby (A and B)

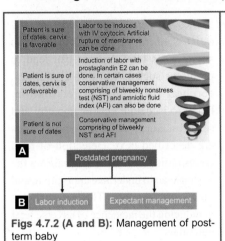

Figs 4.7.2 (A and B): Management of post-term baby

Two management options can be mainly employed in cases of post-term babies: labor induction or expectant management. Prior to any decision, it is important to establish the patient's accurate gestational age.

If the cervix is ripe, labor can be induced with help of oxytocin. In case of unripe cervix, it can be ripened with help of prostaglandins (PGE2). Expectant management includes antepartum fetal surveillance with twice weekly NST, BPP, etc.

4.7.3: Complications of Post-term Pregnancy

4.7.3.1: Consequences of a Post-term Pregnancy (A and B)

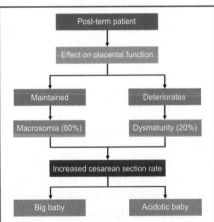

Fig. 4.7.3.1A: Consequences of post-term pregnancy on placental function

In case of postdated pregnancy if the placental function remains maintained, it results in a macrosomic baby. In case the deterioration of placental function occurs, it is likely to result in fetal distress and/or acidosis.

For the conditions, like fetal macrosomia as well as fetal acidosis/fetal distress, cesarean section is most commonly performed.

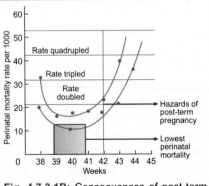

Fig. 4.7.3.1B: Consequences of post-term pregnancy on perinatal outcome

This graph illustrates the effect of post-term pregnancy on maternal and fetal outcome. With an increase or decrease in the duration of pregnancy on weekly basis, the perinatal mortality increases exponentially.

At 42 weeks of gestation, the risk of perinatal mortality is double of that at 40 weeks. Lowest perinatal mortality is between 39 weeks and 41 weeks. Both in cases of preterm and post-term pregnancy, the rate of perinatal mortality and morbidity increases exponentially.

4.7.3.2: Fetal Distress (A to F)

Picture	Medical/Surgical Description	Management/Clinical Highlights
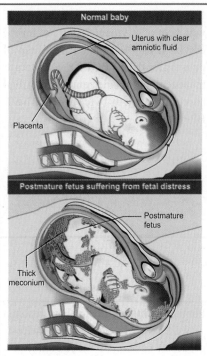 **Fig. 4.7.3.2A:** Postmaturity as a cause of fetal distress	Fetal distress indicates intrauterine fetal compromise implying that the fetus is at risk. Postmaturity as a cause of fetal distress is illustrated in the adjacent figure. Fetal distress during labor is assessed mainly on the basis of two parameters: fetal heart rate pattern and the presence or absence of meconium in the liquor.	Babies with fetal distress are generally delivered in good health, but in some cases fetal distress can lead to problems such as learning disabilities, cerebral palsy, mental retardation, hypoxic ischemic encephalopathy and seizures. Some of these complications are described next. Detection of fetal compromise at an early stage allows the obstetrician to undertake appropriate and timely interventions. This greatly helps in reducing the incidence of adverse fetal outcomes.
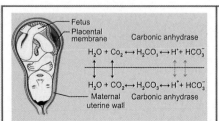 **Fig. 4.7.3.2B:** Biochemical abnormalities in fetal distress	Biochemical evidence of fetal distress in the form of abnormal fetal acid-base balance may sometimes also be observed. This has been illustrated in the adjacent figure.	Placenta plays an important role in maintaining the acid-base balance in the fetus by allowing free passage of H_2O and CO_2. Combination of CO_2 and H_2O results in formation of carbonic acid under the action of the enzyme carbonic anhydrase. Under the action of the same enzyme, carbonic acid dissociates to form hydrogen (H^+) and bicarbonate (HCO_3^-) ions. In presence of hypoxia, initially there is accumulation of CO_2 due to reduced exchange of gases in the fetal blood, resulting in the development of respiratory acidosis. Later, as the hypoxic insult continues there is accumulation of lactic acid and hydrogen ions, and deficiency of bicarbonate ions resulting in the development of metabolic acidosis.

Picture	Medical/Surgical Description	Management/Clinical Highlights
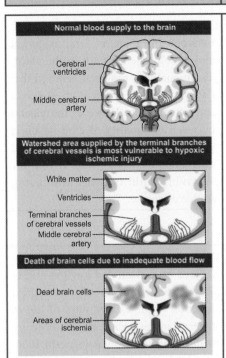 **Fig. 4.7.3.2C:** Mechanism of brain injury	Mechanism of brain injury as a result of hypoxia due to fetal distress is illustrated in Figure 4.7.3.2C. Often, this injury may involve the motor cortex, resulting in the development of spasticity in upper and lower extremities. Injury to the deeper brain substance is rare and may follow a severe hypoxic/hypotensive insult.	In the term fetus, hypoxic injury typically occurs in the subcortical white matter and cerebral cortex. These represent the "watershed" areas supplied by the terminal branches of the cerebral vessels and hence are at the highest risk of ischemic injury.
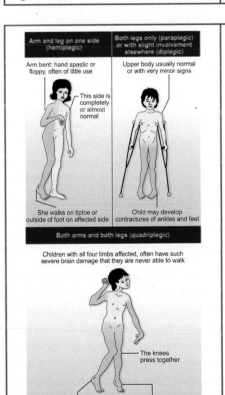 **Fig. 4.7.3.2D:** Types of spastic cerebral palsy	Cerebral palsy (CP) is another complication thought to be related to fetal distress. Mutch et al. (1992) has defined cerebral palsy as an umbrella term covering a group of nonprogressive, but often changing, motor impairment syndromes secondary to lesions or anomalies of the brain arising in the early stages of development. Cerebral palsies are most commonly classified on the basis of the motor abnormality as well as the diagnosed movement disorders present. Cerebral palsies can be most commonly classified into three types: spastic type, ataxic type and athetoid type.	Spastic type of CP is characterized by development of increased tone or tension in a muscle due to an insult to the cerebral cortex. Spastic CP also limits stretching of muscles in daily activities, and causes the development of muscle and joint deformities. As shown in the Figure 4.7.3.2D, depending on the part of the body affected, spastic type of CP can be hemiplegic (both arm and leg on one side of the body are affected), diplegic (both legs are affected) or quadriplegic (all four limbs are affected).

Picture	Medical/Surgical Description	Management/Clinical Highlights
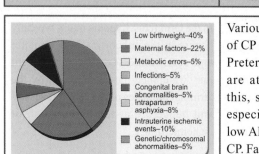 **Fig. 4.7.3.2E:** Risk factors for cerebral palsy	Various risk factors for development of CP are described in Figure 4.7.3.2E. Preterm and low birthweight babies are at a high risk for CP. Besides this, several other obstetric factors, especially intrapartum asphyxia and low APGAR scores are associated with CP. Factors like infections, inborn errors of metabolism, chromosomal/genetic abnormalities are also responsible for producing CP.	There appears to be an association between intrapartum fetal asphyxia and development of CP in the child. Traditionally, it has been believed that CP is related to intrapartum asphyxia and difficult labor. However, the relation between the quality of care which is given to a mother during labor and delivery and the risk of CP in her surviving child is still a continuing source of debate.
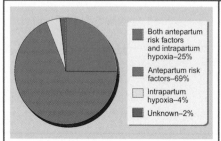 **Fig. 4.7.3.2F:** Risk factors for hypoxic-ischemic encephalopathy	Hypoxic-ischemic encephalopathy (HIE) is a complication related to intrapartum asphyxia and may cause acute or subacute brain injury. Various risk factors for development of HIE are shown in Figure 4.7.3.2F. Antepartum risk factors (preeclampsia, abruption placenta, maternal pyrexia, etc.) have been found to be associated with nearly 70% cases of HIE. On the other hand, intrapartum hypoxia has been shown to account for only a small proportion of newborn encephalopathy (about 4%), whereas a combination of both antepartum risk factors and intrapartum hypoxia has been found to be responsible for nearly 25% cases of HIE.	Neonatal encephalopathy is clinically defined by Nelson and Leviton (1991) as syndrome of disturbed neurological function in the earliest days of life in the term infant, manifested by difficulty in initiating and maintaining respiration, depression of tone and reflexes, subnormal level of consciousness, and often by seizures. Criterion for the diagnosis of HIE is as follows: • Profound metabolic or mixed acidemia (pH < 7.00) • Persistence of an APGAR score of 0–3 for longer than 5 minutes after birth • Neonatal neurologic sequelae (e.g. seizures, coma, hypotonia) • Multiple organ involvement (e.g. kidney, lungs, liver, heart, intestines, etc.)

4.7.3.3: Macrosomia

Picture	Medical/Surgical Description	Management/Clinical Highlights
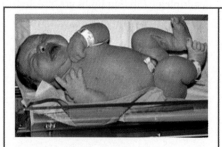 **Fig. 4.7.3.3:** Macrosomia (*Courtesy*: Rajiv Khandelwal)	Macrosomia can be defined as expected fetal weight between 90–95 percentile of gestational age. Birthweight is usually more than 4,000–4,500 g or greater. Besides postdated pregnancy, other risk factors for development of macrosomia include gestational diabetes mellitus, prolonged gestation, maternal obesity, excessive pregnancy weight gain, etc.	Presently there is no method for predicting macrosomia. The woman must be posted for an elective cesarean delivery in case the expected fetal weight is more than 4,500 g in a diabetic mother and more than 5,000 g in a nondiabetic mother. Early induction has been tried in some cases. However, it is associated with an increased rate of failed induction.

| Picture | Medical/Surgical Description | Management/Clinical Highlights |

4.7.3.4: Meconium Aspiration Syndrome (A to E)

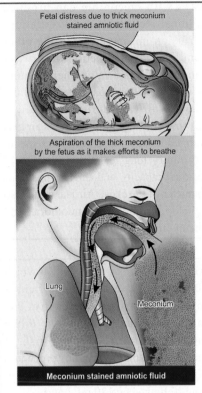

Fig. 4.7.3.4A: Aspiration of meconium by the newborn baby as it makes efforts to breathe

It is believed that hypoxia and acidemia stimulate the parasympathetic system. This causes the anal sphincter to relax, whilst at the same time increasing the production of motilin, which promotes intestinal peristalsis resulting in passage of meconium into the amniotic cavity. Postnatal inhalation can occur late in the second stage or immediately after delivery if the infant gasps or makes breathing movements while the oropharynx, nasopharynx or trachea contains meconium stained liquor.

Meconium aspiration syndrome (MAS) is a disease of term and post-term infants, and its severity is linked to coexisting fetal asphyxia.

Meconium has a number of adverse effects on the neonatal lung, which may ultimately result in the development of MAS that can lead to respiratory failure and hypoxemia.

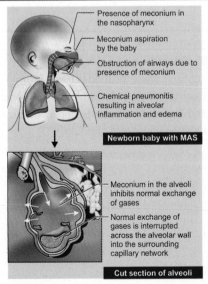

Fig. 4.7.3.4B: Consequences of meconium aspiration

The ways through which presence of meconium inside the fetal lungs can result in adverse effects are shown in Figure 4.7.3B.

Aspiration of meconium can result in mechanical blockage of airways, chemical irritation and secondary bacterial infection. Chemical irritation may produce an inflammatory reaction resulting in pneumonitis, alveolar collapse and cell necrosis. This can eventually result in respiratory failure and hypoxemia.

Picture	Medical/Surgical Description	Management/Clinical Highlights
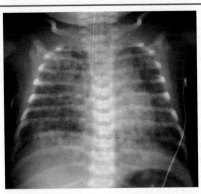 **Fig. 4.7.3.4C:** Chest X-ray of a 2-days-old infant showing signs of meconium aspiration syndrome	Figure 4.7.3.4C shows the classic radiographic findings of MAS namely, atelectasis, pneumothorax, and hyperexpanded areas of the lung.	Complete obstruction of small airways with meconium can produce regional atelectasis and ventilation-perfusion mismatches. On the other hand, partial obstruction of airways can create a ball valve phenomenon, in which air flows past the meconium into the airways during inspiration. However during expiration, this air gets trapped distally, leading to increase in expiratory lung resistance, functional residual capacity, and anterior-posterior diameter of the chest. Air leaks can also develop leading to pneumothorax and pneumomediastinum.
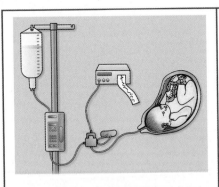 **Fig. 4.7.3.4D:** The procedure of amnioinfusion	The technique of amnioinfusion as described by Weismiller is outlined below: • Attach the drip administration set to a bottle of normal saline or Ringer's lactate at one end and to the sterile catheter at the other end. • While maintaining strict aseptic precautions, the tip of the catheter must be passed through the cervix into the uterine cavity, preferably beyond the presenting part and the saline must be allowed to run through the system.	Amnioinfusion is a procedure in which 500–1,000 mL of an isotonic fluid is infused into the uterine cavity. The infusion of fluid is thought to dilute meconium and reduce the risk of meconium aspiration. In this procedure 500 mL of saline is infused over half an hour, followed by 180 mL hourly.
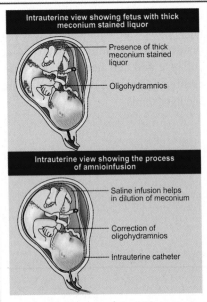 **Fig. 4.7.3.4E:** Intrauterine view of the procedure of amnioinfusion	The process of amnioinfusion has been described in 4.7.3.4D. In the original technique described by Weismiller (1998), saline was infused through an intrauterine pressure catheter using an infusion pump. However, this expensive equipment is beyond the reach of most hospitals in the developing world. In this part of the world amnioinfusion is mainly done by equipment like inexpensive infant feeding tubes and gravity infusion. Intrauterine view of the procedure of amnioinfusion is described in Figure 4.7.3.4E.	Evaluation of fetal wellbeing must continue while the fluid is being infused. During the procedure, uterine pressure and fetal heart rate (via scalp electrode) must be monitored constantly.

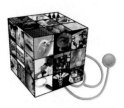

EVIDENCE-BASED BREAKTHROUGH FACTS

1. USE OF VAGINAL VS. INTRAMUSCULAR PROGESTERONE FOR PREVENTION OF PRETERM LABOR

In a prospective randomized trial, vaginal progesterone (90 mg of vaginal progesterone gel once daily) has been found to be more effective than intramuscular progesterone (250 mg of intramuscular progesterone weekly) for the prevention of preterm birth and is also associated with fewer side-effects. Treatment is begun between 14 and 18 weeks gestation and continued until 36 complete weeks of gestation, delivery or the occurrence of premature rupture of membranes.

Source: Maher MA, Abdelaziz, Ellaithty M, et al. Prevention of preterm birth: a randomized trial of vaginal compared to intramuscular progesterone. Acta Obstet Gynecol Scand. 2012. [Epub ahead of print].

2. HEALTH CONSEQUENCES OF PROPHYLACTIC EXPOSURE TO ANTENATAL CORTICOSTEROIDS AMONG CHILDREN BORN LATE PRETERM

Infants born after 34 weeks of gestation seem to benefit from earlier antenatal corticosteroid administration because this strategy is associated with reduced risks of respiratory distress syndrome. However, the treatment with antenatal corticosteroids has been shown to be less beneficial for term infants, because this has been found to be associated with an increased risk of low APGAR scores.

Source: Eriksson L, Haglund B, Ewald U, et al. Health consequences of prophylactic exposure to antenatal corticosteroids among children born late preterm or term. Acta Obstet Gynecol Scand. 2012. [Epub ahead of print]

3. USE OF TOCOLYTIC THERAPY FOR PRETERM DELIVERY

Tocolytic agents such as prostaglandin inhibitors and calcium channel blockers have been found to be the most effective, having the highest probability for delaying delivery and improving neonatal and maternal outcomes.

Source: Haas DM, Caldwell DM, Kirkpatrick P, et al. Tocolytic therapy for preterm delivery: systematic review and network meta-analysis. BMJ. 2012;345:e6226.

4. PESSARY FOR SHORT CERVIX

Use of cervical pessary is likely to prevent preterm birth amongst pregnant women with cervical length less than or equal to 25 mm at 20–23 weeks of gestation. However, presently the use of pessary has not been recommended as the treatment modality of choice in pregnant women with shortened cervical length.

Source: Goya M, Pratcorona L, Pesario Cervical para Evitar Prematuridad (PECEP) Trial Group, et al. Cervical pessary in pregnant women with a short cervix (PECEP): an open-label randomised controlled trial. Lancet. 2012;379(9828):1800-6.

5. DELAYED UMBILICAL CORD CLAMPING MAY HELP PREEMIES: ACOG

According to an opinion issued by ACOG Committee on Obstetric Practice, delay in clamping the umbilical cord by approximately 30–60 seconds is likely to improve outcomes amongst preterm infants by causing a slight increase in the blood volume. This is likely to reduce the requirement for blood transfusion and bring about a reduction in the incidence of intracranial hemorrhage amongst the preterm infants.

Source: The American College of Obstetricians and Gynaecologists Committee opinion. Timing of umbilical cord clamping after birth. Obstet Gynecol. 2012;120:1522-6.

The Committee Opinion is presently available online and is scheduled for publication in the December issue of Obstetrics and Gynecology.

6. PROGESTOGENS FOR PRETERM BIRTH PREVENTION

A systemic review and meta-analysis has shown that use of progestogens help prevent preterm birth when used in singleton pregnancies for women with a history of prior preterm births. However, there is limited evidence related to its effectiveness for prevention of preterm birth in case of multiple gestations.

Source: Likis FE, Edwards DR, Andrews JC, et al. Progestogens for preterm birth prevention: a systematic review and meta-analysis. Obstet Gynecol. 2012;120(4):897-907.

7. VAGINAL PROGESTERONE VERSUS CERVICAL CERCLAGE FOR THE PREVENTION OF PRETERM BIRTH IN WOMEN

An adjusted indirect meta-analysis of randomized controlled trials has shown that vaginal progesterone or cerclage are equally efficacious in the prevention of preterm birth in women with sonographic evidence of short cervix in the mid trimester, singleton gestation and history of previous preterm birth.

Source: Conde-Agudelo A, Romero R, Nicolaides K, et al. Vaginal progesterone vs cervical cerclage for the prevention of preterm birth in women with a sonographic short cervix, previous preterm birth, and singleton gestation: a systematic review and indirect comparison metaanalysis. Am J Obstet Gynecol. 2012;pii: S0002-9378(12)01977-1. doi: 10.1016/j.ajog.2012.10.877. [Epub ahead of print].

Obstetrics

Section 5

Medical Conditions During Pregnancy

SECTION 5 ❖ MEDICAL CONDITIONS DURING PREGNANCY

5.1: ANEMIA IN PREGNANCY

5.1.1: Iron Deficiency Anemia

5.1.1.1: Characteristics of Iron Deficiency Anemia in Pregnancy

Picture	Medical/Surgical Description	Management/Clinical Highlights
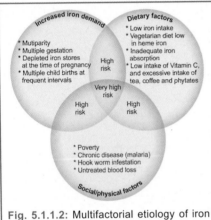 **Fig. 5.1.1.1:** Iron deficiency anemia	Anemia can be defined as reduction in circulating hemoglobin mass below the critical level. WHO defines anemia as presence of hemoglobin of less than 11 g/dL and hematocrit of less than 0.33 g/dL. Center of Disease Control (CDC, 1990) have defined anemia as hemoglobin levels below 11 g/dL in the pregnant woman in first and third trimester, and less than 10.5 g/dL in the second trimester.	Anemia due to deficiency of iron is common during pregnancy due to increased physiological requirement of pregnancy (1,000 g of iron), depleted iron stores and deficient dietary intake. Iron deficiency anemia is usually associated with high red cell distribution width (RDW > 15%) and low mean corpuscular volume (MCV < 80 fL). Treatment comprises of prescription of oral or parenteral iron preparations.

5.1.1.2: Multifactorial Etiology of Iron Deficiency Anemia During Pregnancy

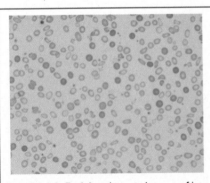 **Fig. 5.1.1.2:** Multifactorial etiology of iron deficiency anemia during pregnancy	Anemia in pregnancy has a multifactorial etiology. Interplay of various factors, such as increased iron demand, dietary factors and poor socioeconomic status play a role in the pathogenesis of anemia. Various other factors responsible for anemia during pregnancy include the following: • Prior history of menorrhagia • Multiple gestations • Vegetarian diet, low in meat • Chronic blood loss due to hookworm infestation, schistosomiasis, etc. • Chronic infection (e.g. malaria) • Chronic aspirin use	Treatment of the patient diagnosed with iron deficiency basically depends on the period of gestation (POG). If the POG is less than 30 completed weeks of gestation, oral iron preparations (containing 200–300 mg of elemental iron with 500 μg of folic acid) must be prescribed in divided doses. If the patient is not compliant with oral therapy or other causes for ineffective oral treatment are present, parenteral therapy may be considered. If POG is between 30 and 36 weeks, parenteral therapy must be administered. If the patient presents with severe anemia beyond 36 weeks, blood transfusion may be required.

5.1.1.3: Peripheral Smear in Case of Iron Deficiency Anemia

Picture	Medical/Surgical Description	Management/Clinical Highlights
Fig. 5.1.1.3: Peripheral smear in case of iron deficiency anemia	In case of iron deficiency anemia, peripheral smear of blood shows microcytic and hypochromic picture. There is presence of pale looking RBCs with large central vacuoles (hypochromic RBCs).	The peripheral smear shows the following features: • *Anisocytosis (abnormal size of cells)*: The RBCs are small and deformed (microcytosis). • *Poikilocytosis (abnormal shape of cells)*: Presence of pencil cells and target cells. There is presence of ring or pessary cells with central hypochromia (large central vacuoles).

5.1.2: Sickle Cell Anemia

5.1.2.1: Characteristic Features of Sickle Cell Anemia (A to C)

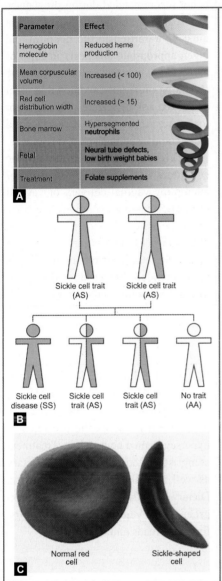

Parameter	Effect
Hemoglobin molecule	Reduced heme production
Mean corpuscular volume	Increased (< 100)
Red cell distribution width	Increased (> 15)
Bone marrow	Hypersegmented neutrophils
Fetal	Neural tube defects, low birth weight babies
Treatment	Folate supplements

A

Sickle cell trait (AS) — Sickle cell trait (AS)

Sickle cell disease (SS) — Sickle cell trait (AS) — Sickle cell trait (AS) — No trait (AA)

B

Normal red cell — Sickle-shaped cell

C

Figs 5.1.2.1 (A to C): (A) Characteristic features of sickle cell anemia; (B) Inheritence pattern of sickle cell anemia; (C) Development of abnormal sickle-shaped cells

Sickle cell disease belongs to a group of autosomal recessive disorders, which affect the structure of hemoglobin. Sickle cell anemia is a homozygous condition belonging to the spectrum of sickle cell disease, which is associated with the mutation of hemoglobin gene. This causes the RBCs to take an abnormal sickle or crescent shape, thereby delivering reduced supply of oxygen to the tissues. Moreover, the sickle cells are fragile and more prone to rupture, resulting in anemia.

Men and women with sickle cell disease should be encouraged to have hemoglobin status of themselves and their partners determined before embarking upon pregnancy. If identified as an "at risk" pregnancy, they should receive counseling about their reproductive options. The methods of preimplantation genetic diagnosis, prenatal diagnosis and termination of pregnancy must be discussed with the patients.

The following precautions must be taken in the antepartum period:
- The woman should be advised to avoid risk factors such as exposure to extreme temperatures, dehydration, overexertion, etc., which are likely to precipitate an acute sickling crisis.
- Women should be screened for pulmonary hypertension with echocardiography.
- Daily penicillin prophylaxis is given to all patients with sickle cell disease (in accordance with the guidelines for all hyposplenic patients).
- Women should be given Hemophilus influenza type b and conjugated meningococcal C vaccine as a single dose, if they have not received it as a part of primary vaccination.
- Pneumococcal vaccine should be given after every 5 years.
- Folic acid (5 mg) should be given once daily both preconceptionally and throughout the pregnancy.
- Hydroxycarbamide (hydroxyurea) should be stopped 3 months prior to conception due to the risk of teratogenicity.
- Iron supplementation needs to be given only if there is laboratory evidence of iron deficiency.
- Low-dose aspirin (75 mg) must be prescribed daily from 12 weeks of gestation to reduce the risk for developing preeclampsia.
- Women should receive prophylactic low-molecular weight heparin during each antenatal care (ANC) hospital admission to prevent the risk of thromboembolism.
- Serial fetal biometry for growth evaluation must be offered every 4 weeks starting from 24 weeks of gestation.

5.1.2.2: Peripheral Smear in Case of Sickle Cell Anemia

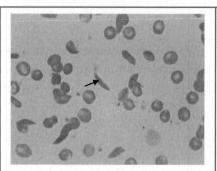

Fig. 5.1.2.2: Peripheral smear in case of sickle cell anemia (arrow points toward a sickle-shaped cell)

Peripheral smear in case of sickle cell anemia shows presence of crescent-shaped, long or target cells. There may be presence of characteristic sickle-shaped cells. If the patient is asplenic, there may be presence of RBCs containing nuclear material (Howell Jolly bodies).

Screening of the newborn for presence of sickle cell anemia has been introduced in the US. Children who are found to be positive undergo hemoglobin electrophoresis. Individuals homozygous for hemoglobin S (HbS) are recognized by the presence of a single band of HbS. Fetal hemoglobin may be less than 30%, with sickle cell hemoglobin being the predominant hemoglobin.

Routine prophylactic blood transfusion is not recommended during pregnancy. In case of acute painful crisis, the patient must be admitted to the hospital and given appropriate analgesia in form of paracetamol or weak opioids. Pethidine should be preferably avoided due to an associated risk of seizures. Requirement for fluids and oxygen must be assessed and they should be administered, if required.

Sickle cell anemia must not be considered as a contraindication for attempting vaginal delivery or vaginal birth after cesarean (section). Delivery should be preferably undertaken between 38 to 40 weeks of gestation. Continuous electronic fetal heart rate monitoring is recommended during labor due to an increased risk for fetal distress.

5.1.3: Megaloblastic Anemia

5.1.3.1: Characteristics of Folate Deficiency Anemia in Pregnancy

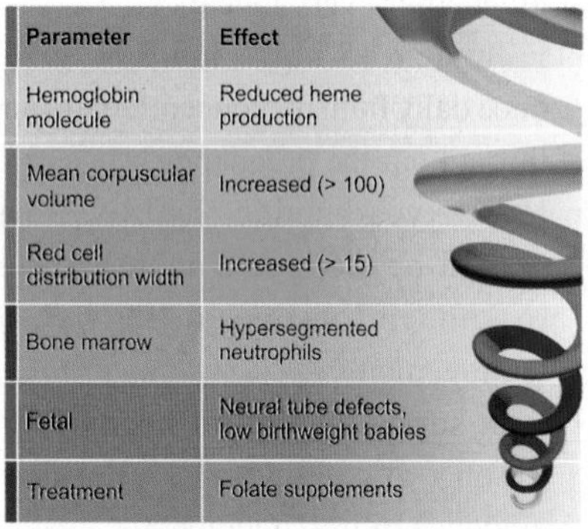

Parameter	Effect
Hemoglobin molecule	Reduced heme production
Mean corpuscular volume	Increased (> 100)
Red cell distribution width	Increased (> 15)
Bone marrow	Hypersegmented neutrophils
Fetal	Neural tube defects, low birthweight babies
Treatment	Folate supplements

Fig. 5.1.3.1: Characteristics of folate deficiency anemia in pregnancy

Folate deficiency is often associated with megaloblastic anemia, which is characterized by presence of macrocytes and megaloblasts, cells larger than normal in size. In megaloblastic anemia, similar to iron deficiency anemia, there is reduced heme production. The effect on the fetus in case of folate deficiency anemia in pregnancy can be in the form of neural tube defects and low birthweight babies.

In case of folate deficiency anemia, the MCV as well as the RDW is increased (MCV > 100 fL; RDW> 15%). Bone marrow shows the presence of hypersegmented neutrophils. Treatment comprises of administration of dietary as well as oral supplements of folate. Dietary sources of folate include dark-green leafy vegetables, citrus fruits, fortified breads and cereals.

5.1.3.2: Peripheral Smear in Case of Megaloblastic Anemia

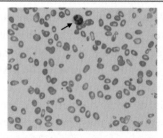

Fig. 5.1.3.2: Peripheral smear in case of megaloblastic anemia (arrow points toward a hypersegmented neutrophil)

Peripheral smear in case of megaloblastic anemia shows the following features:
- Presence of macrocytes and mega-loblasts
- Hypersegmentation of neutrophils
- Fully hemoglobinized RBCs.

Treatment of folate deficiency comprises of prescribing a folate rich diet (broccoli, asparagus, chickpeas, brussels sprouts, etc.) Oral folate supplements (400 µg daily) must be prescribed in the preconceptional as well as for the first 12 weeks of pregnancy.

Picture	Medical/Surgical Description	Management/Clinical Highlights

5.1.4: Thalassemia

5.1.4.1: Pathogenesis of β Thalassemia

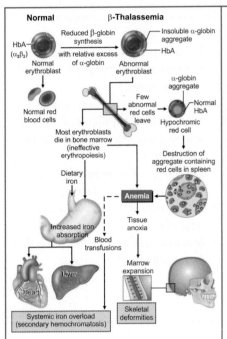

Fig. 5.1.4.1: Pathogenesis of β thalassemia

Thalassemia includes a group of genetically inherited disorders, which are characterized by impaired or defective production of one or more normal globin peptide chains. Abnormal synthesis of globin chains can result in ineffective erythropoiesis, hemolysis and varying degrees of anemia. Depending on whether the synthesis of α or β-chains is affected, thalassemia can be classified into two types: α-thalassemia or β-thalassemia.

Iron deficiency anemia has to be differentiated from other causes of hypochromic anemia including thalassemia and anemia due to chronic diseases.

Anemia due to thalassemia can be differentiated from other types of anemia on the basis of various parameters. Although RBC indices, such as MCV, mean corpuscular hemoglobin (MCH) and mean corpuscular hemoglobin concentration (MCHC) are reduced in proportion to the severity of anemia in cases of iron deficiency, these indices may be reduced to very low values (disproportionate to the severity of anemia) in cases of thalassemia.

Serum iron concentration is usually normal or increased in thalassemic syndromes, while it is usually low in iron deficiency anemia. Marrow examination and hemoglobin electrophoresis also help in differentiating between iron deficiency anemia and thalassemia by respectively showing normal bone marrow iron stores and increased proportions of Hb F and Hb A2 in cases with thalassemia.

5.1.4.2: Peripheral Smear in Case of Thalassemia

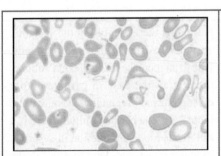

Fig. 5.1.4.2: Peripheral smear in case of thalassemia

Peripheral smear in case of thalassemia shows microcytic hypochromic anemia, which is similar to that seen in iron deficiency anemia (5.1.1.3).

Various parameters for differentiating iron deficiency anemia from thalassemia are discussed in 5.1.4.1. Treatment of moderate to severe anemia comprises of transfusion of red cells. Repeated blood transfusions may be required to maintain healthy supply of red cells. Chelation therapy with desferrioxamine may be required to remove excessive iron, which has accumulated in the body as a result of iron overload. Folic acid supplements are also often prescribed.

5.1.5: Prevention of Anemia

5.1.5.1: Healthy Diet (A and B)

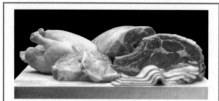

Fig. 5.1.5.1A: Sources of heme iron

Consumption of a healthy diet containing iron-rich food is important for treatment and prevention of anemia. Two types of iron are present in food: heme iron and non-heme iron. Heme iron is principally found in animal products and is mainly derived from myoglobin and hemoglobin present in meat (beef, lamb, poultry, fish, etc). Heme iron is better absorbed (up to 35% more) than non-heme iron. However heme iron forms smaller fraction of the diet. Sources of heme iron include animal blood, flesh and viscera. The daily requirement of iron in pregnant women is about 27 mg per day. These women can benefit from consumption of heme iron rich food sources.

Prevention of anemia comprises of the following steps:
- Routine determination of hemoglobin or hematocrit, starting from the time of adolescence.
- Routine screening for anemia and provision of supplements to adolescent girls, starting right from the school days.
- Encouraging consumption of diet containing iron-rich foods.
- Fortification of widely consumed food with iron.
- Management of endemic infection (e.g. malaria).

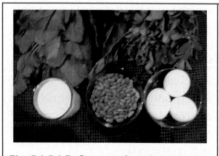

Fig. 5.1.5.1 B: Sources of non-heme iron

Non-heme iron is mainly found in the plant products. During the course of pregnancy as the iron stores decrease, the absorption of dietary non-heme iron increases. Non-heme iron is mostly available in ferric form, and needs to be reduced to ferrous form for absorption. Therefore, absorption of non-heme iron is less than that of heme iron.

Non-heme sources of iron include cereals, seeds, vegetables, milk and eggs. Non-heme iron forms 60% of iron in animal food (remaining 40% of iron in animal food is heme iron) and all iron in vegetarian food. Since the absorption of non-heme iron is less than heme iron, iron recommendations in vegetarians are higher than those in nonvegetarians.

5.2: HYPERTENSIVE DISORDERS OF PREGNANCY

5.2.1: Changes in Blood Pressure During Normal Pregnancy

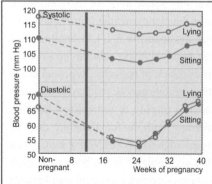

Fig. 5.2.1: Changes in blood pressure during normal pregnancy

Preeclampsia can be considered as a potentially serious disorder, which is characterized by development of high BP (> 140/90 mm Hg) and proteinuria (> 300 mg/L or >1 + on the dipstick) after the 20th week of gestation in a previously normotensive woman. The condition usually disappears following the delivery of the baby.

Normally, there is a fall in the systemic vascular resistance during pregnancy. Due to an increase in the plasma volume, there is an increase in cardiac output during normal pregnancy. Despite of an increase in the cardiac output, there is a fall in BP due to a reduction in systemic vascular resistance. Due to a fall in the systemic vascular resistance there is an overall fall in the diastolic pressure and mean arterial pressure during pregnancy.

5.2.2: Pathogenesis of Preeclampsia (A and B)

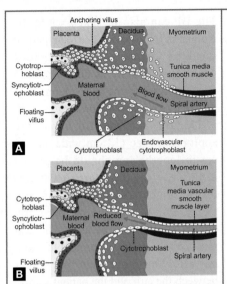

Figs 5.2.2 (A and B): Inadequate trophoblastic invasion: (A) Trophoblastic invasion of spiral arterioles in normal pregnancy; (B) Reduced trophoblastic invasion of spiral vessels in preeclampsia

The exact pathophysiology of preeclampsia is not yet understood. An important mechanism behind the development of preeclampsia is inadequate trophoblastic invasion of the spiral arterioles (as shown in the figure). The maternal arterioles are the main source of blood supply to the fetus and inadequate trophoblastic invasion of these spiral vessels can interfere with normal villous development, resulting in placental insufficiency. Some of the other likely causes of preeclampsia are as follows:

Maternal inflammatory response: This could be due to cytokines such as tumor necrosis factor (TNF-α) and interleukins.

Hereditary factors: The exact genetic defect or preeclampsia gene has not yet been identified.

Immunological factors: Risk of development of preeclampsia is especially decreased in when there is impairment in the production of blocking antibodies to various placental antigenic sites.

Endothelial dysfunction and vasospasm: In preeclampsia, there is also increased production of vasoconstrictors like thromboxane A2 and reduced production of vasodilatory prostaglandins like prostacyclins.

Clinically, preeclampsia can be classified as "severe" when severe hypertension, severe proteinuria or other signs/symptoms of end-organ injury are present. Some indicators of severe preeclampsia during pregnancy include the following:

- Diastolic BP $\geq$ 110 mm Hg and/or systolic BP $\geq$ 160 mm Hg
- Proteinuria 2 + or more on the dipstick
- Presence of symptoms like headache, visual disturbances, oliguria (urine volume $\leq$ 500 mL/24 hours), convulsions, etc.
- Evidence of HELLP syndrome: hemolysis, elevated liver enzyme levels and a low platelet count.

In the absence of any of these findings, preeclampsia can be classified as "mild".

5.2.3: Clinical Features of Preeclampsia

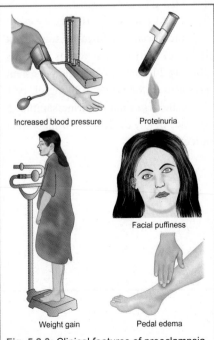

Increased blood pressure

Proteinuria

Weight gain

Facial puffiness

Pedal edema

Fig. 5.2.3: Clinical features of preeclampsia

As previously discussed, the two characteristic features of preeclampsia are development of high BP (> 140/90 mm Hg) and proteinuria (> 300 mg/L or >1 + on the dipstick). Differentiation between mild and severe eclampsia has been previously described. Other clinical features which may be sometimes observed in cases of preeclampsia, but are not diagnostic of preeclampsia include edema of the hands and face, and significant weight gain.

Edema of the hands and face: Since edema is a universal finding in pregnancy, it is not considered as a criterion for diagnosing preeclampsia.

Weight gain: Weight gain of more than 2 pounds per week or 6 pounds in a month or a sudden weight gain over 1–2 days can be considered as significant.

Management of preeclampsia depends on whether the condition is mild or severe. In mild cases of preeclampsia, if the maternal condition stabilizes and the fetal condition remains good, pregnancy must be continued until term. The patient may undergo a normal vaginal delivery unless there is some obstetric indication for cesarean delivery. In cases of severe preeclampsia, the maternal condition must be stabilized first, following which the fetal assessment is done. If the maternal condition does not stabilize or there is occurrence of fetal distress, the patient must be delivered by the fastest route. If the maternal condition stabilizes, the further course of action depends on the POG. In case of POG between 26 weeks and 34 weeks, conservative management must be done until fetal maturity has been reached.

5.2.4: Correct Method of Measuring Blood Pressure

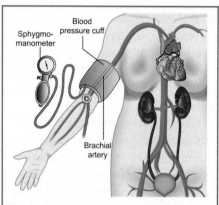

Fig. 5.2.4: Method of measuring BP correctly

Presence of increased BP (> 140/90 mm Hg) for the first time during pregnancy, after 20 weeks of gestation, is one of the diagnostic features of preeclampsia. When taking BP, the woman should lie on her right side with a 30° lateral tilt or she can be made to sit on a chair.

The right upper arm must be used and the arm must be taken out of the sleeve. The BP should be taken after 5 minutes of rest. Royal College of Obstetricians and Gynaecologists recommends that mercury sphygmomanometers should be used at least to establish baseline BP as a reference, since this reading is supposed to be most accurate.

The BP can also be taken while the woman is lying on the bed. The patient should be advised not to lie on her back while taking her BP as this can give a false low reading due to development of supine hypotension syndrome.

The BP cuff should be of the appropriate size (12 cm wide and 35 cm in length) and should be placed at the level of the heart. A BP cuff that encompasses about 80% of arm length and 40% of the width of arm circumference must be used. The cuff must be applied firmly around the arm, not allowing more than one finger between the cuff and the patient's arm.

5.2.5: Method of Measuring Proteinuria Using Dipstick (A and B)

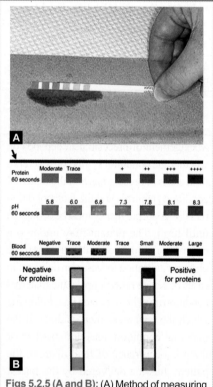

Figs 5.2.5 (A and B): (A) Method of measuring proteinuria using dipstick; (B) Measurement of proteinuria through visual assessment of dipstick

The usual screening test for proteinuria is visual assessment of dipstick or a reagent strip. Dipstick is a device in which a strip of paper impregnated with a reagent (used for testing proteins) is dipped into urine in order to measure the quantity of proteins present there in. The reagent strips for measuring proteins in the urine have the markings for "trace", 1+, 2+, etc. A reading of trace protein is relatively common and usually not a cause for concern. A 1+ dipstick measurement can be taken as evidence of proteinuria. However, this must be confirmed by a 24-hour urine collection for protein estimation.

Though visual dipstick assessment is associated with both false positive and false negative test results, this test is most commonly used for estimation of proteinuria. The approximate equivalence of the dipstick result with the amount of proteinuria is as follows:
1 + = 0.3 g/L; 2 + = 1 g/L;
3 + = 3 g/L; and 4 + = 10 g/L.

Proteinuria is defined as significant if the excretion of proteins exceeds 300 mg/24 hours or there is persistent presence of the protein (30 mg/dL or 1 + dipstick) in random urine sample in absence of any evidence of urinary tract infection.

5.3: GESTATIONAL DIABETES

5.3.1: Diabetic Diet (A and B)

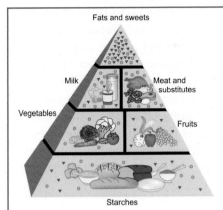

Fig. 5.3.1A: Diabetes food pyramid

The first line therapy for the women with gestational diabetes is exercise and diet therapy. Proper nutritional advice is one of the most important components of the care of women with gestational diabetes. The objective of nutritional treatment is to provide a healthy diet, which contains the necessary calories and nutrients, to both mother and the fetus without causing postprandial hyperglycemia. The meal plan for a diabetic individual can be based on the "Diabetes Food Pyramid" which is shown in the adjacent figure. The women should be advised to eat more from the groups at the bottom of the pyramid and less from the groups at the top.

This diabetes meal plan looks very much like the US Department of Agriculture's (USDA) food guide pyramid. Similar to the USDA's food guide pyramid, the diabetes food pyramid suggests that the individual must try to obtain the bulk of calories from fruits, vegetables, whole grains and low-fat dairy products. The food must be low in saturated fats, transfats, cholesterol, salt and added sugars. The diabetes food pyramid differs from the standard food guide pyramid in the way it groups different foods together. The diabetes food pyramid focuses on the way in which certain foods affect blood glucose levels. For example, in the standard pyramid, beans and legumes are grouped with meats, due to their protein content. In the diabetes pyramid, however, beans are grouped with starches, because they affect blood glucose in the same way that starchy foods do.

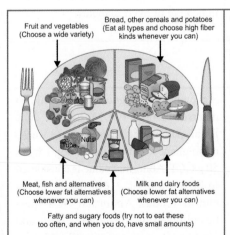

Fig. 5.3.1B: Components of a healthy diet for a diabetic patient

The blood glucose levels are of primary concern to people with diabetes. The healthy meal of a diabetic individual should comprise of one-third carbohydrates (grains, beans, etc.), one-third vegetables and one-third should be in form of proteins, fats, low fat dairy products and refined sugars.

Under this plan, 60–70% of the total daily calories should come from grains, beans and starchy vegetables, with the rest coming from meat, cheese, fish and other proteins. Fats, oils and sweets should be used sparingly.

Picture	Medical/Surgical Description	Management/Clinical Highlights

5.3.2: Sites of Insulin Injection

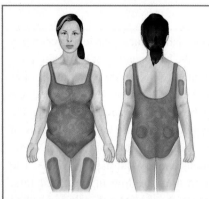

Fig. 5.3.2: Sites of insulin injection

Hypoglycemic therapy in the form of subcutaneous insulin injections should be considered for women with gestational diabetes if diet and exercise fail to maintain blood glucose targets during a period of 1–2 weeks. The common sites in the body for injecting insulin include the following:

- The upper lateral area of the thighs
- The upper outer area of the back of the arms
- The buttocks.

If it is safely achievable, women with diabetes should aim to keep their fasting blood glucose levels between 3.5 mmol/L and 5.9 mmol/L, and 1 hour postprandial blood glucose levels below 7.8 mmol/L during pregnancy. During pregnancy, women are usually prescribed four daily insulin injections (three injections of regular insulin to be taken before each meal and one injection of isophane insulin to be taken at night time).

5.3.3: Hundred Grams Glucose Load by O'Sullivan and Mahan: Criteria Modified by Carpenter and Coustan

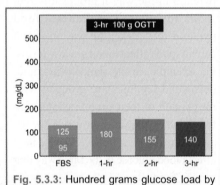

Fig. 5.3.3: Hundred grams glucose load by O'Sullivan and Mahan: Criteria modified by Carpenter and Coustan
(*Source*: Carpenter MW, Coustan DR. Criteria for screening tests for gestational diabetes. Am J Obstet Gynecol. 1982;144:768-73)

In cases of suspected gestational diabetes, an abnormal result on glucose challenge test (GCT) should be followed by an oral glucose tolerance test (GTT). This test involves measurement of blood glucose levels at fixed time intervals following the intake of prefixed quantities of glucose. While a 100 g, 3-hour GTT is a standard in the US, in the UK a 75 g, 2-hour GTT is preferred. If the 100 g 3-hour GTT is used, the diagnosis can be made either using the Carpenter and Coustan criteria (as described in adjacent figure) or criteria defined by the National Diabetes Data Group.

If two or more of these values on GTT are abnormal, the patient has gestational diabetes. Even patients who show no abnormal values in their 3-hour GTT have risks of 6.6% and 3.3% for development of macrosomia and preeclampsia-eclampsia respectively. Thus, the obstetrician needs to maintain strict glycemic control in order to decrease the frequency of the abnormal outcomes to both the mother and fetus at the time of pregnancy. Fasting blood glucose value of 125 mg/dL or greater is indicative of overt diabetes.

5.3.4: Management of Gestational Diabetes

Strategy	Management
Diet as recommended by American Diabetes Association	The calories to be spread evenly over frequent small meals throughout the day
Target values	Fasting blood sugar < 90 mg/dL 1 hour postprandial value < 140 mg/dL
Insulin prescription (dosage of 0.8,1.0,1.2 U/kg body weight)	Insulin to be prescribed if glucose values are out of range despite dietary restrictions
Oral hypoglycemic agents	Must not be prescribed due to the risk of fetal hypoglycemia
Gestational age for delivery	40 weeks
Complications	Arrest of labor, shoulder dystocia, postpartum hemorrhage, neonatal problems such as hypoglycemia, hypocalcemia, polycythemia, hyperbilirubinemia, respiratory distress syndrome, etc.

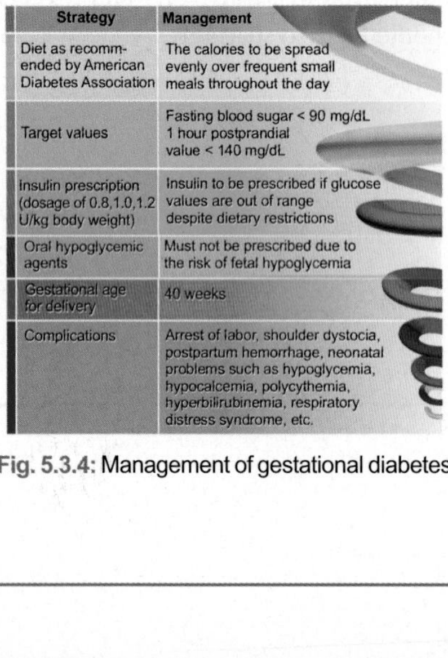

Fig. 5.3.4: Management of gestational diabetes

Management of cases of gestational diabetes is summarized in Figure 5.3.4. The first line therapy for the women with gestational diabetes is exercise and diet therapy. If the changes in diet and lifestyle over a period of 1–2 weeks are unable to bring blood glucose values under control, insulin injections must be prescribed. American College of Obstetricians and Gynecologists does not recommend the use of oral hypoglycemic agents during pregnancy because most of the oral hypoglycemic agents are capable of crossing placenta and causing fetal hypoglycemia.

Screening and diagnosis for gestational diabetes mellitus (GDM) is to be done for all patients between 24 to 28 weeks of pregnancy. This is done using 1-hour, 50 g GCT. Abnormal value is considered to be a value of > 140 mg/dL at the end of 1 hour. Abnormal GCT must be followed by a 3-hours, 100 g oral glucose tolerance test (OGTT). If at the time of GCT, fasting blood glucose value > 125 mg/dL, it is indicative of overt diabetes. No further testing is required. A criterion of abnormal OGTT is any two abnormal values out of four.

5.3.5: Complications of Gestational Diabetes

5.3.5.1: Macrosomia

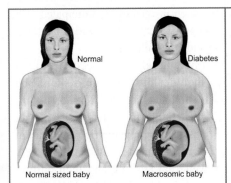

Fig. 5.3.5.1: Risk of development of macrosomia in diabetic patients

The term macrosomia is often used to describe birthweight over 4,000 g or birthweight ≥ 90th percentile for gestational age. This is also referred to as large for gestational age or LGA fetuses. Fetal macrosomia occurs in 17–30% of the pregnancies with gestational diabetes as compared with 10% in nondiabetic population. There are two types of macrosomia: symmetric and asymmetric. Asymmetric macrosomia is characterized by thoracic and abdominal circumference that is relatively larger than the head circumference. In symmetric macrosomia, the baby is symmetrically large on the whole.

The macrosomia baby is at an increased risk of shoulder dystocia, clavicular fracture, brachial palsy, and an overall increased rates of cesarean section.

The management of macrosomia is controversial. The ACOG recommends a primary cesarean section if the expected fetal weight (EFW) at the end of pregnancy is 4,500 g or more. The controversy arises when the EFW is between 4,000 g and 4,500 g. Some investigators argue that a cesarean section must be performed in these cases. However, if trial of vaginal delivery is being performed, the clinician must remain extremely vigilant regarding the development of shoulder dystocia and must immediately perform a cesarean delivery, with the development of any abnormality of labor. Assisted vaginal delivery in form of vacuum or forceps application should not be used in these patients.

5.3.5.2: Sacral Agenesis (A and B)

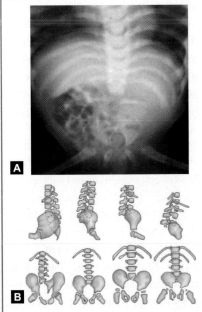

Figs 5.3.5.2 (A and B): Sacral agenesis: (A) X-ray appearance: anterior-posterior view; (B) Renshaw staging system for sacral agenesis

Sacral agenesis, also known as caudal regression syndrome or sacral hypoplasia, is associated with abnormal development of the sacral bone. Renshaw (1978) has classified sacral agenesis on the basis of amount of sacrum remaining and the characteristics of articulation between the spine and pelvis and is as follows:

Type 1: Unilateral sacral agenesis (partial or unilateral)

Type II: Bilateral symmetrical partial sacral agenesis. The sacral vertebra may be normal or hypoplastic. There is stable articulation between the ilium and first sacral vertebra.

Type III: There may be variable amount of sacral agenesis. The ilia may be articulating with the sides of the lowest vertebra present.

Type IV: There may be variable amount of lumbar and total sacral agenesis with the caudal endplate of the lowest vertebra either articulating or fused with the ilia or iliac amphiarthrosis.

Minor abnormalities may not cause any deformity and hence do not require any correction. Severe cases may present with spinal-pelvic instability and/or severe knee contractures with popliteal webbing of the knees. Reconstruction of limbs may be required in type IV defects which may not be entirely successful. Bilateral subtrochanteric amputation may be done in some cases. Some surgeons have advocated spinal-pelvic fusion in order to protect the viscera from unphysiological compression and angulation. Knee flexion and foot deformities can be corrected at an early age using a combination of surgical release procedures, supracondylar femoral extension osteotomies and serial casting.

5.3.5.3: Shoulder Dystocia

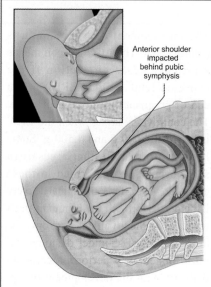

Anterior shoulder impacted behind pubic symphysis

Fig. 5.3.5.3: Shoulder dystocia

Shoulder dystocia can be defined as the inability to deliver the fetal shoulders after the delivery of the fetal head without the aid of specific maneuvers (other than the gentle downward traction on the head). Shoulder dystocia usually results when the diameter of the fetal shoulders (bisacromial diameter) is relatively larger than the biparietal diameter. Low shoulder dystocia results due to the failure of engagement of the anterior shoulder and impaction of anterior shoulder over the maternal symphysis pubis.

There can be a high perinatal mortality and morbidity associated with the complication, and needs to be managed appropriately. There are two main signs that indicate the presence of shoulder dystocia:

- The baby's body does not emerge out even after the application of routine traction and maternal pushing after delivery of the fetal head.
- The "turtle sign": The fetal head suddenly retracts back against the mother's perineum after it emerges from the vagina.

The immediate steps which need to be taken in case of an anticipated or a recognized case of shoulder dystocia include the following:

- Immediately after recognition of shoulder dystocia, help should be summoned instantly. This should include further midwifery assistance, an obstetrician, a pediatric resuscitation team and an anesthetist.
- Maternal pushing and fetal pulling and pivoting should be discouraged, as this may lead to further impaction of the shoulders.
- The woman should be maneuvered to bring the buttocks to the edge of the bed.
- Fundal pressure should not be employed.
- Routine use of episiotomy is not necessary for all cases.
- Management of shoulder dystocia needs to be done within 5–7 minutes of the delivery of the fetal head.
- *McRoberts maneuver:* If the above mentioned steps do not prove to be useful, the McRoberts maneuver is the single most effective intervention.
- *Suprapubic pressure:* Suprapubic pressure in conjunction with McRoberts maneuver is often all that is needed to resolve 50–60% cases of shoulder dystocias.
- *Maneuvers for internal manipulation:* If these simple measures (the McRoberts maneuver and suprapubic pressure) fail, then maneuvers for internal manipulation including Wood's Screw maneuver and delivery of posterior arm must be used.
- *Third line maneuvers:* Third line maneuvers such as cleidotomy, symphysiotomy, Zanavelli's maneuver, etc. can help if nothing seems to work. For details regarding the various maneuvers refer to section 2.

Picture	Medical/Surgical Description	Management/Clinical Highlights

5.3.5.4: Injury to the Brachial Plexus (A and B)

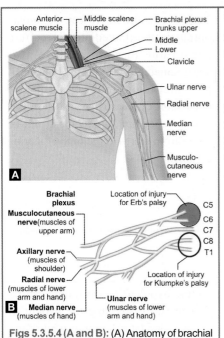 **Figs 5.3.5.4 (A and B):** (A) Anatomy of brachial plexuses; (B) Areas of brachial plexus injury due to shoulder dystocia	The brachial plexus consists of the nerve roots of spinal cord segments C5, C6, C7, C8 and T1. These nerve roots form three trunks, upper, middle and lower, which further divide into anterior and posterior divisions. The upper trunk is made up of nerves from C5 and C6, the middle trunk from undivided fibers of C7 and the lowermost trunk is made up of nerves from C8 and T1.	Injury to the upper part of the brachial plexus is called Erb's palsy (C5 to C7) while injury to the lower nerves of the plexus is called Klumpke's palsy (C8 to T1). Both can cause significant, lifelong disability. Erb's palsy affects the muscles of the upper arm and shoulders causing "winging" of scapula. This type of injury causes adduction and internal rotation of humerus with the forearm extended. This has also been described as the "waiters tip" position.

5.4: HEART DISEASE DURING PREGNANCY

5.4.1: Cardiovascular Changes During Pregnancy (A and B)

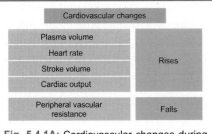 **Fig. 5.4.1A:** Cardiovascular changes during pregnancy	Typical physiological changes occurring in the cardiovascular system during pregnancy in a normal woman have been summarized in Figure 5.4.1A.	Normal physiological changes in pregnancy include the following: 50% increase in plasma volume, 15% increase in heart rate, 25% increase in stroke volume and 45–50% increase in cardiac output. There is a reduction in peripheral resistance by 30%.
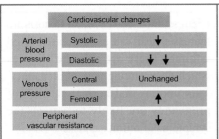 **Fig. 5.4.1B:** Effect of cardiovascular changes during pregnancy on various cardiovascular parameters	Figure 5.4.1B summarizes the effect of various physiological changes (5.4.1A) on the various cardiovascular parameters in a pregnant woman.	As a result of the above-described cardiovascular changes during pregnancy, there is a reduction in BP (systolic, diastolic as well as the mean BP). The central venous pressure remains unchanged, whereas the femoral venous pressure increases.

5.4.2: Changes in Cardiac Output

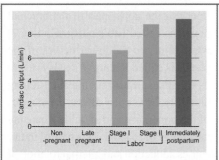

Fig. 5.4.2: Changes in cardiac output with increasing duration of pregnancy (*Source*: Sakala EP. Obstetrics and Gynecology, 2nd editon: Lippincott Williams and Wilkins; 2000)

Figure 5.4.2 shows an increase in cardiac output with increasing POG throughout the pregnancy. This increase in cardiac output starts occurring from 5th week of gestation and continues till 30–34 weeks, following which it plateaus till term. This increase is related to an increase in plasma volume and heart rate, which normally occurs during pregnancy.

There is a sudden increase in the cardiac output in the immediate postpartum period due to autotransfusion of approximately 600–800 mL of utero-placental blood into the peripheral circulation. Cardiac output also increases during labor due to squeezing out of blood from uterus at the time of uterine contractions.

5.4.3: Supine Hypotension Syndrome (A and B)

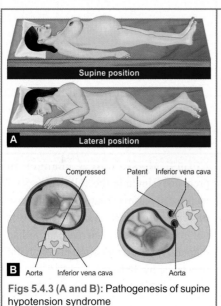

Figs 5.4.3 (A and B): Pathogenesis of supine hypotension syndrome

Also known as aortocaval compression, supine hypotension syndrome refers to the development of sudden hypotension in a pregnant woman who lies flat on the bed. When the woman assumes a supine position while lying down, uterine contents of the gravid uterus press upon the inferior vena cava and aorta, thereby partially occluding them. This may result in the development of hypotension and symptoms such as pallor, reduced heart rate, sweating, dizziness, loss of consciousness, etc.

Supine hypotension syndrome can be prevented by advising the patient to assume a left lateral position while lying down rather than lying flat on a surface. In case the woman accidently lies flat on a surface and experiences symptoms suggestive of supine hypotension syndrome, she should be advised to immediately assume left lateral position. Change to left lateral position and simple reassurance explaining the benign nature of the condition seems to work in most of the cases.

5.4.4: Most Common Heart Disease During Pregnancy

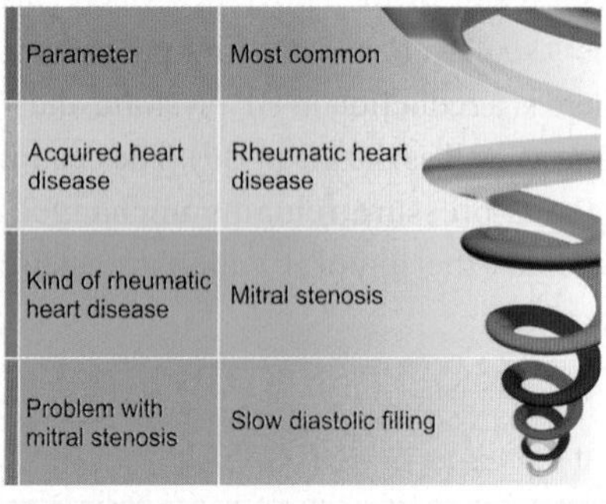

Parameter	Most common
Acquired heart disease	Rheumatic heart disease
Kind of rheumatic heart disease	Mitral stenosis
Problem with mitral stenosis	Slow diastolic filling

Fig. 5.4.4: Most common heart disease during pregnancy

Most common acquired heart disease during pregnancy is rheumatic heart disease, particularly rheumatic stenosis. This is associated with reduced diastolic filling.

Factors which worsen mitral stenosis are increased heart rate and increased blood volume. These are also the changes which occur during normal pregnancy. This implies that normal changes of pregnancy are likely to worsen the symptoms of mitral stenosis.

Picture	Medical/Surgical Description	Management/Clinical Highlights

5.4.5: High-Risk Cardiac Conditions

Cardiac condition	Characteristics
Eisenmenger's syndrome	• Pulmonary hypertension • Bidirectional intracardiac shunt • Avoid hypotension
Marfan's syndrome	• Dilatation of aorta > 40 mm • Risk of aortic dissection • Treatment comprises of surgical reconstruction
Peripartum cardiomyopathy	• Idiopathic biventricular cardiac failure • Treatment comprises of supportive care

Fig. 5.4.5: High-risk cardiac conditions

Some high-risk cardiac conditions, which are associated with high rates of mortality (25–50%) during pregnancy are as follows:

Eisenmenger's syndrome: This syndrome is associated with bilateral intracardiac shunt. In this syndrome, deoxygenated blood instead of moving through pulmonary artery into the lungs, (due to presence of a ventricular septal defect) moves through the intracardiac shunt into the aorta through left ventricle.

Marfan's syndrome: This syndrome is associated with the dilation of aortic root to a size greater than 4 cm. Due to an increased risk of tension on the vessel wall, there is an increased risk of aortic dissection.

Peripartum cardiomyopathy: This is often associated with biventricular cardiac failure in which both sides of the heart are affected.

Treatment of Eisenmenger's syndrome comprises of avoidance of hypotension. In cases of Marfan's syndrome, treatment comprises of surgical reconstruction. Treatment of peripartum cardiomyopathy mainly comprises of provision of supportive care. This usually comprises of using ionotropic agents and maintenance of systemic perfusion.

5.4.6: New York Heart Association Functional Classification of Heart Failure

Class	Symptoms at rest	Symptoms with activity
I	None	None
II	None	Mild
III	None	Marked
IV	Present	Worsened

Fig. 5.4.6: New York Heart Association functional classification of heart failure

The functional classification of heart failure as described by New York Heart Association (NYHA) is as follows:

Class I patients: In these patients, ordinary physical activity does not cause fatigue, palpitations, dyspnea or anginal pain.

Class II patients: These patients are comfortable at rest. Ordinary physical activity results in fatigue, palpitations, dyspnea or anginal pain.

Class III patients: These patients are comfortable at rest. Less than ordinary physical activity results in fatigue, palpitations, dyspnea or anginal pain.

Class IV patients: In these patients, symptoms of cardiac insufficiency may even be present at rest. If any physical activity is undertaken, discomfort is increased.

Patients with class I and class II heart disease can be delivered normally in labor room without requiring admission to the ICU or insertion of invasive lines. The main objective of management in pregnant patients with heart disease should be to minimize any additional load on the cardiovascular system from delivery and the puerperium. This is usually best achieved with the help of the following:

- Aiming for spontaneous onset of labor
- Providing effective pain relief with low-dose regional analgesia
- Assisting vaginal delivery with instruments such as the ventouse or forceps
- Limiting or even avoiding active maternal bearing down ("pushing")
- Vaginal delivery over cesarean section is the preferred mode of delivery for most women with heart disease.

Patients in NYHA class III and IV need to be admitted to the ICU and require insertion of invasive lines.

5.5: THYROID DISORDERS DURING PREGNANCY

5.5.1: Levels of TSH and hCG During Pregnancy

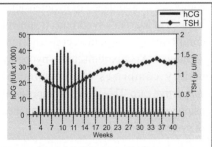

Fig. 5.5.1: Levels of thyroid stimulating hormone (TSH) and human chorionic gonadotropin (hCG) during gestation

(*Source*: Adapted from Glinoer D. The regulation of thyroid function in pregnancy: pathways of endocrine adaptation from physiology to pathology. Endocrine Reviews. 1997;18:404-33.)

The major changes related to thyroid function during normal pregnancy are an increase in serum thyroxine-binding globulin (TBG) concentrations and stimulation of the thyrotropin receptor by chorionic gonadotropin. TBG excess results in an increase in the concentration of both serum total thyroxine (T4) and triiodothyronine (T3). On the other hand, free serum T4 and T3 concentrations remain within normal range.

Thyroid stimulating hormone levels normally decrease during the first trimester. At the same time, there is an increase in the serum hCG levels. Increased levels of hCG stimulate the thyroid glands and cause suppression of TSH levels. Despite the stimulation of thyroid glands caused by hCG, free (unbound) serum levels of thyroid hormone generally remain within, or slightly above, the normal range during the first trimester. This implies that the stimulatory effects of hCG on normal pregnancy are not substantial enough to cause an increase in the levels of thyroid hormones.

In presence of certain pathological conditions, such as hyperemesis gravidarum trophoblastic tumors, hCG concentrations may increase substantially, sufficient enough to induce biochemical hyperthyroidism.

5.5.2: Thyroxine (T4) Concentrations During Gestation

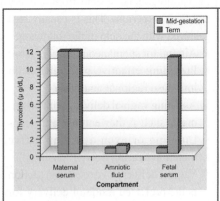

Fig. 5.5.2: Thyroxine (T4) concentrations during gestation
(*Source*: Adapted from Burrow GN, Fisher D, Larsen PR. Maternal and fetal thyroid function. N Engl Med. 1994;331:1072.)

Maternal thyroxine is transferred to the fetus throughout pregnancy. This hormone is important for normal fetal brain development especially before the development of fetal thyroid glands. Level of total T4 increase in the maternal serum throughout the pregnancy. However due to simultaneous rise in the levels of TBG, free T4 levels do not increase during pregnancy. At birth sudden surge of TSH in the baby results in increased secretion of thyroid hormones at birth.

Serum TSH is the most reliable indicator of genuine hypothyroidism during pregnancy. Hypothyroidism is diagnosed when TSH levels are high and T4 levels are either in normal range or low. Overt hypothyroidism in pregnancy can result in complications such as miscarriage, anemia, preeclampsia, abruption placenta, PPH, etc.

Picture	Medical/Surgical Description	Management/Clinical Highlights

5.5.3: Changes in TSH and Thyroxine (T4) at Term

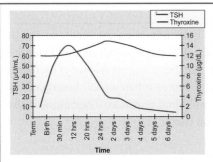

Fig. 5.5.3: Changes in TSH and thyroxine (T4) at birth

(*Source*: Adapted from Fisher D, Klein A. Medical progress. Thyroid development and disorders of thyroid function in the newborn. N Engl J Med. 1981;304:702.)

Figure 5.5.3 demonstrates the levels of TSH and thyroxine in the newborn baby in the immediate postpartum period. At the time of birth, as the fetus emerges in the extrauterine environment, it stimulates an acute release of TSH from the pituitary glands in the immediate postpartum period. TSH levels decrease rapidly during the first 24 hours of life, with a more gradual decrease over the next 2 days. The TSH surge at the time of birth provokes increased secretion of thyroid hormones.

As a result of TSH surge, there is an increase in the levels of total and free T4 concentrations at birth. Reverse T3 concentrations are also elevated at birth. In contrast, serum T3 concentrations are low at birth and increase dramatically thereafter during the first postpartum month.

5.6: ASTHMA AND PREGNANCY

5.6.1: Treatment of Asthma During Pregnancy

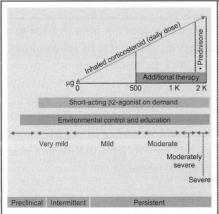

Fig. 5.6.1: Treatment of asthma during pregnancy

Management of asthma during the antenatal period comprises of the following steps:
- Advising the women to avoid having an exposure to any potential asthma triggers
- Fetal surveillance with regular ultrasound scans and daily fetal movement count
- In case of mild asthma (less than two attacks per week), short acting beta agonists (albuterol) may be administered for providing symptomatic relief.
- In mild persistent cases (≥ 2 attacks per week), daily-inhaled steroids (budesonide) may be administered. Short-acting β agonists may be administered for short-term relief.
- In moderate cases, daily inhaled steroids (in moderate-high dosage) plus long-acting β agonists (salmeterol) may be given. Short-acting β agonists may be administered for providing symptomatic relief. Monitoring of peak expiratory flow rate (PEFR) must be done on daily basis.

In case of severe asthmatic attacks, daily administration of inhaled steroids in high dosage may be required. Besides this, daily low-dosage oral steroids (prednisolone) and daily long acting β agonists (salmeterol) may also be administered. Regular monitoring of PEFR may be required.

Management of asthma during labor comprises of the following steps:
- Maternal oxygenation must be well maintained and oxygen saturation must be monitored with pulse oximetry and arterial blood gas determination.
- Opiate analgesics must be avoided due to their bronchoconstrictor and respiratory depressant effect. Labetalol must also be avoided due to its risk of precipitating asthma.
- Use of syntocinon is preferred over ergometrine due to the bronchoconstrictor effect of the latter. Use of carboprost ($PGF_{2\alpha}$) should be avoided due to the risk of bronchospasm. On the other hand, PGE1 and PGE2 compounds can be used locally for induction of labor or abortion.
- Epidural anesthesia is preferred over general anesthesia.

5.7: TUBERCULOSIS IN PREGNANCY

5.7.1: Global Burden of Tuberculosis

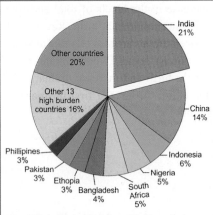

Fig. 5.7.1: Global burden of tuberculosis (*Source*: WHO Geneva; WHO Report 2006: Global Tuberculosis Control; Surveillance, Planning and Financing)

India has the highest worldwide burden of tuberculosis, amounting to nearly 21% (which is approximately equal to one-fifth of global incidence). In the year 2009, the global annual incidence of tuberculosis was estimated to be 9.4 million cases. Out of these, 2 million cases were estimated to occur in India. While tuberculosis is rare in European countries, patients with HIV infection may be particularly susceptible to develop tuberculosis infection.

There has been an increase in the incidence of tuberculosis worldwide due to an increasing prevalence of multidrug resistance tuberculosis. Emergence of multidrug resistance tuberculosis is also on rise.

5.7.2: Mantoux Test

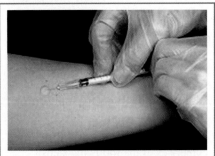

Fig. 5.7.2: Mantoux test

Mantoux test is diagnostic for tuberculosis. Also known as the tuberculin skin test, it is performed by subdermal injection of 0.5 mL of 5 tuberculin units of liquid tuberculin. The tuberculin used in Mantoux test is also known as purified protein derivative. The area of induration upon injection and not that of erythema is measured. A size ≥ 10 mm is considered to be positive.

Pregnancy does not have any adverse effect on the course of tuberculosis, nor does the disease have any adverse effect on the course of pregnancy. Untreated cases of tuberculosis during pregnancy may be associated with increased incidence of complications such as preterm labor, IUGR, increased perinatal mortality, etc.

5.7.3: Medication for Treatment of Tuberculosis

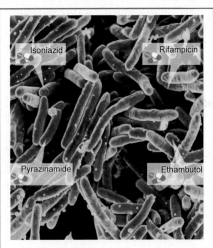

Fig. 5.7.3: Medication for treatment of tuberculosis

The multidrug regimen for treatment of active tuberculosis include the following:
- Isoniazid (5mg/kg) up to 300 mg with 50 mg of pyridoxine
- Rifampicin (10 mg/kg) up to 600 mg
- Ethambutol (15 mg/kg) up to 2.5 mg
- Pyrazinamide (25−30mg/kg) up to 2 g, Treatment is continued up to a period of 9 months. It may be difficult to maintain adherence to treatment in pregnancy because of the general fear against use of any medication during pregnancy and occurrence of pregnancy-related nausea. These drugs have not been found to cause any teratogenic effects during pregnancy.

Basic obstetric management in cases of tuberculosis is same as that in other pregnant patients. Breast-feeding is not contraindicated if the woman is taking antitubercular drugs. Breast-feeding is to be avoided if the infant is also taking drugs to avoid an excessive increase in the levels of drugs. Breast-feeding is also contraindicated if the woman has an active lesion. Moreover in these cases, the baby must be isolated from mother following delivery and administered isoniazid in the dosage of 10–20 mg/kg/day for 3 months. There is no need to isolate the baby if the mother has been on effective chemotherapy for at least 2 weeks.

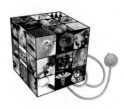

EVIDENCE-BASED
BREAKTHROUGH FACTS

1. RELATIONSHIP BETWEEN SERUM LEVELS OF VITAMIN D AND DEVELOPMENT OF GESTATIONAL DIABETES

Women with lower serum levels of vitamin D during the first trimester of pregnancy are at a greater risk for developing GDM later in pregnancy. This is probably related to the fact that lower vitamin D levels are associated with insulin resistance. On the other hand, higher levels of 25 (OH)D levels are likely to result in greater sensitivity to insulin.

Source: Abstracts of the 48th EASD (European Association for the Study of Diabetes) Annual meeting of the European Association for the Study of Diabetes. October 1–5, 2012. Berlin, Germany. Diabetologia. 2012;55(Suppl 1):S7-537.

2. PREECLAMPSIA: NO LONGER SOLELY A PREGNANCY DISEASE

Preeclampsia, the leading cause of maternal and perinatal morbidity and mortality, not only affects the woman during pregnancy, but also acts as a risk factor for developing diseases later in life, including ischemic heart disease and hypertension, fatal and nonfatal stroke, venous thromboembolism, renal failure, type 2 diabetes mellitus, hypothyroidism and cognitive defects. Furthermore, preeclampsia is also likely to affect the children's adult health. Children born from preeclamptic mothers are more likely to develop disorders, such as hypertension, insulin resistance and diabetes mellitus, neurological problems, stroke and mental disorders later in their life.

Source: Andrea LT, Landi B, Stefano R, et al. Preeclampsia: No longer solely a pregnancy disease. Pregnancy Hypertension: An International Journal of Women's Cardiovascular Health. 2012;2(4):350-7.

3. OUTCOME OF PREGNANCY IN PATIENTS WITH STRUCTURAL OR ISCHEMIC HEART DISEASE

According to the new data from the first-ever formal registry on pregnancy and heart disease, pregnant women who have heart disease are likely to have a 100 times higher rate of mortality in comparison to the normal pregnant population. However, if a woman with pre-existing heart disease receives good specialist care during the antenatal and intrapartum period, the complication rate is likely to be very low.

Source: Roos-Hesselink JW, Ruys TP, Stein JI, et al. Outcome of pregnancy in patients with structural or ischaemic heart disease: Results of a registry of the European Society of Cardiology. *Eur Heart J.* 2012; doi:10.1093/eurheartj/ehs270. [online] Available from www.eurheartj.oxfordjournals.org. [Accessed November, 2012]

4. SCREENING FOR GESTATIONAL DIABETES

Research has demonstrated that even mild forms of hyperglycemia may cause significant adverse health consequences for pregnant women and their children. Thus, it is expected that lowering the presently existing diagnostic criteria for GDM is likely to significantly reduce morbidity and healthcare costs in the long term. However, such a change is also likely to cause an increase in the number of women identified as having this disease, thereby incurring increased healthcare costs. Moreover, changing the diagnostic criteria for GDM is also likely to cause an increase in the rate of cesarean delivery. Therefore, the dilemma remains whether to change or not to change the pre-existing screening and diagnostic criteria for GDM.

Source: Reece EA, Moore T. The diagnostic criteria for gestational diabetes: to change or not to change? Am J Obstet Gynecol. 2012. doi:pii: S0002-9378(12)02034-0 10.1016/j.ajog.2012.10.887. [Epub ahead of print]

5. HAPO STUDY

According to the supporters of HAPO (hyperglycemia and adverse pregnancy outcome) study, all pregnant women should be screened for gestational diabetes, and the HAPO criteria, which uses the lower threshold values of blood glucose to diagnose diabetes, seems to be more acceptable than the existing criteria.

HAPO criteria for the 75 gram, 2-hour OGTT are that any one or more of the following thresholds be met or exceeded:

Timing of plasma glucose	Glucose levels
Fasting plasma	92 mg/dL (5.1 mmol/L)
One hour plasma glucose	180 mg/dL (10 mmol/L)
Two hour plasma glucose	153 mg/dL (8.5 mmol/L)

The 100 grams glucose load by O'Sullivan and Mahan criteria as modified by Carpenter and Coustan has been described in 5.3.3.

Source: Lowe LP, Metzger BE, HAPO Study Cooperative Research Group, et al. Hyperglycemia and adverse pregnancy outcome (HAPO) study: associations of maternal A1C and glucose with pregnancy outcomes. Diabetes Care. 2012;35:574-80.

6. PREGNANCY PLANNING DURING DIABETES

An Irish study has shown that pregnancy planning had an enormous impact on the woman's glycemic control during pregnancy and in significantly improving both neonatal and maternal outcomes. Pregnant patients with type 1 diabetes must be encouraged to plan their pregnancy and to participate in an educational program to ensure adequate glycemic control in the pre-pregnancy period and the first trimester.

Source: Mustafa E, Khalil S, Kirwan B, et al. Pre-pregnancy and first trimester glycaemic control determines foetal and maternal outcomes in women with type 1 and type 2 diabetes. Diabetologia. 2012;55:S437.

7. INSULIN PUMPS

A French study has shown achievement of excellent glycemic levels with the use of insulin pumps in patients with type 1 diabetes. However, this study has also emphasised the importance of pregnancy planning for achieving adequate glycemic control.

Source: 1. Lorenzini F, Boileau BG, Melki V, et al. Insulin pump is effective to reduce macrosomia in pregnancies complicated by type 1 diabetes. Diabetologia. 2012;55:S438.
2. Klupa T, Matejko B, Cyganek K, et al. Efficacy and safety of insulin pump treatment in young adult patients with type 1 diabetes mellitus. Diabetologia. 2012;55:S421.

8. INSULIN DETEMIR ASSIGNED TO PREGNANCY CATEGORY B

Since March 2012, the US Food and Drug Administration (FDA) has approved that insulin detemir be reclassified from pregnancy category C to pregnancy category B, based on data from a randomized trial that reported the safety and efficacy of insulin detemir. However, the data available from this study is not sufficient to recommend the routine use of insulin detemir over neutral protamine Hagedorn (NPH) amongst pregnant women. However, if a patient has well-controlled glucose levels on insulin detemir prior to pregnancy, the clinician may continue using it, with ongoing assessment of glycemic control during pregnancy.

Source: Mathiesen ER, Hod M, Ivanisevic M, et al. Maternal efficacy and safety outcomes in a randomized controlled trial comparing insulin determir with NPH insulin in 310 pregnant women with type 1 diabetes mellitus. Diabetes Care. 2012;35(10):2012-7. Epub 2012.

Obstetrics

Section 6

Postnatal Period

6.1: LACTATION

6.1.1: Let Down Reflex

Picture	Medical/Surgical Description	Management/Clinical Highlights
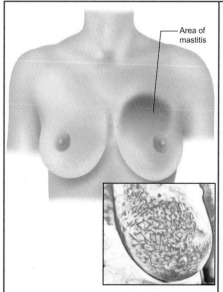 Baby's suckling stimulates nerve endings in areola ⬇ Hypothalamus neural reflex (message) is passed to pituitary gland via hypothalmus ⬇ Posterior pituitary Oxytocin contracts muscle wall of alveoli to release milk during feeding ⬇ Anterior pituitary Prolactin stimulates alveoli to produce breastmilk for future feedings **Fig. 6.1.1:** Let-down reflex	Release of milk from the breast ducts and alveoli as a result of suckling of the breasts by the baby is known as the let-down reflex. It is an involuntary reflex activity, which forms an important part of the breast-feeding process.	Suckling of the breasts by the baby stimulates nerve endings in the areola. This neural reflex is passed onto the pituitary gland by the hypothalamus. Stimulation of posterior pituitary releases oxytocin, which contracts the walls of the breast alveoli to release milk. Prolactin released from the anterior pituitary stimulates the alveoli to produce milk for future feeds.

6.2: ABNORMALITIES OF LACTATION

6.2.1: Mastitis

Picture	Medical/Surgical Description	Management/Clinical Highlights
Area of mastitis **Fig. 6.2.1:** Mastitis (*Source*: Computerized generation of the image)	Mastitis can be defined as the parenchymatous infection of the mammary glands. The most important causative organism is *Staphylococcus aureus*, most commonly community-acquired methicillin-resistant *Staphylococcus aureus* (CA-MRSA). The infection is usually unilateral, commonly occurs on the postpartum day 14 and is associated with marked swelling, inflammation and redness of a single breast lobe. Fever may be present and is associated with chills or rigors. There may be hardening and reddening of the breast tissue and intense pain. Development of abscesses may result in presence of fluctuation. The following investigations need to be done: *Ultrasound examination*: This helps in detecting the presence of breast abscess. *Culture and sensitivity*: Culture and sensitivity of the breast milk help in identifying the causative organism.	Treatment mainly comprises of antibiotic treatment after bacterial identification and sensitivity. Infection usually resolves within 48 hours with treatment.

Picture	Medical/Surgical Description	Management/Clinical Highlights

6.2.2: Blocked Ducts

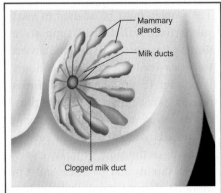

Fig. 6.2.2: Blocked/plugged ducts

Blocked/plugged ducts can occur due to the blockage of nipple pore or due to obstruction further back in the ductal system. The back-pressure by this retained milk is likely to result in inflammation and blockage of ducts, which can cause pain and swelling. Though the skin over the blocked ducts may become reddened and inflamed similar to that in mastitis, the pain is much less than in mastitis. Moreover, the systemic symptoms as observed in mastitis are also absent.

Most of the times, the blocked ducts may resolve on their own within 24–48 hours. Though the blocked duct may be painful, the mother must be advised to continue breast-feeding her child. While feeding the baby, the baby's chin must be positioned to point toward the area of firmness to help emptying of the breast ducts. In cases where breast-feeding is not possible, the milk must be expressed out manually or a breast pump be used. The inflamed area must be frequently massaged, starting from the periphery working toward the nipples. Use of warm compresses (warm, wet towel, warm shower, hot water bottle, etc.) may also help in opening the blocked ducts, providing relief from swelling and pain. Over-the-counter pain killers such as ibuprofen, etc. may help in providing relief from pain.

6.2.3: Breast Abscess (A and B)

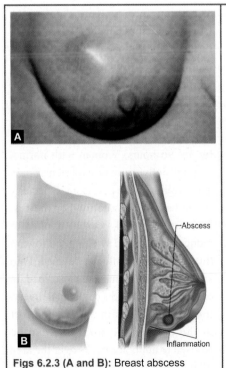

Figs 6.2.3 (A and B): Breast abscess

The bacteria most commonly involved in the causation of breast abscess is *S. aureus*. It usually occurs as a result of severe mastitis and can commonly occur in women who breast-feed. The bacteria can commonly enter through a crack in nipples. Symptoms of breast abscess may include pain, swelling, redness and warmth over the skin overlying the abscess, nipple discharge and tenderness, and fever. The lymph nodes of the affected side may also be tender and enlarged. There is presence of a painful, fluctuant, pus-filled swelling in the breast tissue.

Treatment with antibiotics and painkillers may be required. Though treatment with antibiotics is usually successful, surgical drainage is commonly required. In case of a small abscess (< 3 cm), pus can be sometimes aspirated with help of a needle. In case of large (> 3 cm), deep abscesses, incision and drainage under local/general anesthesia may be required. Some commonly used antibiotics include nafcillin for treatment of penicillinase producing bacteria; vancomycin for treatment of bacteria resistant to nafcillin; clindamycin for treatment of both aerobic and anaerobic bacteria, etc. Breast-feeding should be continued even after drainage.

6.2.4: Breast Engorgement

Picture	Medical/Surgical Description	Management/Clinical Highlights
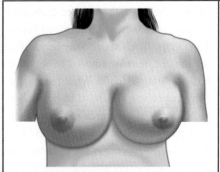 **Fig. 6.2.4:** Breast engorgement	If the process of milk ejection does not occur or is slower than that of its production, the milk may be forcefully trapped inside, resulting in breast engorgement. This condition is associated with an imbalance between milk supply and its consumption by the infant, and fever commonly occurs on postpartum day 3. The condition is usually bilateral and may result in the development of swelling and tenderness of the entire breast and mild to extreme pain. The breast may appear lumpy in some cases. In extreme cases, the breasts may become swollen, hard, shiny and warm.	The woman must be advised to use a supportive, well-fitting, supportive, feeding, brassiere. She should be advised to breast-feed after every 2–3 hours, lasting for 15–20 minutes each. Breast pumps can be also used to express out excessive breast milk. Massaging the breasts while the baby is feeding encourages the flow of milk. Use of nipple shields and pacifiers must be avoided. Use of painkillers such as paracetamol and application of ice packs provide pain relief.

6.3: PUERPERIUM

6.3.1: Normal Puerperal Period

Picture	Medical/Surgical Description	Management/Clinical Highlights
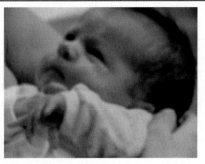 **Fig. 6.3.1:** Baby with mother few hours after birth	Puerperium can be defined as the time from the delivery of placenta until 6 weeks after delivery. During this phase, most of the changes related to pregnancy, labor and delivery have regressed, and the woman has returned to a nonpregnant state. The immediate postpartum period for most women (who undergo a hospitalized delivery) occurs in the hospital setting. Even after normal vaginal delivery, the women are usually kept in the hospital for at least 2 days. In case of a cesarean delivery, the women may require hospital admission for 3–5 days following the delivery.	During this time, the woman is taught how to take routine care of the baby such as bathing, feeding, using diapers, etc. Breast-feeding is encouraged soon after birth and the woman is taught to breast-feed the baby. In the beginning, the woman must be encouraged to breast-feed the baby after every 2–3 hours to encourage milk production. Milk production is usually well established by 36–96 hours. Women with normal vaginal delivery may experience pain and swelling in the perineum, especially if she has an episiotomy. For the first 24 hours, ice packs can be applied to reduce the pain and swelling. Following this, warm Sitz bath can be used. Pain killer medications may be prescribed. In case the woman had a cesarean delivery, there might be pain and discomfort in the area of incision. She can be advised to apply ice packs over the area of incision or prescribed painkillers [nonsteroidal anti-inflammatory drugs, narcotics, etc.]

Picture	Medical/Surgical Description	Management/Clinical Highlights

6.3.2: International Symbol for Breast-Feeding

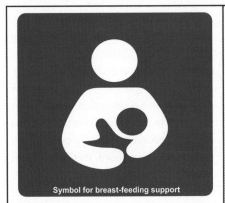 Symbol for breast-feeding support **Fig. 6.3.2:** International symbol for breast-feeding	The international symbol for breast-feeding was created by Matt Daigle, a graphic artist. This symbol has been created in a style of American Institute of Graphic Arts (AIGA) symbols. This symbol can be understood at a glance without having any written description explaining its meaning. The symbol is a graphical representation of the mother nursing a child.	This has now become a universally accepted and understood symbol for breast-feeding, especially at public places. It promotes the culture of breast-feeding over artificial feeding. It is likely to remove fear from the minds of the mothers and encourage them to breast-feed in public places.

6.3.3: Uterine Involution (A and B)

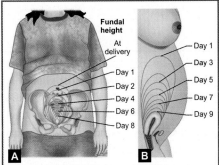 **Figs 6.3.3 (A and B):** Uterine involution following birth of the baby: (A) Front view; (B) Side view	Uterine involution can be defined as a process in which the uterus attempts to return to its prepregnancy shape and size. The process of involution can be clinically assessed by regular measurement of the fundal height and palpation of the consistency of uterine fundus. The woman should be instructed to empty the bladder before taking measurements. Immediately following the delivery of placenta and baby, the fundus lies about 14 cm above the pubic symphysis.	The normal process of involution is associated with a reduction in the uterine height at the rate of 1 cm/day so much so that at the end of second postpartum week it may not be possible to palpate the uterine fundus through abdominal examination. Moreover, the uterus which was previously boggy in consistency now becomes firm and contracted. The uterus usually attains its normal size by 6 weeks.

6.3.4: Involution at the Placental Site

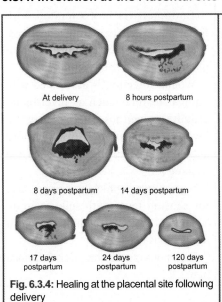 **Fig. 6.3.4:** Healing at the placental site following delivery	The adjacent figure demonstrates uterine involution and healing at the placental site following birth of the baby. Clinical estimation of uterine involution has been described in Figures 6.3.3A and B.	Following the expulsion of placenta and its membranes, there is a shedding of the major part of decidua, especially that from the placental site. Regeneration gradually starts occurring, with epithelialization first occurring over the mouth of uterine glands and interglandular stromal cells. While the entire endometrium is restored by day 16, healing at the placental site completes by about 6 weeks.

6.3.5: Discharge of Lochia

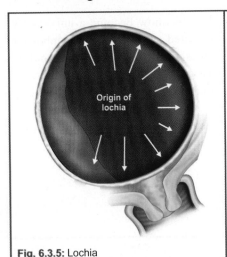

Fig. 6.3.5: Lochia

Changes occurring in the color of lochia after delivery are as follows:
- *Lochia rubra (bright red)*: First few days after birth
- *Lochia serosa (light red)*: Up to the second week of delivery
- *Lochia alba (white)*: After the second week of delivery

Lochia can be defined as the discharge, which occurs for a few days following birth and indicates the process of endometrial regeneration and healing. During the first few days after birth, this discharge is bright red in color and is known as lochia rubra. Over the next few days, it becomes serous in consistency and reduces in amount. It is then known as lochia serosa. Eventually, by 7–10 days postpartum, the discharge becomes yellowish-whitish in consistency and decreases in amount. This may continue for another 2–3 weeks.

6.4: COMPLICATIONS OF PUERPERIUM

6.4.1: Puerperal Pyrexia

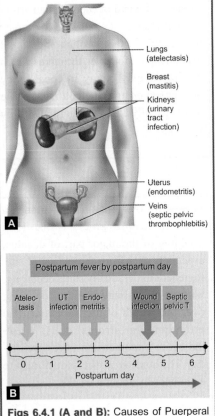

Figs 6.4.1 (A and B): Causes of Puerperal pyrexia
(UT, Urinary tract; T, Thrombophlebitis)

This is characterized by a rise in temperature of 38°C (100.4°F) or higher in the puerperium. This temperature rise must be observed on two separate occasions, 24 hours apart, usually within the first 10 days following delivery excluding the first 24 hours after delivery. Various causes of puerperal pyrexia include atelectasis (day of delivery), urinary tract infection (postpartum days 1–2), endometritis (postpartum days 2–3), wound infection (postpartum days 4–5), septic thrombophlebitis (postpartum days 5–6) and infectious mastitis (postpartum days 7–21).

Atelectasis is also associated with the presence of rales on clinical examination. Its treatment involves early ambulation and pulmonary exercises. Urinary tract infection may be associated with clinical features such as fever, costovertebral angle tenderness, and presence of pus cells and/or bacteria on urine analysis and culture. Treatment usually involves single agent antibiotic based on the sensitivity reports.

Endometritis is associated with fever and exquisite uterine tenderness. Treatment involves administration of multiagent intravenous antibiotics.

Wound infection is associated with clinical features such as fever, pain, cellulitis, wound abscess, etc. Treatment involves administration of intravenous antibiotics, and opening the wound and packing it.

Septic thrombophlebitis is responsible for causing fever with spiky pattern. Treatment involves administration of intravenous heparin.

Infectious mastitis has been described in 6.2.1.

6.4.2: Uterine Infection

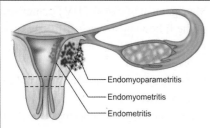

Fig. 6.4.2: Uterine infection

- Endomyoparametritis
- Endomyometritis
- Endometritis

Uterine infection can commonly occur during the postpartum period. This can occur in various forms such as: endometritis (involvement of the endometrium only); endomyometritis (infection spreads from the endometrium into the myometrium); and in the extreme cases endomyoparametritis (involvement of endometrium and myometrium along with that of parametrium). Endometritis is commonly associated with occurrence of fever on second and third postpartum day. The most commonly associated risk factor is emergency cesarean delivery for prolonged rupture of membranes and prolonged labor. Amongst the women who have had a vaginal delivery, those who have had an assisted vaginal delivery are at a higher risk than those who had a spontaneous normal vaginal delivery. Clinical examination reveals fever, abdominal pain and extreme uterine tenderness. There may be presence of an offensive, foul-smelling, greenish-yellow, pus-mixed vaginal discharge. The amount of bleeding may be heavier than before.

Treatment involves administration of multiagent antibiotics (e.g. IV gentamycin and IV clindamycin). In order to prevent the occurrence of endometritis in women undergoing cesarean delivery, it has become a routine practice to administer intravenous prophylactic dosage of 2 g ampicillin or 1 g cefazolin after the cord has been clamped and cut. If the woman shows signs of infection, e.g. fever, urinary tract infections, sepsis, etc., antibiotics must be continued until the woman becomes fever free for at least 48 hours.

6.4.3: Death due to Endometritis

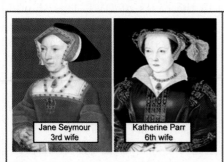

Jane Seymour 3rd wife

Katherine Parr 6th wife

Fig. 6.4.3: Death due to endometritis
[*Source*: Pictures by unknown artists (web collection)]

Henry the VIII King of England in the 16th century had six wives, two of which, Jane Seymour (third wife) and Katherine Parr (sixth wife), died due to puerperal fever, endometritis.

In the 16th century, before the discovery of antibiotics and bacteria had occurred, puerperal fever, typically endometritis was an important cause of mortality amongst the postpartum women.

6.4.4: Deep Vein Thrombosis (A to E)

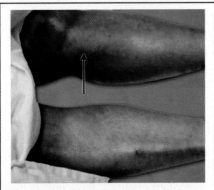

Fig. 6.4.4A: Clinical appearance in case of deep vein thrombosis (indicated by arrow)

Extension of puerperal infection along venous route can result in thrombosis and thrombophlebitis of the affected vein. Thrombosis usually originates as an aggregation of platelets and fibrin on the valves in the veins of the lower extremities (especially calf veins). The thrombus can break-off and embolize to other veins or cause total occlusion of the veins.

Factors which predispose to the formation of thrombus include: endothelial injury, blood stasis and hypercoagulability of blood. The adjacent photograph shows normal leg on right side and left leg with swollen, red and painful calf. A tentative diagnosis of deep vein thrombosis (DVT) was established.

Management of cases of DVT comprises of the following steps:
- Bed rest with foot elevation above the level of heart
- Analgesics can be used to provide pain relief
- Antimicrobial therapy must be started
- Anticoagulants, such as heparin, low molecular weight heparin and oral anticoagulants, such as warfarin, can also be used
- Knee-length or thigh-length graduated elastic compression stockings help in reducing the risk of thrombosis
- Early ambulation helps in reducing the risk
- Vena cava filters can be used in the cases where anticoagulant therapy is contraindicated.

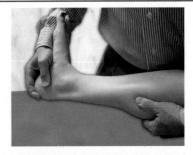

Fig. 6.4.4B: Method of eliciting Homan's sign, which helps in making the diagnosis of deep vein thrombosis

For elicitation of Homan's sign, the patient is instructed to lie supine on the bed with the knee (of the leg to be tested) in a flexed position. The clinician then holds the foot of this leg and forcibly dorsiflexes it. The Homan's sign is said to be positive, if there is pain in the calf upon performing this maneuver.

Besides a positive Homan's sign, other clinical features which may be present in cases of DVT include the following:
- Pain in the calf muscles and edema of leg on the affected side
- Rise in the skin temperature
- Difference in the circumference between the affected and the normal leg may be more than 2 cm.

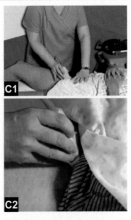

Figs 6.4.4 (C1 and C2): Procedure of ultrasound examination for studying the thigh veins

Before performing the ultrasound, the patient must lie supine and the leg (on which the ultrasound is to be performed) to be exposed up to the level of inguinal ligament. The hip and the knee must then be extended, with the hip slightly abducted. If possible, attainment of 30–40° Trendelenburg position facilitates the examination by increasing venous distension. The study must begin with the examination of common femoral vein, which is just inferior to the inguinal ligament between pubic symphysis and anterior superior iliac spine.

In the cases of DVT, legs should be elevated and graduated elastic compression stocking should be worn to reduce edema. Also the calf circumference should be measured daily to help monitor the response to treatment. Treatment of cases of DVT is described in Figure 6.4.4A.

Picture	Medical/Surgical Description	Management/Clinical Highlights
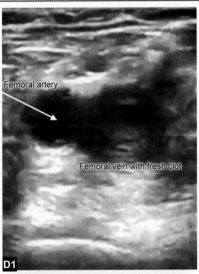Femoral artery Femoral vein with fresh clot **D1** **D2** **D3** **Figs 6.4.4 (D1 to D3):** (D1) Gray scale ultrasound examination showing presence of a possible clot in the femoral vein; (D2) Doppler ultrasound shows a cross section of the thrombus in femoral vein; (D3) Color Doppler showing thrombus in the superficial femoral vein (longitudnal view)	Ultrasound examination is the investigation of choice in cases of DVT, which helps in detecting changes related to compression of the femoral veins. Normal veins show augmentation of blood flow with compression of the vessel walls. Also, increased flow is likely to occur during expiration. Filling defects in the vessels may occur due to an onsite or upstream flow obstruction. Doppler sonography is not a formal component of lower extremity compression examination for DVT.	Various other investigations, which may be required in cases of DVT are as follows: • Duplex Doppler ultrasound: This is highly sensitive and specific for detection of femoral DVT • CT or MRI • I-125 fibrinogen scanning: This is not recommended for diagnosis of DVT in pregnancy due to the risk of radiation exposure to the fetus.
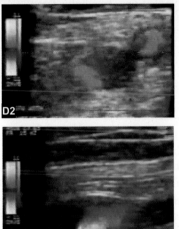Femoral artery — Collapsed walls of the vein **Fig. 6.4.4E:** Ultrasound examination showing coaptation of the walls of a patent vein as a result of compression with the transducer; the artery, on the other hand does not compress	In a normal vein, compression applied with an ultrasound transducer is likely to cause coaptation of the vessel walls. The walls of a thrombosed vein or a patent artery do not coapt with each other even on the application of pressure with a transducer.	In normal circumstances, application of pressure causes compression of the walls of a vein, but not that of an artery. If the vein gets compressed on application of pressure by a transducer, no DVT is present. On the other hand, inability to completely compress a vein could be due to DVT.

6.4.5: Pulmonary Embolism

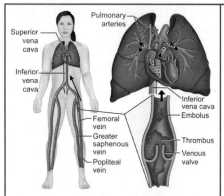

Pulmonary embolism most commonly arises from the calf veins. The venous thromboemboli travel through the right side of the heart to reach the lungs.

Fig. 6.4.5: Pathogenesis of pulmonary embolism

Pulmonary embolism is characterized by partial or complete blockage of pulmonary vessels resulting in acute respiratory and/or hemodynamic compromise. Acute respiratory consequences of pulmonary embolism include increased alveolar dead space, hypoxemia and hyperventilation.

Pulmonary embolism can be either acute or chronic. There may be presence of other symptoms such as tachypnea, dyspnea, hemoptysis, pleuritic chest pain, cough, tachycardia and temperature of greater than 37°C.

The following investigations may be done in the suspected cases: X-ray chest, electrocardiogram, arterial blood gases, venous perfusion scanning, pulmonary angiography, Doppler ultrasound, etc.

Treatment comprises of the following:
- *Patient resuscitation*: This comprises of cardiac massage and oxygen therapy
- *Heparin therapy*: Heparin is usually administered in a bolus dose of 5,000 IU, followed by 40,000 IU/day to maintain a clotting time over 12 minutes in the first 48 hours. Thereafter, heparin levels are regulated so as to maintain activated partial thromboplastin time of twice the normal
- Maintenance of blood pressure using dopamine or adrenaline
- Thrombolytic therapy using streptokinase may be administered
- Tachycardia can be counteracted using digitalis
- *Surgical treatment*: Procedures such as implantation of vena caval filters, ligation of inferior vena cava and ovarian veins can be done.

6.4.6: Amniotic Fluid Embolism

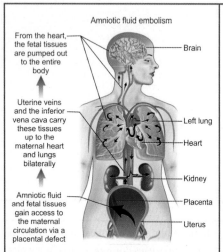

Fig. 6.4.6: Amniotic fluid embolism

Amniotic fluid embolism is a catastrophic syndrome occurring during labor and delivery or in the immediate postpartum period. This condition occurs when amniotic fluid, fetal cells, hair or other debris enter the maternal circulation via the placental bed of the uterus and trigger an allergic reaction. This reaction then results in cardiorespiratory collapse and disseminated intravascular coagulation. It may be associated with the following symptoms: dyspnea, nonreassuring fetal status (in case of pregnant women), altered mental status followed by sudden cardiovascular collapse, profound respiratory failure with deep cyanosis, etc.

The following investigations need to be done in these cases, echocardiography, electrocardiography, complete blood count including the coagulation parameters, arterial blood gases, chest X-ray and ventilation-perfusion scanning.

The goals of management are to restore cardiovascular and pulmonary equilibrium by maintaining the systolic blood pressure > 90 mm Hg; urine output > 25 mL/hour; arterial PO_2 > 60 mm Hg and correction of coagulation abnormalities.
- In case of uterine atony, efforts must be made to re-establish uterine tone
- Control of the airway is done with tracheal intubation and administration of 100% O_2 with positive pressure ventilation
- Infusion of crystalloids must be started to treat hypotension, and increase the circulating volume and cardiac output. Dopamine infusion may be started, if patient still remains hypotensive
- An immediate cesarean delivery is required in patients who have yet not delivered
- Blood and blood products: This may include use of fresh frozen plasma, platelets, cryoprecipitate, recombinant factor VIIa, etc.

Picture	Medical/Surgical Description	Management/Clinical Highlights

6.5: INJURIES TO THE BIRTH CANAL

6.5.1: Perineal Injuries (A to D)

Picture	Medical/Surgical Description	Management/Clinical Highlights
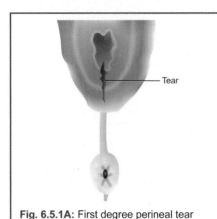 **Fig. 6.5.1A:** First degree perineal tear	First degree perineal tear as shown in Figure 6.5.1A involves only the vaginal mucosa and not the perineal muscles.	In case of presence of vaginal tears or lacerations, their repair is performed essentially in the same manner as that of the episiotomy (Figures 6.6.2 and 6.6.3) in order to achieve hemostasis and to obliterate the dead space. In case of first degree tear, the repair of mucosa is performed using continuous sutures with chromic catgut.
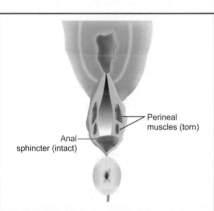 **Fig. 6.5.1B:** Second degree perineal tear involving the perineal muscles as well	Second degree perineal tear as shown in Figure 6.5.1B involves the perineal muscles along with that of vaginal mucosa. However, the anal sphincters remain intact in these cases.	While repairing the perineal tears, utmost importance must be given toward the maintenance of hemostasis and anatomical restoration without excessive suturing.
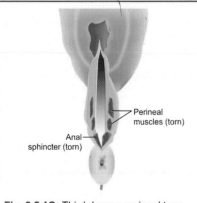 **Fig. 6.5.1C:** Third degree perineal tear	Third degree perineal tear as shown in Figure 6.5.1C involves the anal sphincter complex. It can be classified into three subtypes: 1. 3a: Less than 50% of external anal sphincter is torn 2. 3b: More than 50% of external anal sphincter is torn 3. 3c: Internal anal sphincter also gets involved.	In case of lacerations, the steps of repair are essentially the same as that of an episiotomy except in the cases of third degree and fourth degree lacerations where there might be an extension up to the anal sphincters and rectal mucosa respectively.

Picture	Medical/Surgical Description	Management/Clinical Highlights

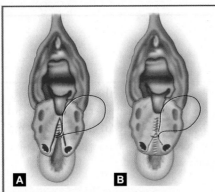

Fig. 6.5.1D: Fourth degree perineal tear

Fourth degree perineal tear as shown in Figure 6.5.1D involves the rectal mucosa along with the anal sphincter complex (external and internal anal sphincters).

Method of repair of a fourth degree perineal tear is described in 6.5.2 (A to G).

6.5.2: Repair of a Third/Fourth Degree Laceration (A to G)

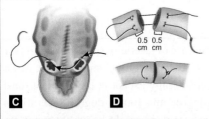

Figs 6.5.2 (A and B): (A) Approximation of anorectal mucosa and submucosa using continuous sutures; (B) Second layer of sutures placed through the rectal muscularis

In case of fourth degree laceration, it is important to approximate the torn edges of the anorectal mucosa with the fine absorbable sutures. Approximation of the anorectal mucosa and submucosa is done using 3-0 or 4-0 chromic catgut or vicryl sutures in a running or an interrupted manner.

The superior extent of the anterior anal laceration is identified and sutures are placed through the submucosa of the anorectum starting above the apex of the tear and extending down until the anal verge.

- A second layer of sutures is placed through rectal muscularis using 3-0 vicryl or catgut sutures in a running or interrupted fashion.

  This layer of sutures acts as a reinforcing layer and incorporates the anal sphincter at the distal end. Finally, the torn edges of the anal sphincter are isolated, approximated and sutured together with three or four interrupted stitches.

Figs 6.5.2 (C and D): (C) End-to-end approximation of the external anal sphincter. Sutures being placed through the posterior wall of external anal sphincters (these would be tied in the end); (D) Close-up view of the external anal sphincters showing end-to-end approximation

0.5 cm   0.5 cm

The anal sphincters need to be repaired in case of fourth degree tears as well as some third degree tears. The internal anal sphincter is identified as the thickening of the circular smooth muscle layer at the distal 2–3 cm of the anal canal. It appears as the glistening white fibrous structure lying between the anal canal submucosa and the fibers of external anal sphincter.

Following the repair of internal anal sphincters, the torn edges of external anal sphincters are identified and grasped with Allis clamp. The repair of these sphincters can be performed either using end-to-end repair (Figure 6.5.2E) or the overlap method (Figure 6.5.2G).

Picture	Medical/Surgical Description	Management/Clinical Highlights
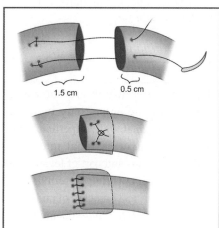 **Figs 6.5.2 (E and F):** (E) End-to-end sutures taken through the interior of external anal sphincter (shown in whitish blue); (F) Approximation of the anterior wall of external anal sphincter	For end-to-end approximation of the external anal sphincters, four to six simple interrupted sutures using 2-0 or 3-0 vicryl are placed through the edges of external anal sphincter and its connective tissue capsule at 3, 6, 9 and 12 O'clock positions.	The sutures are first placed through the inferior and posterior portions of the sphincter; these stitches are tied last in order to facilitate the repair.
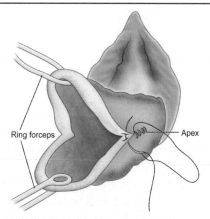 **Fig. 6.5.2G:** Overlap method of suturing the anal sphincters	The overlap method of suturing the anal sphincters involves taking two sets of sutures: the first row of sutures is taken 1.5 cm from the edge on one side and 0.5 cm on the other side in such a way that when the sutures are tied, the free ends overlap one another. The free end is then sutured to the rest of the sphincter.	The overlap method was considered to be superior to the end-to-end method as it was thought to be associated with fewer postoperative complications such as fecal urgency and anal incontinence.

6.5.3: Cervical Tear and its Repair

Picture	Medical/Surgical Description	Management/Clinical Highlights
Fig. 6.5.3: Cervical tear and its repair	The procedure of cervical tear repair comprises of the following steps: • Direct visualization and inspection of the cervix is done using three sponge holding forceps. • The anterior lip of cervix is grasped with one forceps at 12 O'clock position, the second forceps is placed at 2 O'clock position and the third one is placed at 4 O'clock position. • The position of these three forceps is progressively changed, until the entire cervical circumference has been inspected.	Small, nonbleeding lacerations of the cervix can be left unsutured. Lesions larger than 2 cm in size or those with a bleeding vessel need to be sutured. • The lacerations can be stitched with the help of continuous interlocking chromic catgut sutures. • The stitch must begin 1 cm above the apex of the tear. If the apex cannot be visualized, gentle traction must be applied to bring the apex into the view. The stitch must be placed as high as possible. • After stitching the laceration, the obstetrician must look for any continuing bleeding.

Ring forceps — Apex

6.6: EPISIOTOMY

6.6.1: Procedure of Giving an Episiotomy

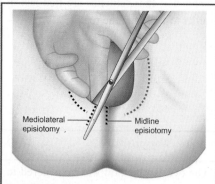

Fig. 6.6.1.1: Direction of giving different types of episiotomies

An episiotomy is a surgical incision given through the perineum in order to enlarge the vagina for assisting the process of childbirth. Episiotomy can be given in different directions: mediolateral or median direction.

An episiotomy given in the mediolateral direction (on either left or right side) is most commonly performed in our set-up. In many centers a median episiotomy is also performed extending from the center of fourchette toward the anus. A mediolateral episiotomy, on the other hand, extends from the lowest edge of the vaginal opening laterally either to the left or right side.

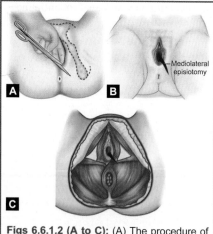

Figs 6.6.1.2 (A to C): (A) The procedure of giving a mediolateral episiotomy; (B) Cut in the skin after giving a mediolateral episiotomy; (C) Cut in the perineal muscles after giving a mediolateral episiotomy

The procedure of episiotomy comprises of the following steps:
- Under all aseptic precautions, two fingers of the clinician's left hand are placed between the fetal presenting part and the posterior vaginal wall.
- The incision in a mediolateral or midline direction is made using a curved scissors at the point when the woman is experiencing uterine contractions; the perineum is being stretched by the maternal presenting part and is at its thinnest.

The structures which are cut while performing the episiotomy include: posterior vaginal wall; superficial and deep transverse perineal muscles; bulbospongiosus and part of levator ani muscle; fascia covering these muscles; transverse perineal branches of pudendal nerves and vessels; and subcutaneous tissues and skin.

6.6.2: Repair of an Episiotomy Incision (A to C)

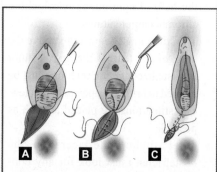

Figs 6.6.2 (A to C): (A) Vaginal mucosa being repaired using continuous stitches; (B) Muscle layer being repaired using interrupted stitches; (C) Skin being repaired using interrupted matrix sutures

The repair of an episiotomy incision is performed in three layers: first layer comprising of the vaginal mucosa and submucosal tissues; second layer comprising of the perineal muscles; and the third layer comprising of the skin and subcutaneous tissues.

Prior to the repair of an episiotomy incision or a perineal or a cervical tear, the patient is placed in a lithotomy position with a good source of light, illuminating the area of incision. The area to be repaired must be cleaned with an antiseptic solution. The surgeon must also examine the cervix, the vaginal walls, the vulval outlet and paraurethral areas for any suspected injuries or tears, which also need to be repaired.

Picture	Medical/Surgical Description	Management/Clinical Highlights

6.6.3: Procedure of Giving an Episiotomy and its Repair during the Process of Normal Vaginal Delivery (A to F)

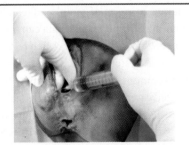 **Fig. 6.6.3A:** Administration of local anesthesia	An episiotomy incision is usually given after administration of local anesthesia as shown in the Figure 6.6.3A. Under all aseptic precautions after cleaning and draping the perineum, the proposed site of repair is infiltrated with 10 mL of 1% lignocaine solution.	Anesthesia in the form of nerve block (paracervical block) or local injection of anesthetic drug is given at the site of incision if the patient had not previously received regional anesthesia (e.g. epidural anesthesia) for the delivery.
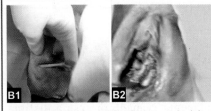 **Figs 6.6.3 (B1 and B2):** Giving an incision mediolaterally	The episiotomy incision should be made starting from the center of fourchette extending laterally either to the right or left. This type of episiotomy is known as the mediolateral type of episiotomy.	An episiotomy is a surgical incision, usually made with sterile scissors, in the perineum as the baby's head is being delivered. Following the delivery of the baby after the placenta has been expelled, the episiotomy incision is repaired.
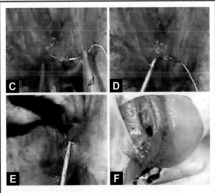 **Figs 6.6.3 (C to F):** Repair of the episiotomy incision	The vaginal mucosa is repaired using continuous sutures with chromic 2-0 and 3-0 chromic catgut sutures (Figure 6.6.3C). Next the fascia and the muscles of incised perineum are reapproximated with interrupted sutures of 2-0 or 3-0 chromic catgut (Figure 6.6.3D). Lastly the skin is closed using interrupted stitches with silk or subcuticular stitches (Figure 6.6.3E). Figure 6.6.3F shows the appearance of perineum following the repair of episiotomy.	The first vaginal suture is placed just above or at the apex of the incision. After closing the vaginal incision and reapproximating the cut margins of the hymenal ring, the sutures are tied and cut. Following the repair of first two layers, the next two layers, i.e. muscles and skin are repaired.

6.7: PLACENTA AND ITS ABNORMALITIES

6.7.1: Abnormal Placental Attachment (A and B)

Fig. 6.7.1A: Types of morbidly adherent placenta	If the placenta has yet not separated from the myometrium, the condition is known as an adherent placenta. Adherent placenta could be due to two causes: simple adhesion and morbid adhesion. Morbidly adherent placenta can be of three types: placenta accreta, placenta increta and placenta percreta.	In case of simple adhesion, although the placenta remains attached to the uterine wall, the placental attachments are not abnormal. On the other hand, in case of morbid adhesion, the placental attachment is definitely abnormal with chorionic villi being attached directly to the uterine muscle.

Picture	Medical/Surgical Description	Management/Clinical Highlights
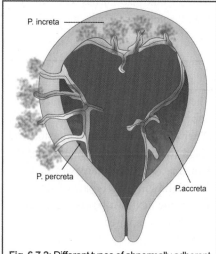*(see below)* **Fig. 6.7.1B:** Diagrammatic representation of level of penetration of different types of adherent placenta	Pathological adherence of the placenta to the myometrium is termed as morbidly adherent placenta. In these cases, the anchoring placental villi attach to the myometrium, rather than being contained by decidual cells. The mechanism for the abnormal implantation in cases of morbidly adherent placenta is probably due to thin, poorly formed, or absent decidua basalis that does not resist deep penetration by trophoblast.	Manual removal of placenta may be required in cases of simple adhesions. Abnormally adherent placenta can result in severe bleeding and may often require cesarean hysterectomy. Conservative management can be tried in a few selected cases where the patient is stable, is not having any active bleeding and wants to conserve her future fertility.

Figure content for 6.7.1B:

Penetration beyond the myometrium: placenta percreta

Myometrium: site of implantation of placenta increta — Myometrium

Deep layer of decidua basalis: site of implantation of placenta accreta — Nitabuch layer

Superficial layer of decidua basalis: site of normal placental implantation

Decidua

6.7.2: Diagrammatic Representation of Different Types of Placental Invasions

Picture	Medical/Surgical Description	Management/Clinical Highlights
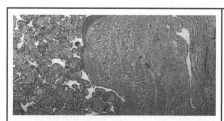 P. increta P. percreta P. accreta **Fig. 6.7.2:** Different types of abnormally adherent placenta (P, Placenta)	Different types of abnormally adherent placenta include placenta accreta, placenta increta and placenta percreta. While the term "accreta" refers to abnormal attachment of the placenta to the uterine myometrium, the terms "increta" and "percreta" refer to much deeper invasion of the placental villi into the uterine musculature.	The diagnosis of morbidly adherent placenta is made in case a distinct cleavage plane between the placenta and the uterine wall cannot be located and the tissue plane between the uterine wall and the placental edge cannot be developed through blunt dissection with the edge of the gloved hand at the time of manual removal of placenta.

6.7.3: Histological Specimen Showing Placenta Increta

Picture	Medical/Surgical Description	Management/Clinical Highlights
Fig. 6.7.3: Histological specimen showing placenta increta	Figure 6.7.3 shows histopathological appearance of placenta increta. Placental villi can be observed on the right side. The myometrial tissue can be observed on the left side, and it can be noticed of being invaded by the placental tissue. The placental invasion is however confined only to the inner layers of myometrium and not the whole thickness of myometrium.	In placenta increta, the invasion by the placental villi is limited to approximately half the myometrial thickness.

6.7.4: Hysterectomy Specimen Showing Placental Invasion of Myometrium

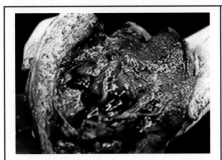

Fig. 6.7.4: Hysterectomy specimen showing placental invasion of myometrium

Figure 6.7.4 shows hysterectomy specimen of uterus in a 34-years-old G_3 P_2L_2 patient (previous lower segment cesarean section with present baby in transverse lie). Hysterectomy was perfomed because the patient was having uncontrollable postpartum hemorrhage (PPH) after delivery of the baby. Invasion of placental tissue in the myometrium was observed on histopathology examination. Therefore, diagnosis of placenta increta was made.

In this patient, the diagnosis of placenta increta was made later, after the performance of cesarean hysterectomy. History of a previous cesarean section acted as a risk factor for the development of placenta increta in the present pregnancy.

6.7.5: Ultrasound Based Diagnosis of Adherent Placenta

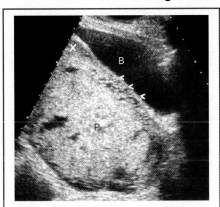

Fig. 6.7.5: Abdominal sonography at 27 weeks' gestation showing a morbidly adhering placenta (B, Bladder; P, Placenta)

Ultrasound imaging has now become a useful tool for diagnosing morbidly adherent placenta in the second and third trimester of pregnancy. Prenatal ultrasound has been reported to have a sensitivity of 94% and specificity of 79% for diagnosis of cases of placenta accreta.

In the adjacent Figure, the normal hypoechogenic retroplacental zone ("clear space") is reduced in thickness (upper part X). The hyperechoic uterine serosa bladder interface is interrupted (<). Note also the prominent lacunar vascular spaces. The final diagnosis established following hysterectomy was that of placenta percreta.

The various sonographic criteria for the detection of morbidly adherent placenta are as follows:
- Absence of a normal, hypodense retroplacental myometric zone
- A reduced surface area between uterine serosa and urinary bladder
- The presence of focal exophytic masses with the same echogenicity as placenta beyond the uterine serosa
- Presence of unusual, prominent, lacunar vascular spaces within the placental parenchyma

6.7.6: Color Doppler Scanning

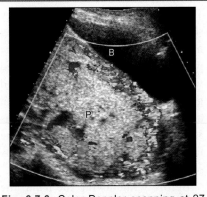

Fig. 6.7.6: Color Doppler scanning at 27 weeks' gestation in a case of placenta percreta demonstrating prominent placental vessels extending across the myometrium into the bladder wall (B, Bladder; P, Placenta)

Doppler sonography has been found to be quite sensitive for the detection of morbidly adherent placenta. Ultrasonography, especially with color flow Doppler, serves as a useful investigation in making a prenatal diagnosis of morbidly adherent placenta because Doppler sonography can help in detection of abnormal vascularization of the myometrium. Color Doppler sonography helps in improving the diagnostic accuracy of gray-scale ultrasound techniques, with sensitivity and specificity for moderately adherent placenta being 82% and 97% respectively.

The features on Doppler ultrasound which are highly predictive of myometrial invasion by the placenta are as follows:
- Distance of less than 1 mm between the interface of urinary bladder and uterine serosa
- Presence of large intraplacental lakes.

6.7.7: Magnetic Resonance Imaging of the Patient with Placenta Percreta

Picture	Medical/Surgical Description	Management/Clinical Highlights
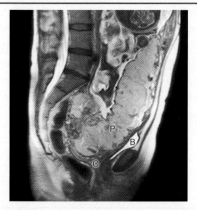 **Fig. 6.7.7:** Magnetic resonance imaging of the patient with placenta percreta at 27 weeks of gestation (P, Placenta; C, Cervix; B, Bladder)	Magnetic resonance imaging (MRI) is often used as an adjunct to sonography in cases with strong clinical suspicion of morbidly adherent placenta.	The MRI findings which help in the diagnosis of placenta percreta include the following: • Uterine bulging • Heterogeneous signal intensity within the placenta • Presence of dark intraplacental bands on T2 imaging.

6.7.8: Magnetic Resonance Imaging of Placenta Increta

Picture	Medical/Surgical Description	Management/Clinical Highlights
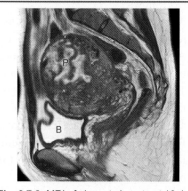 **Fig. 6.7.8:** MRI of placenta increta at 10 days postpartum (P, Placenta; B, Bladder)	Axial T2-weighted magnetic resonance image in this case demonstrates a retained placental mass as well as focal thinning of the fundus. Diagnosis of placenta increta was established in this case.	Being a costly investigation, MRI is usually used as a supplementary diagnostic procedure in cases where the placenta cannot adequately be assessed by sonography and where there is an increased risk of abnormal placentation.

6.7.9: Manual Removal of Retained Placenta

Picture	Medical/Surgical Description	Management/Clinical Highlights
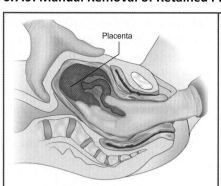Placenta **Fig. 6.7.9:** Procedure of manual removal of the placenta	The steps of surgery for manual removal of placenta are as follows: • The patient is placed in a lithotomy position. One of the surgeon's hands must be placed over the patient's abdomen in order to steady the fundus and push the uterus downward. • At the same time, the surgeon's right hand, smeared with antibiotics, is introduced inside the vagina in a cone-shaped manner. • It is then passed into the uterine cavity along the course of the umbilical cord. Once the placental margin is reached, The ulnar border of the hand is used to gradually separate the placenta.	The placental tissue is gradually separated by using the sideways slicing movements of the fingers. Once the placenta has separated, it can be grasped with the help of the entire hand and gradually taken out. The abdominal hand helps in stabilizing the uterine fundus and in guiding the movements of the fingers inside the uterine cavity until the placenta has completely separated out. Before withdrawing the hand, the surgeon must also look for any possible placental remnants or damage to the uterine wall. Bimanual compression of the uterus must also be done until the uterus becomes firm.

Picture	Medical/Surgical Description	Management/Clinical Highlights

6.8: UMBILICAL CORD

6.8.1: Normal Umbilical Cord

6.8.1.1: Cut Section of the Normal Umbilical Cord

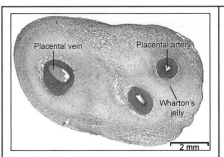 Fig. 6.8.1.1: Cut section of the normal umbilical cord	This is a histological cut-section of umbilical cord following parturition.	A normal umbilical cord has two umbilical arteries and one vein. Wharton's jelly is seen to be surrounding the umbilical vessels. There also may be presence of allantois. Wharton's jelly, composed of mucopolysaccharides, fibroblasts and macrophages, is derived from extraembryonic mesoderm and provides insulation to the umbilical vessels. Allantois, on the other hand, is a tubular extension from the endoderm of yolk sac and plays an important role in the formation of umbilical cord and placenta in humans.

6.8.1.2: Clamping the Umbilical Cord

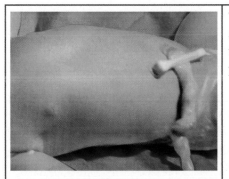 Fig. 6.8.1.2: Clamping of the umbilical cord	The umbilical cord acts as a physical and physiological connection between the developing fetus (embryo) and the placenta.	After parturition, there occur physiological changes involving closure of placental circulation. There is a physiological expansion of Wharton's jelly after birth and the resultant closure of umbilical vessels, which eventually occlude and fibrose.

6.8.1.3: Healing of the Umbilical Cord

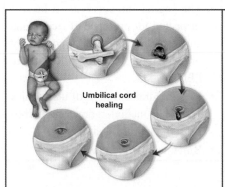 Fig. 6.8.1.3: Healing of the umbilical cord stump	At the time of delivery, the umbilical cord is clamped, cut and ligated. Shortly after birth, the umbilical cord occludes physiologically. The remnant stump of umbilical cord dries and falls off within 1−3 weeks.	The cord stump (before it dries and falls off) should be kept clean and dried. The baby's diaper should be tied in such a way that it is below the umbilical cord stump. This helps in ensuring that the cord stump does not get contaminated with urine and remains exposed to air. The mother should avoid bathing the baby in a tub before the stump falls off.

6.8.2: Abnormalities of Umbilical Cord

6.8.2.1: Central Insertion of Umbilical Cord (A to C)

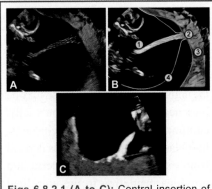

Figs 6.8.2.1 (A to C): Central insertion of umbilical cord: (A) Transvaginal ultrasound image showing umbilical cord attached centrally to the placenta; (B) Diagrammatic representation of the same; (C) Doppler ultrasound showing centrally attached umbilical cord (1: Umbilical cord; 2: Cord insertion; 3: Placenta; 4: Amnion)

(*Source*: Computerized generation of image B)

Under normal circumstances, the umbilical cord inserts into the center of placenta. A normal umbilical cord has a length of 50–60 cm, thickness of 1–2 cm and present with 10–15 helices. However there may be a wide variation in the shape and size of the umbilical cord.

This type of cord insertion occurs in most cases of normal pregnancies and does not present any danger to the fetus or mother and is normally managed.

6.8.2.2: Velamentous Insertion of the Cord (A and B)

Refer to Section 1

6.9: POSTPARTUM HEMORRHAGE

6.9.1: Definition

6.9.1.1: Mechanism of Bleeding in an Atonic Uterus

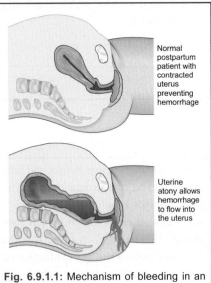

Normal postpartum patient with contracted uterus preventing hemorrhage

Uterine atony allows hemorrhage to flow into the uterus

Fig. 6.9.1.1: Mechanism of bleeding in an atonic uterus

Uterine atony is one of the most important causes for PPH, responsible for nearly 90% cases. Separation of the placenta from the wall of the uterus results in shearing off of the maternal blood vessels, which supply blood to the placenta. Under normal circumstances, the contraction of the uterine musculature causes compression of these blood vessels. However, the bleeding would continue to occur if the uterine musculature does not effectively contract and the uterus remains atonic.

If the placenta has delivered, but the uterus is not hard and contracted, instead appears to be atonic and flabby, the PPH is of atonic type. In this case the following steps need to be carried out:
- The urinary bladder must be emptied.
- The uterine cavity must be explored for any retained placental bits.
- The vagina and cervix must be still inspected for presence of lacerations and tears (traumatic PPH is commonly present in association with atonic PPH).
- Repeat administration of uterotonics (oxytocin, methylergometrine, carboprost, misoprostol, etc.).
- Bimanual uterine massage.

6.9.2: Nonsurgical Steps for Control of Postpartum Hemorrhage (A to C)

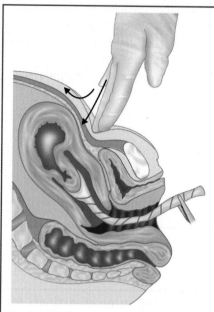

Fig. 6.9.2A: Controlled cord traction

Controlled cord traction or Brandt-Andrews maneuver comprises of the following steps:

- The cord must be clamped as close to the perineum as possible.
- The clinician must look for the signs of placental separation such as appearance of a suprapubic bulge due to hardening and contracting of uterus; sudden gush of blood; a rise in the height of the uterus (as observed over the abdomen) due to the passage of placenta to the lower uterine segment; and irreversible cord lengthening.
- Once one of the signs of placental separation occur, the clinician must hold the cord with the right hand and place the left hand over the mother's abdomen just above the pubic bone.
- The clinician must apply slight tension on the cord with right hand in downward and backward direction. At the same time the uterus must be stabilized by applying counterpressure in upward and backward direction.

- While applying controlled cord traction, the cord should never be pulled without applying counter traction above the pubic bone.
- As the placenta delivers, it should be held in two hands and gently turned, until the membranes are twisted and stripped off intact from the uterine wall.
- If the membranes tear, gentle examination of the upper vagina and cervix must be carried out to look for torn bits of membrane. These, if present, can be removed with the help of a sponge forceps.
- The entire placenta and membranes must be examined carefully to look for any missing lobe/membrane bit.

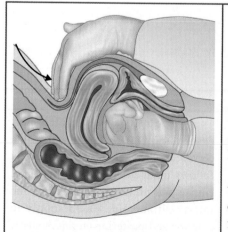

Fig. 6.9.2B: Bimanual uterine compression

If the clinician finds the uterus to be soft upon bimanual examination, a bimanual uterine massage must be performed to contract the myometrial muscles. The maneuver involves the massage of the posterior aspect of the uterus with the abdominal hand and that of the anterior aspect of the uterus with the vaginal hand. Uterus must be massaged every 15 minutes during the first 2 hours. If this maneuver controls the bleeding, the clinician must maintain this compression for at least 30 minutes.

The procedure of bimanual uterine compression comprises of the following steps:

One of the clinician's hands is formed into a fist and placed inside the vagina, with the back of the hand directed posteriorly and knuckles in the anterior fornix so as to push against the body of the uterus. The other hand compresses the fundus from above through the abdominal wall. The fundus of the uterus must be immediately massaged, until the uterus has well contracted.

Picture	Medical/Surgical Description	Management/Clinical Highlights

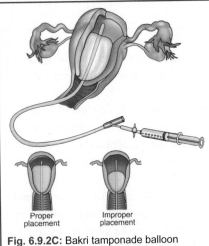

Fig. 6.9.2C: Bakri tamponade balloon

Balloon tamponade is another nonsurgical method to control PPH using a large bulb Foley's catheter, Sengstaken-Blakemore tube or an SOS Bakri tamponade balloon. A Foley's catheter with a balloon of 30 mL (which may be inflated up to 100 mL) is quite effective in controlling postpartum bleeding. However, the shape of the balloon may not correspond to that of elongated uterine cavity. The recently available SOS Bakri tamponade balloon (as shown in the adjacent figure) has been specifically designed to deal with PPH.

The Bakri balloon catheter helps in temporary control of PPH, potentially avoiding a hysterectomy. The balloon portion of the catheter is inserted past the cervical canal and internal ostium into the uterine cavity under ultrasound guidance.

6.9.3: Surgical Steps for Control of Postpartum Hemorrhage

6.9.3.1: Surgical Anatomy (A to C)

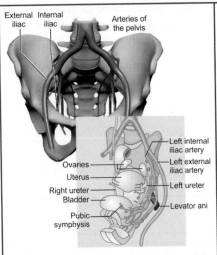

Fig. 6.9.3.1A: Blood supply to the pelvis (front view)

The blood supply to the pelvic structures is mainly by the common iliac vessels, which give rise to internal as well as the external iliac arteries. The internal iliac artery has an anterior division and a posterior division. Anterior division gives rise to five visceral branches and three parietal branches. The visceral branches are as follows: uterine; superior vesical; middle hemorrhoidal; inferior hemorrhoidal and vaginal arteries, whereas the parietal branches are: obturator artery; inferior gluteal and internal pudendal arteries. The posterior division on the other hand gives rise to the following branches: collateral branches to the pelvis, iliolumbar, lateral sacral and superior gluteal arteries.

Most of the surgical methods for controlling PPH aim at controlling the blood supply to the uterus by ligation of some of the vessels, which supply blood to the uterus. These commonly include the ligation of internal iliac artery, and/or uterine or ovarian vessels.

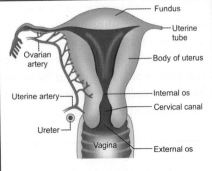

Fig. 6.9.3.1B: Blood supply to the uterus

The blood supply to the uterus is mainly via the uterine and ovarian vessels. The ovarian arteries are direct branches of the aorta, which arise beneath the renal arteries. The uterine artery is the branch of internal iliac vessel.

The uterine artery also gives off a small descending branch that supplies the cervix and the vagina. The uterine vein follows the uterine artery all along its course and ultimately drains into the internal iliac vein. Blood supply to anterior and posterior uterine walls is provided by the arcuate arteries, which run circumferentially around the uterus.

Picture	Medical/Surgical Description	Management/Clinical Highlights
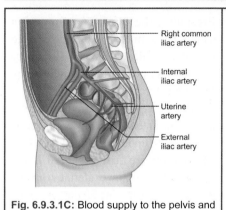 **Fig. 6.9.3.1C:** Blood supply to the pelvis and uterus (side view)	Figure 6.9.3.1C shows the side view of uterus, illustrating the supply of blood to the uterus through uterine and ovarian vessels.	The uterine artery passes inferiorly from its origin into the pelvic fascia. It runs medially in the base of broad ligament to reach the uterus. It then reaches the internal os by passing superiorly. While taking such a course, the uterine artery passes above the ureter at right angles. It then ascends along the lateral margin of the uterus within the broad ligament. It continues to move along the lower border of the fallopian tubes where it ends by anastomosing with the ovarian artery, which is a direct branch from the abdominal aorta.

6.9.3.2: Surgical Procedures for Control of Postpartum Hemorrhage (A to E)

Picture	Medical/Surgical Description	Management/Clinical Highlights
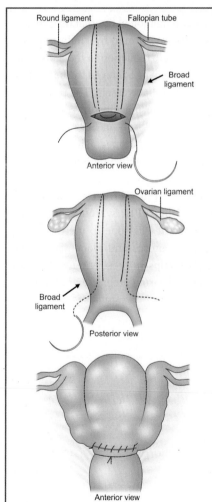 **Fig. 6.9.3.2A:** Diagrammatic representation of B-Lynch suture	Procedure of application of B-Lynch sutures is as follows: • A number 2 or number 0 plain or chromic catgut absorbable sutures using a number 2-sized needle are used for this procedure. Using these sutures, a puncture is made in the uterus about 3 cm below the right hand corner of the lower uterine segment incision and brought out 3 cm above the incision. The suture is then passed 3–4 cm medial to the right cornu of the uterus. • The suture is then placed posteriorly and brought down vertically to the same level where the suture had previously left the uterine cavity from the anterior side. • The suture is passed through the posterior uterine wall into the cavity and back through the posterior wall for about 4–5 cm to the left of the previous site of entry. • Then the suture is passed outside and posteriorly over the uterine cavity 3–4 cm medial to the left cornual border and is brought out anteriorly and vertically down to the left of the left corner of the lower segment. The needle is then passed through the left corner in the same fashion as on the right hand side to emerge below the incision on the left side.	Compression sutures can be considered as the best form of surgical approach for controlling atonic PPH as it helps in preserving the anatomical integrity of the uterus. After application of suture, when the sutures are in place, the assistant bimanually compresses the uterus while the chromic catgut sutures are pulled tightly by the surgeon. Thus, these sutures acts as uterine bracing suture which when tightened and tied help in compressing the anterior and posterior uterine walls together. This technique is safe, effective and helps in retaining future fertility. Before using the B-Lynch suture, a bimanual compression must be performed to assess the effectiveness of these sutures. If the bleeding is controlled temporarily in this fashion, the B-Lynch sutures are likely to be effective.

Picture	Medical/Surgical Description	Management/Clinical Highlights
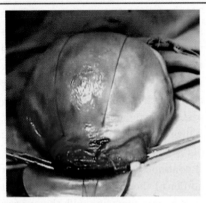 **Fig. 6.9.3.2B:** B-Lynch suture	The application of B-Lynch brace-like, compression sutures has been found to be safe and effective, and there have been reports of successful pregnancy following its use. These sutures help in controlling bleeding by causing hemostatic compression of the uterine fundus and lower uterine segment. A few complications, such as uterine ischemic necrosis with peritonitis, have been described with its use.	Presently, the uterine compression sutures have almost completely replaced uterine artery ligation, hypogastric artery ligation and postpartum hysterectomy for surgical treatment of atonic uterus. The sutures are secured vertically around the anterior and posterior uterine walls giving appearance of suspenders. The sutures are first anchored in the anterior aspect of lower uterine segment, passed over the uterine fundus, anchored in the posterior aspect of the lower uterine segment, then again brought back anteriorly passing over the fundus of the uterus.
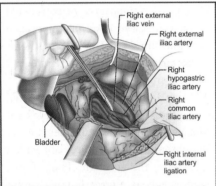 **Fig. 6.9.3.2C:** Internal iliac artery (hypogastric artery) ligation	Procedure of ligation of internal iliac vessels is as follows: • The peritoneum between the fallopian tube and the round ligament is incised to enter the retroperitoneal space. • The common, internal and external iliac arteries must then be clearly identified. • The external iliac artery on the pelvic sidewall is identified and followed proximally until the bifurcation of common iliac artery. The ureter passes over the bifurcation of common iliac artery. • The ureter must be identified and reflected medially along with the attached peritoneum. • The peritoneum is opened over the common iliac vessels and dissection is continued for approximately 5 cm from the point of origin (i.e. the level of bifurcation of common iliac vessels). This site is ideal for ligation because the posterior division arises within 3 cm of the bifurcation and the ligature must be placed distal to the posterior division of the artery in order to reduce the risk of subsequent ischemic buttock pain.	Bilateral ligation of internal iliac vessels was first performed by Kelly in 1894. Appreciable reduction in the amount of bleeding can be achieved by the ligation of internal iliac vessels. The procedure, however, is technically difficult and may be successful only in 50% of cases in whom it is performed. This procedure helps in accomplishing hemostasis via the process of simple clot formation and is a highly effective method of controlling PPH, which is indicated in cases of PPH due to uterine atony, ruptured uterus and placenta accreta. It also helps in preserving fertility of women desiring pregnancy in future.

Picture	Medical/Surgical Description	Management/Clinical Highlights
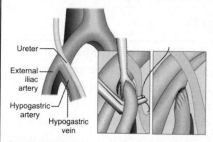 **Fig. 6.9.3.2D:** Internal iliac artery ligation (magnified view)	Figure 6.9.3.2D shows a magnified view, illustrating internal iliac artery ligation. Following the dissection of the peritoneum over the internal iliac artery, a blunt-tipped, right-angled clamp is gently placed around the hypogastric artery, 5.0 cm distal to the bifurcation of the common iliac artery. The hypogastric artery is double-ligated with nonabsorbable sutures (1-0 silk or No. 2 chromic catgut) at two sites 1 cm apart. For this, a nonabsorbable suture is inserted into the open clamp, the jaws are locked and the suture is carried around the vessel. The vessel is then securely ligated. The vessel, however, must not be divided.	The ligation of internal iliac vessel is also performed on the contralateral side in the same manner. Once the surgical process of ligation is complete, the dorsalis pedis and femoral vessels must be palpated to ensure that external or common iliac arteries have not been inadvertently ligated.
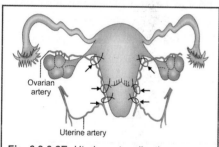 **Fig. 6.9.3.2E:** Uterine artery ligation	The procedure of uterine artery ligation comprises of the following steps: • The uterus is grasped and tilted in order to expose the blood vessels coursing through the broad ligament immediately adjacent to the uterus. • The most common site of ligation is 2 cm below the level of transverse lower uterine incision site. • While taking the stitch, maximum amount of myometrial thickness must be included in order to ensure complete occlusion of the artery and vein. • The needle is then placed through an avascular portion of the broad ligament and tied anteriorly. • There is no need for opening the broad ligament and the uterine artery ligation must be performed bilaterally. • Following the ligation of uterine artery, ligation of the cervical branch must also be performed.	Since approximately 90% of the blood supply to the uterus is via the uterine artery, ligation of this vessel through the uterine wall at the level of uterine isthmus above the bladder flap is likely to control the amount of bleeding. If, despite of bilateral ligation of uterine vessels, bleeding remains uncontrollable, ligation of utero-ovarian anastomosis is also done just below the ovarian ligament. However, this method may not prove useful to control bleeding in case of placenta previa or ruptured uterus. Bilateral ligation of the uterine vessels has not been observed to interfere with future reproduction.

6.10: UTERINE RUPTURE

6.10.1: Uterus Rupture Following Vaginal Birth after Cesarean Section (A and B)

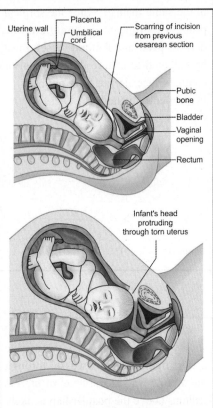

Fig. 6.10.1A: Attempted vaginal birth after cesarean section associated with subsequent rupture of previous lower segment uterine scar

Figure 6.10.1A shows a rupture of the previous lower segment uterine scar in a patient who was given a trial of vaginal birth after previous cesarean delivery. Uterine rupture is defined as a disruption of the uterine muscle extending to and involving the uterine serosa. The uterine rupture can be of two types: (1) complete rupture and (2) incomplete rupture. Complete rupture describes a full-thickness defect of the uterine wall and serosa, resulting in direct communication between the uterine cavity and the peritoneal cavity.

On the other hand, incomplete rupture (also known as uterine dehiscence) describes a defect of the uterine wall that is contained by the visceral peritoneum or broad ligament. Incomplete rupture is associated with minimal bleeding, with the peritoneum and fetal membranes remaining intact.

The identification or suspicion of uterine rupture is a medical emergency and must be followed by an immediate and urgent response from the obstetrician. An emergency laparotomy with repair of the transverse incision is usually required to save the patient's life. Complete uterine rupture is very unlikely today and occurs in much less than 1% of women attempting vaginal birth after cesarean section (VBAC). Due to the risk of rupture recurrence in a subsequent pregnancy, women with previously repaired uterine ruptures are advised not to attempt vaginal delivery in the future. In case of future pregnancy, a repeat cesarean section should be performed prior to the onset of uterine contractions.

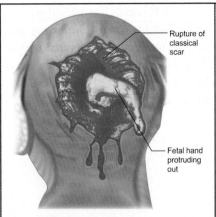

Fig. 6.10.1B: Rupture of a previous classical uterine scar

Figure 6.10.1B shows rupture in case of a previous classical uterine scar. Classical cesarean section involves administration of a vertical scar in the upper uterine segment and is associated with the highest risk of rupture in case of trial with VBAC. Though steps must be taken to resuscitate the patient, surgery should not be delayed owing to hypovolemic shock because it may not be easily reversible, until the hemorrhage from uterine rupture has been controlled.

Uterine rupture of a classical scar may be associated with massive PPH.

Since nowadays, classical caesarean is rarely performed, rupture of a previous classical scar is even rarer. Moreover according to recommendations by American College of Obstetricians and Gynecologists, women with a previous classical scar should have a repeat cesarean birth and not be given trial with VBAC. While in the previous days, most cases of classical rupture were managed with hysterectomy, nowadays some cases are also managed by controlling the bleeding surgically and repairing the defect.

6.11: UTERINE INVERSION

6.11.1: Definition and Classification (A to C)

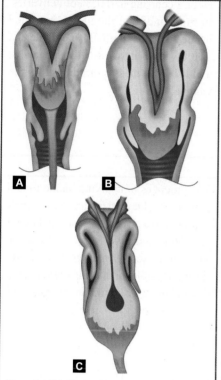

Figs 6.11.1 (A to C): Degrees of uterine inversion: (A) First degree; (B) Second degree; (C) Third degree

Uterine inversion during the acute postpartum period is a relatively rare complication in which the uterus is turned inside out either partially or completely. The uterine endometrium with or without attached placenta may be visible. Uterine inversion can be classified as follows:

- *First degree*: Dimpling of the uterine fundus, which remains well above the level of internal os
- *Second degree*: Uterine fundus passes through the cervix, but lies inside the vagina
- *Third degree (complete)*: The uterus protrudes completely out of the vaginal introitus. The uterine endometrium with or without the attached placenta may be visible.

In terms of onset of the inversion, it can be classified as acute, subacute and chronic.

Diagnosis of uterine inversion is based on the following:

Abdominal Examination: There is an absence of uterine fundus or presence of an obvious defect of the fundus upon abdominal palpation.

Bimanual Examination: This helps in confirming the diagnosis and degree of prolapse. This may reveal the following:
- Profuse bleeding through the cervical os
- Palpation of the inverted fundus at the cervical os or vaginal introitus
- In cases of incomplete inversion, the fundal wall may be palpated in the lower uterine segment and cervix.

Imaging Studies

Ultrasound: On transverse scans, a hyperechoic mass in the vagina with a central hypoechoic H-shaped cavity may be visualized. A depressed longitudinal groove, extending from the uterine fundus to the center of the inverted part may be observed on the longitudinal scans.

Magnetic resonance imaging: Appearance of the uterus is similar to that found on sonographic imaging.

6.11.2: Procedure of Correction (A to C)

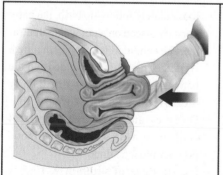

Fig. 6.11.2A: Grasping the protruding fundus

The Johnson's method of manual reposition for uterine inversion involves the steps as described in Figures 6.11.2 A to C. The protruding fundus is grasped by the obstetrician with the help of palms of the hand in such a way that the fingers of the clinician are directed toward the posterior fornix (Figure 6.11.2A).

The mainstay of treatment of uterine inversion is urgent manual replacement of the uterus, preferably under general anesthesia. The placenta often is still attached to the uterus and it should be left in place until after reduction. Every attempt should be made to replace the uterus quickly. Acute inversion can be managed with manual reposition (Johnson's method) or hydrostatic replacement (O'Sullivan's method). Tocolysis or general anesthesia is usually required to facilitate uterine reposition.

Picture	Medical/Surgical Description	Management/Clinical Highlights
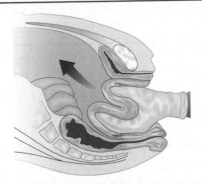 **Fig. 6.11.2B:** Gentle repositioning of the uterus	The uterus is returned to its original position by lifting it up through the pelvis and into the abdomen (Figure 6.11.2B). The part of the uterus that has inverted last must be replaced first. While the uterus is returned back, counter support must be applied with the hand placed over the abdomen.	Uterine inversion is rare, but may be sometimes present in the third stage of labor, occurring in 0.05% of deliveries. In this condition, the uterus is turned inside out, either partially or completely. The inverted uterus usually appears as a bluish-gray mass protruding from the vagina.
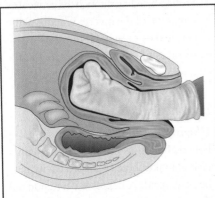 **Fig. 6.11.2C:** The clinician's hand must remain inside the uterine cavity, until the uterus has contracted	Once the uterus is reverted, uterotonic agents should be given to promote uterine tone and to prevent recurrence. In order to ensure that the uterus has been properly repositioned and the inversion does not return back, following the manual replacement, the clinician's hand should also remain inside the uterine cavity until the uterotonic agents have taken their effect (Figure 6.11.2C).	The practices of applying undue fundal pressure, undue cord traction and Crede's expression of placenta have been thought to be the causative factors for uterine inversion. Active management of the third stage of labor may also help reduce the incidence of uterine inversion.

6.12: NEWBORN INFANT AND ITS CARE

6.12.1: Care of a Newborn (A to I)

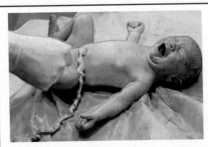 **Fig. 6.12.1A:** A newborn baby immediately after delivery in the labor room *Courtesy:* Rajiv Khandelwal	Examination of a newborn baby allows the midwife or pediatrician or the obstetrician to assess and monitor the baby's condition and promptly provide appropriate care and treatment as soon as possible. Every newborn must be examined thoroughly within 24 hours of the birth. A neonate which has delivered vaginally, has a gestational age greater than 38 weeks, is a singleton birth having birthweight appropriate for gestational age, has normal vitals, has passed stools and urine, feeds successfully and is normal on general physical examination, can be discharged by 48 hours of birth.	The following steps need to be taken immediately after birth of the baby: • Immediately following birth, the baby must be placed on a cot where neutral thermal condition is being maintained. Hypothermia must be avoided and the baby must be thoroughly dried. Early breast-feeding must be encouraged. • Daily cleansing of the umbilical cord stump with spirit and antibiotic powder must be done. • Single dose of vitamin K (0.5–1 mg) is given to all newborn babies within 6 hours of birth. This helps in preventing bleeding due to the deficiency of vitamin K. • Hepatitis B vaccine is administered at birth.

Picture	Medical/Surgical Description	Management/Clinical Highlights
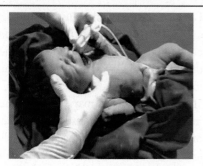 **Fig. 6.12.1B:** Suctioning the mouth and nose of a newborn baby *Courtesy:* Rajiv Khandelwal	As shown in Figure 6.12.1B, following the birth of the baby, the clinician must clear the oropharynx and nasopharynx by either wiping the mouth and nose with a clean towel or suctioning using a suction catheter (Figure 6.12.1B). The suction machine should be set at the negative suction pressure of about 100 mm Hg.	The baby's mouth must be suctioned first and then the nose so that in case the baby grasps at the time of nasal suction, it does not accidently aspirate the secretions present in the mouth. Besides cleaning the airways, suctioning also provides some amount of tactile stimulation.
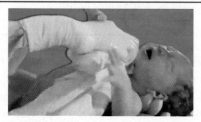 **Fig. 6.12.1C:** Cleaning the newborn baby *Courtesy:* Rajiv Khandelwal	As shown in Figure 6.12.1C, the baby must be dried immediately after birth from head to toe with a prewarmed towel. The excessive blood, vernix or meconium must be wiped off from the baby's skin using sterile moist swabs, following which the skin is dried using a soft towel.	Drying the baby helps in providing stimulation. Tactile stimulation helps in causing resumption of breathing in cases of primary apnea. This step also helps in avoiding hypothermia. Since the newborn child may be susceptible to develop hypothermia, the aim should be to maintain the axillary temperature of 36.5°C. In order to avoid hypothermia, routine baby bath must also be delayed..
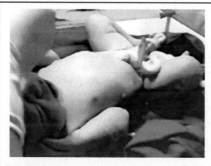 **Fig. 6.12.1D:** Extra length of the cord is cut *Courtesy:* Rajiv Khandelwal	While taking care of the baby immediately at birth, the extra length of the umbilical cord is cut. Umbilicus is examined for any discharge, redness or infection and presence of any hernia. The cut end of the cord must also be inspected for the number of umbilical arteries and veins.	Daily cleansing of the umbilical cord stump with spirit and antibiotic powder must be done in order to prevent infection. The umbilical cord stump normally heals naturally within 1–3 weeks, if allowed to dry naturally.
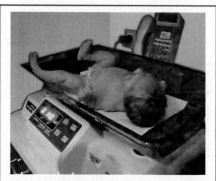 **Fig. 6.12.1E:** Taking the weight of a newborn *Courtesy:* Rajiv Khandelwal	The weight of the newborn baby is taken immediately after birth as shown in Figure 6.12.1E. Average weight of a normal baby at birth is about 3.25 kg. Weight less than 2.5 kg in a newborn child is classified as a low birthweight. The infant must be weighed every fortnightly or once a month to assess the gradual progress in weight. Most newborn infants lose up to 10% of their birthweight during the first week of life. However, most of them regain this weight by the time they are 10–14 days old.	The child's weight usually doubles by 4 months and triples by 1 year. The Weech's formula may be used for calculating expected normal weight for children as follows: • Weight between 3 months and 12 months: (Age in months + 9) ÷ 2. • Weight between 1 year and 6 years: (Age in years × 2) × 8 • Weight between 7 years and 12 years: [(Age in years × 7) – 5] ÷ 2

Picture	Medical/Surgical Description	Management/Clinical Highlights
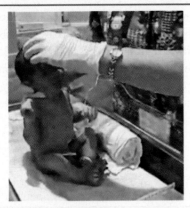 **Fig. 6.12.1F:** Assessing the head and the fontanels *Courtesy:* Rajiv Khandelwal	The baby's head is assessed and the fontanels are palpated. The head circumference is measured with a paper tape. The head fontanels and sutures are palpated. The baby's head must also be examined for the presence of any abnormal swellings such as caput succedaneum, cephalohematoma, chignon, molding, etc. The anterior fontanel is diamond shaped (2.5 × 2.5 cm) and has not ossified at birth. It usually ossifies 9−18 months after birth. If it fails to ossify even by 2 years, it can be considered pathological.	Large fontanels may be present in cases of hypothyroidism, various congenital malformations, etc. On the other hand, small fontanels may be due to hyperthyroidism, microcephaly, etc. Bulging fontanels may be due to the increased intracranial pressure, meningitis or hydrocephalus. Depressed fontanels are seen with dehydration. Delayed closure of fontanels may be associated with hypothyroidism, rickets, Down's syndrome, etc. Posterior fontanel usually closes by 2−4 months of life.
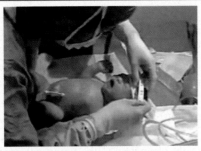 **Fig. 6.12.1G:** Measurement of head circumference *Courtesy:* Rajiv Khandelwal	While assessment of the baby's head, its circumference is also measured. The size of the head is an indicator of the size of its contents viz. the brain and the ventricles. The head circumference is measured from the external occipital protuberance to the glabella.	Head circumference on average is 33–38 cm at birth and normally increases by 0.5–0.8 cm/week during the first few months of life to allow for normal increase in the size of the baby's brain. The adult head size is reached between 5 years and 6 years of age. Formula for estimating head circumference in the 1st year of life is as follows: Normal range of head circumference in cm = [(length in cm + 9.5) + 2.5] ÷ 2
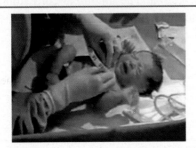 **Fig. 6.12.1H:** Measurement of chest circumference *Courtesy:* Rajiv Khandelwal	Chest circumference is measured at the level of the nipples as shown in Figure 6.12.1H.	At birth, chest circumference is usually less than head circumference by about 2.5 cm. The head circumference becomes equal to chest circumference by 1 year of age, following which the chest circumference exceeds the head circumference.
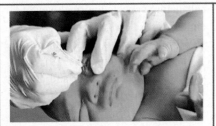 **Fig. 6.12.1I:** Eye care in a newborn child *Courtesy:* Rajiv Khandelwal	Eyes of a newborn child must be wiped with a cotton wool swab soaked with sterile isotonic saline or a soft towel. Antibiotic ointment is instilled in the baby's eye to prevent the occurrence of ophthalmia neonatorum.	In order to protect against ophthalmia neonatorum due to gonococcal and *Chlamydia trachomatis* infection, gentamycin or erythromycin (0.5%) or 1.0% solution of silver nitrate or 1.0% tetracycline ointment is routinely instilled in the eyes of all newborn infants (U.S. Preventive Services Task Force, 1996). The ointment is instilled immediately after birth and thereafter every 6 hours.

Picture	Medical/Surgical Description	Management/Clinical Highlights

6.12.2: Skin-to-skin Contact

	Skin-to-skin contact is initiated immediately after birth by placing the newborn baby either between the mother's breast or over her abdomen.	This is likely to facilitate bonding between the mother and child by encouraging breast-feeding and also helps in providing protection against hypoglycemia.

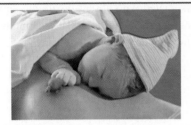

Fig. 6.12.2: Initiating skin-to-skin contact between the mother and the baby

6.12.3: Initiating Breast-feeding in a Newborn Child

	World Health Organization has recommended initiation of breast-feeding within 1 hour of giving birth amongst all women who have given birth to a live baby. Breast-feeding is likely to reduce neonatal mortality by 22%. Exclusive breast-feeding is recommended up to 6 months of age and can be given along with complementary foods until 2 years of age.	Breast-feeding ensures adequate supply of nutrients to the newborn infants, which are essential for its normal growth and development. Colostrum, a sticky, yellowish discharge produced from the breasts, a few days after birth must be definitely fed to the newborn child because it is rich in immunoglobulins and therefore helps in providing immunity to the newborn.

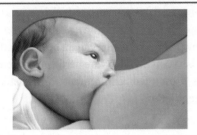

Fig. 6.12.3: Initiating breast-feeding in a newborn child

6.12.4: Infant with a Low APGAR Score (A to F)

	If the baby's APGAR (Activity, pulse, grimace, appearance and respiration) score at birth is between 4 and 6, tactile stimulation in the form of slapping of the soles of feet or rubbing the back may be given. The clinician must perform an immediate suction of the oropharynx and nasopharynx. If there is no response, the clinician must progress to positive pressure ventilation by providing lung inflation using infant self-inflating bag. If even this does not work, endotracheal intubation may be required.	APGAR score helps in the assessment of fetal condition and ranges in values from 0 to 10. Baby's APGAR score between 4 and 6 at birth may be associated with irregular or inadequate breathing, slow heart rate (less than 100 beats/minute), blue color, and normal or reduced tone. The basic approach to resuscitation in cases with low APGAR score is airway, breathing and circulation.

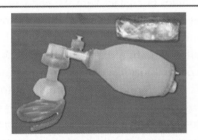

Fig. 6.12.4A: Infant self-inflating bag

	Ventilatory support with bag and mask ventilation must be continued until regular breathing is established. Oxygen by bag and mask ventilation at a pressure of 30–40 cm of H_2O must be given.	Once the lungs have inflated and the heart rate has increased ($\geq$ 100 beats/minute) or if the chest has been seen to move in response to passive inflation, then ventilation should be continued at a rate of 30–40/minute.

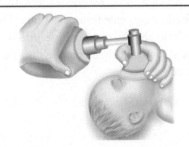

Fig. 6.12.4B: Bag and mask ventilation

Picture	Medical/Surgical Description	Management/Clinical Highlights
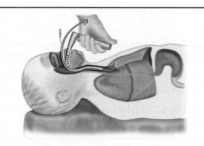 **Fig. 6.12.4C:** Tracheal intubation	Tracheal intubation may be required in cases with low APGAR scores (< 4). In these cases, the airways are opened and then the lungs inflated.	APGAR score of less than 4 may be associated with absent breathing, slow or absent heart rate (< 100 beats/minute), blue or pale and/or floppy baby.
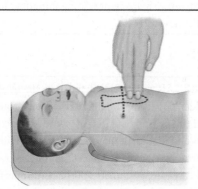 **Fig. 6.12.4D:** Magnified view of endotracheal intubation	Tracheal intubation remains the gold standard of airway management in cases with low APGAR scores. Figure 6.12.4D shows a magnified view of endotracheal intubation.	Endotracheal intubation is especially required in cases where direct tracheal suctioning is required (in case of meconium aspiration); effective bag and mask ventilation cannot be provided; chest compressions are performed; there is prolonged requirement for assisted ventilation.
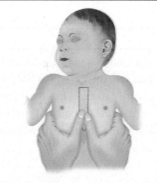 **Fig. 6.12.4E:** Infant chest compression using two finger compression	Once the lungs have inflated, still if the heart rate remains slow (< 60 beats/minute) then chest compressions must be started. Chest compressions can be given using two-finger compression technique or using an encircling method. In the two-finger technique of chest compression, the tips of middle finger and either ring or index fingers of one hand are used for application of compression. The fingers must be placed perpendicular to the chest and fingertips must be pressed down.	Compression must be applied for up to one-third of the anterior-posterior diameter of the chest. The fingers must remain in contact with the chest wall at all times both during compression and release. The chest must be allowed to fully expand in between the compressions. Current recommendation is to perform three compressions for each ventilation breath (3:1 ratio) for a total of 30 breaths and 90 compressions per minute. Once the heart rate increases above 60 beats/minute chest compression can be discontinued.
Fig. 6.12.4F: Chest compression using chest encircling technique	The most effective technique of giving chest compressions comprises of encircling the chest with both hands, so that the fingers lie behind the baby's back and the thumbs are opposed on the sternum just below the inter-nipple line and the chest is compressed by one-third of its depth. Pressure is applied on the lower third of sternum.	If after adequate lung inflation and chest compressions the heart rate has not responded, drug therapy (adrenaline, bicarbonate, naloxone, etc.) needs to be considered, and positive pressure ventilation and chest compression must be continued.

Picture	Medical/Surgical Description	Management/Clinical Highlights

6.12.5: Endotracheal Intubation (A to E)

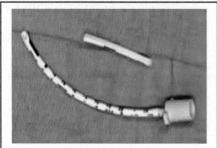

Fig. 6.12.5A: Endotracheal tube

The endotracheal tube is a device, which is passed between the vocal folds in such a way that the tip of the tube lies above the bifurcation of trachea (carina). Most endotracheal tubes have a black line near the tip called "vocal cord guide", which should be placed at the level of vocal cords. Cuffed tubes are usually not recommended for neonates. The tube may be cut to a shorter length, about 15 cm (as shown in the picture). The extra length is likely to increase resistance to airflow. For infants weighing less than 1 kg, endotracheal tube having an inside diameter of 2.5 mm should be used. In an infant weighing above 3.0 kg, the size of endotracheal tube should be 3.5–4.0 mm.

Endotracheal intubation may be required in the following situations:
- A nonvigorous meconium stained baby
- Cases where positive pressure ventilation needs to be given for a longer time
- Chest compression needs to be simultaneously given
- Administration of epinephrine when intravenous access is not easily available
- Situations like extreme prematurity, diaphragmatic hernia, etc.

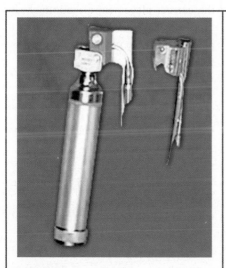

Fig. 6.12.5B: Laryngoscope

Laryngoscope with Miller blade (size No. 1) should be used for endotracheal intubation in a newborn term infant. A straight Miller blade is used so that it keeps the floppy epiglottis out of the way.

The laryngoscope blade must be held next to the infant's face and must be gently introduced inside the infant's mouth so that it reaches between the lips and the larynx.

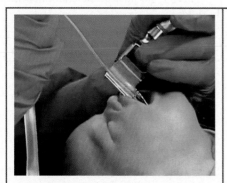

Fig. 6.12.5C: Insertion of laryngoscope

The laryngoscope is inserted in the infant's mouth with the help of clinician's left hand as shown in the Figure 6.12.5C.

The laryngoscope must be held between the thumb and the index finger of the left hand. Middle and the ring finger must be used for holding the chin and the little finger must be used for pushing down the larynx. Endotracheal tube is inserted with the right hand.

Picture	Medical/Surgical Description	Management/Clinical Highlights
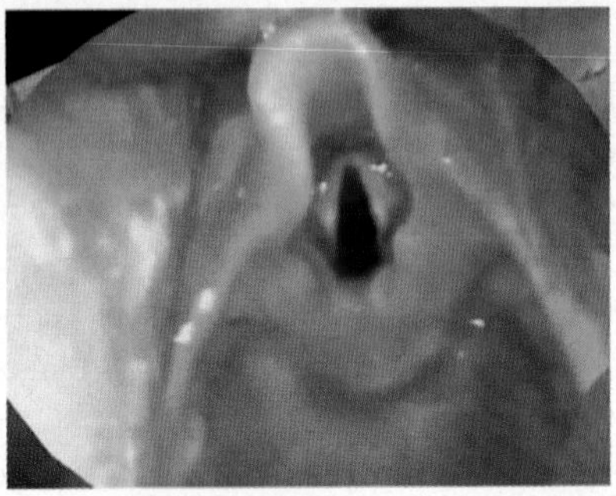 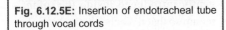 **Fig. 6.12.5D:** View through laryngoscope showing vocal cords	Figure 6.12.5D illustrates the view observed through laryngoscope, showing the vocal cords. The endotracheal tube is passed between the vocal cords.	The blade of the laryngoscope is extended into the mouth so that the tip is over the epiglottis.
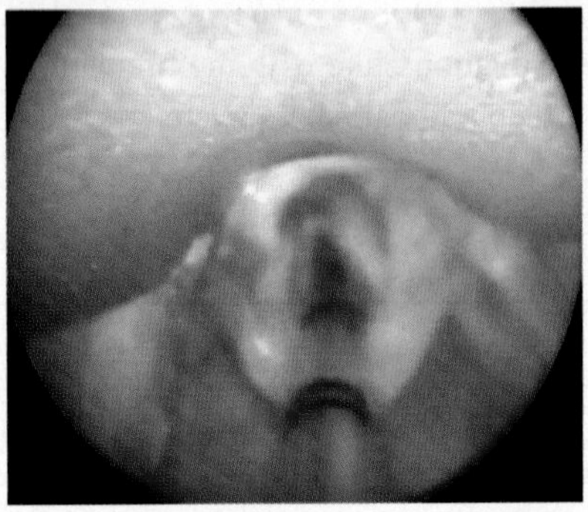 **Fig. 6.12.5E:** Insertion of endotracheal tube through vocal cords	Once the vocal cords are visualized through the laryngoscope, the endotracheal tube should be advanced between the vocal cords so that the black marker on the endotracheal tube is placed at the level of vocal cords. This helps in positioning the tip of the endotracheal tube above the tracheal bifurcation. Approximate depth of insertion of endotracheal tube from lips (in cm) = infant's weight (in kg) + 6	Once the endotracheal tube has been passed between the vocal cords, the clinician must observe the baby's chest movements and listen to the breath sounds. An increasing heart rate and detection of CO_2 on capnography and colorimetric device helps in confirming the correct placement of endotracheal tubes. Signs which indicate incorrect placement of the tube in trachea are as follows: • The newborn remains cyanotic and there is bradycardia despite positive pressure ventilation. • Capnograph reading does not display level of CO_2. • Colorimetric device does not display change in color related to presence of CO_2. • Good breath sounds are not present over the chest. • Abdomen appears to be distended and there is presence of noise over the stomach. • There is no mist in the endotracheal tube. • Chest does not symmetrically move with each positive pressure ventilation

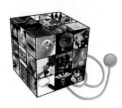

EVIDENCE-BASED BREAKTHROUGH FACTS

1. CIRCUMCISION OF THE MALE INFANT

The American Academy of Pediatrics (AAP) task force on circumcision of the male infant has recommended that "the health benefits of newborn male circumcision outweigh the risks; furthermore, the benefits of newborn male circumcision justify access to this procedure for families who choose it". Specific benefits associated with circumcision include the prevention of urinary tract infections, penile cancer and transmission of some sexually transmitted infections, such as HIV. However, the routine use of circumcision has not been recommended by the AAP. The health benefits and risks of newborn circumcision must be weighed in light of the family's own religious, cultural, and personal preferences, as the medical benefits alone may not outweigh these other considerations for individual families.

Source: American Academy of Pediatrics Task Force on Circumcision. Circumcision policy statement. Pediatrics. 2012;130(3):585-6. Epub 2012.

2. USE OF BENZODIAZEPINES DURING LACTATION

Benzodiazepines should be used cautiously during lactation because it can cause sedative withdrawal amongst the nursing infants. Although sedation in infants (and mothers) is a potential problem, the risk appears to be low and the studies support the continued recommendation to initiate breast-feeding while taking benzodiazepines in the postpartum period.

Source: Kelly LE, Poon S, Madadi P, et al. Neonatal benzodiazepines exposure during breastfeeding. J Pediatr. 2012;161(3):448-51. Epub 2012.

3. EFFECT OF BREAST-FEEDING DURING THE POSTPARTUM ORAL GLUCOSE TOLERANCE TEST

Amongst the postpartum women with recent gestational diabetes mellitus, breastfeeding an infant during the 2-hour 75-g OGTT may modestly lower plasma 2-hour glucose (5% lower on average), as well as insulin concentrations in response to ingestion of glucose.

Source: Gunderson EP, Crites Y, Chiang V, et al. Influence of breastfeeding during the postpartum oral glucose tolerance test on plasma glucose and insulin. Obstet Gynecol. 2012;120(1):136-43.

4. LOW LEVELS OF OMEGA-3 FATTY ACIDS MAY INCREASE THE RISK OF POSTPARTUM DEPRESSION

According to a literature review, low levels of omega-3 polyunsaturated fatty acids (PUFAs) may moderately increase the woman's risk for developing postpartum depression. This can be probably related to a chemical reaction initiated by omega-3 fatty acids in pregnant women which cause release of serotonin, a mood regulator. Therefore, it is likely that supplementation with omega-3 fatty acid during pregnancy would help in preventing or treating perinatal depression. However, this assumption yet needs to be proved by good quality clinical trials.

Source: Shapiro GD, Fraser WD, Séguin JR. Emerging risk factors for postpartum depression: serotonin transporter genotype and omega-3 fatty acid status. Can J Psychiatry. 2012;57:704-12.

Obstetrics

Section 7

Imaging in Obstetrics

7.1: INSTRUMENTATION

7.1.1: Principle of Ultrasound

Picture	Management/Clinical Highlights
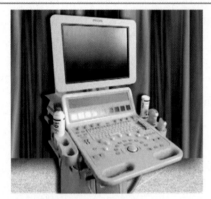 Fig. 7.1.1: Principle of ultrasound	Ultrasonography is a procedure, which uses high-frequency sound waves to view internal organs. The ultrasound probe has piezoelectric crystals in it, which convert the electric current into sound waves. These sound waves pass through the mother's abdomen as the clinician moves the transducer over the body part, which needs to be assessed. As these sound waves pass through the internal structures and hit various body's structures, they get reflected back which can be used to identify distance between body parts and their size and shape. When the sound waves hit a high density structure like bone, they are reflected back in form of high velocity waves, giving a white appearance on the screen. However when these sound waves hit a less dense structure, reflected waves are of a lower velocity. These waves give a black appearance on the screen.

7.1.2: Ultrasound Machine

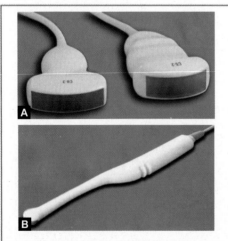 Fig. 7.1.2: Ultrasound machine	An ultrasound machine comprises of the following components: *Central processing unit*: This is the computer unit which does all the calculations and converts electrical signals into the image on the display and screen. It also sends electric signals to the transducer probes and stores processed information on the disc. *Transducer probes*: These house the piezoelectric crystals which send and receive the sound waves. *Display screen/monitor*: The processed images are displayed on the monitor so that they can be visualized and interpreted by the clinician. *Transducer pulse control*: This is used for changing the amplitude, pulse frequency and duration of the pulses emitted by the transducer probe. *Printer*: It prints images from the displayed data.

7.1.3: Ultrasound Probes (A and B)

Figs 7.1.3 (A and B): Ultrasound probes: (A) Transabdominal ultrasound probe; (B) Transvaginal ultrasound probe	Transducer is a hand-held device held against the surface of skin. It helps convert electric signals into high-frequency sound waves. These sound waves emitted by the transducer are focused into a narrow beam, which passes through various body structures and tissues and is then reflected back. The transducer, therefore, also acts as a receiver and converts these reflected sound waves into an electrical signal which is converted into an image on the screen. The transvaginal ultrasound probe shown in the adjacent picture is a straight-type probe, which is easier to manipulate in comparison to a bending-type probe. The head of the transvaginal probe either houses mechanical sector type or convex (curved-array) type probe.

7.1.4: Cover for Ultrasound Probes

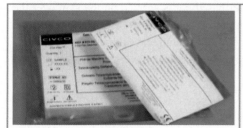

Fig. 7.1.4: Cover for ultrasound probes

Probe covers are made typically from latex or latex-free material, nontoxic polyethylene material or thin polymer foil, which have been cut to appropriate size and shape in accordance with the probe to be used. Use of cover helps in maintaining sterility of this equipment to highest degree, since most of these equipment or devices cannot be easily sterilized or autoclaved. Probe covers, both sterile and nonsterile, are used with ultrasound transducers. Use of sterile probe covers help in providing protection against cross-contamination, thereby protecting both the patient and hospital staff from the risk of hospital-acquired infection. Sterile probe covers are used for sterile scanning and puncture procedures.

7.1.5: Ultrasound Gel

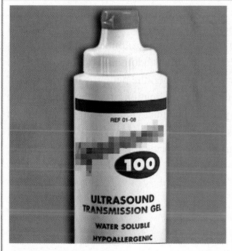

Fig. 7.1.5: Ultrasound gel

Ultrasound gel is a water-based conducive medium for transmission of sound waves and is applied to the area of skin to be examined. Since the ultrasound waves travel poorly through air, presence of gel allows easy transmission of sound waves from the probe to the skin and thereby to the tissues lying beneath it. An ultrasound gel is usually applied over the skin before performing the ultrasound examination. The gel also acts as a lubricant facilitating easy movement of transducer over the skin.

7.2: TECHNIQUE

7.2.1: Set Up of an Ultrasound Examination Room

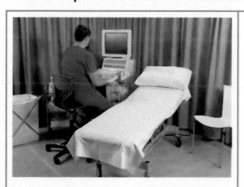

Fig. 7.2.1: Set up of an ultrasound room

This picture shows an ultrasound examination room with an ultrasound machine, examination bed and a chair for the patient's attendant, nurse or a female chaperone (especially if the examining doctor is a male).

7.2.2: Applying Gel over the Abdomen before Performing a Scan

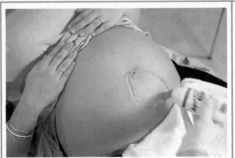

Fig. 7.2.2: Application of gel before performing a scan

Before performing the scan, a water based gel is applied on the skin over the site where the ultrasound examination is to be performed. Besides acting as the conductive medium for the passage of ultrasound waves, presence of gel also helps in lubricating the skin, thereby facilitating easy movement of the ultrasound probe over the skin.

7.2.3: Transabdominal Ultrasound (A to C)

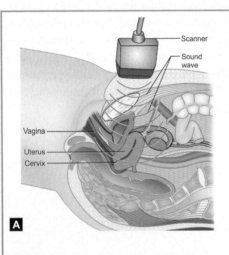

Scanner

Sound wave

Vagina

Uterus

Cervix

A

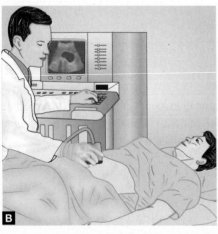

B

Figs 7.2.3 (A and B): (A) Technique of doing transabdominal ultrasonography; (B) Performing transabdominal ultrasound on a patient

The technique of performing transbdominal ultrasound is illustrated in Figures 7.2.3 (A to C). Before performing a transabdominal examination, the patient is instructed to come with a full bladder because transabdominal sonography (TAS) gives a clearer visualization of pelvic details when the patient's bladder is full, especially until 28 weeks of gestation. After application of a lubricant over the patient's abdomen, the transducer is placed in contact with the patient's abdomen and moved around over the patient's abdomen in order to visualize the fetus and determine its viability, its organs, placenta, and cervix for length and competence.

Picture	Medical/Surgical Description
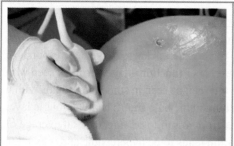 Fig. 7.2.3C: Performing a third trimester ultrasound scan	While the first and second trimester ultrasound scans respectively help in dating the pregnancy and assessment of congenital anomalies, third trimester ultrasound scan is helpful in assessment of fetal well-being. It is usually performed between 32 weeks and 36 weeks of gestation. It helps in assessment of baby's head and abdominal circumference. Ultrasound scan at 37 weeks helps in assessment of the baby's position (cephalic, breech or transverse) and helps the clinician in taking the decision for elective cesarean delivery in cases of noncephalic presentation. It may also help in monitoring multifetal gestation, assessment of placental position, estimating the amount of amniotic fluid and assessing the presence of nuchal cord. However, third trimester scan is not able to provide much information regarding estimation of the baby's weight or dating of pregnancy.

7.2.4: Transvaginal Ultrasound

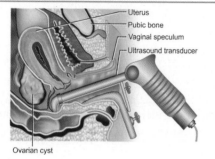 Fig. 7.2.4: Technique of transvaginal ultra-sonography	Figure 7.2.4 illustrates the technique of transvaginal sonography. Transvaginal ultrasound examination is performed after the woman has emptied her bladder. While performing the examination, a specially designed transducer, covered with a well-lubricated condom is placed inside the vagina, after having the women empty her bladder. The transducer is then moved around the vagina and pressed up on either sides of the cervix to allow visualization inside the uterus and pelvis.

7.3: NORMAL ANATOMY ON ULTRASOUND

7.3.1: Anatomy in the Proliferative Phase (A and B)

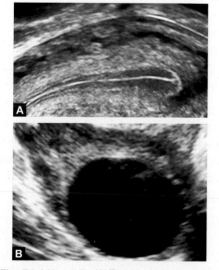 Figs 7.3.1 (A and B): (A) Transvaginal sonography of the uterus in the proliferative phase, showing presence of a well-defined "three line sign"; (B) Ovary showing presence of a dominant follicle	In the proliferative phase on TVS, there is presence of a well-defined "three-line sign", which is formed by the central hyperechoic reflection representing the endometrial cavity and the additional hyperechoic reflections representing the thin developing layer of the endometriumin on either side. The outer lines represent the interface between endometrium and myometrium. There is a hypoechogenic functional layer. The general hypoechogenic character of the functional layer of the proliferative endometrium is related to the simple configuration of the glands and blood vessels. There is minimal or absent posterior acoustic enhancement. The ovary may show presence of a dominant follicle with several other follicles in different stages of development.

Picture	Medical/Surgical Description

7.3.2: Normal Anatomy in the Luteal Phase (A to C)

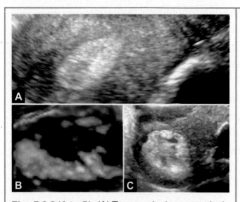

Figs 7.3.2 (A to C): (A) Transvaginal sonography in the luteal phase showing uniformly hyperechogenic endometrium; (B and C) Two small pictures in the bottom half show corpus luteum, which appears as an echogenic structure within the ovary with prominent peripheral vascularization

In the immediate pre and postovulatory period (2 days postovulation), an additional inner hyperechogenicity of variable thickness, which corresponds to a relatively high fluid content of these inner functional layers, can be seen with TVS. A small amount of fluid (1–2 mL) can be seen in some individuals within the lumen of the endometrium resulting in the halo sign. The total double layer thickness in the luteal phase ranges from 4 mm to 12 mm with an average of 7.5 mm. The luteal phase endometrium tends to be hyperechoic and maximum in thickness. There is presence of posterior acoustic enhancement and "three line sign" is also absent.

7.3.3: Transabdominal Scan (A and B)

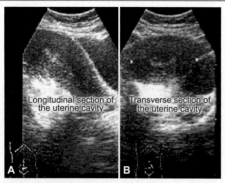

Figs 7.3.3 (A and B): Normal uterus as visualized on transabdominal scan: (A) Longitudinal section; (B) Transverse section

Figure 7.3.3A shows sagittal section of the uterus showing hyperechogenic endometrium. Figure 7.3.3B shows transverse section of the uterus on transabdominal scan.

7.3.4: Normal Ovary as Visualized on the Transabdominal Scan

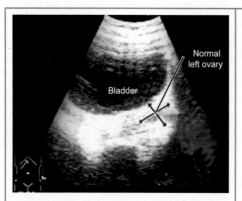

Fig. 7.3.4: Normal ovary as visualized on the transabdominal scan

Figure 7.3.4 shows normal ovary as visualized on transabdominal scan. Multiple follicles of different sizes in various stages of development can be visualized. Since the image was captured in early proliferative phase, when the ovulation was not about to occur immediately, the dominant follicle was not visualized.

Picture	Medical/Surgical Description

7.3.5: Maternal Liver

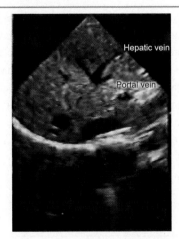

Fig. 7.3.5: Liver as visualized on transabdominal scan

The adjacent figure shows normal maternal liver as visualized on transabdominal scan. There is presence of normal hepatic parenchyma along with the presence of hepatic and portal veins. Although assessment of the liver does not form a routine part of ultrasound examination performed during pregnancy, it may be required for women presenting with gastrointestinal problems to rule out liver or gall bladder pathology.

7.4: EARLY PREGNANCY SCANNING

7.4.1: Gestational Sac at Four Weeks and Three Days of Pregnancy

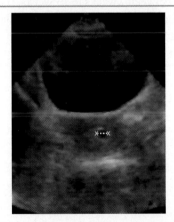

Fig. 7.4.1: Intrauterine gestational sac at 4 weeks and 3 days of gestation

Ultrasound examination in the first trimester is crucial in establishing intrauterine pregnancy, gestational age, early pregnancy failure, and to exclude other causes of bleeding such as ectopic and molar pregnancy, missed abortion, incomplete abortion, etc. During normal pregnancy, at the time of TVS, the gestational sac appears first by 4.5−5 weeks; the yolk sac by 5−5.5 weeks; the fetal pole by 5.5−6 weeks and fetal heartbeat by 6 weeks. All these findings are likely to appear 1 week later on the transabdominal scan.

7.4.2: Gestational Sac at Five Weeks Pregnancy

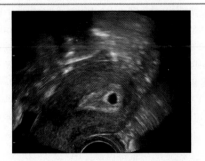

Fig. 7.4.2: Transvaginal scan demonstrating an intrauterine pregnancy at 5 weeks of gestation showing a double-rimmed gestational sac

Transvaginal ultrasound is most useful in the first trimester and is of great help especially in fat women and in those with retroverted uterus, in whom transabdominal ultrasound may not be able to visualize pelvic details clearly. Double rimmed gestational sac can be considered as a sign of intrauterine pregnancy during early weeks of gestation (4−6 weeks) in cases where the embryo or yolk sac has yet not made its appearance. In cases of normal intrauterine pregnancy, hyperechogenic ring of decidua capsularis is surrounded by another hyperechogenic ring (decidua parietalis). The gestational sac appears double rimmed because these two layers of decidua are separated by an anechoic space and fluid within the uterine cavity.

7.4.3: Yolk Sac

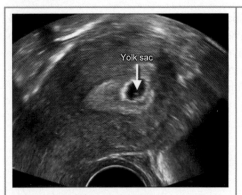

Fig. 7.4.3: Appearance of yolk sac (shown by arrow) on transvaginal sonography at 6 weeks of gestation

In a normal intrauterine pregnancy, the yolk sac normally appears by 5−6 weeks of gestation whereas the embryo appears at about 6 weeks of gestation. The yolk sac appears as a round sonolucent structure surrounded by a bright rim. Yolk sac does not increase to a size more than 6 mm in case of a normal pregnancy. The pregnancy may be considered to be abnormal if no yolk sac appears at the gestational sac size of 10 mm or no fetal pole is seen at the gestational sac size of 18 mm.

7.4.4: Measurement of the Crown-rump Length (A and B)

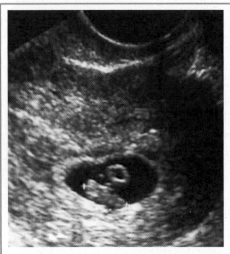

Fig. 7.4.4A: Ultrasound measurement of the crown-rump length

Crown-rump length (CRL) is an ultrasonic measurement, which is made earliest in pregnancy, when the gestational age is between 7 weeks to 13 weeks. It gives the most accurate measurement of the gestational age. CRL is the longest length of the fetus excluding the limbs and the yolk sac. CRL is about 1 mm at 5 weeks and 4 mm at 6 weeks of normal gestation.

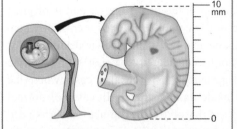

Fig. 7.4.4B: Diagrammatic measurement of the crown-rump length

Crown-rump length helps in measuring the length of human embryo starting from the top of head (crown) to the lowest part of the buttocks (rump). Measurement of CRL can help the obstetrician give an accurate assessment of the woman's expected date of delivery through estimation of her gestational age. Early in pregnancy, the accuracy of determining gestational age though CRL measurement is within ± 4 days but later in pregnancy due to different growth rates of the fetus, the accuracy of determining gestational age with help of ultrasound decreases considerably.

Picture	Medical/Surgical Description

7.4.5: Fetal Heart at Nine Weeks of Gestation

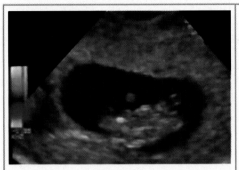

Fig. 7.4.5: Fetal heart at 9 weeks of gestation as observed on color Doppler examination

Fetal heart can be observed on ultrasound by 6–7 weeks of gestation. A detailed four-chamber view (with or without Doppler) can help in delineation of various cardiac defects. In most of the cases, by the time the embryo measures 2 mm, fetal heart activity may be clearly seen and is as high as 85 beats per minute (BPM), which may increase to 100–175 BPM by 5–9 weeks of gestation. If the fetal pole measures 5 mm or more with no heartbeat, diagnosis of miscarriage is usually made.

7.4.6: Normal Cervical Length on Transvaginal Sonography

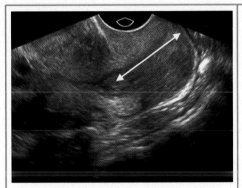

Fig. 7.4.6: Normal cervical length as measured on transvaginal sonography

Measurement of cervical length is useful in predicting preterm labor. Ultrasound should be used for assessing the length of cervix in women who are at an increased risk of preterm birth usually on two occasions at 14–24 weeks of gestation. The whole length of cervical canal between the external and internal os must be measured with help of ultrasound. TVS is more accurate than TAS in measuring the length of cervical canal.

7.4.7: Normal Cervical Length on Transabdominal Sonography

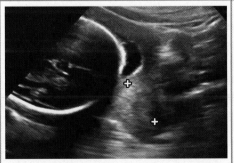

Fig. 7.4.7: Normal cervical length as measured on transabdominal sonography

At 20 weeks of gestation, the average length of cervical canal is 40 mm, whereas at 34 weeks, it is about 34 mm. Cervical length less than 15 mm at 24 weeks on ultrasound examination can be considered as abnormal. Besides dilatation and shortening of cervix on ultrasound examination, funneling of membranes into the cervical canal is also suggestive of probable preterm labor.

7.5: NORMAL THIRD TRIMESTER PREGNANCY SCAN

7.5.1: Fetal Head

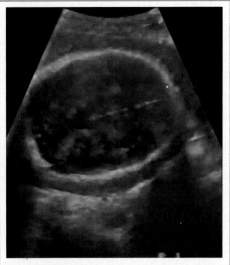

Fig. 7.5.1: Fetal head as observed on transabdominal ultrasound

While performing an ultrasound examination in the third trimester of pregnancy, it is important to identify the fetal head. After locating the fetal head, correct plane for measuring the biparietal diameter must be identified (See 7.5.3).

7.5.2: Measuring the Biparietal Diameter (A and B)

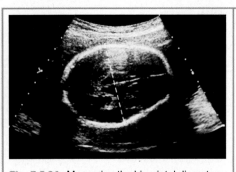

Fig. 7.5.2A: Measuring the biparietal diameter

Biparietal diameter is the distance between the two sides of the head. It can be measured at the level of the plane defined by the frontal horns of the lateral ventricles and the cavum septum pellucidum anteriorly, falx cerebri in the midline, the thalami symmetrically positioned on either side of the falx in the center, and occipital horns of the lateral ventricles, Sylvian fissure, cisterna magna and the insula posteriorly. Septum pellucidum can be visualized at one third of the fronto-occipital distance. The measurement is taken from outer table of the proximal skull to the inner table of the distal skull with the cavum septum pellucidum perpendicular to the ultrasound beam.

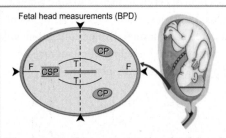

Fig. 7.5.2B: Diagram showing fetal head measurement

Biparietal diameter is usually measured after 13 weeks of pregnancy for dating of pregnancy. It increases from about 2.4 cm at 13 weeks to about 9.5 cm at term. An obstetrician maintaining a chart showing serial measurements of BPD is able to efficiently monitor the fetal growth (refer to 4.4.2.3). The BPD remains the standard against which other parameters of gestational age assessment are compared. At 20 weeks of gestation, accuracy of BPD is within 1 week.

Picture	Medical/Surgical Description

7.5.3: Transthalamic Scan (A and B)

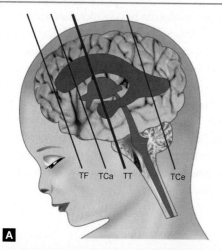

A

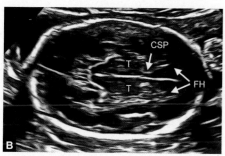

B

Figs 7.5.3 (A and B): (A) Different planes in which the fetal head scan is taken (TF, Transfrontal; TCa, Transcaudate; TT, Transthalamic; TCe, Transcerebellar); (B) Computerized generation of image showing the plane of transthalamic scan (CSP, Cavum septum pellucidum; T, Thalami; FH, Frontal horn)

Scans of the fetal head can be taken in various planes as shown in Figure 7.5.3A. Transthalamic scan (Fig. 7.5.3B) is the one in which the thalami, cavum septum pellucidum and the femoral horns of the lateral ventricles can be identified. This is the plane in which the BPD and occipitofrontal diameter (OFD) are measured.

7.5.4: Occipitofrontal Diameter

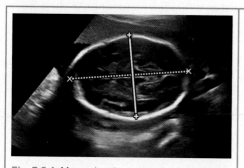

Fig. 7.5.4: Measuring the occipitofrontal diameter (dotted line in the photograph represent the occipitofrontal diameter)

Occipitofrontal diameter (OFD) extends from a point above the root of the nose (most prominent point on the frontal bone) to the most prominent point on the occipital bone (external occipital protuberance). OFD is measured in the same plane as the BPD. However instead of taking measurement from outer table to inner table, the measurement is taken from outer table of proximal skull to outer table of the distal skull. The plane of OFD corresponds to the greatest circumference of fetal head and is on an average 34.5 cm.

Picture	Medical/Surgical Description

7.5.5: Fetal Spine (A and B)

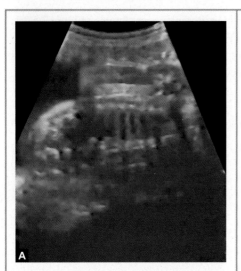

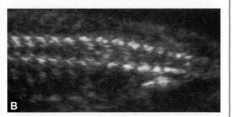

Figs 7.5.5 (A and B): (A) Fetal spine in longitudinal section; (B) Coronal view of fetal spine

Neural tube defects of the central nervous system can be considered as one of the most common congenital malformation. Most scans aimed toward diagnosing the neural congenital anomalies are done around midgestation (at about 20 weeks of pregnancy). Longitudinal section of the fetal spine must be performed because it helps in revealing various spinal malformations such as vertebral anomalies and sacral agenesis. Longitudinal section of the spine (at about 14 weeks) demonstrates three ossification centers (one inside the body and one at the junction between the lamina and pedicle on each side). These appear as three parallel lines depending upon the orientation of ultrasound beams. Attempts must also be made to demonstrate the intactness of the skin overlying the spine. Presence of a mass bulging out must also be observed.

7.5.6: Fetal Abdomen and Heart

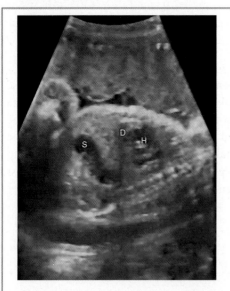

Fig. 7.5.6: Visualization of fetal heart (H), stomach (S) and diaphragm (D) on transvaginal ultrasound examination

The fetal heart can be visualized and it appears to be rhythmically contracting on real time ultrasound examination. Size, location and arrangement of stomach and diaphragm can also be determined. Fetal abdomen shows presence of stomach bubble. Diaphragm can be visualized as a thin line separating the chest from abdomen

Picture	Medical/Surgical Description

7.5.7: Measuring the Fetal Abdominal Circumference (A and B)

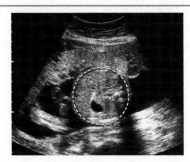

Fig. 7.5.7A: Ultrasound measurement of abdominal circumference

Abdominal circumference is a measure of fetal abdominal girth. The abdominal circumference is measured in an axial plane at the level of the stomach and the bifurcation of the main portal vein into the right and left branches.

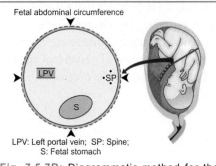

Fetal abdominal circumference

LPV

•SP

S

LPV: Left portal vein; SP: Spine;
S: Fetal stomach

Fig. 7.5.7B: Diagrammatic method for the measurement of abdominal circumference

While measuring the abdominal circumference, the radiologist must be careful about keeping the section as round as possible and not letting it get deformed by the pressure from the probe.

7.5.8: Fetal Femur

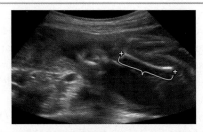

Fig. 7.5.8: Fetal femur on transvaginal sonography

Femur length is the length of femoral diaphysis, the longest bone in the body and represents the longitudinal growth of the fetus. Femur appears as an echogenic structure on ultrasound examination.

7.5.9: Measuring the Femoral Length (A and B)

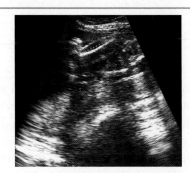

Fig. 7.5.9A: Measurement of femur length

At the time of measuring femur length, the femoral diaphysis should be horizontal showing a homogeneous echogenicity.

Picture	Medical/Surgical Description
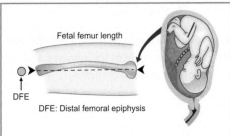 Fig. 7.5.9B: Diagrammatic method for the measurement of femur length	Femur length is measured from the origin of the shaft to the distal end of the shaft, i.e. from greater trochanter to the lateral femoral condyle. The femoral head and distal femoral epiphysis, which present after 32 weeks are not included in the measurements. Femur length increases from about 1.5 cm at 14 weeks to about 7.8 cm at term.

7.5.10: Measurement of Transcerebellar Diameter (A to C)

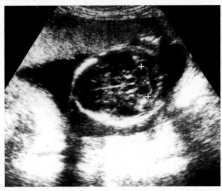 Fig. 7.5.10A: Measurement of transverse cerebellar diameter	Another parameter which is gaining increasing importance in measurement of gestation age is the transverse cerebellar diameter. This diameter refers to the widest diameter of the cerebellum. The major advantage of measuring cerebellar diameter is that this parameter allows for the estimation of gestational age that is independent of the shape of the fetal head, throughout the pregnancy.
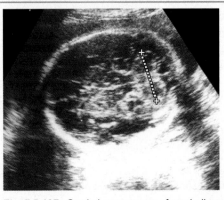 Fig. 7.5.10B: Grade I appearance of cerebellum	The ultrasound appearance of the cerebellum seems to change progressively from an "eyeglass" (grade I), to a "dumbbell" (grade II), and finally to a "fan" shape (grade III) with advancing gestation. A gradual change in ultrasound appearance of the fetal cerebellum is seen with advancing gestation. Grade I criteria is as follows: cerebellar appearance on the ultrasound is that of "a pair of eyeglasses". On ultrasonography each cerebellar hemisphere appears round and gives appearance of two fluid-containing cysts. The vermis has not developed well and therefore acts as a connection between the two round hemispheres.
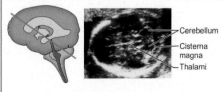 Fig. 7.5.10C: Grade III appearance of the cerebellum	The vermis, with increasing gestational age becomes more prominent and therefore appears as echogenic rectangular tissue connecting the two cerebellar hemispheres, which changes the whole cerebellar appearance from "a pair of eyeglasses" to that of a "dumbbell (grade II)". This changes into grade III (hyperechoic, "fan shape") with increasing period of gestation. The vermis becomes more echogenic thereby giving the cerebellum a "fan shape".

Picture	Medical/Surgical Description

7.5.11: Anteriorly Placed Placenta in Fundal Region

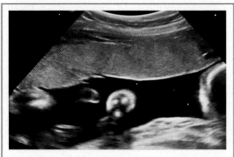

Fig. 7.5.11: Grade 0 placenta on the ultrasound, placed in the fundal region

Placenta is recognized by the presence of chorionic plate. The adjacent figure shows a grade 0 placenta.

Grading of placenta is as follows:

- Grade 0 placenta (first and second trimester): It has uniform echogenicity with smooth chorionic plate without indentations.
- Grade I placenta (mid second trimester to early third trimester): The chorionic plate shows subtle indentations. There are small diffuse calcifications randomly dispersed throughout the placenta.
- Grade II placenta (late third trimester): The indentations throughout the chorionic plate become larger and calcifications also become more prominent.
- Grade III placenta (39 weeks to postdated): Complete indentations of the chorionic plate reaching all the way to the basilar plate are present. This results in the formation of cotyledons with a significant increase in the number of calcifications.

7.5.12: Measurement of Fetal Heart Rate

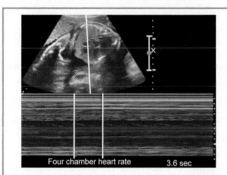

Fig. 7.5.12: Measurement of fetal heart rate using M-mode ultrasound

M-mode is a type of ultrasound which records moving echoes from the heart. The depth of echo-producing interface is displayed along one axis and time is displayed along the second axis. This information is then interpreted in form of fetal heart rate. The fetal heart rate at term usually varies between 120 BPM to 160 BPM.

7.5.13: Four-Chamber View of Fetal Heart

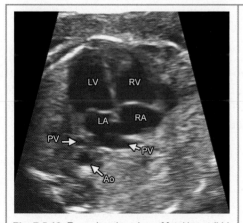

Fig. 7.5.13: Four-chamber view of fetal heart (LV, Left ventricle; RV, Right ventricle; LA, Left atrium; RA, Right atrium; PV, Pulmonary vein; Ao, Aorta)

Detailed assessment of the four chambers of fetal heart is usually performed routinely on ultrasound examination in the second trimester. In the fetuses at risk of congenital heart disease (previous history of heart disease in a parent or sibling or presence of noncardiac structural defect), this view may be particularly required. The four-chambered view is obtained in a horizontal section, just above the level of diaphragm.

7.5.14: Measurement of Amniotic Fluid Index

For measurement of amniotic fluid index and evaluation of disorders associated with abnormalities of amniotic fluid, kindly refer to Section 4.

7.5.15: Term-Fetuses on Two-Dimensional Sonography Scan

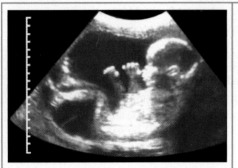

Fig. 7.5.15: Fetus at term as observed on two-dimensional ultrasound scan

Figure 7.5.15 shows a term fetus at 40 weeks of gestation in a normal pregnancy. At this time all the organ systems are mature enough to facilitate its survival in the extrauterine environment. During this time the fetal weight varies between 2.7 kg and 4.0 kg and fetal length between 50 cm and 55 cm. The placenta has attained grade 3 maturity and the amount of amniotic fluid appears normal.

7.5.16: Two-Dimensional Scan Showing Fetal Hands and Elbow

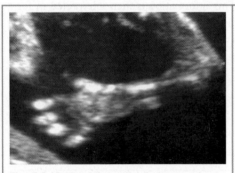

Fig. 7.5.16: Two-dimensional ultrasound scan showing fetal hands and elbow

The adjacent two-dimensional ultrasound image shows fetal arm with fingers and wrist extended and the elbow slightly flexed. Second trimester ultrasound evaluation of fetal fingers at 18–20 weeks of gestation helps in evaluation of various types of congenital anomalies in fetal fingers. Three-dimensional ultrasound of fetal hand in these cases is not essential, but it does enable the parents to identify and understand the lesion, and also enabled exploration of future surgical plan by the plastic surgeons.

7.5.17: Two-Dimensional Scan Showing Fetal Lower Limb

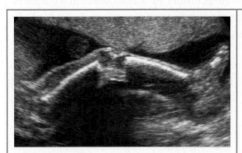

Fig. 7.5.17: Two-dimensional scan showing lower limb

The adjacent photograph shows two-dimensional ultrasound scan demonstrating left lower limb of a 24 weeks fetus with the hip and knee semi-extended and feet showing presence of five toes. Toes of the feet are examined for presence of abnormalities similar to those found in fingers as described in 7.5.18.

Picture	Medical/Surgical Description

7.5.18: Two-Dimensional Scan Showing Fetal Hand

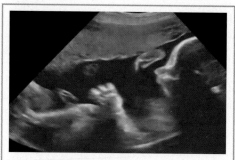

Fig. 7.5.18: Two-dimensional ultrasound scan showing fetal hand

Ultrasound examination performed in the second trimester helps in detailed evaluation of fetal fingers and hand. Any congenital anomaly in the fingers ranging from subtle finger deformities to the complete amputation can be identified. Some of the abnormalities in the fingers may include abnormalities in alignment, thumb anomalies, abnormalities in size and number of fingers, abnormality in echogenicity patterns associated with abnormal calcifications, constriction band sequence, etc. The adjacent figure shows ultrasound examination of a fetus at 24 weeks of gestation with elbow of left arm flexed and the wrist folded and hand closed.

7.6: THREE-DIMENSIONAL IMAGING

7.6.1: Nine-weeks-old Fetus (A and B)

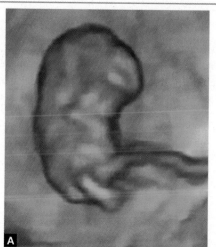

Figs 7.6.1 (A and B): (A) Nine-weeks-old fetus as observed on three-dimensional ultrasound scan; (B) Computerized generated graphic showing a nine-weeks-old fetus

At 9th week of gestation, the fetal head becomes rounded and forms nearly half of the embryo. During this period, the development of upper and lower limbs is occurring with the development of upper limbs being faster than that of lower limbs. By the end of 9th week, fingers have been completely formed. Physiological midgut herniation occurs, which becomes normal by 10th week. By 9th week of pregnancy, the facial image becomes well defined. External ear can also be appreciated. There also occurs rapid increase in the size of lateral ventricles. The early spine is also visible in the entire length.

7.6.2: Twelve-weeks-old Fetus

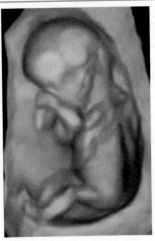

Fig. 7.6.2: Twelve-weeks-old fetus

During the 12th week of gestation, the fetal neck becomes well-defined; the face becomes broader and the eyes are widely separated. By 12 weeks of gestation, fetal sex can also be distinguished. Three-dimensional ultrasound examination provides more detailed analysis of fetal anomaly at this stage and it becomes possible to count the number of fetal fingers and toes. The lateral ventricle starts dominating the brain and the growing cerebellum can also be clearly observed.

7.6.3: Fourteen-weeks-old Fetus

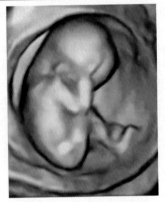

Fig. 7.6.3: Fourteen-weeks-old fetus

Further development of the central nervous system occurs during this phase. Complete development of the cerebellum usually occurs by 17 weeks of gestation.

7.6.4: Sixteen-weeks-old Fetus

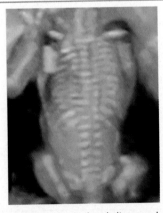

Fig. 7.6.4: Three-dimensional ultrasound scan of a 16-weeks-old fetus showing fetal spine

The optimal time for evaluation of fetal spine is 12–16 weeks of gestation. Features of a normal spine as visualized on ultrasound examination have been described in 7.5.5.

Picture	Medical/Surgical Description

7.6.5: Twenty-weeks-old Fetus

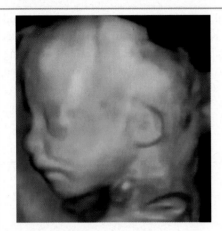

Fig. 7.6.5: Twenty-weeks-old fetus

During the second trimester, further development of fetal morphology occurs and facial features become more clearly identifiable. Therefore, second trimester scan for fetal morphology is usually performed between 18 weeks and 20 weeks of gestation.

7.6.6: Fetal Leg of a Twenty-three-weeks-old Fetus

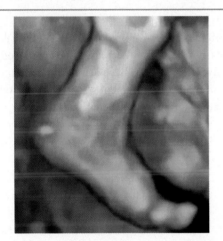

Fig. 7.6.6: Fetal leg of a 23-weeks-old fetus as observed on three-dimensional ultrasound

Evaluation of fetal leg in the second trimester can help in delineation of anatomical abnormalities in the fetal leg and foot. Abnormalities in either toes or fingers could be indicative of an underlying chromosomal abnormality.

7.6.7: Twenty-five-weeks-old Fetus

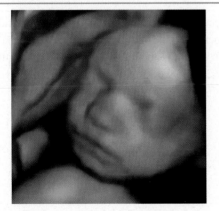

Fig. 7.6.7: Twenty-five-weeks-old fetus

Fetus between 25 weeks and 27 weeks of gestation weighs about 700–800 g and measures about 35–40 cm in length. At 26 weeks of gestation, the fetal lungs start producing surfactant, which helps in the expansion of lung alveoli by reducing the surface tension. The baby also starts blinking and closing its eyes, and hearing sounds during this period.

7.6.8: Twenty-nine-weeks-old Fetus

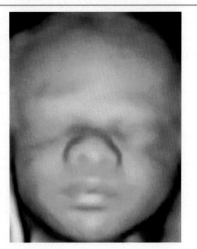

Fig. 7.6.8: Twenty-nine-weeks-old fetus

During 29 weeks of gestation, the fetal length becomes approximately 40 cm and the fetal weight becomes about 1−1.1 Kg. There is accumulation of subcutaneous fat. Further maturation of the baby's brain helps in better control of breathing and body temperatures. There is also an increase in the fetal movements, and increased perception of stimuli such as light, sound, taste and smell.

7.6.9: Thirty-two-weeks-old Fetus

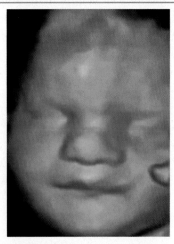

Fig. 7.6.9: Thirty-two-weeks-old fetus

At 32 weeks of gestation, the fetal weight is about 1.7−1.8 kg and fetal length is about 42−44 cm. The fetal movements may be slightly decreased due to reduced space within the uterine cavity. All five sense organs have started functioning and the baby's brain shows periods of rapid eye movement sleep. The nails of the toes have formed completely and the hair on the head continues to grow.

7.6.10: Thirty-five-weeks-old Fetus

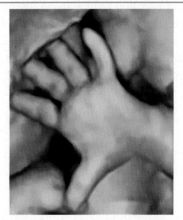

Fig. 7.6.10: Hand of a 35-weeks-old fetus

At 35 weeks of gestation, further accumulation of fat occurs on the arms and legs to help the baby regulate its temperature. The baby now occupies the uterine cavity almost completely. The baby's weight is about 2.3–2.5 kg and the length is about 45–48 cm. In the male babies, by 35 weeks of gestation, the testes have descended into the scrotum.

Picture	Medical/Surgical Description

7.6.11: Thirty-nine-weeks-old Fetus

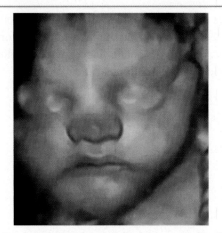

Fig. 7.6.11: Thirty-nine-weeks fetus as visualized on transvaginal sonography

By 39 weeks of gestation, most of the lanugo hair has disappeared with a little amount remaining over the shoulders, arms and legs. During this period, the lungs are maturing and the amount of surfactant is increasing. Accumulation of fat (particularly that of brown fat, required for thermogenesis) continues. The baby's length becomes about 50–52 cm and weight becomes about 3.0–3.2 kg.

7.6.12: Fetal Face along with Fetal Hand at Thirty-three Weeks of Gestation

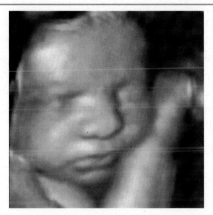

Fig. 7.6.12: Three-dimensional ultrasound image showing fetal face along with fetal hand at 33 weeks

At 33 weeks of gestation, the fetal length is about 43–45 cm, and the weight varies between 1.9 kg and 2.0 kg. The brain is rapidly developing and ossification of most bones of the limbs is complete during this time. During this period in a male fetus, the testicles start descending from the abdomen into the scrotum.

7.6.13: Fetal Face

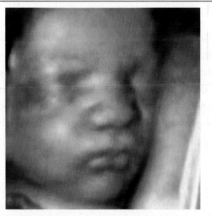

Fig. 7.6.13: Three-dimensional ultrasound image showing fetal face

Visualization of the baby's three-dimensional images facilitates bonding between the parents and the baby. The best time to obtain such images is between 24 weeks and 34 weeks of gestation, when the baby's face can be quite clearly visualized.

Picture	Medical/Surgical Description

7.6.14: Fetal Foot

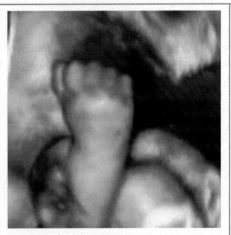

Fig. 7.6.14: Visualization of fetal feet on three-dimensional ultrasound

Three-dimensional ultrasound serves as a noninvasive method for evaluation of fetal feet and legs. This ultrasound examination is useful in identification of various anomalies and malformations in fetal toes and/or fingers, which could be associated with the presence of underlying chromosomal anomalies.

7.6.15: Fetal Ear

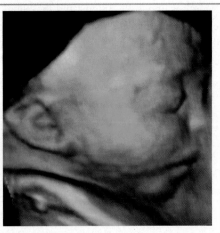

Fig. 7.6.15: Visualization of fetal ears on three-dimensional ultrasound

Three-dimensional ultrasound examination is a noninvasive method for detection of fetal ear anomalies, which may be associated with some underlying chromosomal anomaly. Three-dimensional ultrasound helps in determination of the ear position, location and ear morphology. Due to complexities in the shape of fetal ear, examination with two-dimensional ultrasound is only able to provide limited information. In this context, three-dimensional ultrasound provides better delineation of ear morphology.

7.6.16: Fetal Fingers

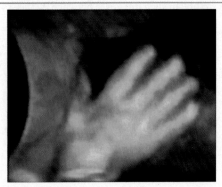

Fig. 7.6.16: Visualization of fetal fingers on three-dimensional ultrasound

Two-dimensional ultrasound examination performed in the second trimester may provide detailed information about anatomy of fetal fingers and presence of any anomalies. Though examination by three-dimensional ultrasound is not mandatory, it may be performed in cases where there is suspicion regarding presence of some anomaly on two-dimensional ultrasound. Three-dimensional ultrasound examination is likely to provide greater information during the evaluation of fetal hands and fingers in both normal and abnormal cases.

Picture	Medical/Surgical Description

7.6.17: Comparison of a Newborn Image with that of the Three-Dimensional Image (A to C)

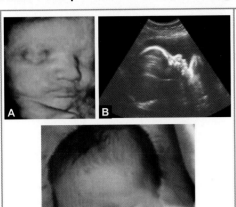

Figs 7.6.17 (A to C): Three-dimensional and two-dimensional images of the baby at term in comparison with actual photograph of the baby, taken a few hours after birth

Three-dimensional image of the baby taken at term shows close resemblance to the baby's face as observed after birth. Visualization of the baby's face at term on three-dimensional ultrasound help the parents to develop close bonding with the baby even before the baby's delivery.

7.6.18: Fetal Eye Opening

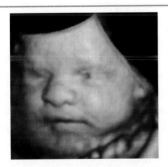

Fig. 7.6.18: Opening of fetal eyes at 26 weeks of gestation

Fetal movements can be observed on three-dimensional/four-dimensional ultrasound examination, typically starting from the second trimester. The most active fetal behavioral pattern can be considered to be "hand movements" and the least active as the "mouth movements". Fetal eye blinking and the facial grimaces can be observed between 24 weeks and 26 weeks of gestation. Two types of facial expressions, which can be easily observed, include smiling and scowling.

7.6.19: Thirty-eight-weeks-old Fetus Opening its Mouth

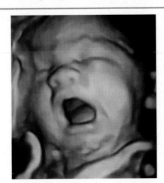

Fig. 7.6.19: Thirty-eight-weeks-old fetus opening its mouth

During third trimester, the fetal motor behavior increasingly becomes more variable and frequent. There is an increase in the facial movements such as opening and closing of jaws, swallowing and chewing. The quality of these movements can be observed to improve over time due to the maturation process.

Picture	Medical/Surgical Description

7.6.20: Fetus Protruding its Tongue

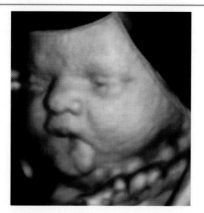

By the time the pregnancy approaches term, the number of general movements decrease due to the maturation of cerebrum. At this time, specific movements such as yawning and protrusion of tongue can be observed.

Fig. 7.6.20: Three-dimensional ultrasound at term showing the fetus protruding its tongue out

7.7: DOPPLER ULTRASOUND

7.7.1: Principle of Doppler Ultrasound

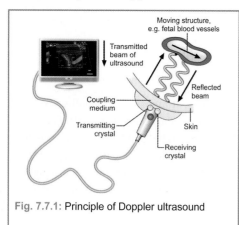

Fig. 7.7.1: Principle of Doppler ultrasound

In Doppler ultrasound, the ultrasound waves are targeted at a particular object (reflector), which they strike before getting reflected. If the reflector does not move, the frequency of the reflected wave is equal to that of transmitted wave. If the reflector moves toward the transceiver, the reflected frequency would be higher than that of the transmitted wave, while if the reflector moves away from the probe, the frequency of the reflected wave would be less than that of the transmitted wave. This frequency change is known as the Doppler shift and is proportional to the velocity of the reflector. This forms the principle behind the Doppler ultrasound. The Doppler ultrasound probe is able to transmit ultrasound waves into the body, directed toward a particular blood vessel and receive their reflections from the body. The apparatus then measures the difference between the transmitted and received frequencies. The frequency difference (expressed in hertz) is proportional to the velocity of movement along the line that connects the wave transceiver and the moving reflector. In obstetric applications, the Doppler wave is produced by insonating the moving blood vessels with ultrasound waves.

7.7.2: Doppler Blood Flow Indices

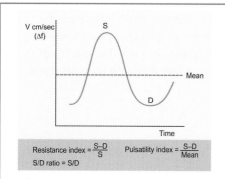

Fig. 7.7.2: Description of various Doppler indices

The most commonly used Doppler blood flow indices for pregnancy assessment are as follows:

- Systolic/diastolic (S/D) ratio: $\dfrac{\text{Peak systolic blood flow}}{\text{End diastolic velocity}}$

- Pulsatility index (PI): $\dfrac{\text{Peak systolic velocity} - \text{end diastolic velocity}}{\text{Mean systolic velocity}}$

- Resistance index (RI): $\dfrac{\text{Peak systolic velocity} - \text{end diastolic velocity}}{\text{Peak systolic velocity}}$

Picture	Medical/Surgical Description

7.7.3: Normal Blood Flow within the Ovary

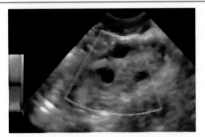

Fig. 7.7.3: Blood flow within the ovary as visualized on color Doppler ultrasound

On Doppler ultrasound examination of ovaries, perifollicular vascularity can be observed around a preovulatory follicle. Several follicles in various stages of development can be observed. It may be difficult to visualize the complete path of vascular flow around the larger follicles due to the tortuosity of the ovarian vessels and its branches.

7.7.4: Normal Uterine Perfusion

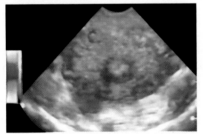

Fig. 7.7.4: Normal uterine perfusion in pregnancy

The adjacent figure shows uterine perfusion on Doppler ultrasound in presence of 7-weeks-sized intrauterine gestational sac. During a normal pregnancy, there is an increase in the uterine size and vascularity, particularly in the third trimester. The increased uterine vascularity is related to dilatation of uterine vessels and increase in terminal vascular branches. In normal pregnancy, the perfusion of the entire uterofetoplacental circulation is supplied by the uterine vessels.

7.7.5: Three-Vessel Umbilical Cord (A and B)

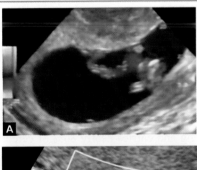

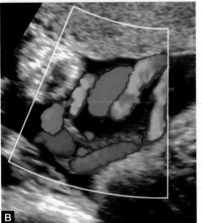

Figs 7.7.5 (A and B): Three-vessel umbilical cord

Normal umbilical cord normally has three vessels: two arteries and one vein. These vessels can be identified on Doppler ultrasound examination as shown in the adjacent figures.

Picture	Medical/Surgical Description

7.7.6: Two-Vessel Umbilical Cord

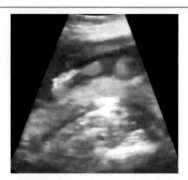

Fig. 7.7.6: Two-vessel umbilical cord

Two vessels in the umbilical cord may be present in nearly 1% patients. In these cases, there is a single umbilical artery and single vein. Two-vessel umbilical cord is indicative of underlying chromosomal disorders in the fetus. Nearly 20% of babies with two vessels in the umbilical cord would have some form of fetal malformations. In these cases a more detailed ultrasound examination may be required for evaluation of fetal anomalies.

7.7.7: Color Doppler Evaluation of Fetal Aorta

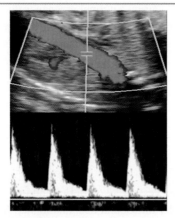

Fig. 7.7.7: Color Doppler evaluation of fetal descending aorta

The fetal descending aorta (FDA) is routinely scanned along with the umbilical arteries. The Doppler waveforms of the fetal aorta show forward flow both during systole and diastole throughout the cardiac cycle. In the fetal aorta, diastolic flow velocity is lower in relation to systolic flow velocity in comparison to umbilical arteries. As a result, S/D values for fetal aorta are higher than that of umbilical arteries. With the falling peripheral resistance and increasing diastolic flow in fetal aorta, throughout pregnancy, there is a fall in S/D ratio, PI and RI with increasing period of gestation.

7.7.8: Color Doppler Evaluation of Middle Cerebral Artery (A and B)

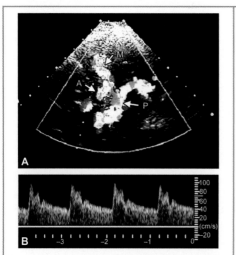

Figs 7.7.8 (A and B): Color Doppler evaluation of middle cerebral artery (MCA) showing circle of Willis; (B) Doppler velocity waveforms in MCA (A, Anterior cerebral artery; M, Middle cerebral artery; P, Posterior cerebral artery)

Middle cerebral artery is a major lateral branch of the circle of Willis, which is most accessible to ultrasound imaging and carries nearly 80% of cerebral blood. On Doppler imaging, MCA can be seen to be running anterolaterally at the borderline between the anterior and the middle cerebral fossae.

Picture	Medical/Surgical Description

7.7.9: Middle Cerebral Artery Pulsatility Index with Increasing Period of Gestation

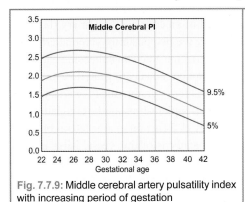

Fig. 7.7.9: Middle cerebral artery pulsatility index with increasing period of gestation

The blood velocity in MCA increases with advancing gestation in normal pregnancy. In the early stages of the pregnancy, the diastolic flow velocities in the cerebral vessels are small or absent, but toward the end of the gestation these velocities increase. This increase has been observed to be significantly associated with the decrease in PI.

7.7.10: Color Doppler Evaluation of Umbilical Cord

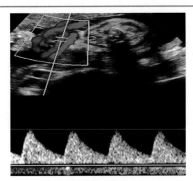

Fig. 7.7.10: Color Doppler evaluation of umbilical cord

As previously discussed, normal umbilical cord normally has two arteries and one vein. Doppler ultrasound examination in the adjacent figure demonstrates these three vessels. The Doppler waveform exhibits blood flow pattern through both the umbilical arteries and umbilical vein.

7.7.11: Normal Blood Flow in Ductus Venosus

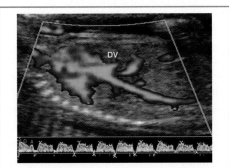

Fig. 7.7.11: Normal blood flow in the ductus venosusn (DV)

The ductus venosus (DV) is a very important part of fetal venous circulation. This vessel acts as a shunt and helps in directly connecting the umbilical vein to the inferior vena cava. The fetus receives oxygenated blood from the mother through placenta in form of umbilical veins. As this oxygenated blood bypasses DV, some of the oxygenated blood goes to the liver, but most of it bypasses the liver and empties directly into the inferior vena cava, which enters the right atrium. This highly oxygenated and nutrient-rich umbilical venous blood is eventually supplied to the fetal brain and myocardium instead of the fetal liver. Normal blood flow through ductus venosus has been shown in the adjacent figure and comprises of the following waves: S wave (related to peak systolic velocity); D wave (related to ventricular diastole) and A wave (related to atrial contraction).

7.7.12: Reversed Blood Flow in Ductus Venosus (A and B)

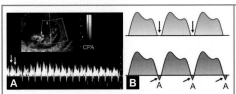

Figs 7.7.12 (A and B): Reversed blood flow in the ductus venosus (arrow pointing upward direction)

Abnormal blood flow in the DV is associated with either absence of A wave or reversal of blood flow in the A wave [as shown in Figures 7.7.12 (A and B)]. Abnormal DV flow could be indicative of IUGR or cardiac abnormality or underlying Down's syndrome. During the periods of fetal hypoxia, a compensatory mechanism occurs, causing transient dilatation of the ductus, which is supposed to increase oxygenated blood flowing through it during these periods of hypoxia or reduced umbilical flow.

Picture	Medical/Surgical Description

7.7.13: Circle of Willis (A and B)

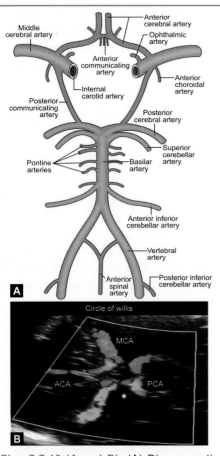

Anteriorly the circle of Willis is composed of anterior cerebral artery (branch of internal carotid artery) and posteriorly by the two posterior cerebral arteries (branches of the basilar artery). These are interconnected on either side with the internal carotid artery with the help of posterior communicating arteries. Anterior cerebral arteries are connected with help of anterior communicating artery. The vessel which is placed most favorably for Doppler ultrasound examination is middle cerebral vessel (See 7.7.8). This vessel forms the major lateral branch of the circle of Willis. Doppler ultrasound analysis of this vessel helps in the evaluation of brain perfusion. In Figure 7.7.13 B, the abbreviations stand for the following: ACA, Anterior cerebral artery; MCA, Middle cerebral artery; and PCA, Posterior cerebral artery.

Figs 7.7.13 (A and B): (A) Diagrammatic representation of circle of Willis; (B) Doppler ultrasound visualization of circle of Willis

7.7.14: Color Doppler Evaluation of Umbilical Artery (A and B)

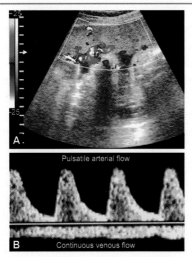

The assessment of umbilical blood flow provides information regarding blood perfusion of the fetoplacental unit. The deoxygenated blood from the fetus is delivered by two umbilical arteries whereas the oxygenated blood moves to the fetus via umbilical vein. These vessels are connected to the mother via the placenta and to the fetus via the umbilical cord. In a normal pregnancy, the impedance to the blood flow in umbilical vessels continuously decrease throughout the gestation. The blood flow during the diastole is often absent in the first trimester. The diastolic component becomes evident with advancing gestational age. Characteristic umbilical blood flow has saw-toothed appearance of pulsatile arterial flow in one direction and continuous umbilical venous blood flow in the other.

Figs 7.7.14 (A and B): (A) Umbilical artery circulation on color Doppler ultrasonography; (B) Umbilical artery Doppler ultrasound waveforms

Picture	Medical/Surgical Description

7.7.15: Umbilical Artery Pulsatility Index

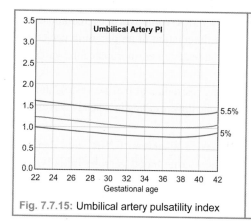

Fig. 7.7.15: Umbilical artery pulsatility index

There is an increased blood flow in umbilical vessels both during the systole and diastole with increasing gestation in a normal pregnancy. As a result, the impedance to the blood flow continuously decreases throughout the gestation, thereby causing a reduction in the umbilical artery PI.

7.7.16: Systolic/Diastolic Ratio in Umbilical Vessels

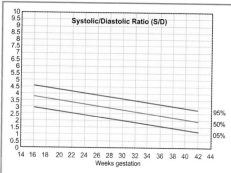

Fig. 7.7.16: Systolic/diastolic ratio in umbilical vessels decreasing with increasing gestational age

The S/D ratio of umbilical vessels serves as an index of measurement, which compares the systolic with the diastolic flow in the umbilical arteries and identifies the amount of resistance in the placental vasculature. Increased vascular resistance in the fetal placental unit has been associated with reduced end-diastolic umbilical artery velocities. In normal pregnancy, the end diastolic blood flow in umbilical artery increases with advancing gestation. As a result there is a decline in both PI and S:D ratio with increasing gestation.

7.7.17: Color Doppler Evaluation of Uterine Artery

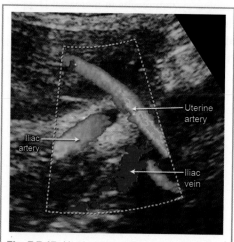

Fig. 7.7.17: Uterine artery Doppler analysis

Uterine artery Doppler helps in evaluating the uteroplacental perfusion. Doppler ultrasound of the uterine arteries is a noninvasive method for assessing the resistance of vessels supplying the placenta. In normal pregnancies, due to the trophoblastic invasion of spiral vessels, there is an increase in blood flow velocity and a decrease in resistance to flow.

Picture	Medical/Surgical Description

7.7.18: Uterine Artery Blood Flow Patterns (A to C)

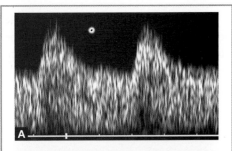

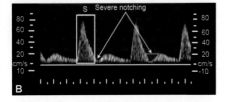

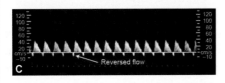

Figs 7.7.18 (A to C): Uterine artery blood flow patterns: (A) Normal uterine artery blood flow; (B) Diastolic notching in the uterine vessels; (C) Reversed flow on uterine artery Doppler

The normal uterine artery waveform (Fig. 7.7.18A) comprises of two components:

- *A pulsatile component*: Formed by the interaction of an outgoing wave and reflected wave. The outgoing wave upon reaching the uteroplacental vascular bed is reflected back to the heart.
- *A steady waveform*: Due to a fall in the resistance of uterine vessels during pregnancy, there occurs increased diastolic flow resulting in a steady waveform pattern.

In pregnancies complicated by hypertensive disorders, IUGR, etc., there is increased resistance to blood flow in the uterine blood vessels. Initially, the Doppler ultrasound of the uterine artery shows increased resistance to flow (decreased mean velocity) and reduced diastolic blood flow. This results in an elevated PI and RI. With an increase in vascular resistance, there occurs an early diastolic notch (Fig. 7.7.18B). With further worsening of situation, the blood flow in the diastole stops completely (absent end diastolic flow) or blood starts flowing in revere direction (Fig. 7.7.18C). Reversed end diastolic velocity is an ominous finding warranting close monitoring and mandates immediate delivery depending on the clinical situation of the patient.

7.7.19: Doppler Analysis of Venous Blood Flow (A and B)

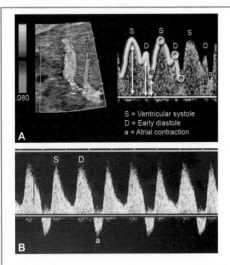

Figs 7.7.19 (A and B): (A) Doppler analysis of venous blood flow; (B) Normal blood flow through ductus venosus

The typical waveform for the blood flow in the venous vessels consists of three phases related to cardiac cycle (Fig. 7.7.19A and B). Peak S wave corresponds to ventricular systole, peak D wave to early diastole and peak A wave to atrial contraction. In normal fetuses, the blood flow in the venous system is always in the forward direction throughout the cardiac cycle. Forward blood flow in the venous system is a function of cardiac compliance, contractibility and afterload. A decline in forward velocities in venous system results in increased Doppler indices and suggests impaired preload handling. Absence or even reversal of the A wave is the hallmark of the advancing circulatory deterioration since this documents the inability of the heart to accommodate venous return.

7.8: CONGENITAL ABNORMALITIES

7.8.1: Down's Syndrome (A to H)

Nuchal Translucency

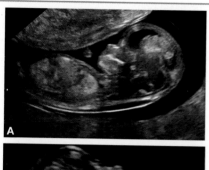

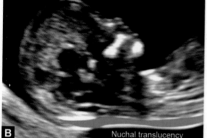

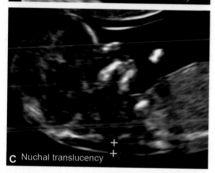

Figs 7.8.1 (A to C): Measurement of nuchal translucency

Nuchal thickening was one of the first nonstructural sonographic markers which was identified and till date remains the single most predictive sonographic marker for identification of fetuses at risk of Down's syndrome. Nuchal means the neck. Therefore, nuchal translucency (NT) refers to the normal subcutaneous fluid-filled areas between the back of fetal neck and the overlying skin. The measurement of NT is usually performed, when the CRL is about 45 mm to 84 mm. Most of the examinations are performed transabdominally. The fetus is imaged in a midsagittal plane with the head in a neutral position. The amnion should be distinguished from the fetal skin. The calipers are placed on the inner border of the NT and perpendicular to the long axis of the fetal body. The largest of three measurements is taken into consideration.

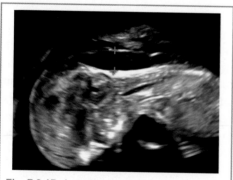

Fig. 7.8.1D: Increased nuchal translucency (6.4 mm in this photograph)

Nuchal translucency increases with the gestational age. A value of NT 3 mm or more is considered as abnormal, and genetic counseling and/or amniocentesis are advisable in these cases.

Picture	Medical/Surgical Description

Nasal Bone

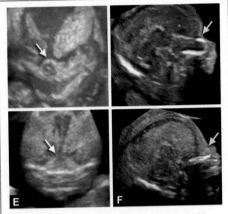

Figs 7.8.1 (E and F): (E) Presence of nasal bone (white arrow); (F) Absence of nasal bone (shown by yellow arrow)

Absence of nasal bone can be considered as a useful ultrasound parameter for identifying fetuses with trisomy 21 because such fetuses may often suffer from hypoplasia or delayed ossification of the nasal bone.

Hyperechogenic Bowel

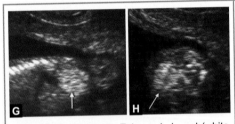

Figs 7.8.1 (G and H): Echogenic bowel (white arrows)

Fetal echogenic bowel refers to the presence of hyperechoic bowel, which has the same echogenicity as that of the adjacent iliac bone. The diagnosis of echogenic bowel is made when the bowel appears to be at least as echogenic as adjacent bone at the time of second trimester ultrasound. Slotnick et al. categorized echogenicity of the bowel into three grades based on the echogenicity of the bowel in relation with that of the iliac crest. These include grade 1 (echogenicity of the bowel that is less than that of the iliac crest); grade 2 (echogenicity of the bowel is similar to that of the iliac crest) and grade 3 (echogenicity of the bowel is greater than that of the iliac crest). The association of echogenic bowel with aneuploidy (especially Down's syndrome) and adverse pregnancy outcome is strongest with moderate to severe echogenicity (grades 2 and 3). Amniocentesis may be required in these cases. Finding of echogenic bowel must prompt a detailed ultrasound examination for evaluation of other anomalies (renal and cardiac).

7.8.2: Micrognathia and Low Set Ears (A and B)

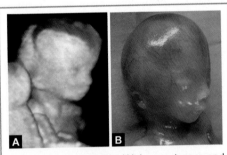

Figs 7.8.2 (A and B): (A) Low set ears and micrognathia at 15 weeks gestation as observed on three-dimensional imaging; (B) Aborted fetus in the same case showing the defect. Underlying chromosomal anomaly in this patient was detected as trisomy 18 (*Courtesy:* Ritsuko K Pooh)

As previously discussed, three-dimensional ultrasound is able to provide a better description of ear morphology, structure and position in comparison to two-dimensional ultrasound. By determining the line between the orbits and peak point of auricles, diagnosis of low set ears can be made. Low set ears and micrognathia (under-sized jaws) are commonly associated with anomalies such as aneuploidies (especially Down's syndrome). Further evaluation may be required in these cases.

Picture	Medical/Surgical Description

7.8.3: Cleft Lip (A and B)

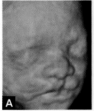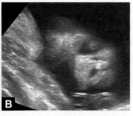

Figs 7.8.3 (A and B): Unilateral cleft lip on left side as observed on (A) Three-dimensional ultrasound and (B) Two-dimensional ultrasound

Diagnosis of cleft lip or palate can be made on ultrasound examination, before the baby's birth, usually on the second trimester scan. Babies with cleft lis or palate may require further evaluation for presence of other anomalies. Amniocentesis may be required to rule out the presence of an underlying chromosomal anomaly. However, cleft lip can also occur commonly as an isolated defect. Surgery for the repair of cleft lip is commonly performed between 1 month and 4 months of age.

7.8.4: Anencephaly (A to C)

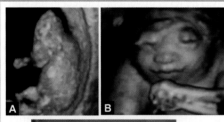
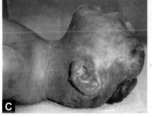

Figs 7.8.4 (A to C): (A and B) Three-dimensional ultrasound showing an anencephalic fetus; (C) Aborted fetus in same case at 18 weeks gestation (*Courtesy*: Ritsuko K Pooh and Kyonghon Pooh)

Anencephaly is a type of neural tube defect occurring due to the deficiency of folic acid. It refers to the spectrum of various destructive changes in the cranial vault mainly due to its failed development. The changes may range from exencephaly (in the first trimester) to frank anencephaly (in the second trimester). On ultrasound examination, there is absence of cranial vault. There might be exencephaly where the brain hemispheres are intact, though they are abnormally developed. In exencephaly, cerebral hemispheres are visible above the fetal face and they are in direct contact with the amniotic fluid. In the second trimester, the orbits may show a frog appearance with the cerebral hemispheres being destroyed. Though the risk of associated chromosomal anomalies is low (2–11%), the outcome is usually fatal.

7.8.5: Spina Bifida

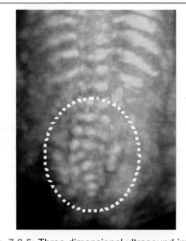

Fig. 7.8.5: Three-dimensional ultrasound image showing lumbar spina bifida occulta at 20 weeks (*Courtesy*: Ritsuko K Pooh and Kyonghon Pooh)

Spina bifida, another neural tube defect, results due to the failure of posterior vertebral arches to fuse during the early first trimester. The various types of abnormalities, which may be present are as follows:
- *Spina bifida occulta*: This is the mildest type of spina bifida, which is usually asymptomatic and no neural elements are usually involved. The defect in the spine is covered with the skin, and the spinal cord and meninges remain in place.
- *Meningocele*: There is a defect in the spine through which the meninges protrude out, but the spinal cord remains in place.
- *Meningomyelocele*: See 7.8.6

Ultrasound Features
- *Fetal head assessment*: In cases of spina bifida, on assessment of fetal head, there may be secondary ventriculomegaly and frontal scalloping sign (Lemon sign) as seen on transventricular scan. On transcerebellar scan, Chiari II malformation (banana sign) due to obliteration of cisterna magna may be present.
- *Fetal spine assessment*: In a normal spine by 20–21 weeks of gestation, both the vertebral bodies and posterior processes are seen. In case of an open spinal defect, the posterior processes may be missing.

Picture	Medical/Surgical Description

7.8.6: Meningomyelocele (A and B)

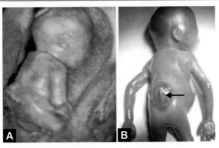

Figs 7.8.6 (A and B): (A) Three-dimensional ultrasound showing a large meningomyelocele at 20 weeks gestation; (B) External appearance of the aborted fetus of the same patient as in A. Central canal of the spinal canal has been delineated with a black arrow (*Courtesy*: Ritsuko K Pooh)

Meningomyelocele is the commonest type of spina bifida. There is a defect in the spine because the bones have not fused properly. Both the meninges and the spinal cord protrude through this defect and bulge out to form a mass at the baby's back. This defect is more dangerous than the defects where herniation of meninges and spinal cord does not occur because it is more likely to cause neurological disability.

Prenatal detection of this condition is based on the sonographic recognition of the disrupted ossification centers. Three main ossification centers (two posterior and one anterior) can usually be observed by 16 weeks of gestation, though the spine is fully formed by 22–24 weeks. Posterior ossification centers refer to the lamina-pedicle junction on two sides, whereas the anterior ossification center refers to the developing vertebral body. The level of vertebral defect in the spine where the fusion of the ossification has not occurred can be identified on three-dimensional sonography.

7.8.7: Club Feet (A and B)

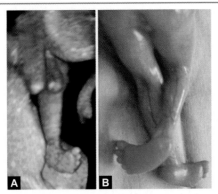

Figs 7.8.7 (A and B): (A) Three-dimensional image showing club foot at 15 weeks of gestation; (B) Aborted fetus of the same case as in A. Karyotype analysis revealed an underlying chromosomal anomaly (*Courtesy*: Ritsuko K Pooh)

Clubfoot or congenital talipes equinovarus is a commonly occurring birth defect. The prenatal diagnosis of clubfoot is established on ultrasound examination. The three main abnormalities identified on ultrasound include hindfoot equinus, hindfoot varus and forefoot varus. On the posterior sagittal view, the distal tibia, talus and calcaneus are properly aligned. The distance between the distal ossified tibia and superior ossified calcaneus decreases on plantar flexion in normal cases, but not in cases with club foot. On abduction, there is a smaller increase in the distance between medial malleolus and navicular bone in comparison to that in the normal foot.

7.8.8: Polydactyly (A and B)

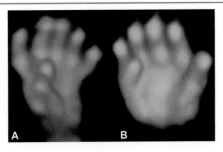

Figs 7.8.8 (A and B): Polydactyly of fetal hands as observed on three-dimensional ultrasound images

Three-dimensional ultrasound is a noninvasive method for assessment of fetal fingers. Polydactyly or an abnormal number of digits (6 or more) is the commonest abnormality of fetal digits. It can be classified as preaxial (affecting the thumbs), postaxial (affecting the little finger) or rarely central (where three central digits are affected). It may frequently occur as an isolated anomaly or may be associated with an underlying chromosomal abnormality or syndrome (e.g. Laurence Moon Biedl syndrome, trisomy 13, etc.). In case of diagnosis of polydactyl on a second trimester scan, a complete fetal ultrasound evaluation and genetic counseling may be required. As previously discussed, three-dimensional imaging is not mandatory, but helps in better delineation of anatomical and morphological details.

7.8.9: Scoliosis (A and B)

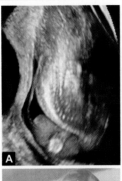
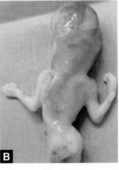

Scoliosis is a spinal deformity associated with both lateral deformity and vertebral rotation. Ultrasound examination appears to be lucrative alternative for the assessment of fetal deformity associated with scoliosis. The landmarks such as lamina and spinous processes can be identified on the ultrasound images. The diagnosis of fetal scoliosis mandates a detailed assessment for other anomalies and genetic counseling regarding the likely fetal outcome.

Figs 7.8.9 (A and B): (A) Three-dimensional image showing scoliosis at 12 weeks of gestation; (B) Aborted fetus in the same case showing severe scoliosis. No underlying chromosomal abnormality was detected in this case (*Courtesy:* Ritsuko K Pooh)

7.8.10: Omphalocele (A to D)

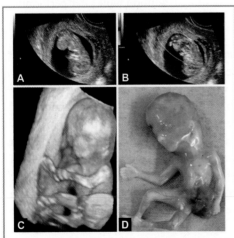

Omphalocele can be defined as the herniation of the intra-abdominal contents into the base of umbilical cord. A membrane almost always covers an omphalocele and the umbilical cord usually inserts onto the membranes in midposition. However, sometimes, the umbilical cord may be eccentrically placed in case of large defects.

Figs 7.8.10 (A to D): (A) Two-dimensional ultrasound image showing omphalocele at 12 weeks gestation; (B) Color Doppler ultrasound image showing omphalocele at 12 weeks gestation; (C) Three-dimensional ultrasound image in the same patient;(D) Aborted fetus showing the ruptured omphalocele sac. No underlying chromosomal anomaly was found in this case (*Courtesy*: Ritsuko K Pooh)

7.9: CASE STUDIES IN OBSTETRICS

7.9.1: Ectopic Pregnancy (A to D)

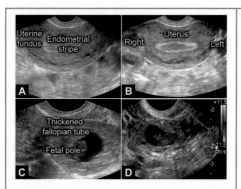

Figs 7.9.1 (A to D): (A) Longitudinal section of uterus showing an empty endometrial cavity with a triple line endometrial stripe; (B) Transverse scan of uterus showing an empty uterine cavity with absence of gestational sac; (C) Thickened fallopian tube on left side showing a gestational sac with fetal pole; (D) Doppler ultrasound showing low-resistance, increased blood flow around the gestational sac

A 24-year-old nulliparous woman married since last 1 year, presented with 3 months amenorrhea to the accident and emergency department with vaginal bleeding and severe abdominal pain particularly confined to the left iliac fossa. She had done a home pregnancy test, which was positive. Vaginal examination revealed cervical motion tenderness and a normal-sized uterus. An ultrasound examination and urine hCG levels were ordered. Urine hCG levels were found to be raised, and TVS examination revealed a left adnexal mass (about 2.5 cm in size) and an empty uterus. Diagnosis of a left sided ectopic pregnancy was made. Since the patient was nulliparous, wanted to conserve her future fertility, there was no active bleeding and the patient's vitals were stable, laparoscopic salpingotomy was performed.

7.9.2: Hydatidiform Mole (A to C)

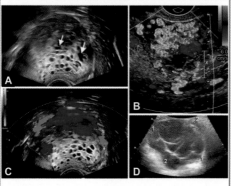

Figs 7.9.2 (A to C): (A) Cluster of grape appearance on TVS (white arrows); (B1 and B2) Doppler ultrasound showing highly vascularized tissues; (C) Left sided ovary with theca lutein cyst (size of the left ovary is about 10.58 × 9.65 cm)

A 20-years-old primigravida patient presented with bleeding at 9 weeks of gestation. She was diagnosed as a case of hydatidiform mole after performing an ultrasound examination. Transvaginal sonographic examination showed cluster of grape appearance. There was presence of numerous anechoic cysts with intervening hyperechoic material. Doppler ultrasound examination showed presence of highly vascularized tissues with low-resistance blood flow. The ovary on right side was perfectly normal, whereas left sided ovary showed presence of a large theca lutein cyst. Serum and urine β hCG titers were performed and were found to be elevated. The case was diagnosed as molar pregnancy and suction evacuation was performed. The evacuated products were sent for histopathological examination, which revealed the presence of hydatidiform mole. Serial β hCG measurements after evacuation ensured that complete sustained remission of hydatidiform mole had occurred. Serial assays of serum and urine β hCG levels were carried out on two weekly-basis until three negative levels were obtained.

Picture	Medical/Surgical Description

7.9.3: Triplet Gestation (A and B)

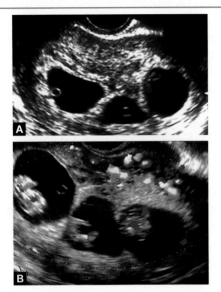

Figs 7.9.3 (A and B): (A) Triplets at 6 weeks of gestation; (B) Color doppler showing triplets at 8 weeks of gestation

A 34-year-old primigravida with 36 completed weeks of gestation and previous history of in vitro fertilization presented for an antenatal care check-up. She gives history of being diagnosed with triplet pregnancy on an ultrasound examination done at 6 weeks. Since fetal heart was not detected on this scan, a repeat ultrasound was performed at 8 weeks to confirm fetal viability and diagnosis of triplet gestation.

7.9.4: Cystic Hygroma (A to C)

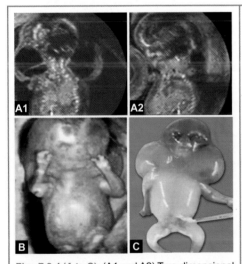

Figs 7.9.4 (A to C): (A1 and A2) Two-dimensional images demonstrating the orthogonal views showing cystic hygroma in a patient at 14 weeks of gestation; (B) Three-dimensional image in the same patient as A; (C) Aborted fetus in the same patient. Fetal karyotype was found to be 45X (*Courtesy*: Ritsuko K Pooh)

A 34-years-old G3P2L2 with 14 completed weeks of gestation presented to the gynecological emergency with complaints of reduced fetal movements since last 3–4 days. An ultrasound examination was performed in the patient, which showed absent fetal heart sounds. Two-dimensional images demonstrating the orthogonal views showed presence of multiple, discreet and circumscribed cystic areas in the neck region. A tentative diagnosis of cystic hygroma was made. Three-dimensional ultrasound examination was performed to further confirm the diagnosis. In lieu of dead baby, the labor was induced. Aborted fetus demonstrated the presence of cystic hygroma. Fetal karyotype analysis revealed 45X karyotype (Turner's syndrome) in this patient. Also known as cystic lymphangioma, cystic hygroma is characterized by cystic dilation of the lymphatic tissue in the neck region.

Picture	Medical/Surgical Description

7.9.5: Placenta Increta (A and B)

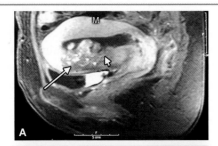

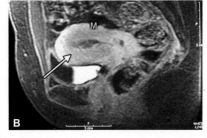

Figs 7.9.5 (A and B): (A) Arrow showing placental invasion of myometrium (M); (B) Same case showing almost normal looking myometrium following treatment with methotrexate

A 30-year-old G2P1L1 patient, with a previous history of cesarean delivery for breech presentation was given a trial for vaginal birth. She had a normal vaginal delivery in the morning at the hospital. A live healthy baby weighing 4.5 kg was delivered. Following the birth of the baby, no signs of placental separation appeared. Since the placenta failed to deliver even 1 hour after birth of the baby, the patient was posted for manual removal of placenta under general anesthesia. The placenta failed to get separated even at the time of manual removal. No distinct cleavage plane could be located between the placenta and the uterine wall. Therefore, no forceful attempts were made to separate the placenta. The umbilical cord was trimmed as close to vaginal introitus as possible and placenta was left in position. This was followed by the administration of antibiotics and uterotonic agents. Since there was no active bleeding and her condition was stable, she was shifted to the ward. When the patient continued to experience intermittent bleeding in the postpartum period, an MRI examination was performed which confirmed the diagnosis of placenta increta. The patient did not want hysterectomy. Therefore, she was administered single dose of 75 mg intramuscular methotrexate. MRI examination performed 1 week following treatment showed normal looking myometrium and regression of symptoms.

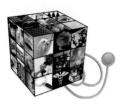

EVIDENCE-BASED BREAKTHROUGH FACTS

1. **ABSENT INTRACRANIAL TRANSLUCENCY AS A MARKER OF OPEN SPINA BIFIDA**

A new, first trimester, ultrasound marker for detection of open spina bifida (at the 11–13 ± 6 weeks transvaginal ultrasound scan) has been described as an absence of intracranial translucency in the midsagittal plane of the fetal face.

Source: Markov D, Pavlova E, Markov P. Three-dimensional transvaginal ultrasound diagnosis of open spina bifida at 13 ± 2 weeks of gestation with an absent intracranial translucency. Ultrasound in Obstetrics & Gynecology. 2010;36 (Suppl. 1): 168-305.

Section 8

General Gynecology

Gynecology

8.1: GYNECOLOGICAL ANATOMY

8.1.1: Organ System

8.1.1.1: Appearance of Female Internal Genitalia on Laparoscopic Examination

Picture	Medical/Surgical Description	Management/Clinical Highlights
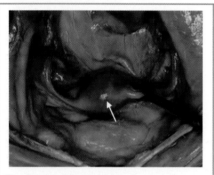 Fig. 8.1.1.1: Laparoscopic examination showing the female internal genitalia	Figure 8.1.1.1 shows normal laparoscopic view of the pelvis demonstrating the female internal genitalia present in the true pelvis.	The female internal genitalia comprises of a pear-shaped, muscular organ, the uterus, cervix, vagina, two fallopian tubes, emerging from the uterine cornu each and two ovaries. Each of the internal genital organ has been described in details below.

8.1.1.2: Uterus

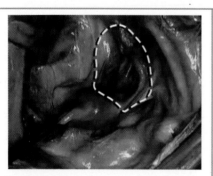 Fig. 8.1.1.2: Uterus (shown by arrow)	The uterus is a thick-walled, muscular, pear-shaped organ located in the middle of the pelvis, in which the development of fetus occurs. The adult uterus comprises of two main parts: body (uterine corpus) and cervix. The nongravid uterus lies in the lesser pelvis, with its body lying on the urinary bladder and cervix between the urinary bladder and rectum.	The uterus is a very dynamic structure, the size and proportions of which change during the various stages of life. The adult uterus is usually anteverted and anteflexed so that its mass lies over the bladder. When the bladder is empty, the uterus lies in a transverse plane. The nongravid uterus is approximately 7.5 cm long, 5 cm wide and 2 cm thick. It weighs about 90 g.

8.1.1.3: Fallopian Tube and Ovary

Fig. 8.1.1.3: Fallopian tube and ovary (shown by dotted circle)	Also known as the oviduct or the uterine tube, each fallopian tube is about 2–3 inches long and extends from the upper edge of the uterus towards the ovaries. The two fallopian tubes end by flaring into a funnel-shaped structure called infundibulum having finger-like projections (fimbriae). The fallopian tubes are lined with cilia, which along with the muscles of the tube's wall help in propelling an oocyte downward through the fallopian tube into the uterine cavity where it ultimately implants in form of a blastocyst. Starting from the lateral to medial side, the fallopian tube can be divided into four parts, which are as follows: infundibulum, ampulla, isthmus and the uterine part.	The ovaries are almond-shaped, pearl-colored, female gonads responsible for producing the oocytes (female gametes or the germ cells). The developing egg cells (oocytes) are contained in the fluid-filled cavities called follicles in the wall of the ovaries. Each ovary is suspended by a short fold of peritoneum known as the mesovarium, which arises from the broad ligament. The oocyte expelled at the time of ovulation passes into the peritoneal cavity. However, its intraperitoneal life is short because it is soon trapped by the fimbriae of the infundibulum of the uterine tube. Eventually, the ovum is carried to the ampulla where it is fertilized.

Picture	Medical/Surgical Description	Management/Clinical Highlights

8.1.1.4: Round Ligament

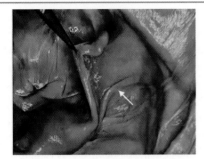

Fig. 8.1.1.4: Round ligament (shown by arrow)

The uterus is anchored in its position by several ligaments. One of these includes the round ligaments (as shown in the Figure 8.1.1.4). Situated below the fallopian tubes, these ligaments are 10–12 cm long and extend from the lateral aspect of uterus, passing anteriorly between the layers of the broad ligament. They leave the pelvis through the deep inguinal ring by passing through the inguinal canal and eventually get inserted into the labia majora.

Round ligaments along with the cardinal ligaments help in maintaining the uterus in an anteverted position. Due to the growth of the uterus during pregnancy, stretching of the round ligaments can cause pain.

8.1.1.5: Mesosalpinx (A and B)

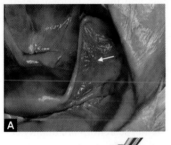

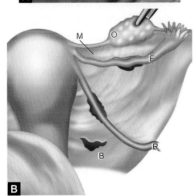

Figs 8.1.1.5 (A and B): Mesosalpinx

Mesosalpinx as shown in Figures 8.1.1.5 (A and B) can be considered as the portion of broad ligament, which stretches from the ovary to the level of fallopian tube and encloses it. In figure 8.1.1.5A, the arrow points towards the mesosalpinx. In the figure 8.1.1.5B, abbreviations stand for following: M, Mesosalpinx; O, Ovary; F, Fallopian tube; R, Round ligament; B, Broad ligament.

Since the mesosalpinx encloses the fallopian tubes, it also supports it.

8.1.1.6: Infundibulopelvic Ligament

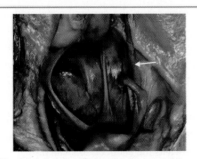

Fig. 8.1.1.6: Infundibulopelvic ligament (shown by arrow)

Known as the suspensory ligament of the ovary, the infundibulopelvic ligament extends from the ovary to the pelvic side wall.

It is a part of broad ligament and contains ovarian vessels, which enter the ovary at its hilum.

8.1.1.7: Vagina (A and B)

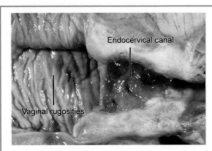

Fig. 8.1.1.7A: Macroscopic specimen showing vagina and cervix

The vagina is a narrow, muscular but elastic organ, having a length of about 4–5 inches in an adult woman. It connects the external genital organs to the uterus. Figure 8.1.1.7A demonstrates the macroscopic specimen of the cervix and vagina. The vagina is the main female organ for sexual intercourse. It acts as the passageway for transportation of sperms and for the expulsion of the menstrual blood. It also helps in the delivery of the baby.

The lower end of vagina lies at the level of hymen and at this level, it is surrounded by erectile tissues which correspond to the corpus spongiosum of males. The vaginal portion of the cervix projects into the upper part of the vagina, resulting in the formation of anterior, posterior and lateral fornices. The depth of the fornices depends upon the development of the portio vaginalis of the cervix. The attachment of the vagina to cervix is at a higher level on the posterior aspect in comparison to the other regions. As a result, the posterior vaginal fornix is the deepest and the posterior vaginal wall longest in comparison to the anterior or lateral walls. The posterior wall is about 4.5 inches long, whereas the anterior wall is about 3.5 inches.

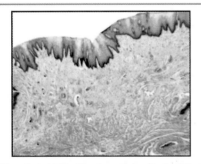

Fig. 8.1.1.7B: Nonkeratinized stratified squamous epithelium

The vaginal mucosa is lined by nonkeratinized stratified squamous epithelium as shown in the Figure 8.1.1.7B.

There are no glands in the vagina and the vaginal secretions are mainly derived from the mucus discharge of the cervix and transudation through the vaginal epithelium. The vaginal secretions are acidic due to the presence of lactic acid.

8.1.1.8: Cervix (A and B)

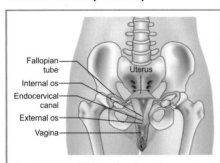

Fig. 8.1.1.8A: Different parts of the cervix

The cervix forms lower third of the uterus and is approximately 2.5 cm in length in an adult nonpregnant woman.

As shown in the adjacent figure, the cervix is composed of two parts: supravaginal part (between the uterine isthmus and the vagina) and the vaginal part (which protrudes into the vagina). The portion of cervix projecting into the vagina is known as ectocervix or portio vaginalis. The part of cervix within the uterine cavity is known as the endocervix.

The sperms enter the uterine cavity through the cervical canal. It also serves as a passage for the exit of menstrual blood. During labor, the cervical canal widens to form the lower uterine segment, the contractions of which help in the expulsion of the fetus. The opening of the ectocervix is known as the external os. The opening of the cervix inside the uterine cavity is known as the internal os. The passage between the external os and internal os is known as the endocervical canal.

Picture	Medical/Surgical Description	Management/Clinical Highlights
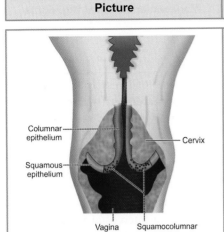 Fig. 8.1.1.8B: Epithelium of the cervix	The epithelium of cervix is varied. The ectocervix is composed of stratified squamous epithelium; whereas the endocervix which lies within the uterus is composed of simple columnar epithelium. The area adjacent to the junction of ectocervix and endocervix is known as the transformation zone.	The endocervical glands are responsible for producing mucus, whose consistency varies during various phases of the menstrual cycle. This mucus is thick and impenetrable to sperm until just before ovulation. At ovulation, the consistency of the mucus changes and it becomes more thin and stretchable so that sperms can penetrate through it and fertilization can occur. The cervix is mostly composed of fibrous tissue, which mainly comprises of collagen and a small amount of elastin.

8.1.1.9: Female Perineum (A and B)

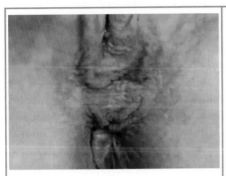 Fig. 8.1.1.9A: The female perineum	As shown in the adjacent photograph, perineum can be defined as the surface region in both males and females, which lies between the pubic symphysis and the coccyx.	The perineum lies inferior to the pelvic diaphragm, between the individual's legs.
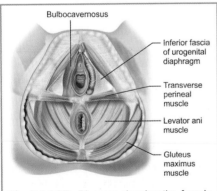 Fig. 8.1.1.9B: Diagram showing the female perineum	The adjacent picture showing the diagram of female perineum demonstrates three layers of pelvic muscles, which are as follows: • *Muscles of the pelvic diaphragm*: these include the levator ani muscle of both the sides • *Muscles of the urogenital diaphragm*: deep transverse perineal muscle • *Superficial muscles of the pelvic floor*: superficial transverse perineal muscle, external anal sphincter and bulbospongiosus.	Female perineum is a diamond-shaped area, present on the inferior surface of trunk including the vagina anteriorly and the anus posteriorly.

8.1.2: Blood/Nerve/Lymphatic Supply

This has been described in details in Section 1.

8.1.3: Anterior Abdominal Wall

8.1.3.1: Arteries

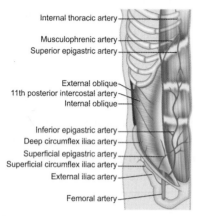

Fig. 8.1.3.1: Arteries of the anterolateral abdominal wall

The primary blood supply to the abdominal wall is from the superficial and deep blood vessels, which is demonstrated in Figure 8.1.3.1. The superficial blood vessels originate from the femoral artery and include the superficial epigastric, the superficial circumflex and the superficial external pudendal arteries. The deep vessels on the other hand, originate from the external iliac and the internal thoracic artery. These include the inferior epigastric artery, the deep circumflex artery and the superior epigastric artery, which is the terminal branch of the internal thoracic artery.

The main blood vessels supplying the anterolateral abdominal wall are as follows:
- Superior epigastric vessels and the branches of musculophrenic artery
- Inferior epigastric and deep circumflex iliac arteries
- Superficial circumflex iliac and superficial epigastric arteries
- Posterior intercostal vessels of the 11th intercostal space and the anterior branches of the subcostal vessels

Anastomosis between the various vessels of abdominal wall helps in ensuring an excellent blood supply to all areas of the abdominal wall.

8.1.3.2: Nerves

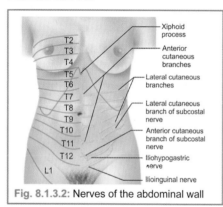

Fig. 8.1.3.2: Nerves of the abdominal wall

The nerves supplying the anterolateral abdominal wall are described in Figure 8.1.3.2.

The major nerves supplying the anterior abdominal wall include the thoracoabdominal nerves, subcostal nerve, the ilioinguinal nerves, the iliohypogastric nerves, the lateral cutaneous branches of the thoracic spinal nerves, subcostal nerves, and anterior abdominal cutaneous branches of thoracoabdominal nerves.

8.1.3.3: Rectus Sheath

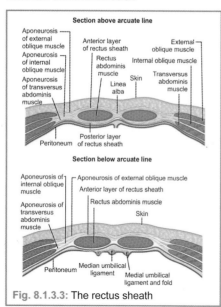

Fig. 8.1.3.3: The rectus sheath

The rectus sheath as shown in Figure 8.1.3.3 is formed by the conjoined aponeuroses of the flat abdominal muscles. It is formed by the decussation and interweaving of the aponeurosis of these muscles. The composition of the rectus sheath above and below the arcuate line is described in this figure.

The aponeurosis of external oblique muscle contributes to the formation of the anterior wall of the sheath throughout its length.

Above the arcuate line, the superior two-thirds of the internal oblique aponeurosis splits into two layers (anterior and posterior) at the lateral border of rectus abdominis, The anterior and posterior lamina respectively join the aponeurosis of external oblique muscle, and internal oblique and transversus abdominis nuscles to form the anterior and posterior layers of the rectus sheath.

Below the arcuate line, the aponeuroses of the three flat muscles pass anterior to the rectus abdominis to form the anterior layer of the rectus sheath.

Picture	Medical/Surgical Description	Management/Clinical Highlights

8.1.4: Pelvic Floor

8.1.4.1: Muscles of Pelvic Floor

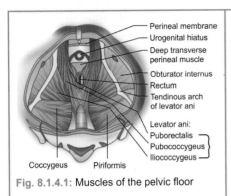

Fig. 8.1.4.1: Muscles of the pelvic floor

Figure 8.1.4.1 illustrates the three layers of the muscles of pelvic floor.

The muscles of the pelvic floor can be grouped into three layers, which are as follows:
1. Muscles of the pelvic diaphragm (levator ani muscle)
2. Muscles of the urogenital diaphragm (deep transverse perineal muscle)
3. Superficial muscles of the pelvic floor (superficial transverse perineal muscle, external anal sphincter and bulbospongiosus).

8.1.4.2: Levator Ani Muscle (A to E)

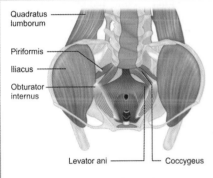

Fig. 8.1.4.2A: Levator ani muscle

The origin of levator ani muscles is fixed on the anterior end because the muscle arises anteriorly either from the bone or from the fascia which is attached to the bone. On the other hand, the levator ani muscles posteriorly get inserted into the anococcygeal raphe or into the coccyx, both of which are movable.

Due to the fixed anterior attachment and the mobile posterior attachment, the contraction of levator ani muscles tends to pull the posterior attachment towards the pubic symphysis.

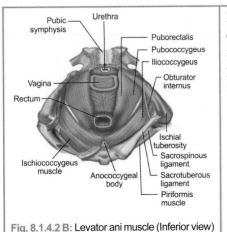

Fig. 8.1.4.2 B: Levator ani muscle (Inferior view)

Figure 8.1.4.2B shows the inferior view of levator ani muscle. Each levator ani muscle consists of three main divisions: pubococcygeus, iliococcygeus and ischiococcygeus.

The pubococcygeus originates from the posterior surface of the pubic bone and gets inserted into the anococcygeal raphe. The iliococcygeus is fan-shaped muscle, which arises from a broad origin along white line of pelvic fascia. It passes backward and inward to be inserted into the coccyx. The ischiococcygeus muscle takes its origin from the ischial spine and spreads out posteriorly to be inserted into the front of coccyx.

Picture	Medical/Surgical Description	Management/Clinical Highlights
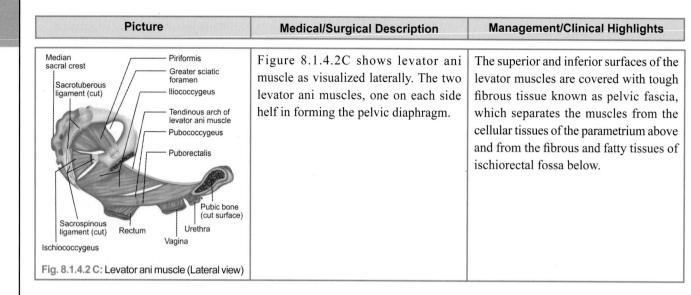 Fig. 8.1.4.2 C: Levator ani muscle (Lateral view)	Figure 8.1.4.2C shows levator ani muscle as visualized laterally. The two levator ani muscles, one on each side helf in forming the pelvic diaphragm.	The superior and inferior surfaces of the levator muscles are covered with tough fibrous tissue known as pelvic fascia, which separates the muscles from the cellular tissues of the parametrium above and from the fibrous and fatty tissues of ischiorectal fossa below.
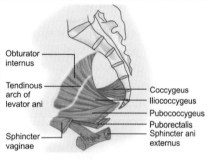 Fig. 8.1.4.2D: Sagittal section of female pelvis showing the levator ani muscle	The levator ani muscle constitutes the pelvic diaphragm and supports the pelvic viscera. The levator ani muscle creates a hammock-like structure by extending from the left tendinous arch to the right tendinous arch.	The muscle has openings through which the vagina, rectum and urethra traverse. Contraction of the levator muscles tends to pull the rectum and vagina inward toward the pubic symphysis. This causes narrowing and kinking of both vagina and rectum.
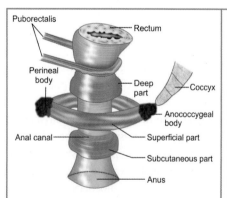 Fig. 8.1.4.2E: Sling formed by levator ani muscles	The pubococcygeus part of levator ani muscle originates from the posterior surface of the pubic bone. It passes backward and lateral to the vagina and rectum to be inserted into the anococcygeal raphe and the coccyx. The inner fibers of this muscle which come to lie posterior to the rectum are known as the puborectalis portion of the muscle. These form a sling around the rectum and support it as shown in the adjacent figure.	Some of the inner fibers of puborectalis fuse with the outer vaginal wall as they pass lateral to it. Other fibers decussate between the vagina and rectum in the region of perineal body. The decussating fibers divide the space between the two levator ani muscles into an anterior portion (hiatus urogenitalis), through which pass the urethra and vagina, and a posterior portion (hiatus rectalis), through which passes the rectum.

8.1.4.3: Ligaments of the Pelvic Floor

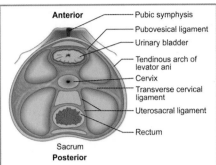

Fig. 8.1.4.3: Different ligamentous supports of the uterus

Figure 8.1.4.3 shows different ligamentous supports of the uterus, which include the cardinal ligaments, the uterosacral ligaments, pubourethral ligaments, the urethropelvic ligaments and the vesicopelvic ligaments.

Level I support comprises of the attachments of the cardinal (transverse cervical ligaments) and uterosacral ligament to the cervix and upper vagina. Together, this dense visceral connective tissue complex helps in maintaining vaginal length and horizontal axis. It allows the vagina to be supported by the levator plate and positions the cervix just superior to the level of ischial spines.

The cardinal ligaments contain the uterine arteries and provide attachment of uterus to the pelvic side walls. The uterosacral ligaments provide attachment of the cervix to the bony sacrum at the level of S2 to S4. The pubourethral ligaments provide support to the middle portion of the urethra by anchoring it to the undersurface of the pubic bone. The urethropelvic ligaments are composed of the levator fascia. This ligament provides support to the urethra by helping in its attachment to the tendinous arc. On the other hand, the vesicopelvic ligament provides support to the bladder by facilitating its attachment to the tendinous arc.

8.1.4.4: Perineal Body

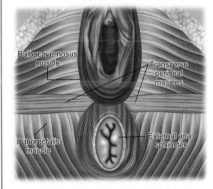

Fig. 8.1.4.4: Perineal body

The perineal body is a pyramid-shaped fibromuscular structure lying at the midpoint between the vagina and the anus. It lies at the level of the junction between the middle third and lower one-third of the posterior vaginal wall.

Perineal body assumes importance in providing support to the pelvic organs as it provides attachment to the following eight muscles of the pelvic floor: superficial and deep transverse perineal muscles, and the levator ani muscles of both the sides, bulbocavernosus anteriorly, and the external anal sphincter posteriorly.

8.2: EXAMINATION

8.2.1: Equipment (A to D)

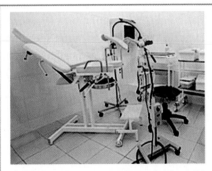

Fig. 8.2.1A: Gynecological examination table

The adjacent figure shows a cluttered gynecological examination room containing gynecological examination table, ultrasound machine and other gynecological equipment.

Adjustable length stirrups are present on the examination table, which enables the patient to be placed in the lithotomy position. The bed also allows the patient to be positioned in a semi-reclined position to facilitate examination.

Picture	Medical/Surgical Description	Management/Clinical Highlights

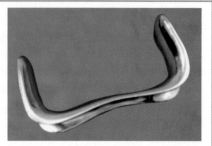

Fig. 8.2.1B: Sim's speculum

Figure 8.2.1B shows a Sim's speculum. Though the Sim's speculum is commonly used, cervical inspection using this speculum is associated with two main disadvantages: the gynecologist needs to bring the patient to the edge of the table, and help of an assistant may also be required while conducting a per speculum examination using a Sim's speculum.

Cervical examination can also be performed using a Sim's vaginal speculum and an anterior vaginal wall retractor. This speculum allows the assessment of vaginal walls and evaluation of presence of uterine prolapse such as cystocele or rectocele.

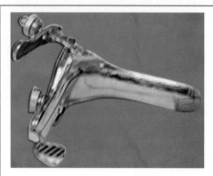

Fig. 8.2.1C: Cusco's speculum

A self-retaining, bivalve speculum such as Cusco's speculum (Fig. 8.2.1C) serves as an ideal equipment for vaginal examination. This speculum on its own allows appropriate vaginal exposure so as to ensure adequate vaginal inspection. Presence of cervical lesions (ectropion, polyps, cervical erosions, etc.) can be visualized. Cervical inspection using this speculum also permits the gynecologist to take Pap's smear at the time of per speculum examination. Once the speculum is inserted and secured in position, the cervical and vaginal walls must be observed for the presence of lesions or discharge. Specimens for culture and cytology must also be obtained.

- Prior to insertion of Cusco's speculum, under all aseptic precautions, the vaginal introitus must be exposed by spreading the labia from below using the index and middle fingers of the left hand.
- The Cusco's bivalve speculum must then be inserted at an angle of 45°, pointing slightly downward. Contact with any anterior structures must be avoided.
- Once past the introitus, the speculum must be rotated to a horizontal position and insertion continued until its handle is almost flush with the perineum.
- The blades of the speculum are opened up for a distance of approximately 2–3 cm using the thumb lever in such a way that the cervix "falls" in between the blades.
- The speculum can be secured in its position by using the thumb nut in case of a metal speculum.

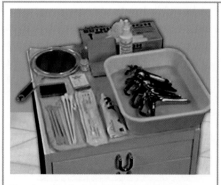

Fig. 8.2.1D: Gynecological examination tray

The adjacent figure shows a gynecological examination tray comprising of speculum (Cusco's), cotton swabs, gloves, Ayre's spatula and K-Y jelly.

Following the completion of gynecological examination, the used speculum is sterilized. The items (such as cotton swabs, gloves, Ayre's spatula, etc.), which have been used are replaced.

8.2.2: Patient's Position for Examination (A to C)

Picture	Medical/Surgical Description	Management/Clinical Highlights
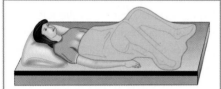 Fig. 8.2.2A: Lithotomy position	In this position, the individual's feet are positioned at the same level as the hips using the stirrups, while the hips and knees are fully flexed, with the patient lying flat on her back. At the same time, the perineum is positioned at the edge of the examination table.	Lithotomy position is commonly used for performing medical examination and minor surgical procedures involving the pelvis and lower abdomen. This is also the position most commonly used at the time of childbirth.
Fig. 8.2.2B: Dorsal recumbent position	In the dorsal recumbent position (as shown in the adjacent figure), the patient lies supine on her back, head and shoulders. The lower limbs are flexed and rotated outward. This position enables the legs to be widely separated with the knees bent and the feet remaining flat.	Dorsal recumbent position is now preferably used in obstetric practice over the lithotomy position. It is commonly used at the time of vaginal examination, application of ventouse or forceps and other obstetric procedures such as IUCD insertion or catheterization.
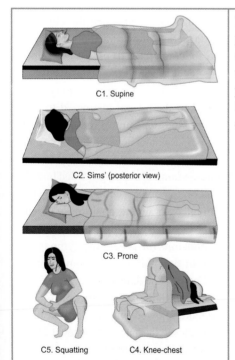 C1. Supine C2. Sims' (posterior view) C3. Prone C5. Squatting C4. Knee-chest Figs 8.2.2 (C1 to C5): Other positions sometimes used: (C1) Supine; (C2) Sim's position (posterior view); (C3) Prone position; (C4) Knee-chest position; (C5) Squatting	Though nowadays the dorsal recumbent position is most commonly used in the obstetric practice, other less commonly used positions in obstetric clinical practice include the supine position, Sim's position, prone position, knee-chest position and the squatting position.	In the supine position, the patient lays flat straight on her head, shoulders and back. In the prone position, the patient lies flat on her abdomen. In the knee-chest position, the patient lies on her knees with her head resting on the pillow and elbows resting on the bed. Patient's head is turned to one side. This position is sometimes adopted for rectal and vaginal examination and also works as a treatment option to bring the uterus into normal position. Sim's position is sometimes used for rectal examination and for administration of enemas. In this position, the patient is placed on her left side with her right (upper) knee flexed against the abdomen and left (lower) knee slightly flexed. Since the thighs and knees are drawn up against the chest, the chest and abdomen falls forward. The patient's left arm is kept behind her body, while her right arm is comfortably placed.

Picture	Medical/Surgical Description	Management/Clinical Highlights

8.2.3: Abdominal Examination

8.2.3.1: Abdominal Quardrants

Picture	Medical/Surgical Description	Management/Clinical Highlights
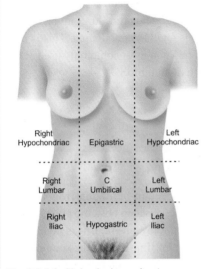 Fig. 8.2.3.1: Abdominal quardrants	Nine abdominal regions which can be identified over the abdominal region are shown in Figure 8.2.3.1. The clinical findings on abdominal examination are described in relation to the various abdominal regions.	The nine abdominal regions are as follows: the umbilical region is around the umbilicus; the region above the umbilical region is epigastric region; whereas the region below the umbilical region is hypogastric region. The six remaining regions are divided into left and right and are named according to the area of the spine: the lumbar regions are on the left and right side of the umbilical region. The regions on either side of the hypogastric are known as the left iliac and right iliac regions. The two regions on either side of the epigastric are termed as the hypochondriac regions.

8.2.3.2: Shifting Dullness (A and B)

Picture	Medical/Surgical Description	Management/Clinical Highlights
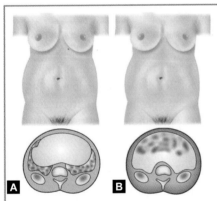 Figs 8.2.3.2 (A and B): Shifting dullness: (A) Shows presence of an ovarian or uterine tumor; (B) Shows ascites	Presence of ascites is basically detected by two tests: fluid thrill and shifting dullness. Dullness in the flanks upon percussion and shifting dullness indicates the presence of free fluid in the peritoneal cavity. Presence of dullness in both flanks when the patient is supine and dullness only in the dependent flank when the patient is on her side indicates the presence of ascites. The ability to demonstrate shifting dullness increases with the volume of ascitic fluid. Shifting dullness may also be absent if the volume of ascitic fluid is only small.	To demonstrate shifting dullness, the patient is laid supine and the clinician starts percussing from the midline of the abdomen towards one of the flanks. The level at which the percussion note changes from tympanitic to dull is noted and then the patient instructed to turn to the side opposite to the one where the percussion is being done. In normal individuals (without presence of any intra-abdominal mass), gas-filled bowels float on top of the ascitic fluid when the patient is in supine position, whereas fluid gravitates in the flanks. This is responsible for producing tympanitic note in the midline of abdomen and a dull note in the flanks. The patient is then turned to her side and allowed time so that the fluid gravitates to the side of dependent flank. Now the clinician performs the percussion once again. The dependent flank where the fluid had gravitated would sound dull to percussion, while the nondependent flank would be tympanitic. The patient is then turned to the other side and the above mentioned step is again repeated.

Picture	Medical/Surgical Description	Management/Clinical Highlights

8.2.3.3: Fluid Thrill

Fig. 8.2.3.3: Fluid Thrill	Another test for ascites is the demonstration of fluid thrill.	The test for fluid thrill comprises of the following steps: • The patient is laid supine and the clinician places one hand flat against her flank on one side. • An assistant (e.g. a nurse) or the patient herself is asked to place the ulnar aspect of her hand firmly in the midline of the abdomen. Without crossing arms, the gynecologist taps the opposite flank of the abdomen with his/her other hand. In case the ascitic fluid is present, the impulse generated by the tap will be transmitted to the clinician's other hand on the flank. The hand on the abdomen helps in preventing the transmission of the impulse over the abdominal wall. Fluid thrill is demonstrable only if a large volume of ascitic fluid is present. Absence of shifting dullness or fluid thrill or both does not rule out the presence of a small volume ascites.

8.2.4: Examination of Genitalia

8.2.4.1: Inspection of Female External Genitalia (A to E)

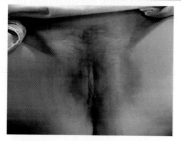 Fig. 8.2.4.1A: Inspection of female external genitalia	The gynecologist examines the external genitalia for the presence of any obvious lesions or signs of inflammation.	Examination of external genitalia in the presence of abnormality may reveal areas of discoloration, ulceration, redness, etc. Ulcerative areas could be indicative of herpetic infection, vulvar carcinoma, syphilis, etc. Vulvar mass at 5'O clock or 7'O clock position may suggest a Bartholin's gland cyst.
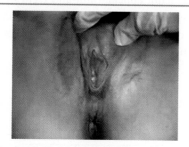 Fig. 8.2.4.1B: Inspection of clitoris	Figure 8.2.4.1B shows method of inspection of clitoris. Clitoris is an erectile organ, which becomes erectile during the coital activity and plays an important role in inducing orgasm.	Clitoris corresponds to the penis in males. It is attached to the pubic symphysis with the help of suspensory ligament. It is a highly vascular organ. It is well supplied by nerves and therefore lesions of clitoris can become extremely painful.

Picture	Medical/Surgical Description	Management/Clinical Highlights
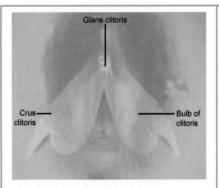 **Fig. 8.2.4.1C:** Full extent of clitoris	Figure 8.2.4.1C shows normal full extent of clitoris. The clitoris consists of a midline shaft lying in the median sagittal plane and is about 1.5–2 cm long and 0.5–1 cm wide which bifurcates internally into paired curved crura 5–9 cm long. The crura are attached to the under surface of the pubic symphysis. Present below the crura on both sides are bulbs of erectile tissue called bulbs of clitoris. Towards the end of clitoris, it is externally capped with glans. The glans is covered by a clitoral hood, which is formed due to the fusion of the upper parts of the labia minora.	Clitoromegaly occurs due to virilism under the effect of excessive androgens. As a result of this abnormality, clitoral length becomes more than 3–4 cm and width more than 1 cm.
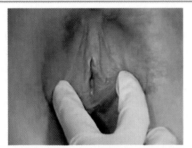 **Fig. 8.2.4.1D:** Inspection of labia minora	Figure 8.2.4.1D shows method of inspection of labia minora. Labia minora are thin folds of skin enclosing the veins and elastic tissues. It lies on the inner aspect of labia majora.	Since labia minora become erectile during the sexual activity, they do not contain any sebaceous glands or hair follicles. Anteriorly labia minora enclose the clitoris and posteriorly they form the fourchette
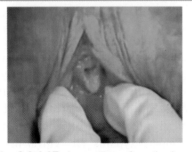 **Fig. 8.2.4.1E:** Inspection of urethral and vaginal orifice	Figure 8.2.4.1E demonstrates the method for inspection of urethral and vaginal orifice.	The urethral orifice lies above the vaginal orifice. The labia majora must be separated using the fingers of gloved hand, following which both urethral and vaginal orifices must be examined for presence of discharge, any masses (caruncles, swellings), excoriation, presence of other lesions, etc.

8.2.4.2: Palpation (A to C)

Picture		
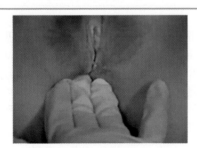 **Fig. 8.2.4.2A:** Palpation of perineum	Perineum can be defined as an area present between the symphysis pubis and coccyx. It is present in both males and females. In females, it includes the perineal body and the surrounding structures.	Perineum appears thin and rigid in a multiparous patient, whereas it is thick, smooth and muscular in a nulliparous patient.

Picture	Medical/Surgical Description	Management/Clinical Highlights
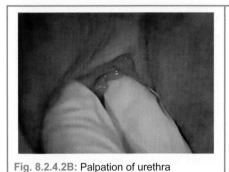 Fig. 8.2.4.2B: Palpation of urethra	In presence of urethral symptoms, the urethra and Skene's glands need to be palpated. For this, the index finger must be placed in vagina and urethra be milked by applying pressure up and down.	Normally there should not be appearance of any discharge or pain. In case of presence of discharge, it should be sent for culture and sensitivity. Also presence of pain mandates further investigations in form of urine analysis, kidney function test, etc.
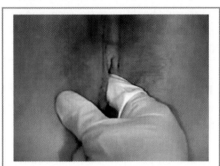 Fig. 8.2.4.2C: Palpation of Bartholin's glands	Bartholin glands and the lesions which can involve them have been described in section 10 (10.4.3A and B).	Bartholin's glands are assessed by palpating the posterior part of labia majora. For this, the examiner inserts his/her index finger in the vagina and thumb over the posterior part of labia majora.

8.2.4.3: Per Speculum Examination (A to D)

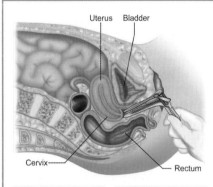 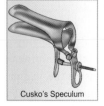 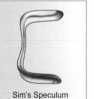 Cusko's Speculum Sim's Speculum Fig. 8.2.4.3A: Per speculum examination	Speculum examination of the vagina and cervix involves inspection of external genitalia, vagina and cervix. The types of speculum which are commonly used include the Sim's speculum and Cusco's speculum.	Per speculum examination may reveal vaginal wall rugosities which is normal or smoothness of vaginal epithelium, which could be suggestive of atrophic vaginitis. Presence of masses, vesicles or any other lesions can also be assessed on per speculum examination. This examination should ideally precede the bimanual examination. This is primarily because the vaginal discharge can be seen and removed for examination before it gets contaminated with the lubricant used for vaginal examination. Moreover, the cellular debris from the cervix and uterus remains undisturbed and can be obtained for cytological studies at the time of per speculum examination. Also, many superficial vaginal lesions may start bleeding following the vaginal examination and may not allow an optimal per speculum examination.

Picture	Medical/Surgical Description	Management/Clinical Highlights
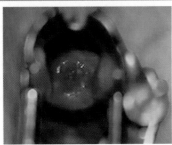 Fig. 8.2.4.3B: Per speculum examination	The adjacent figure shows appearance of cervix on per speculum examination using Cusco's speculum.	Various abnormalities of the cervix, which need to be assessed, include presence of inflammatory lesions and cysts. Some of them such as an ectropion or Nabothian follicles are completely benign. Lesions may be present due to infections such as candidiasis, Trichomonas, bacterial vaginosis, Herpes simplex, etc. These usually respond to appropriate treatment. Presence of irregular lumps, especially those with surface erosion, which bleeds on touch, should raise the suspicion of malignancy. Follow-up must be done in these cases with Pap smear and colposcopy.
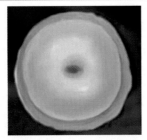 Fig. 8.2.4.3C: Appearance of nulliparous cervical os	A nulliparous cervix appears to have a circular os as shown in the adjacent photograph.	The appearance of the cervix can vary widely, depending on the age, parity and estrogen status of the patient. In this case, the nulliparous cervical os appears normal on per speculum examination and no further treatment is required.
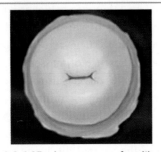 Fig. 8.2.4.3D: Appearance of multiparous cervical os	A multiparous cervical os has a transverse (horizontal) slit as shown in the figure. This appears to be normal features on per speculum examination.	Following child-birth, the outer appearance of extend cervical os changes. It becomes wider and acquires a "fish-mouth" appearance. Moreover, the squamocolumnar junction can also be more easily visualized following normal vaginal delivery.

8.2.4.4: Per Vaginal Examination (A to C)

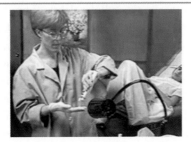 Fig. 8.2.4.4A: Use of water-based, nongreasy lubricant before starting vaginal examination	In clinical scenario, the vaginal examination is immediately followed by a bimanual examination (Fig. 8.2.4.4A) without removing fingers from the vaginal introitus.	While the fingers of the examiner's right hand are still inside the vaginal introitus, the palm of his/her left hand is placed over the abdomen. The success of bimanual examination primarily depends on the ability of the examiner to use the abdominal hand more often than the vaginal fingers.

Picture	Medical/Surgical Description	Management/Clinical Highlights
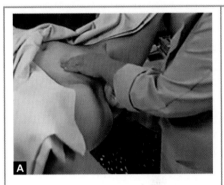 Figs 8.2.4.4 (B and C): Two finger vaginal examination	Two finger vaginal examination is performed by inserting two fingers of right hand inside the vagina.	Cervical shape, size, position, mobility, consistency and tenderness caused by pressure or movement of fingers may be assessed on two-finger vaginal examination.

8.2.4.5: Bimanual Examination (A to C)

Picture	Medical/Surgical Description	Management/Clinical Highlights
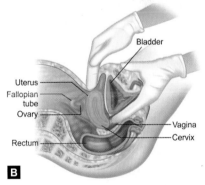 Figs 8.2.4.5 (A and B): Bimanual vaginal examination being performed in a patient	As shown in Figures 8.2.4.5 (A to C) bimanual vaginal examination is performed with the palm of left hand over the abdomen and the fingers of right hand still inside the vagina. Bimanual vaginal examination is usually more informative than per speculum examination and can be performed in most women. The following points are noted on bimanual examination: size of the uterus; its position, (anteverted or retroverted); and mobility (freely mobile or restricted mobility or fixed uterus). *Size of the uterus:* Bulky uterus corresponds to 6 weeks pregnant size and is slightly larger than the normal. When the uterus appears to be filling all the fornices, it corresponds to 12 weeks size. The in-between size could be between 8 weeks and 10 weeks.	Procedure of bimanual examination comprises of the following steps: • A water-based, soluble, nongreasy lubricant must preferably be used. A water soluble jelly is the best and if that is not available, cetrimide solution must be used. • The labia are separated with the thumb and index finger of left hand. • Following this, the two fingers of right hand, first one finger and then the second finger are inserted into the vagina only when the patient relaxes the muscles around the vagina and when it is clear that a two-finger examination would be possible without causing any pain. • The position and direction of the cervix are the guides to the position of the body of the uterus.
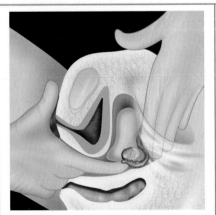 Fig. 8.2.4.5C: Examination of adnexa on bimanual examination	Bimanual vaginal examination is usually more informative than per speculum examination and can be performed in most women. Besides giving information related to the cervix and uterus, bimanual examination also enables the clinician to palpate the adnexa between abdominal and vaginal hands.	While palpation of adnexa, if there is a mass felt, its relation to the uterus is noted, like whether the mass is felt separate to the uterus or is continuous with it. When the mass is felt separate from the uterus, the origin of the mass is most likely from the adnexa or broad ligament. However, if the mass is continuous with the uterus, it probably arises from the uterus, like a fibroid.

Labels in Figure 8.2.4.5 B: Bladder, Uterus, Fallopian tube, Ovary, Rectum, Vagina, Cervix

Picture	Medical/Surgical Description	Management/Clinical Highlights

8.2.4.6: Position of Uterus as Detected on Bimanual Examination (A to E)

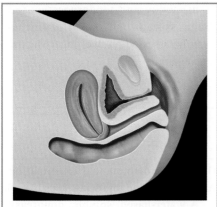

Fig. 8.2.4.6A: Anteverted uterus

In the position of anteversion (Fig. 8.2.4.6A), the external os is directed downwards and backwards. Due to this, the uterus is tilted forward towards the bladder.

The uterus normally lies in the position of anteversion and anteflexion. The position of anteversion results in the examining fingers to find the anterior lips of cervix as the lowest part of the cervix.

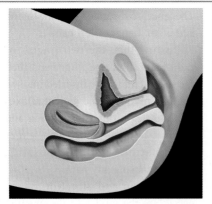

Fig. 8.2.4.6B: Retroverted uterus

Retroversion is a type of uterine displacement in which the cervix is directed downwards and forwards. Due to this, the uterus is tilted backward. This results in the examining fingers to find the posterior lip of cervix as the lowest part of cervix. Retroversion could be either fixed or mobile.

Management of retroverted uterus is described in 12.2.2 (A and B)

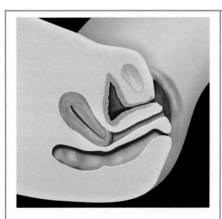

Fig. 8.2.4.6C: Mid-position of uterus

The uterus is considered to be in mid-position, if it lies mid-way between the position of anteversion and retroversion.

The mid-position of the uterus can be commonly encountered in cases of mobile retroversion such as uterine prolapse, anterior myomas, ovarian cysts of the pelvis and physiological causes such as menopause and early pregnancy.

Picture	Medical/Surgical Description	Management/Clinical Highlights
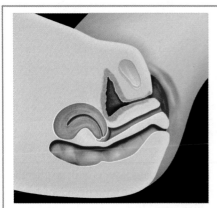 Fig. 8.2.4.6D: Anteflexed uterus	The forward inclination of the body of uterus on cervix is known as anteflexion.	The position of anteflexion causes the body of the uterus to bend forward on the cervix at the level of internal os. As a result, the body of the uterus lies against the bladder.
 Fig. 8.2.4.6E: Retroflexed uterus	The backward inclination of the body of uterus on cervix at the uterocervical junction is known as retroflexion. Retroflexion is usually associated with retroversion.	Fixed retroversion could be related to conditions such as PID (salpingo-oophoritis), pelvic tumors, chocolate cysts of the ovary and pelvic endo-metriosis.

8.2.4.7: Rectovaginal Examination

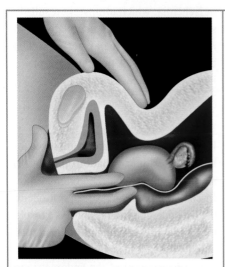 Fig. 8.2.4.7: Rectovaginal examination	Combined rectal and vaginal examination is done when required. Similar to the bimanual examination, the examiner inserts a lubricated, gloved finger into the rectum to feel for tenderness and masses. Per rectum examination also helps in revealing masses in the posterior pelvis.	Presence of nodularity in the Pouch of Douglas and tenderness of uterosacral ligaments on rectovaginal examination are signs of endometriosis. Some practitioners include rectal examination as part of the routine examination, while others do this procedure only in specific cases.

8.3: MENSTRUAL CYCLE

8.3.1: Events in a Normal Menstrual Cycle

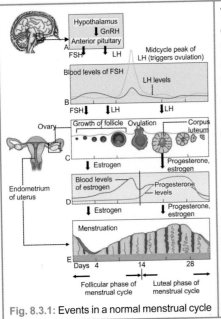

Fig. 8.3.1: Events in a normal menstrual cycle

The events of the normal menstrual cycle are shown in Figure 8.3.1. The first day of a typical menstrual cycle corresponds to the first day of menses. The menstrual phase usually lasts for 5 days and involves the disintegration and sloughing of the functionalis layer of the endometrium. A typical menstrual cycle comprises of 28 days. Ovulation occurs in the middle of the menstrual cycle, i.e. day 14th of a typical cycle.

The first 14 days of the cycle, before the menstruation occurs form the proliferative phase, while the next 14 days of the cycle form the secretory phase. At the midpoint of the cycle, ovulation occurs. Following the process of ovulation, the ruptured ovarian follicle gets converted into corpus luteum (CL); the main hormone produced by CL being progesterone.

8.3.2: Endometrial Layers

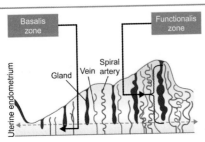

Fig. 8.3.2: Layers of endometrium

Figure 8.3.2 shows two layers of endometrium, which can be distinguished in the endometrial lining of the uterine cavity: functionalis layer (lying adjacent to the endometrial cavity) and the basalis layer (lying adjacent to myometrium). In the first half of cycle, changes are induced under the effect of estrogen, whereas in the second half of the cycle, changes are induced under the effect of progesterone, produced by CL.

The functionalis layer is built up after the menses. This is the layer of endometrium, which gets shed during the menstrual cycles. If pregnancy does not occur, in the absence of progesterone, the vessels of functionalis layer constrict, resulting in ischemia, which ultimately results in sloughing off of the functionalis layer, resulting in menstrual periods. The basalis layer, on the other hand, remains intact during menses.

8.3.3: Endometrial Phases

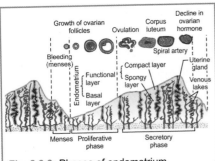

Fig. 8.3.3: Phases of endometrium

Figure 8.3.3 illustrates development of the endometrium through the proliferative and secretory phase. The endometrium during the luteal phase gets transformed for implantation of conceptus in anticipation of the pregnancy.

If pregnancy occurs, the rising levels of human chorionic gonadotropin (hCG) stimulate and rescue the endometrium. In case the pregnancy does not occur, the CL undergoes regression. As a result, the levels of estrogen and progesterone rapidly decline causing withdrawal of the functional support of the endometrium. This results in menstrual bleeding, marking the end of one endometrial cycle and the beginning of the other.

8.3.4: Pathophysiology of Menstruation (A and B)

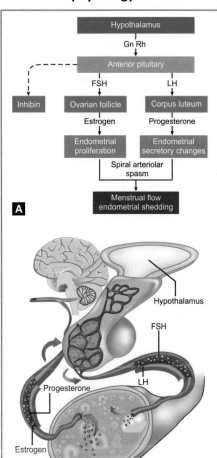

A

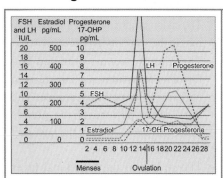

B

Figs 8.3.4 (A and B): Pathophysiology of menstruation

Figures 8.3.4 (A and B) demonstrate the pathophysiology of menstruation, which is under the regulation of hormones produced by hypothalamus and pituitary gland.

Hypothalamus produces gonadotropins (GnRh), which stimulate the production of FSH and LH. FSH stimulates the ovary to produce estrogen whereas LH stimulates the ovary to produce progestogens. Estrogen stimulates the endometrium to progress into the proliferative phase, whereas progestogens stimulate the endometrium to progress into luteal phase. If pregnancy does not occur, the CL ceases to produce progestogens, which causes the spasm of arteriolar vessels, which eventually results in menstrual flow and shedding of endometrium.

Initial follicular development is independent of hormonal influence. However, soon FSH, which is produced by pituitary takes control and stimulates a cohort of follicles in the ovary encouraging them to develop into preantral stage. FSH causes aromatization of the androgens present in the theca cells into estrogen in the granulosa cells. Out of the various follicles, only one single follicle is destined to develop into a dominant follicle, which undergoes ovulation. With the progression of the proliferative phase, there is an increased production of estrogen. Besides causing a decline in FSH levels, the mid-follicular rise in estradiol levels also exert a positive feedback influence on LH secretion. The presence of LH in the follicle prior to ovulation is important for optimal follicular development, which ultimately results in formation of a healthy oocyte.

8.3.5: Changes in Different Hormones During Various Phases of Menstrual Cycle

Fig. 8.3.5: Levels of various hormones during various phases of menstrual cycle

Figure 8.3.5 illustrates changes in levels of hormones during various phases of menstrual cycle. Increased levels of estrogen during the follicular phase exerts a negative feedback effect on FSH production as a result of which growth of all the follicles except one, "the dominant follicle" is inhibited. A surge of LH takes place just prior to ovulation. LH initiates luteinization and progesterone production in the granulosa layer. A preovulatory rise in progesterone facilitates the positive feedback action of estrogen and may be required to induce the midcycle FSH peak.

Ovulation occurs about 10–12 hours after the LH peak and 24–36 hours after the peak estradiol levels have been attained. The onset of LH surge is the most reliable indicator of impending ovulation.

8.3.6: Changes in Ovarian Follicle During Various Phases of Menstrual Cycle

Kindly refer to Section 1 (1.2.1.5).

8.3.7: Dominant Follicle

Kindly refer to Section 1 (1.2.1.6).

8.3.8: Histological Picture of the Endometrium in the Proliferative Phase

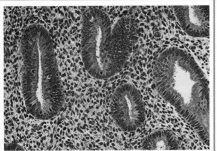

Fig. 8.3.8: Histological picture of the endometrium in the proliferative phase

The proliferative (follicular) phase extends from day 5 to day 14 of the typical cycle. In this phase, the endometrial proliferation occurs under estrogen stimulation. The estrogen is produced by the developing ovarian follicles under the influence of FSH. This causes marked cellular proliferation of the endometrium and an increase in the length and tortuosity of the spiral arteries. Endometrial glands develop and contain some glycogen. This phase ends as ovulation occurs.

The following changes take place during the proliferative phase:
- The functional and the basal layers of endometrium become well defined. The proliferation mainly occurs in the functional layer.
- The basal layer measures 1 mm in thickness, while the functional layer reaches a maximum thickness of about 3.5–5 mm by 14th day.

8.3.9: Histological Picture of the Endometrium in the Secretory Phase

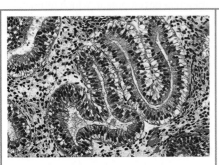

Fig. 8.3.9: Histological picture of the endometrium in the secretory phase

Secretory phase is marked by production of progesterone and less potent estrogens by the CL. It extends from day 15 to day 28 of the typical cycle. The functionalis layer of the endometrium increases in thickness and the stroma becomes edematous. The glands become tortuous with dilated lumens and stored glycogen. If pregnancy occurs, the placenta produces hCG to replace progesterone and the endometrium (and the accompanying pregnancy) is maintained.

If pregnancy does not occur, the estrogen and progesterone levels cause negative feedback at the hypothalamus, resulting in the fall in the levels of the hormones FSH and LH. The spiral arteries become coiled and have decreased blood flow. At the end of this period, they alternately contract and relax, causing disintegration of the functionalis layer and eventually menses.

The endometrial features of the secretory phase include the following:
- The most characteristic feature of this phase is development of subnuclear vacuolation in the glandular epithelial cells. In this, the glycogen filled vacuoles develop between the nuclei and the basement membrane (by the day 17–18).
- The endometrium measures about 8–10 mm in the secretory phase.
- The glands become crenated and tortuous to assume a characteristic corkscrew-shaped appearance. The cork-screw pattern of the glands becomes saw-toothed in the later part of the secretory phase.
- The stroma of the functional layer becomes edematous further.
- The functional layer of the endometrium can be divided into two layers: superficial and deep.
- The spiral vessels become dense and deeply coiled.

Picture	Medical/Surgical Description	Management/Clinical Highlights

8.4: PRINCIPLES OF SURGERY

8.4.1: Anesthesia (A to D)

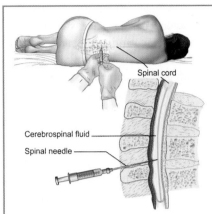

Fig. 8.4.1A: Spinal block

Regional anesthesia has currently become the most effective means of providing analgesia during labor. The two most commonly used procedures for regional anesthesia are the spinal (Fig. 8.4.1A) and epidural block (Fig. 8.4.1B). While administration of regional anesthesia, the patient is not required to be made unconscious.

Use of regional anesthesia can result in complications such as hypotension, spinal headaches, convulsions, and peripheral or central neurological damage.

The patient's consent must be obtained before the administration of regional anesthesia, either spinal or epidural. The procedure of spinal anesthesia involves injection of a local anesthetic agent into the cerebrospinal fluid in the subarachnoid space [lying between the arachnoid mater and the pia mater, through a fine needle, about 9 cm (3.5 inches) long].

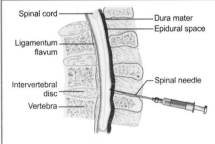

Fig. 8.4.1 B: Epidural block

The regional anesthesia, especially the epidural analgesia is also commonly administered for the purpose of pain relief during labor. In epidural analgesia, the pain killer medicines are instilled inside the epidural space.

These can be either administered in the form of bolus doses or continuous infusion by the medical professionals or by the patient herself in the form of patient-controlled epidural analgesia.

The procedure of epidural anesthesia involves the administration of a dilute amount of local anesthetic either in the form of bupivacaine or ropivacaine combined with a low concentration of short-acting narcotic like fentanyl. These medicines are placed in the epidural space via a catheter. The epidural catheter must be placed after observing complete aseptic precautions. The catheter tip must be placed in the epidural space and not in the intrathecal or intravascular space.

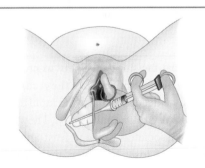

Fig. 8.4.1C: Pudendal nerve block

During the procedure of pudendal nerve block (Fig. 8.4.1 C), the pudendal nerve, which is derived from the second, third and fourth sacral nerve is blocked with local anesthetic administered using a special needle introduced via a needle guide. In order to achieve adequate anesthetic effect, the block needs to be repeated on the opposite side as well. Though the anesthesia may prove excellent for minor surgical procedures of vagina and perineum, the failure rate of the procedure is high, approaching almost 50%.

The procedure of administration of pudendal nerve block comprises of the following steps:

The patient is placed in the lithotomy position, following which a 22-gauge needle is placed through the transducer, with the tip of the needle aiming just medial and posterior to the ischial spine. This is the region where the pudendal nerve is most likely to be situated. Approximately 1 ml of 1% lidocaine solution is injected. Another 3 ml of lidocaine solution is injected near the sacrospinous ligament; another 3–5 ml of the solution is injected in the loose areolar tissues behind the ligament and another 10 ml just above the ischial spine.

Picture	Medical/Surgical Description	Management/Clinical Highlights

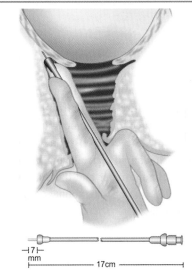

Fig. 8.4.1D: Paracervical nerve block

Paracervical block is an anesthetic procedure in which the local anesthetic agent is injected at several sites along the sides of vaginal portion of the cervix in the vaginal fornices. It has been accepted as a simple, safe and effective method for anesthetic administration. Though this block helps in providing complete relief against the pain of the first stage of labor, additional anesthesia is required at the time of delivery. This is an ideal method of anesthetic administration for dilatation and curettage. Paracervical block can also be used in other minor procedures such as cervical repair, conization, and Shirodkar's or Wurm's operations.

Nowadays with the gaining popularity of epidural and spinal anesthesia, the use of paracervical blocks has greatly declined.

The block comprises of the following steps:
- The woman is placed in a modified lithotomy position under sterile drapes but without surgical preparation.
- The cervicovaginal fornix is located with the examining finger.
- The guide is placed at the 5 O'clock and 7 O'clock positions after sweeping the guide away from the cervix in order to place the needle in the posterior lateral fornix.
- The needle is then inserted through the guide, and approximately 5–10 ml of the local anesthetic solution (1% solution of lidocaine hydrochloride with epinephrine 1:1,000,000) is injected through the lateral vaginal fornix on both sides.

8.4.2: Types of Skin Incisions

8.4.2.1: Vertical Incision (A to C)

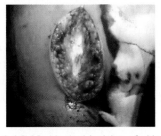

Fig. 8.4.2.1A: Vertical incision of skin and subcutaneous fat

Several types of vertical abdominal incisions have been used in gynecologic surgery including midline, and paramedian incisions. The steps of giving a vertical incision are described in Figures 8.4.2.1 (A to C). The midline or paramedian vertical incision can be considered as the simplest of abdominal incisions, which can be given speedily, especially during gynecologic oncology surgeries.

In the lower abdomen, the vertical incision is made from just above the pubis to below the umbilicus in the midline. The scalpel or electrocautery can be used to incise the skin and subcutaneous fat. The subcutaneous fat should not be dissected from the fascia because this creates unnecessary dead space.

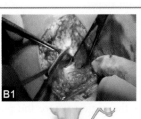

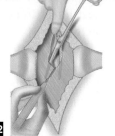

Figs 8.4.2.1 (B1 and B2): Fascial incision

Following incision of the skin, the fascia is incised, and the rectus muscles are separated vertically in the midline.

Vertical incisions are likely to provide excellent exposure as they can be easily extended and provide rapid entry into the abdominal cavity. They are also associated with the least amount of blood loss. However, their use is associated with potential problems such as an increased rate of infection and the possibility of nerve damage and atrophy of the rectus muscle. The use of vertical incisions in clinical practice has considerably declined due to poor cosmetic results.

Picture	Medical/Surgical Description	Management/Clinical Highlights

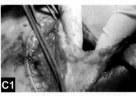

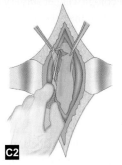

Figs 8.4.2.1 (C1 and C2): Peritoneal incision

Once the rectus muscles are divided, the peritoneum is grasped between two hemostats, opened with a scalpel and incision extended in the vertical direction. The transversalis fascia and peritoneum are also opened in a vertical direction. The entry should begin at the superior extent of the incision to prevent the possibility of bladder injury.

In case the operative findings require that the incision be extended above the umbilicus, the surgeon must avoid cutting through the umbilicus. Involvement of the umbilicus may result in an increased risk of postoperative wound infections due to bacterial colonization of the umbilicus.

8.4.2.2: Pfannenstiel Incision (A to C)

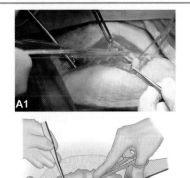

Figs 8.4.2.2 (A1 and A2): Fascial incision

The technique of giving a Pfannenstiel incision is described in Figures 8.4.2.2 (A to C). The slightly curved skin incision is made transversely, approximately 4 cm above the superior border of the pubis, and is carried through the skin and subcutaneous fat to the level of rectus fascia. The incision is usually made 1–2 finger breadths above the pubic crest. An incision length of 10–15 cm is sufficient. Following the incision of skin and subcutaneous tissues, the rectus sheath is incised transversely with the help of a scalpel or electrocautery.

This type of incision can be considered as the gynecological incision having the best wound security. Though the cosmetic results are excellent, the extent of exposure is limited. This incision should not be used in patients with extensive gynecological malignancy or nonmalignant conditions such as widespread endometriosis requiring extensive exposure or in case of extensive pelvic hemorrhage. This type of incision must also not be used in cases where speed is required for entering the abdomen.

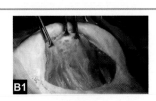

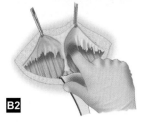

Figs 8.4.2.2 (B1 and B2): Separation of the rectus muscle

Following the incision of rectus fascia, the upper edge of the fascia is grasped with two Kocher clamps on either side of the midline. The rectus muscle is then dissected free from the fascia.

Next, the lower edge of the rectus fascial edge is grasped with Kocher clamps. Electrocautery or blunt dissection with the scissors can be used to dissect the rectus muscles and the pyramidalis muscle from the fascia. The rectus muscles are then separated in the midline by spreading the points of a hemostat between the muscles until the transversalis fascia is encountered.

The use of a Pfannenstiel incision is associated with good exposure to the central pelvis but limited exposure to the lateral pelvis and upper abdomen. As a result, this incision cannot be used for a radical hysterectomy and pelvic lymph node dissection, unless the patient is very thin. This type of incision is also associated with an excellent postoperative strength and good cosmetic result.

Picture	Medical/Surgical Description	Management/Clinical Highlights
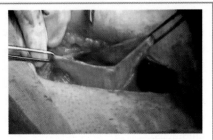 Fig. 8.4.2.2C: Vertical incision of the peritoneum	Following the incision of rectus sheath and muscle, the peritoneum is opened and incised vertically. The entry must be made at the superior extent of exposure, in order to minimize the risk of perforating the urinary bladder.	Pfannenstiel incision is associated with some disadvantages as well. It provides limited exposure of the lateral pelvis and upper abdomen. Due to the limited exposure, the usefulness of this incision for gynecologic cancer surgery is largely limited. Also, there is an increased risk of hematoma or seroma formation due to the large extent of dissection required and greater operating time.

8.4.2.3: Maylard's Incision (A to C)

Picture	Medical/Surgical Description	Management/Clinical Highlights
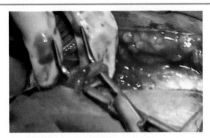 Fig. 8.4.2.3A: Identification and ligation of inferior epigastric vessels	The technique of giving Maylard's incision has been described in Figures 8.4.2.3 (A to C). This muscle cutting incision, first devised by Maylard helps in providing adequate exposure of the pelvic sidewalls due to the incision of rectus muscle. As a result, this incision is used for radical pelvic surgery including radical hysterectomy with pelvic lymph node dissection and pelvic exenteration for cervical cancer, and cytoreductive surgery for ovarian cancer.	The skin incision is made approximately at the level of the anterior superior iliac spine, about 3–8 cm superior to the pubis symphysis. It is extended about 5 cm medial to the iliac spine. Skin, subcutaneous tissue and rectus sheath are divided transversely as described previously for the Pfannenstiel incision. Most surgeons prefer to ligate the deep inferior epigastric vessels in order to reduce the blood loss before transecting the rectus muscles as demonstrated in the adjacent figure. However all the surgeons do not make use of this practice.
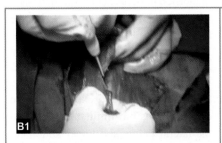 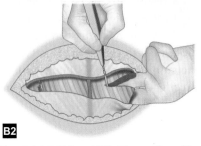 Figs 8.4.2.3 (B1 and B2): Transection of the rectus muscle	The Maylard's incision is different from Pfannenstiel incision in the sense that instead of separating the rectus muscles and fascia, the rectus muscles are cut transversely as shown in the Figure 8.4.2.3B. In order to make the incision safely, the muscle must be elevated off the peritoneum with the hand or using some retractor.	Advantage of Maylard's incision is that it helps in providing extensive pelvic exposure.

Picture	Medical/Surgical Description	Management/Clinical Highlights
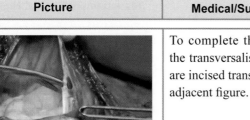 **Fig. 8.4.2.3C:** Peritoneal incision following transection of rectus	To complete the Maylard's incision, the transversalis fascia and peritoneum are incised transversely as shown in the adjacent figure.	Disadvantage of using Maylard's incision is that this incision requires more time to accomplish and can be associated with potential blood loss in comparison to other incisions.

8.4.2.4: Cherney's Incision (A and B)

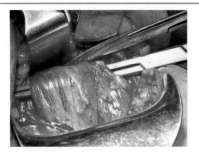 **Fig. 8.4.2.4A:** Identification of rectus muscles prior to their detachment	Cherney's incision begins with a low transverse incision of the abdominal skin and rectus sheath similar to the Pfannenstiel incision.	Cherney's incision is similar to Pfannenstiel incision, except for the fact that in the Pfannenstiel incision the rectus muscles are separated, while in the Cherney's incision, these muscles are detached from their insertion over the pubic bone (as shown in the Figure 8.4.2.4A).
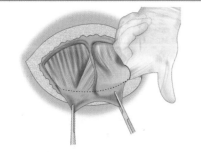 **Fig. 8.4.2.4B:** Diagram showing transection of the tendons of the rectus muscle	Following the incision of the skin and rectus sheath, the sheath is then elevated off the rectus abdominis muscle inferior to the fascial incision until the pubic bone is reached. Next, the rectus muscles are severed approximately 0.5 cm above their insertion from the pubic bone, using electrocautery. The peritoneum is then opened after retracting the cut rectus muscles.	A half centimeter segment of tendon is left on the symphysis for reattachment at the time of closure. The muscles and tendons are retracted caudad, and the peritoneum is incised longitudinally.

8.4.3: Closure of Abdominal Incision

8.4.3.1: Closure of Pfannenstiel Incision (A and B)

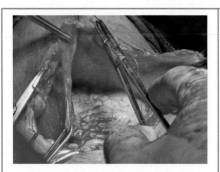 **Fig. 8.4.3.1A:** Closure of peritoneum	Previously, the method of choice for closure of Pfannenstiel was layered closure using interrupted sutures. However in recent times, most surgeons prefer to close the abdominal wall with continuous running stitches using delayed absorbable sutures. Layered closure in case of a Pfannenstiel incision is shown in Figures 8.4.3.1 (A and B). Figure 8.4.3.1A shows closure of peritoneum using continuous stitches.	In layered closure, each of the abdominal layers: peritoneum, rectus fascia, subcutaneous tissue and skin are closed separately.

Picture	Medical/Surgical Description	Management/Clinical Highlights

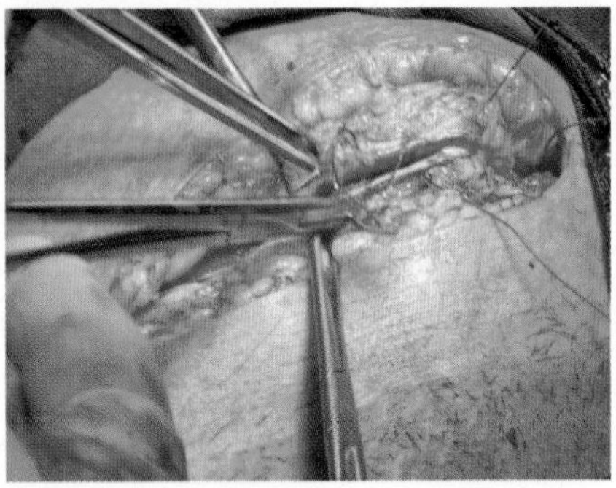

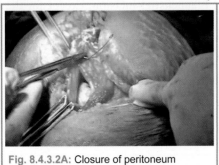

Fig. 8.4.3.1B: Closure of rectus sheath

| | Figure 8.4.3.1B shows closure of rectus sheath using continuous stitches. | Since the strength of closure of rectus sheath is important for maintaining wound strength, some surgeons prefer to use continuous sutures, while locking each stitch. |

8.4.3.2: Closure of Vertical Incision (A and B)

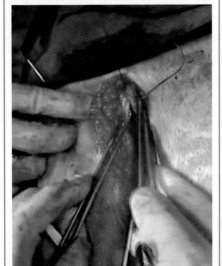

Fig. 8.4.3.2A: Closure of peritoneum

| | Layered closure in case of a vertical incision is shown in Figures 8.4.3.2 (A and B). Figure 8.4.3.2A shows closure of peritoneum using continuous stitches. | As previously described for Pfannenstiel incision, vertical incision is also closed in layers using continuous sutures. |

Fig. 8.4.3.2B: Closure of rectus sheath

| | Figure 8.4.3.2B shows closure of rectus sheath using continuous stitches. | The rates of dehiscence obtained with continuous sutures are same as those obtained with interrupted sutures closures. |

| Picture | Medical/Surgical Description | Management/Clinical Highlights |

8.4.4: Surgical Needles

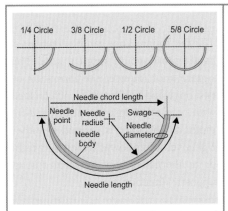

Fig. 8.4.4: Various needle configurations and characteristics of a curved surgical needle

The surgical needles have three components: eye, body and the point of the needle. Eye of the needle is the point of attachment of the suture. The body of the needle is available in different shapes: straight, half-curved, curved or compound. Curved needles are available in various curvatures with 3/8 of the circle being the curvature, which is most commonly used at the time of gynecological surgery.

Point of the needle begins at the widest part of the body of the needle and extends up to the extreme tip. The needle points can be of two types: cutting point and the tapered point.

Curved needles are most commonly used in obstetrics and gynecology. Obstetricians and gynecologists rarely use straight needles, except in cases where skin closure is required. Half-curved needles are often used for skin closure in laparoscopic suturing.

Tapered points needles are commonly used in friable tissues, which are likely to be easily perforated such as bowel and peritoneum. One variation of the taper point is the blunt point where there is a rounded blunt tip at the end of the tapered shaft. Cutting points can be of two types: conventional and reverse. The conventional cutting point needles have a sharp edge on the inside of the curve. In the reverse cutting needles, the sharp edge is on the outer curve of the needle. Cutting needles are more commonly used in cases of tough tissue such as skin.

8.4.5: Surgical Sutures

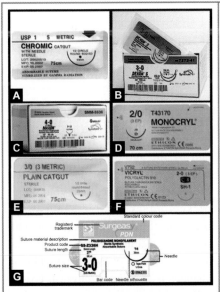

Figs 8.4.5 (A to G): Different types of suture materials: (A) Chromic catgut; (B) Dexon; (C) Maxon; (D) Monocryl; (E) Plain catgut; (F) Vicryl; (G) Polydioxanone monofilament

A suture is any strand of material used to approximate tissue or ligate vessels. Broadly, the various types of suture materials can be of two types: absorbable and nonabsorbable.

Whether absorbable or nonabsorbable, based on the number of strands used in these sutures, they can be of two types: monofilaments and multifilament sutures. Monofilament suture materials comprise of a single smooth strand (e.g. silk and mersilene in case of nonabsorbable sutures and polyglyconate and polydioxanone in case of absorbable sutures).On the other hand, the multifilament suture materials comprise of multiple fibers woven together. Some examples of nonabsorbable multifilament suture materials are nylon and prolene, whereas the absorbable multifilament fibers are vicryl and dexon.

The various qualities, which must be taken into consideration before choosing a particular suture material, include physical properties of the various suture materials such as tensile strength, security of the knot that has been tied, nonallergenic properties of the suture material, etc. and healing characteristics of the tissues.

Picture	Medical/Surgical Description	Management/Clinical Highlights

8.4.6: Surgical Knots

8.4.6.1: Square Knot

	The deciding point for the overall tensile strength of the surgical sutures depends on the fact whether the surgical knot has been tied properly or not. The surgical knots can be of two basic types: flat knots and the sliding knots. Flat knots can be of three types: square, surgeon's and granny's knots. The sliding knot can be either identical or nonidentical.	The flat square knot can be considered as the most secure surgical knot. The square knot requires the formation of two opposing half hitches, each created with help of an instrument or hand-tie method. The knot is formed as either right over left followed by left over right or an alternative knot, performed in an opposite direction.

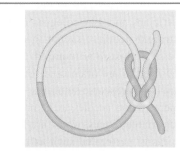
Fig. 8.4.6.1: Square knot

8.4.6.2: Granny's Knot

	Granny's knot is a type of flat knot, illustrated in Figure 8.4.6.2.	Granny's knot is similar to the square knot except that there is no reversal of direction on successive throws as done in case of a square knot. Granny's knots are generally not recommended in clinical practice because they are subject to slippage.

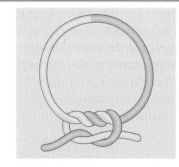
Fig. 8.4.6.2: Granny's knot

8.5: ADOLESCENT AND PEDIATRIC GYNECOLOGY

8.5.1: Puberty

8.5.1.1: Overview of Puberty (A and B)

	Puberty is the process of physical changes which cause transformation of the child's body into that of an adult, capable of reproduction. It can be defined as progression from appearance of sexual characteristics to sexual, reproductive and mental maturity.	The process of puberty typically begins by the age of 10 or 11 years in girls and by the age of 12 or 13 years in boys. During the period of puberty, there are anatomical (development of secondary sexual and genital organs), physical, endocrinological, psychological and emotional changes. The sequence of occurrence of pubertal changes is as follows: physical growth followed by development of secondary sexual characters and thelarche (by 10–12 years). Pubarche occurs after approximately 1 year and lastly there is development of ovaries and genital organs followed by occurrence of menarche.

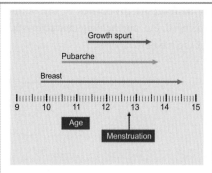
Fig. 8.5.1.1A: Normal changes occurring during puberty

Picture	Medical/Surgical Description	Management/Clinical Highlights

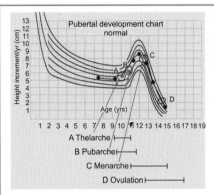

Fig. 8.5.1.1B: Normal pubertal development chart

The sequence of occurrence of pubertal changes is as follows: physical growth followed by development of secondary sexual characters and thelarche (by 10–12 years). Pubarche occurs after approximately 1 year and lastly there is development of ovaries and genital organs followed by occurrence of menarche. Various changes occurring during the normal pubertal development are as follows:

Thelarche: This refers to the breast development and occurs at the average age of 10.5 years. The first physical sign of puberty in girls is appearance of a firm, tender lump under the center of the areola in one or both the breasts

Pubarche: The next noticeable change of puberty is development of pubic hair, usually occurring within a few months of thelarche

Menarche: This refers to the occurrence of first menstrual bleeding and typically occurs about 2 years after thelarche.

On physical examination the following characteristics may be observed:

Breast enlargement: This may initially be unilateral or asymmetric. Gradually, the breast diameter increases, the areola darkens and thickens, and the nipple becomes more prominent.

Examination of the external genitalia: This may reveal presence of pubic hair or enlargement of the clitoris.

Vagina, uterus, ovaries: The mucosal surface of the vagina also responds to the increasing levels of estrogen, changing from a thin, bright red prepubertal vaginal mucosa to a thicker, dull-pink color post-puberty. There also occurs keratinization of skin and transformation of the vaginal epithelium into a multilayered squamous epithelium under the influence of estrogen. Vaginal epithelium turns acidic with the appearance of Doderlein's bacilli.

Body shape, fat distribution and physical development: There is an increase in the girl's height and weight, which is usually completed by 14 years of age. There is broadening of the lower half of the pelvis and hips, thereby resulting in a wider birth canal. Fat deposition occurs in a typical female distribution in the areas of breasts, hips, buttocks, thighs, upper arms and pubis.

8.5.1.2: Changes in Age of Menarche over Time

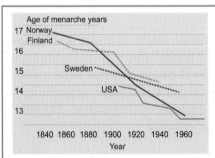

Fig. 8.5.1.2: Changes in age of menarche over time

As shown in the Figure 8.5.1.2, there has been a gradual decline in the age of menarche over the past few decades. Presently, the average age of menarche in girls is 11.75 years. The process of puberty typically begins by the age of 10 or 11 years in girls and by the age of 12 or 13 years in boys. During the period of puberty, there are anatomical (development of secondary sexual and genital organs), physical, endocrinological, psychological and emotional changes.

Puberty is initiated as a result of hormone signals sent from the brain to the gonads (the ovaries and testes). The hormonal signals are responsible for stimulating the growth and function of a variety of organs such as brain, bones, muscles, skin, breast and sex organs. The principal hormone involved in the males is testosterone, while that in females is estradiol. Interaction of various hormones secreted through the hypothalamus-pituitary-ovarian axis and other endocrine organs such as adrenals and thyroid glands play a role.

8.5.1.3: Changes in Height in Both Girls and Boys at the Time of Puberty

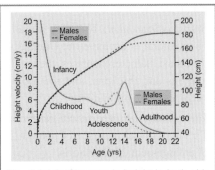

Fig. 8.5.1.3: Changes in height in both girls and boys at the time of puberty

Figure 8.5.1.3 shows changes in the height of both girls and boys at the time of puberty. Maximum height achieved in adulthood is more in males in comparison to that achieved in females. The maximum increase in the height velocity occurs in both males and females during adolescence. This increase in height velocity is more in males in comparison to those in females and occurs about 2 years earlier in females in comparison to males.

In order to assess if the pubertal development is occurring normally in an individual, X-ray of the nondominant hand, elbow and knees is done in order to assess the bone age.

8.5.1.4: Clinical Examination (A to C)

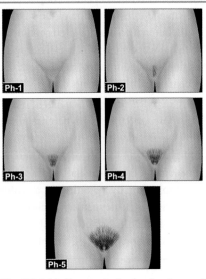

Fig. 8.5.1.4A: Tanner staging for development of pubic hair in females

Figure 8.5.1.4A describes the Tanner staging for the development of pubic hair in females, which is as follows:
Ph-1: Pre-pubertal stage
Ph-2: Sparse growth of long slightly pigmented hair usually slightly curly mainly along the labia
Ph-3: The hair becomes darker, coarser and curlier and spreads over the junction of the pubes
Ph-4: The hair spreads covering the pubes
Ph-5: The hair extends to the medial surface of the thighs and is distributed as an inverse triangle.

Sex education forms an important aspect in relation to the management of normal puberty related changes amongst adolescents. Although puberty is a natural physiological process, sex education regarding the pubertal changes helps in allaying stress and anxiety from the minds of young girls. Young girls need to be educated about sex and sexually transmitted diseases. In case of possibility of sexual intercourse at young age, contraception (barrier methods, initially) must be prescribed. Extra nutrition (especially proteins, iron and calcium) may be required to support their growth.

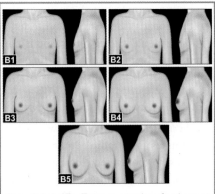

Fig. 8.5.1.4B: Tanner staging for breast development

Figure 8.5.1.4B describes the Tanner stages of breast development, which are as follows:
B-1: Pre-pubertal
B-2: Development of breast bud
B-3: Enlargement of breast and areola with no separation of the breast contour
B-4: Projection of areola and papilla to form a secondary mound above the level of the breast
B-5: Recession of the areola to the general contour of the breast with projection of the papilla only.

Tanner stages of breast development describe the various stages in development of breast tissues, which occur in a predictable sequence at the time of normal physical development in adolescents.

Picture	Medical/Surgical Description	Management/Clinical Highlights
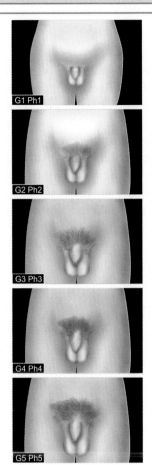 **Fig. 8.5.1.4C:** Tanner stages of pubic hair and genital development in males	Tanner stages of pubic hair and genital development in males are as follows: *G1 Ph1 (Stage I):* This is the prepubertal stage of development. There is no coarse or pigmented hair. Testes are smaller in volume (less than 4 mL). Penis is also in prepubertal stage showing no growth. *G2 Ph2 (Stage II):* Minimum coarse or pigmented hair at the base of penis. Testes increase to about 4 mL in volume. There is a slight increase in the length and width of penis. There also may be some reddening and change in the nature of skin over the scrotum. *G3 Ph3 (Stage III):* Dark colored, pigmented hair spread over until the junction of pubis. Testicular volume increases to about 12 mL. The increase in the length of penis is much more than the width. *G4 Ph4 (Stage IV):* Pubic hair of adult quality is spread all over the pubis and perineum. There also occurs development of glans penis and darkening of the skin over the scrotum. *G5 Ph5 (Stage V):* Male internal and external genitalia achieve the mature adult size. Pubic hair of adult quality also spreads over the medial aspect of thighs.	Tanner stages define physical measurements of external primary and secondary sexual characteristics.

8.5.2: Precocious Puberty

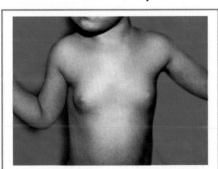 **Fig. 8.5.2:** Precocious breast development in a 7-year-old girl	Precocious puberty refers to the appearance of physical and hormonal signs of pubertal development at an age earlier than is considered normal. Puberty is considered precocious in case there is development of secondary sexual characteristics in girls younger than 8 years (Fig. 8.5.2) or there is onset of menses before the age of 10 years (chronological age). For boys, onset of puberty before the age of 9 years is considered precocious. Precocious puberty can be of two types: (1) Central precocious puberty (CPP) (constitutional/true/complete precocious puberty), which is gonadotropin-dependent and (2) Precocious pseudopuberty, which is gonadotropin-independent.	*Surgical Management:* When CPP is caused by a CNS tumor other than a hamartoma, surgical resection may be attempted. Radiation therapy is often indicated if surgical resection is incomplete. *Medical Management:* Continuous administration of luteinizing hormone-releasing hormone (LHRH) and GnRH agonists provides negative feedback and results in decreased levels of LH and FSH 2–4 weeks after initiating treatment. GnRH analogues in the dosage of 100 µg intranasally BD for 6 months can be used to suppress menstruation because the young girls might not be capable of managing menstrual hygiene.

8.6: TUBERCULOSIS

8.6.1: Diagnosis

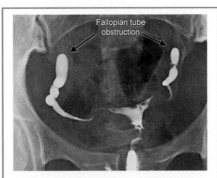

Fig. 8.6.1: Hysterosalpingogram in an asymptomatic patient (later diagnosed as genital tuberculosis) showing lead pipe like appearance of fallopian tubes and bilateral tubal obstruction along with bilateral hydrosalpinx

Other findings suggestive of tubercular salpingitis, if HSG is done in an asymptomatic woman, include the following:

- Lead pipe appearance of the tubes
- Beading and variations in the filling density
- Tobacco pouch appearance
- Calcification of tube and jagged fluffiness of the tubal outline
- Cornual block
- Distorted uterine contour
- Vascular or lymphatic intravasation of the dye

Tubercular infection of the genital tract first affects the fallopian tubes resulting in pelvic inflammatory disease. Later, it spreads downward causing uterine synechiae and Asherman's syndrome. Cervical and vulvar lesions are rare. Infection of genital tract with *Mycobacterium tuberculosis* is almost always secondary to a focus elsewhere in the body.

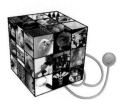

EVIDENCE-BASED BREAKTHROUGH FACTS

1. **USE OF PROPHYLACTIC DEXAMETHASONE AMONGST PATIENTS UNDERGOING LAPAROSCOPIC GYNECOLOGICAL SURGERY**

According to a new meta-analytic review, use of prophylactic dexamethasone amongst patients undergoing laparoscopic gynecological surgery, helps in reducing the incidence of postoperative nausea and vomiting without causing any significant side-effects, such as delayed wound healing, increase in blood glucose levels, etc., amongst these patients.

Source: Pham A, Liu G. Dexamethasone for antiemesis in laparoscopic gynecologic surgery: a systematic review and meta-analysis. Obstet Gynecol. 2012;120:1451-8.

Gynecology

Section 9

Menstrual Disorders

9.1: ABNORMAL MENSTRUAL BLEEDING

9.1.1: Different Types of Menstrual Abnormalities

Picture	Medical/Surgical Description	Management/Clinical Highlights
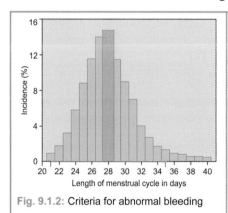 Fig. 9.1.1: Different types of menstrual bleeding	Different types of menstrual bleeding disorders include menorrhagia, hypomenorrhea, polymenorrhea, oligomenorrhea, metrorrhagia, menometrorrhagia, etc.	Menorrhagia can be defined as prolonged or heavy cyclic menstruation, which amounts to menstrual periods lasting for more than 7 days or blood loss exceeding 80 mL in amount. The bleeding despite of being excessive or heavy occurs at regular intervals. Metrorrhagia can be described as intermenstrual bleeding. Diminished blood flow during menstrual cycles is termed as hypomenorrhea. Cycles with intervals ≥ 35 days are termed as oligomenorrhea. In polymenorrhea, cycles occur more frequently at regular intermissions with time intervals ≤ 21 days. In menometrorrhagia, bleeding is either prolonged or excessive, occurs at infrequent intervals with an increased frequency.

9.1.2: Criteria for Abnormal Bleeding

Fig. 9.1.2: Criteria for abnormal bleeding	As shown in the adjacent figure, normal menstrual cycles in most women occur at every 28 ± 7 days duration in which the bleeding lasts for an average of 7 days (ranging between 4 days and 10 days), with flow varying between 25 mL and 80 mL. In most women, however, bleeding occurs at 28 days. The criteria for abnormal uterine bleeding (AUB) comprise of one of the following: • Bleeding occurring < 21 days apart • Bleeding occurring > 35 days apart • Bleeding is unpredictable and irregular. • Amount of bleeding > 80 mL.	The most important reason for assessment of cases of AUB is that the diagnosis of endometrial cancer is usually made during the evaluation of cases with abnormal vaginal bleeding. Abnormal perimenopausal or postmenopausal bleeding is associated with endometrial cancer in approximately 10% of cases. The most commonly used noninvasive investigation for diagnosis of cases of AUB is ultrasonography. This can be followed-up with investigations such as saline infusion sonography (SIS), hysteroscopy and endometrial biopsy (EB) to reach a definitive diagnosis.

9.1.3: Abnormal Uterine Bleeding Due to Endometrial Polyp

Figures 9.1.9 (C and D) demonstrates the role of ultrasound for establishing the diagnosis of endometrial polyps in patients with AUB.

9.1.4: Endometrial Biopsy for Evaluation of Abnormal Uterine Bleeding (A to D)

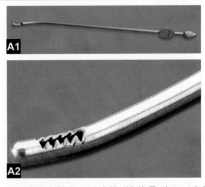

Figs 9.1.4 (A1 and A2): (A1) Endometrial biopsy curette; (A2) Magnified view showing the upper end with serrated edges

The EB curette is a narrow metal cannula having serrated edges with side openings on one end and an opening for syringe to be attached at the other end. Application of suction through the syringe helps in aspiration of endometrial curettings. EB curette is used for performing endometrial biopsy, which facilitates histopathological examination of the endometrium.

In case the endometrial thickness is greater than 4 mm on transvaginal ultrasound examination in a postmenopausal patient with AUB, endometrial studies (endometrial aspiration, biopsy, etc.) should be done in order to exclude endometrial hyperplasia or even malignancy.

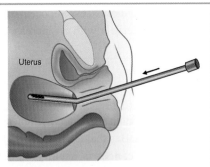

Fig. 9.1.4B: Placement of endometrial biopsy curette inside the uterine cavity

Procedure of endometrial biopsy comprises of the following steps:
- Firstly, the patient is placed in the lithotomy position and then a bimanual examination is conducted in order to assess the uterus.
- The cervix is then visualized with help of a Sim's speculum and a tenaculum.
- The cervical os is cleaned with help of Betadine® solution.
- After the position and size of the uterine cavity have been assessed using a uterine sound, the EB curette is inserted gently inside the uterine cavity until any significant resistance is felt.

Endometrial biopsy helps in providing an adequate sample for diagnosis of endometrial problems in nearly 90–100% of cases. However, it may fail to detect the presence of small masses including polyps and leiomyomas.

Steps for endometrial biopsy have been demonstrated in Figures 9.1.4B to D.

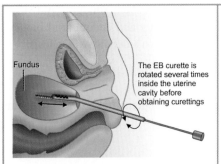

The EB curette is rotated several times inside the uterine cavity before obtaining curettings

Fig. 9.1.4C: Before obtaining the endometrial curettings, the endometrial biopsy curette is rotated several times inside the uterus

While inside the uterine cavity, the cannula is rotated several times in order to scrape off the endometrial lining. This procedure should be repeated at least four times and the device is rotated by 360° to ensure adequate coverage of the area.

Both perimenopausal and menopausal women with bleeding following a period of amenorrhea must have an EB because these women are at a high risk for development of endometrial carcinoma, polyps or hyperplasia in future. Other patients who are at an increased risk of development of endometrial malignancy include patients with triad of hypertension, diabetes and obesity, and those with chronic anovulation.

Picture	Medical/Surgical Description	Management/Clinical Highlights
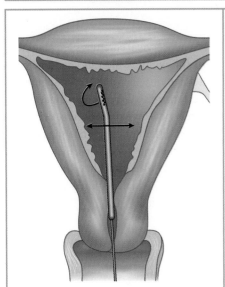 Fig. 9.1.4D: Transverse section of endometrial cavity showing the endometrial biopsy curette	The endometrial scrapings obtained by scraping the EB curette are then sucked in through the syringe. When adequate amount of endometrial curetting have been obtained, the curette is removed and samples are sent for microscopic examination. One set of sample is sent in normal saline for assessment of acid fast bacilli. Other set of sample is sent in acetone for assessment of histopathology.	Endometrial curettage can be performed as an outpatient investigation and does not require general anesthesia as is required for D&C. Thus this procedure has superseded dilatation and curettage, and it has presently become the gold standard for obtaining endometrial tissue and for detecting endometrial diseases.

9.1.5: Endometrial Aspiration (A to D)

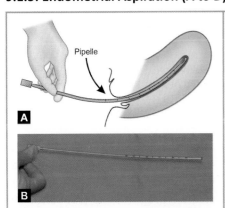 Figs 9.1.5 (A and B): (A) Diagram showing endometrial aspiration; (B) Pipelle® endometrial sampler for doing endometrial aspiration	Endometrial aspiration can be done with the help of devices like Pipelle® curette, Sharman curette, Gravlee jet washer, Isaac cell sampler, Vabra® aspirator, etc. Pipelle® endometrial sampler comprises of a hollow tube, which is about 3 mm in outer diameter. It also comprises of a solid obturator, which fits snugly inside the outer tube. If a Pipelle® device is not available, a size 4 mm Karman's cannula along with a 20 cc syringe can also be used for the procedure.	Since no dilatation of the internal os is required prior to insertion at the time of endometrial aspiration, the procedure can be performed as an outpatient procedure without any requirement of anesthesia. Though the procedure is usually painless, the patient can be prescribed nonsteroidal anti-inflammatory drugs (NSAIDs) in case she experiences pain. Following the procedure, the endometrial sample obtained is sent for histopathological examination.
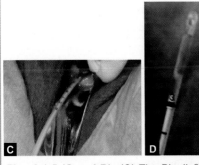 Figs 9.1.5 (C and D): (C) The Pipelle® is negotiated through the internal cervical os; (D) Suction of endometrial tissue inside the Pipelle® as the obturator is pulled out	The diagnostic accuracy of endometrial aspiration using the Pipelle® device is 92–98% when compared with subsequent D&C. The sample produced by the newer slim endometrial suction curettes (Pipelle®) is similar to that produced by older devices, while at the same time causing much less pain and trauma.	The Pipelle® is conveyed through the internal cervical os without requirement of prior dilatation. The obturator/plunger should be withdrawn until adequate vacuum has been created, which helps in suctioning out endometrial aspirates.

Picture	Medical/Surgical Description	Management/Clinical Highlights

9.1.6: Fractional Curettage (A to E)

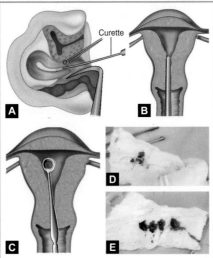

Figs 9.1.6 (A to E): (A) Endocervical curettage is performed; (B) Internal cervical os is dilated; (C) Endometrial curettage is performed; (D) Endocervical curettings; (E) Endometrial curettings

Fractional curettage involves taking three samples, one from endocervical canal, and second and third from lower and upper segments. This procedure is performed when endometrial aspiration is unable to establish the diagnosis in patients with AUB.

The endocervical curettings are obtained first following, which the endometrial curettage of upper and lower segments is performed so that no contamination of endocervical curettings occurs. In case it appears difficult to negotiate the curette through internal cervical os, the clinician may be required to dilate the internal cervical os, which requires some form of anesthesia.

9.1.7: Hysteroscopic Directed Biopsy

Hysteroscopic directed biopsy is considered as the most accurate diagnostic test for diagnosis of endometrial malignancy by some clinicians. However, it is an invasive test. For details related to hysteroscopic directed biopsy, kindly refer to Section 12.

9.1.8: Histopathological Findings (A to D)

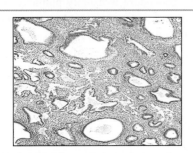

Fig. 9.1.8A: Histopathological appearance of simple endometrial hyperplasia

Simple endometrial hyperplasia is associated with an increase in the number of glands and endometrial stroma. Some glands are cystically dilated. However, epithelium does not show any atypical features.

Most individuals with simple hyperplasia without any atypia can be managed with hormonal manipulation using medroxyprogesterone (Provera), 10 mg daily every 5 days for 3 months or with close follow-up. Progestin may be administered orally, intramuscularly, in form of an intrauterine device (IUD) or as a vaginal cream. A follow-up EB after 3–12 months can be done.

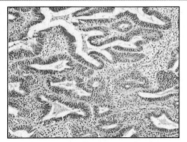

Fig. 9.1.8B: Histopathological appearance of complex endometrial hyperplasia

In complex endometrial hyperplasia, there is an increase in the number of glands, which are aligned back to back. Glandular outlines are irregular. Complex proliferation of the epithelium occurs, but without any associated atypical features.

Some physicians treat complex hyperplasia with hormonal therapy (medroxyprogesterone 10–20 mg daily for up to 3 months). A D&C may be required to exclude the presence of endometrial carcinoma.

Picture	Medical/Surgical Description	Management/Clinical Highlights
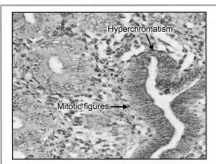 **Fig. 9.1.8C:** Histopathological appearance of complex endometrial hyperplasia with atypia	In cases of complex endometrial hyperplasia with atypia, besides the above mentioned changes associated with complex endometrial hyperplasia, epithelium also shows atypia (hyperchromatism, mitotic figures, etc.). This is a premalignant lesion that may progress to cancer in 30–45% of women. Additionally, atypical endometrial hyperplasia may be associated with a co-existing endometrial cancer in approximately 20% of patients.	Though some physicians treat complex hyperplasia with or without atypia with hormonal therapy (medroxyprogesterone, 10–20 mg daily for up to 3 months), hysterectomy may be considered for complex or high-grade cases of hyperplasia with atypia.
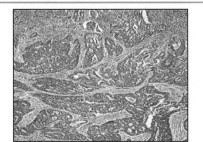 **Fig. 9.1.8D:** Histopathological appearance of frank endometrial Cancer	In these cases there is replacement of normal uterine endometrium with frank invasive cancer showing invasion of the basement membrane.	Laparotomy with total abdominal hysterectomy and bilateral salpingo-oophorectomy along with staging is required in these cases in order to determine the stage of uterine cancer. Treatment is then directed based on the stage of cancer.

9.1.9: Ultrasound (A to D)

Picture	Medical/Surgical Description	Management/Clinical Highlights
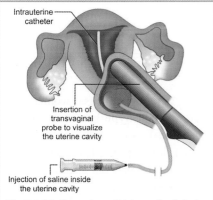 **Fig. 9.1.9A:** Procedure of doing saline infusion sonography	This technique employs the use of sterile saline solution as a negative contrast medium in conjunction with traditional transvaginal ultrasound. Thus, besides imaging the uterine cavity, this technique also helps in evaluating the patency of the fallopian tubes. The advantage of SIS over hysteroscopy is that this technique also helps in scanning the ovaries, pelvis and peritoneal cavity, while imaging the uterine cavity. SIS has been observed to have high sensitivity rate of 94.9% and specificity rate of 89.3%.	Saline infusion sonography serves as an alternative to hysteroscopy and helps in differentiating between various potential etiologies of thickened endometrium, e.g. polyps, submucous myomas, homogenously thickened endometrium, etc. It also helps in determining whether an abnormality is endometrial or subendometrial in origin.
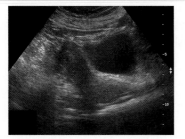 **Fig. 9.1.9B:** TAS showing an enlarged uterine cavity, measuring 77 × 31 mm, with multiple cystic spaces within	In this case, biopsy confirmed the presence of endometrial cancer. Though there are no specific sonographic findings indicative of endometrial cancer, presence of intermingled hypoechoic and hyperechoic areas within the endometrium are indicative of malignancy.	There may be abnormal fluid collections within the endometrial cavity or an irregular endometrial-myometrial junction. In cases with suspected endometrial cancer on ultrasound, even with a normal endometrial thickness, an EB or hysteroscopic-guided EB may be required to exclude malignancy.

Picture	Medical/Surgical Description	Management/Clinical Highlights
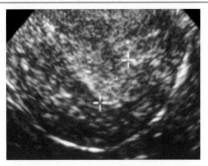 Fig. 9.1.9C: Presence of thickened endometrium (> 4 mm) on TVS in a patient with AUB	Patients presenting with AUB having a history of unopposed estrogen exposure should be first evaluated by transvaginal ultrasound examination. Biopsy is unnecessary when the endometrial thickness is less than 4 mm.	There is no consensus in the literature regarding the cut-off value for normal endometrial thickness. The increased bilayered (double layered) endometrial thickness has been found to vary between 4 mm and 8 mm in various studies. A bi-endometrial (double layer) thickness of 4 mm is considered as a cut-off point by most clinicians and is associated with the sensitivity of 96–98%.
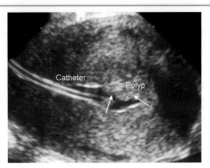 Fig. 9.1.9D: In the same patient whose TVS has been shown above, SIS revealed presence of an endometrial polyp	In this patient though the endometrium was thickened, there was no other risk factor for endometrial cancer. Based on the clinical suspicion of an endometrial polyp, SIS was performed, which revealed presence of an endometrial polyp. SIS is able to clearly delineate the masses or defects inside the uterine cavity. SIS helps in differentiating between focal lesions (polyps and submucosal myomas) and global endometrial thickening. SIS can be used as a second line diagnostic procedure in women with AUB when findings from transvaginal ultrasound are nonconclusive.	Hysteroscopic resection and guided biopsy has been considered as the most effective treatment for management of endometrial polyps. This also facilitates histologic assessment. On the other hand, blind biopsy or curettage has low diagnostic accuracy and therefore need not be performed in these cases.

9.1.10: Management

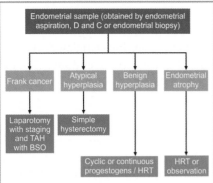

Fig. 9.1.10: Management of endometrial hyperplasia

Lesions without atypia can regress spontaneously. However, prescription of progestins helps in the treatment of underlying etiology, i.e. chronic anovulation and exposure to excessive estrogens.

Premenopausal women with nonatypical endometrial hyperplasia are usually prescribed a course of low-dose progestins for a period of 3–6 months. For example medroxyprogesterone acetate (10–20 mg) may be administered orally for 12–14 days each month. Another frequently used option is to prescribe combined oral contraceptive pills (OCPs) in women who do not have any contraindications for its use. Complex hyperplasia without atypia can also be treated with progestins. Office EB is performed annually in these cases.

Even in postmenopausal women with endometrial hyperplasia, cyclic or continuous low-dose medroxyprogesterone treatment is required. However, in these women, it is important to ensure that an adequate sample has been obtained to exclude atypia. D&C may be required in some cases.

In case of atypical hyperplasia in women at any age, hysterectomy is the best treatment option because of the high risk of malignancy.

9.2: DYSFUNCTIONAL UTERINE BLEEDING

9.2.1: Medical Treatment Used for Controlling Dysfunctional Uterine Bleeding

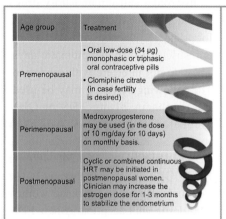

Fig. 9.2.1: Medical treatment used for controlling dysfunctional uterine bleeding

In women belonging to reproductive age groups, OCPs prove useful in controlling DUB. In perimenopausal women, medroxyprogesterone (10 mg/day for 10 days) may be used on monthly basis to regulate bleeding patterns. In postmenopausal women, cyclic or combined continuous hormone replacement therapy (HRT) may be useful in controlling bleeding.

In premenopausal women and women belonging to reproductive age groups, OCPs can regulate cycles, at the same time providing contraception. If contraception is not required, medroxyprogesterone acetate can be used to regulate cycles.

Clomiphene citrate (in the dosage of 50–150 mg per day on days 4th to 9th of the cycle) can induce ovulation in a woman with anovulatory cycles, who desire pregnancy. In a perimenopausal women, OCPs can be continued until a woman has reached menopause and then HRT may be started.

9.3: DYSMENORRHEA

9.3.1: Mechanism of Primary Dysmenorrhea

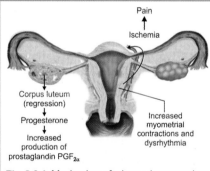

Fig. 9.3.1: Mechanism of primary dysmenorrhea

Figure 9.3.1 illustrates the mechanism of primary dysmenorrhea. In the event pregnancy does not occur, the corpus luteum undergoes regression. This causes a reduction in the level of progesterone in the blood, resulting in an increased production of prostaglandins ($PGF_{2\alpha}$). This causes increased myometrial contractions, dysrhythmia and myometrial ischemia, which is responsible for producing spasmodic pain during menstrual cycles (shedding of uterine endometrium in the event pregnancy does not occur).

It is important to understand the mechanism of primary dysmenorrhea so as to plane the treatment accordingly. Since the abnormal production of prostaglandins is the main pathology involved, treatment strategies must be aimed toward reducing their production. Medicines such as NSAIDs prove to be helpful by decreasing the production of $PGF_{2\alpha}$. Oral contraceptives prove useful by preventing ovulation due to which there is no formation of corpus luteum.

9.3.2: Causes of Secondary Dysmenorrhea

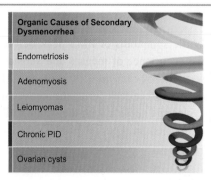

Fig. 9.3.2: Causes of secondary dysmenorrhea

Dysmenorrhea is labeled as primary in the absence of underlying medical disease/pathology. Secondary dysmenorrhea on the other hand, is associated with an underlying medical disease/pathology. Some of the common causes of secondary dysmenorrhea include endometriosis, leiomyomas, adenomyosis, ovarian cysts, pelvic congestion, insertion of copper intrauterine contraceptive devices (IUCDs), etc.

Management of cases of secondary dysmenorrhea comprises of treating the underlying pathology. Pain in these cases must be controlled with the help of first-line medical therapy, comprising of NSAIDs with or without contraception. Continuous use of OCPs is the second option of choice.

9.3.3: Management of Cases of Dysmenorrhea

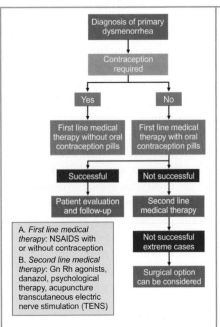

Fig. 9.3.3: Management of cases of primary dysmenorrhea

The diagnosis of dysmenorrhea can be considered in a patient with abdominal pain in whom pain occurs in relation with the menstrual cycles. If there is no relation with menstrual cycles, the patient should be evaluated for other causes of abdominal pain. In cases of dysmenorrhea, it is also important to rule out the presence of any underlying gynecological pathology to establish the diagnosis of secondary dysmenorrhea. In presence of any gynecological pathology, diagnosis of secondary dysmenorrhea is established.

Nonsteroidal anti-inflammatory drugs are the most commonly used medicines for primary dysmenorrhea and their use is restricted to the symptomatic days. They do not interfere with ovulation. The following NSAIDS may be used: indomethacin 24 mg TDS or QID; ibuprofen 400 mg TDS; naproxen sodium 240 mg TDS; ketoprofen 40 mg TDS and mefenamic acid 240–400 mg BD or QID. Hormonal therapy is the treatment of choice for those women who desire contraception. A new FDA approved treatment for premenstrual syndrome (PMS) is a new OCP, Yaz (containing 3 mg drospirenone and 20 μg ethinyl estradiol).

9.3.4: Response of Patients of Primary Dysmenorrhea with NSAIDS

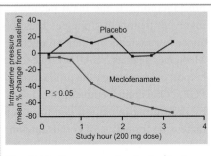

Fig. 9.3.4: Response of patients of primary dysmenorrhea with NSAIDs

The graph shows the response of intrauterine pressure response to NSAIDs when they are administered in cases of primary dysmenorrhea. NSAIDs are able to reduce the intrauterine pressure by nearly 75% within 3 hours in comparison to placebo.

This graph highlights the effectiveness of NSAIDs for treatment of cases with primary dysmenorrhea. Use of NSAIDs causes a reduction in the intrauterine pressure and therefore abdominal pain.

9.3.5: Comparison of Dysmenorrhea with Premenstrual Syndrome

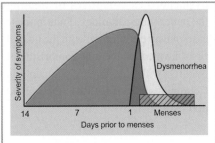

Fig. 9.3.5: Comparison of dysmenorrhea with premenstrual syndrome

There may appear to be a close overlap between the symptoms of dysmenorrhea and PMS. The graph shows comparison of symptoms of PMS with that of dysmenorrhea. There is likely to be an overlap between the two because both occur in relation to the menstrual cycles. However, the fact remains that each is a separate clinical entity.

While symptoms of PMS peak before the occurrence of menses and subside with its occurrence, symptoms of dysmenorrhea peak during the menstrual cycles and subside with the waning off of the menstrual periods.

Picture	Medical/Surgical Description	Management/Clinical Highlights

9.4: PREMENSTRUAL SYNDROME

9.4.1: Spectrum of Premenstrual Symptoms

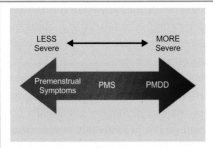

Fig. 9.4.1: Spectrum of premenstrual symptoms

Premenstrual syndrome or premenstrual tension includes a combination of physical, psychological and emotional symptoms, which the women experience for a few days (usually 7–10 days) preceding menstruation.

When the common premenstrual symptoms such as depression, anxiety, irritability, abdominal bloating, breast tenderness, headache, sleeplessness, fatigue, emotional liability, mood swings, depression, irritability, lassitude, insomnia, etc. increase in severity, it is termed as PMS. When the symptoms of PMS attain extreme severity, become debilitating, and include at least one mood related symptom, it is termed as premenstrual dysmorphic disorder (PMDD).

9.4.2: Differential Diagnosis of Premenstrual Syndrome

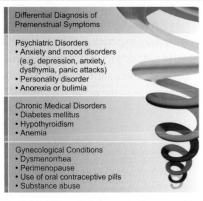

Fig. 9.4.2: Differential diagnosis of premenstrual syndrome

Premenstrual syndrome may show clinical resemblance to numerous medical disorders. Various conditions, which may mimic PMS include psychiatric disorders (such as anxiety and mood disorders, e.g. depression, anxiety, dysthymia, panic attacks, personality disorders, anorexia or bulimia); chronic medical disorders (diabetes mellitus, hypothyroidism, anemia, etc.); gynecological conditions (dysmenorrhea, perimenopause, etc.); use of OCPs; substance abuse disorders; etc.

There is no investigation available to establish the diagnosis of PMS. The diagnosis is established on the basis of clinical presentation. The characteristic feature of PMS is that these symptoms occur a week before the onset of menstruation and improve a few days after the periods start.

9.4.3: Management of Mild and Moderate Premenstrual Syndrome

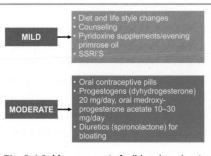

Fig. 9.4.3: Management of mild and moderate premenstrual syndrome

Reassurance, patient counseling, psycho-therapy and selective use of medicines are useful in most of the mild to moderate cases. Use of vitamin B6, magnesium and/or calcium supplements and evening primrose oil may also prove to be useful in mild to moderate cases of PMS.

Conservative management comprises of a well-balanced diet containing high fiber content (whole grain, fruits and vegetables), restriction of salt, alcohol or caffeine, and regular aerobic exercises daily. If the lifestyle modifications are not useful, antidepressants such as selective serotonin reuptake inhibitors (SSRIs) such as fluoxetine may be prescribed. If these do not help, the clinician may prescribe OCPs and progestogen supplements. Diuretics may be useful for bloating.

9.4.4: Management of Severe and Extreme Cases of Premenstrual Syndrome

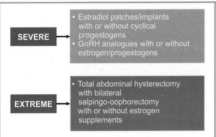

Fig. 9.4.4: Management of severe and extreme cases of premenstrual syndrome

Severe PMS may result in physical discomfort, pain, as well as mental disorders and mood swings. In PMDD, the symptoms may become so severe that the woman may lose control over her social life, relationship, work and everyday activities. In extremely severe cases, she might even experience suicidal tendencies.

Pharmacological treatment of PMDD comprises of using antidepressants (SSRIs) such as fluoxetine (10–20 mg); sertraline (25–50 mg); paroxetine (10–20 mg); citalopram, etc. In severe cases estradiol patches/implants with or without cyclical progestogens and/or GnRH analogues may be useful. Surgery is normally not required but in extremely severe cases of PMDD total abdominal hysterectomy with bilateral salpingo-oophorectomy with or without estrogen supplements may be done.

9.4.5: Premenstrual Syndrome Diary

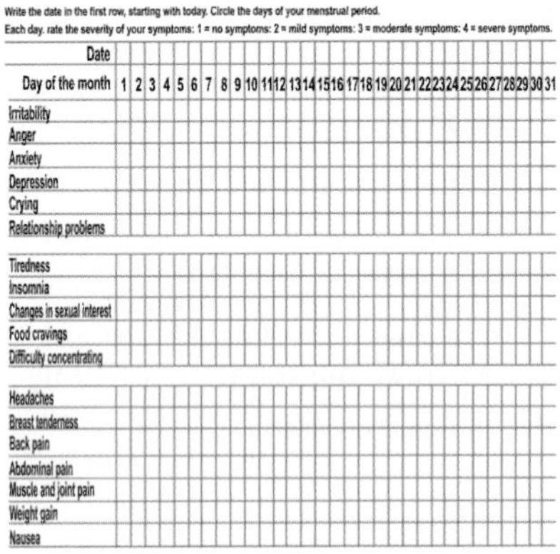

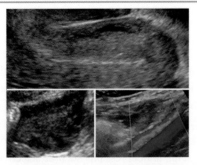

Fig. 9.4.5: Premenstrual syndrome diary

Many health care professionals advise the patient to maintain a premenstrual diary for 2–3 months so that they can determine which symptoms are causing maximum discomfort to the patient. An effective treatment plan can then be formulated based on the symptom pattern observed on premenstrual diary.

The columns in this diary describe day of the cycle, while the rows describe various premenstrual symptoms, which the woman may experience. The woman is asked to note down various premenstrual symptoms, which she experiences on the different days of the cycle. The record is usually maintained for 2–3 months to see if a pattern emerges.

9.5: POSTMENOPAUSAL BLEEDING

9.5.1: Ultrasound Showing Thin Endometrium

Fig. 9.5.1: A patient presenting with PMB in which TVS shows presence of thin hyperechogenic endometrium. Color Doppler demonstrates the presence of iliac vessels adjacent to the ovary with no growing follicle.

Menopause is defined by the WHO as the permanent cessation of menstruation resulting from the loss of ovarian follicular activity. The most serious concern in postmenopausal and perimenopausal women with abnormal PMB is endometrial carcinoma.

The first line of management in these patients is performance of a transvaginal ultrasound to evaluate the endometrial thickness. In a normal postmenopausal women (as shown in the picture), there is a thin hyperechogenic endometrium and empty ovaries with absence of any follicle. Endometrial biopsy is usually not required in these cases. Follow-up may be done to evaluate any further bleeding.

Picture	Medical/Surgical Description	Management/Clinical Highlights

9.5.2: Ultrasound Showing an Increased Endometrial Thickness

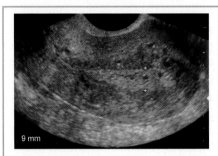

Fig. 9.5.2: Transvaginal sonography in a patient with postmenopausal bleeding showing an endometrial thickness of 9 mm

The most commonly used noninvasive investigation for diagnosis of cases of PMB is ultrasonography.

According to American College of Obstetricians and Gynecologists (ACOG) (2009) recommendations, postmenopausal cases of AUB with endometrial thickness > 4 mm require additional evaluation with investigations such as SIS, hysteroscopy or EB. In premenopausal patients with AUB, no further evaluation is recommended for a normal appearing endometrium ≤ 10 mm.

9.6: TREATMENT OF MENSTRUAL DISORDERS

9.6.1: Various Techniques for Endometrial Ablation (A to F)

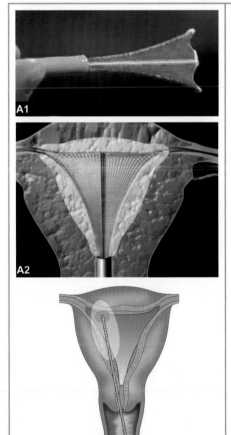

Figs 9.6.1 (A and B): (A1 and A2) (A1) NovaSure® device; (A2) Endometrial ablation with radiofrequency energy; (B) Freezing the endometrium with a special probe

Various methods for endometrial ablation help in treating DUB by destroying the endometrial lining. The methods for endometrial ablation are mainly of two types: first generation (hysteroscopic) methods and second generation (nonhysteroscopic methods). Hysteroscopic methods include laser and electrosurgical resection. On the other hand, nonhysteroscopic methods include procedures such as Thermachoice®, microwave therapy, etc. The pictures here illustrate the procedure of endometrial ablation using application of controlled radiofrequency energy (NovaSure® device) and endometrial ablation using a cryoprobe.

During endometrial ablation by radiofrequency energy, a probe is inserted into the uterus through the cervix. The tip of the probe expands into a mesh-like device that sends radiofrequency energy into the uterine lining. The energy and heat destroys the endometrial tissue, while suction is applied to remove it. In this method, electromagnetic radiations having frequency of 27 MHz with power of 550 W are applied for a time period lasting for 20 minutes.

In cryoablation, the cryoprobe is inserted under ultrasound guidance up to the level of uterine fundus and cooled to –90°C. The tip of the probe freezes the uterine lining by perfusing liquid nitrogen. A cycle of 2 minutes freeze followed by 2 minutes thaw leads to endometrial destruction until the depth of approximately 4–5 mm.

Picture	Medical/Surgical Description	Management/Clinical Highlights

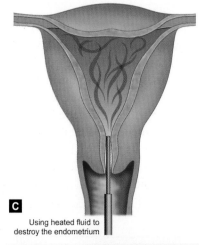

C Using heated fluid to destroy the endometrium

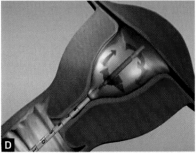

D

Figs 9.6.1 (C and D): (C) Using heated fluid to destroy the endometrium; (D) Use of heated balloon to destroy the endometrium

Various second generation procedures used for endometrial ablation include: cryoablation, hydrothermal ablation, laser thermoablation, microwave ablation, thermal balloon ablation, electrosurgical ablation, photodynamic ablation, radiofrequency induced thermal ablation, etc. The pictures here illustrate the procedure of endometrial ablation using heated fluid (hydroablation) and using a heated balloon (Thermachoice™) to destroy the endometrium.

The Hydrothermablator® (HTA) is the device used for performing hydrothermal ablation. This is performed as an office procedure under local anesthesia in which preheated normal saline is infused into the uterus via the hysteroscope and is allowed to circulate freely in the endometrial cavity. Since this procedure is done under direct vision through a hysteroscope, it differs from other second generation techniques by virtue of not being a blind procedure. Before infusion, the solution is heated to 194°F/90°C; once the proper temperature is reached, the hot water circulates for 10 minutes inside the uterine cavity to destroy the endometrial cells.

During endometrial ablation using a thermal balloon, the endometrium may be hysteroscopically ablated via the insertion of a thermal uterine balloon. In this procedure, a balloon catheter, filled with isotonic sodium chloride solution is inserted inside the endometrial cavity, inflated, and heated to 87°C for 8 minutes. The fluid is usually instilled until the pressure reaches between 160–180 mm Hg. The device is kept inside for 8 minutes following which it is removed.

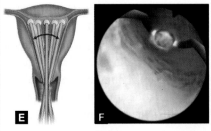

E **F**

Figs 9.6.1 (E and F): (E) Endometrial ablation with microwave energy; (F) Electrosurgery with a roller ball-tipped resectoscope

The pictures here show endometrial ablation using microwave energy and electrosurgical ablation using a roller ball-tipped resectoscope. Microwave endometrial ablation (MEA) uses high-frequency microwave energy to cause rapid, but shallow heating of the endometrium. MEA requires 3 minutes of time and only local anesthesia. Its use is now proving to be as effective as transcervical resection of the endometrium (TCRE).

In the procedure of endometrial ablation using a roller ball-tipped resectoscope, the endometrium is ablated via electrosurgical energy using a roller ball. See Figure 9.6.2 for further details.

Microwave endometrial ablation device consists of the software controlled unit, which provides microwave energy of fixed 9.2 GHz frequency at 30 W power. These microwaves are released into the uterine cavity by means of a 15 cm long, 8 mm diameter applicator, which also has a thermocouple at the tip to record the abdominal temperature. The local heating effect by the microwaves (75–80°C) leads to ablation.

Microwaves are selected so that they do not cause destruction beyond 6 mm.

9.6.2: Roller Ball Endometrial Ablation

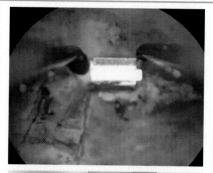

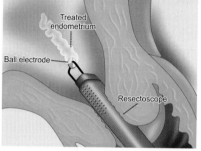

Fig. 9.6.2: Roller ball endometrial ablation

Electrosurgical technique that uses a heated roller ball to burn away the endometrial tissue is called roller ball ablation. The roller ball is a ball about 2 mm in diameter that rotates freely on its handle.

In this procedure, the endometrium is ablated via electrosurgical energy using a roller ball. This type of endometrial ablation essentially is the same as TCRE, except that instead of a wire loop, a heated roller ball is used to destroy the endometrium. Roller ball electrodes are available in two sizes: small (2.5 mm) and large (5 mm). Roller ball endometrial ablation is an easier technique in comparison to the TCRE, and it is associated with a lower risk of complications including uterine perforation, fluid absorption and hemorrhage.

9.6.3: Transcervical Resection of the Endometrium (A and B)

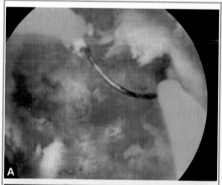

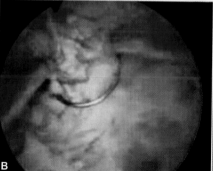

Figs 9.6.3 (A and B): Transcervical resection of the endometrium: (A) Wire loop touching the endometrial surface; (B) Wire loop resecting out the endometrium

Transcervical resection of the endometrium is the first generation endometrial ablation procedure, which has been considered the standard cure for menorrhagia since many years. In this method, a heated wire loop is used to resect out the endometrial lining. The wire loop is around 6 mm long and is attached at an angle to a pencil-shaped handle. Success rates as high as 80–90% can be achieved with this method. The resectoscope has the advantage of being able to remove polyps and some fibroids at the time of ablation. The main risk associated with TCRE is uterine perforation.

This procedure is usually done in an operating room under general anesthesia and comprises of the following steps:
- After dilating the cervix, a hysteroscope is inserted inside the uterine cavity, following which a heating device composed of a wire loop is placed inside the uterine cavity.
- Using a wire loop, the surgeon cuts away the endometrial lining.
- Fluid is continuously pumped inside the uterine cavity in order to keep it distended while the endometrial resection is being carried out.

SECTION 9 ❖ MENSTRUAL DISORDERS

9.7: MENOPAUSE

9.7.1: Etiology (A to C)

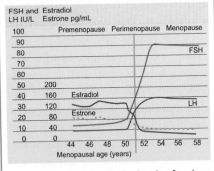

Fig. 9.7.1A: Changes in the levels of various hormones at the time of menopause

Menopause occurs due to decline in ovarian activity. There is failure of ovulation, failure of formation of corpus luteum and failure of secretion of progesterone by the ovaries. Estrogenic activity is reduced and there occurs endometrial atrophy, resulting in amenorrhea. Initially, there is a rebound increase in the secretion of FSH and LH by the anterior pituitary. However, with further advancing years, the gonadotropic activity of pituitary glands also cease and a fall in FSH levels eventually occurs.

These aberrations in the endocrine balance in the menopausal women are likely to result in numerous symptoms. Nearly 60–70% of women remain asymptomatic; others may experience symptoms, which are described in Figure 9.7.1B. Management of various menopausal symptoms is also described there. In the long term, menopause is likely to result in complications such as arthritis, osteoporosis, fracture, cerebrovascular accidents, ischemic heart disease, myocardial infraction, atherosclerosis, stroke, skin changes, Alzheimer's disease, etc.

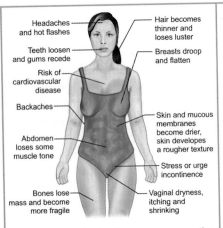

Fig. 9.7.1B: Effects of menopause on the female body

Anatomical changes occurring during menopause include atrophy and retrogression of the genital organs. Menopausal changes may result in the following symptoms:

Vaginal symptoms: These include genital symptoms such as dryness of vagina, dyspareunia and genital prolapse.

Cessation of periods: There could be a sudden cessation or gradual diminution in the amount of blood loss for each successive menstrual period, until the menstrual flow eventually ceases.

Hot flashes: This commonly occur as a result of vasomotor disturbances.

Osteoporosis: There is likely to be reduction in bone mineral mass, resulting in osteopenia and/or osteoporosis, which may predispose to fracture development.

Mental symptoms: Mental depression may occur. There may also be irritability and loss of concentration. Neurological symptoms such as paresthesias may also occur.

Libido: Most women experience reduced libido.

Urinary symptoms: These may include dysuria, stress and urge incontinence, and recurrent urinary tract/vaginal infections.

Management of menopause comprises of the following steps:

Counseling: This involves explaining the normal menopause-related changes to the patient, giving her advice related to contraception, and asking her to eat a well-balanced nutritious diet (rich in vitamin A, C, D and E). She must be advised to do weight-bearing exercises, which may help to prevent or delay osteoporosis.

Antidepressants or antianxiety agents: These may be prescribed to relieve the woman of her anxiety and depression.

Hormone replacement therapy: There are three routes of estrogen administration available: (1) oral; (2) transdermal and (3) vaginal. Nonhormonal alternatives, such as black cohosh, soy or isoflavones, red clover, vitamin E, etc., can also be used.

Picture	Medical/Surgical Description	Management/Clinical Highlights

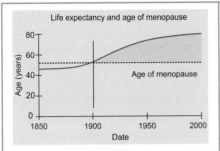

Fig. 9.7.1C: Average age at menopause

Menopause normally occurs between the age of 40 years and 60 years, with the average age being about 51 years. Unlike the average age of menarche, which has progressively increased over the past years, the average age of menopause has remained constant over the past years. At the same time, there is an increase in the average life expectancy. Therefore, while in the past, most women died before attaining menopause, now, with an increase in life expectancy, there has been an increase in number of menopausal women.

Menopause can be defined as the cessation of ovarian function resulting in permanent amenorrhea (lasting for at least 1 year). Climacteric (perimenopause) is the phase of waning ovarian activity, and it may begin 2–3 years before menopause and may continue 2–5 years after it. The onset of menopause involves the women to make physical, sexual and psychological adjustments.

9.7.2: Treatment for Menopausal Symptoms (A to D)

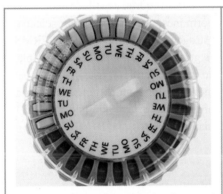

Fig. 9.7.2A: Pills of hormone replacement therapy in a circular dispenser

Hormone replacement therapy refers to a woman taking supplements of hormones such as estrogen alone or estrogen in combination with progesterone (progestin in its synthetic form). HRT can be taken in the form of a pill, patch, gel, vaginal cream or slow-releasing suppository, which can be placed in the vagina. The figure shows pills of HRT in a circular dispenser. HRT pills contain synthetic hormones such as estrogen and progestogen, and these are arranged in the slots of a circular dispenser. The slots are marked by days of the month so that the woman is reminded to take them on a regular basis. The color of pills change depending on the composition of its constituents.

Hormone replacement therapy must be selectively prescribed to women who are at high risk for menopausal abnormalities. Indications for the use of HRT are as follows:

Menopausal and postmenopausal patients: These include symptomatic patients suffering from vasomotor, urinary symptoms or symptoms related to genital atrophy such as dryness, itching, dysuria, dyspareunia, etc.

Individuals at high risk for cardiovascular diseases, osteoporosis, Alzheimer's disease, etc. may also require HRT.

Premature menopause: Women suffering from premature menopause, such as premature ovarian failure, or those who have undergone surgical oophorectomy may require HRT.

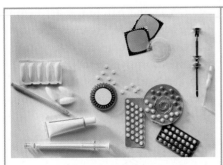

Fig. 9.7.2B: Different types of preparations for hormone replacement therapy

Besides being available in form of pills, HRT is available in various forms such as transdermal patches, gel, vaginal cream or slow-releasing suppositories, which can be placed in the vagina.

Some commonly available HRT preparations are as follows:
- Pills containing conjugated estrogen and progesterone
- Vaginal creams
- Transdermal skin patches

Picture	Medical/Surgical Description	Management/Clinical Highlights
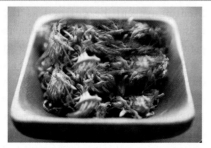 **Fig. 9.7.2C:** Black cohosh, natural remedy for treatment of menopause	Black cohosh is a herb (*Actaea racemosa*), member of buttercup family. This is a perennial plant, which is native to North America. It is commonly prescribed nonhormonal natural preparation for hot flashes and other menopausal symptoms. Commercial preparations of black cohosh are commonly made from its roots and rhizomes. Presently, there is no definite evidence available in literature regarding its efficacy. As of now, the effect of black cohosh is not thought to be any better than that of placebo.	According to the opinion by ACOG (2001), black cohosh must be used for 6 months or less in women with menopausal symptoms. The mode of action of black cohosh is probably related to its estrogenic activity. According to the US pharmacopeia, women using black cohosh must discontinue using it and consult their health care practitioners in case they experience symptoms of liver dysfunction.
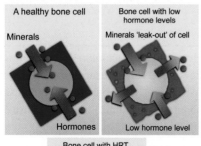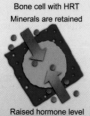 **Fig. 9.7.2D:** Effect of hormone replacement therapy on osteoporosis	Due to lack of estrogen, minerals such as calcium are not retained inside the bone. Due to this, the bone is not able to retain its strength and it wastes away. HRT provides additional hormones, which help in locking the receptors on cell surface and repairing the balance between the minerals absorbed and minerals retained in the blood stream.	Besides the hormonal replacement therapy, medicines, such as bisphosphonates (etidronate, tiludronate, etc.), hormones, such as estrogen, selective estrogen-receptor modulators (SERMS) (e.g. raloxifene), calcitonin, etc. play an important role in osteoporosis treatment. Dietary modifications such as high intake of calcium and vitamin D may also help.

9.7.3: Osteoporosis: Complication of Menopause (A to I)

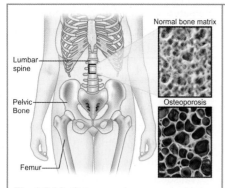 **Fig. 9.7.3A:** Osteoporosis	Osteoporosis is characterized by low bone mass and loss of bone (typically trabecular bone) resulting in weak and fragile bones. As a result, it is associated with an increased risk of fractures in the bones. Some risk factors for development of osteoporosis include female gender, age greater than 65 years, vertebral compression fractures, fragility fractures after the age of 40 years, Caucasian or Asian race, thin or small body frames, family history of osteoporosis, cigarette smoking, excessive alcohol consumption, lack of exercise, diet low in calcium, low estrogen levels, amenorrhea, etc.	In order to reduce the risk of development of osteoporosis later in life, lifestyle modifications such as regular weight-bearing exercises and high intake of vitamin D and calcium must begin during adolescence. Presently, the most effective medications for osteoporosis are antiabsorptive agents, which are FDA approved. Some of these include HRT, bisphosphonates, calcitonin, SERMS, etc.

Picture	Medical/Surgical Description	Management/Clinical Highlights
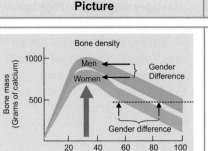 Fig. 9.7.3B: Changes in bone marrow density with age and gender	Peak bone density in women normally occurs at about 25 years of age, following which the bone loss starts to occur. After the age of 35 years, men and women normally lose 0.3–0.5% of their bone density per year as a part of normal ageing process.	Menopause results in falling estrogen levels, which may result in the development of primary osteoporosis. As the regulatory effect of estrogen on bone resorption is lost, it is accelerated and not adequately balanced by compensatory bone formation.
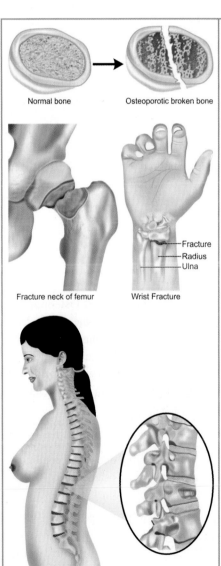 Fig. 9.7.3C: Fractures due to osteoporosis	The fractures most commonly occurring with osteoporosis include compression fractures in vertebral bones, hip, radius, etc. These fractures are responsible for considerable pain, decreased quality of life, loss of work days and disability.	Hormone replacement therapy (combination of estrogen and progestogens) must be prescribed for the prevention of osteoporosis. For prevention and treatment of osteoporosis related fractures, the following therapeutic options are available: • SERMS such as raloxifene (evista) has been approved by the FDA • Bisphosphonates: Bisphosphonates, which are presently available for treatment of osteoporosis include alendronate, risedronate and ibandronate. These drugs reduce the risk of fracture development by suppressing bone resorption by osteoclasts. They however do not reduce osteoblast formation. • New therapeutic agents such as calcitonin, injectable recombinant parathyroid hormone and a monoclonal antibody (denosumab) have also been approved for the treatment of osteoporosis.

Picture	Medical/Surgical Description	Management/Clinical Highlights

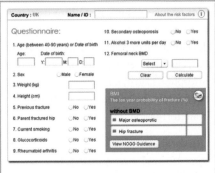

Fig. 9.7.3D: FRAX tool for evaluating fracture risk
Source: (http://www.shef.ac.uk/FRAX/)

The FRAX tool developed by the WHO helps in assessing an individual's 10-year risk for developing fractures. This tool is accessible online. It incorporates 11 risk factors and femoral neck raw bone mineral density (BMD) in g/cm². This helps in calculating the 10-year fracture risk probability. This tool also helps in identifying the patients who may benefit from pharmacotherapy.

FRAX tool gives the 10-year probability of hip fracture development and also a 10-year probability of development of a major osteoporotic fracture (spine, forearm, hip or shoulder)

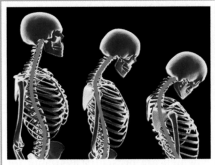

Fig. 9.7.3E: Changes in vertebral column due to osteoporosis

During menopause, there is likely to be deterioration of the bones of vertebral column resulting in a stooped posture or kyphosis. This is also known as dowager's hump. Due to osteoporotic changes in the vertebral bones, they are likely to become weaker and thinner. The intervertebral discs also lose their fluid content, undergo degeneration and become compressed. As a result, the spine loses its normal S-shape and becomes kyphotic.

Management of osteoporosis has been discussed previously in the section.

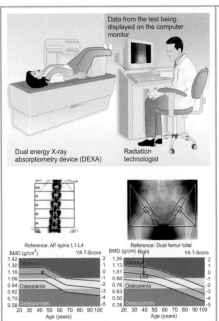

Fig. 9.7.3F: Process of bone densitometry

Using a dual energy X-ray absorptiometry (DEXA) scan, the patient's bone density is compared to the average bone density in young adults of same sex and race. The score is called the T-score and it expresses the bone density in terms of standard deviations (SDs) below the peak young adult bone mass. Osteoporosis can be defined as the bone density score of –2.5 SD or below.

Osteopenia, on the other hand, can be defined as a bone density T-score between –1 and –2.5 SD amongst all women who are aged 65 years or older. Severe osteoporosis is used to describe those patients who have a T-score below –2.5 SD and have suffered a fragility fracture. Normal BMD is defined as a T-score between + 2.5 and –1.0 SD.

According to National Osteoporosis Foundation Guidelines, there are several groups of people who must be considered for DEXA scan. These are as follows:

- All postmenopausal women below the age of 65 years who have risk factors for osteoporosis
- Women aged 65 years and older
- Postmenopausal women with fractures
- Women having one of the conditions associated with osteoporosis

Picture	Medical/Surgical Description	Management/Clinical Highlights
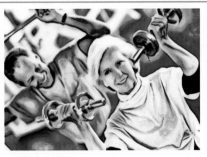 **Fig. 9.7.3G:** Exercises for prevention of osteoporosis (*Source*: Computerized generation of image)	Moderate-level exercises such as brisk walking and lifting of moderate weights has been commonly recommended for prevention for osteoporosis. Quitting smoking and curtailing alcohol consumption also helps in prevention of osteoporosis.	Goal of treatment of osteoporosis is prevention of bone damage by stopping bone loss and increasing bone strength and density. Although early detection and timely treatment of osteoporosis can reduce the risk of fractures in future, none of the treatment options provide complete cure. It is difficult to completely rebuild the bone, which has been weakened by osteoporosis. Therefore prevention of osteoporosis is more important. Exercise does not bring about an increase in bone density, but it helps in improving balance and increasing muscle strength.
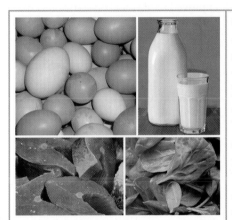 **Fig. 9.7.3H:** Calcium rich diet for prevention of osteoporosis	Once osteoporosis is present, high dietary intake of calcium or calcium supplements is not sufficient for treatment of osteoporosis. However, high intake of calcium in the diet during childhood and adolescence helps in building up strong bones. Moreover, adequate body stores of vitamin D help in ensuring adequate calcium absorption. Vitamin D along with adequate calcium (1,000–1,200 mg of elemental calcium daily) is likely to increase bone density and reduce the risk of fracture development in premenopausal and perimenopausal women. HRT or menopausal hormone therapy also helps in preventing bone loss, increasing bone density and preventing the development of fractures.	For women between 31 years and 50 years of age, recommended dietary intake of calcium is 1,000 mg every day, whereas for those 51 years or older, the recommended intake is 1,200 mg per day. The recommended intake of vitamin D is 600 IU daily for a postmenopausal woman who is not at a high risk for fracture development, whereas that for a postmenopausal woman who is more than 70 years of age or is at an increased risk for osteoporosis, it is 800 IU/day.
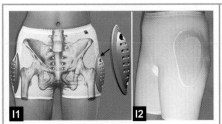 **Figs 9.7.3I (I1 and I2):** Hip protector garments for prevention of osteoporosis	The hip protector garment is an elasticated roll-on girdle with shock absorbing pads, which are placed along the sides of the hip bones. This acts as a valuable tool for prevention of hip fractures amongst individuals who are prone to falls or have significant osteoporosis. These pads help in absorbing the energy related to a fall. However, the effectiveness of these garments in fracture prevention is still a matter of controversy.	FDA has approved use of hip protector garments for prevention of hip fractures in unstable elderly people with osteoporosis. It is available under the brand names of Hipsaver® and Safehip®. The protective effect of these garments is immediate as opposed to that of various pharmacological therapies.

9.8: MÜLLERIAN ABNORMALITIES

9.8.1: Classification of Müllerian Abnormalities

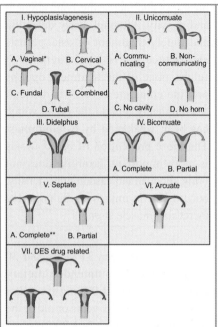

Fig. 9.8.1: Classification of the uterine anomalies by the American Society for Reproductive Medicine (1998)

The most commonly used classification system for categorizing Müllerian duct anomalies is the American Fertility Society classification (1988). This system arranges various Müllerian anomalies on the basis of the major uterine anatomic defect involved. This classification system helps in standardizing various reporting systems. It is based on the clinical classification scheme as proposed by Buttram and Gibbons (1979).

Most of the Müllerian anomalies are corrected surgically, which has been described with each individual anomaly. Surgical correction of various Müllerian anomalies (such as vaginal agenesis and aplasia) have enabled many women to have normal sexual relationships. Development in assisted reproductive technology have also allowed these women to conceive and have normal babies. Surgical treatment of other Müllerian defects (septate uterus/ bicornuate uterus, etc.) has resulted in an improved fertility and obstetric outcome.

9.8.2: Types of Müllerian Anomalies (A to G)

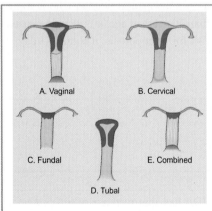

Fig. 9.8.2A: Hypoplasia/agenesis

Vaginal agenesis/hypoplasia is often associated with absence of uterus or in some cases with uterine hypoplasia. Müllerian hypoplasia/aplasia can be either partial or complete. Müllerian aplasia is usually diagnosed when the adolescent girl presents with primary amenorrhea. On physical examination, there is age appropriate development of secondary sexual characteristics. External genitalia appears normal in appearance. Appearance of introitus and vagina can vary depending upon the extent of defect. In complete cases vaginal vault may be completely absent or a short vaginal dimple may be present. A uterus is usually not palpable on per rectal examination. Ultrasound examination shows absence of uterus and fallopian tubes in presence of normal ovaries. MRI is another useful investigation, which helps in confirming the diagnosis.

The aim of treatment is to help create a neovagina. This can be done through surgical or nonsurgical means. Nonsurgical method comprises of using serially graduated dilators for creation of a neovagina. Surgical technique comprises of vaginoplasty: Mc Indoe's vaginoplasty or laparoscopic Vecchietti's procedure.

Picture	Medical/Surgical Description	Management/Clinical Highlights
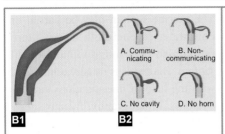 **Figs 9.8.2(B1 and B2):** Unicornuate uterus	This is a congenital anomaly where the uterus is formed from only one Müllerian duct. The other duct does not develop or becomes rudimentary. As a result, there is a hemiuterus with only one fallopian tube. There is a single cervix and a single vagina. Unicornuate uterus may occur alone or along with a rudimentary horn, which may or may not have a uterine cavity with or without functional endometrium. In some cases, a communication may exist with the main endometrial cavity. This can result in complications such as hematometra. Obstetric outcome may be poor in cases of unicornuate uterus.	Hysterosalpingography is able to establish the diagnosis of unicornuate uterus. This is however unable to detect the presence of a noncommunicating horn, if present. MRI and/or high resolution ultrasound is able to reveal this diagnosis. On imaging studies, only one fallopian tube is present. The uterus is normally placed, though the uterine volume is reduced. Accessory horn can be excised at the time of laparoscopic hemihysterectomy. In case of symptomatic hematometra associated with a functioning rudimentary horn, endometrial ablation can be performed through hysteroscopic route.
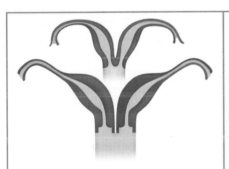 **Fig. 9.8.2C:** Didelphus uterus	Didelphus uterus occurs due to arrest in the midline fusion of Müllerian ducts. This results in the formation of two hemiuterei and two endocervical canals. Each hemiuterus is connected to one fallopian tube. There can be single or double vaginas. There might be a complete or partial longitudinal vaginal septum, which divides the vaginas. The most important presenting complaint is that the use of tampon at the time of menses is unable to completely obstruct the blood flow. There might be a history of second trimester, spontaneous abortions.	Diagnosis is established on the basis of clinical examination, hysterosalpingography, ultrasonography and MRI. No treatment may be required in the asymptomatic cases of didelphus uterus. Treatment may be however required in cases of poor obstetric outcome. Unification of the two hemiuterei is done with help of Strassman's metroplasty. In case of obstruction in one of the hemiuterus, there might be development of hematometra and/or hematosalpinx. In case of obstruction, resection of vaginal septum and removal of hemiuterus and/or tube may be required.
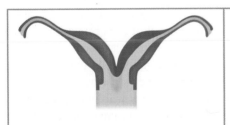 **Fig. 9.8.2D:** Bicornuate uterus	Bicornuate uterus is formed as a result of incomplete fusion of the Müllerian ducts in the region of fundus. The lower uterus and cervix are usually completely fused. As a result, there are two separate, but communicating endometrial cavities and a single chambered cervix and vagina. Women with this anomaly may present with obstetric problems at the time of labor.	Diagnosis is established by hysterosalpingography, ultrasound and MRI. Strassman's metroplasty is a commonly performed procedure for unification of bicornuate uterus (for details related to surgery, kindly refer to Section 12).

Picture	Medical/Surgical Description	Management/Clinical Highlights
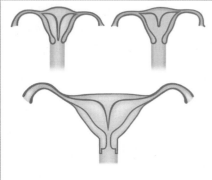 Fig. 9.8.2E: Septate uterus	Septate uterus is one of the most common structural abnormalities amongst the various Müllerian abnormalities. It occurs due to incomplete resorption of the medial septum following the complete fusion of Müllerian ducts. The uterine septum is usually located in the midline in the fundal region.	The uterine septum may be partial or complete. In complete cases, there might also be a longitudinal vaginal septum. Diagnosis is usually established with the help of investigations such as hysterosalpingography, hysteroscopy and laparoscopy. The diagnosis is usually confirmed on laparoscopy, which shows a normal smooth contour of the uterine fundus. MRI and ultrasound are two other useful investigations. Hysteroscopic resection of uterine septum is the most commonly performed strategy.
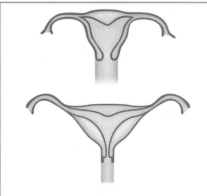 Fig. 9.8.2F: Arcuate uterus	Arcuate uterus occurs due to near complete absorption of the utero-vaginal septum. There may be a small intrauterine indentation (smaller than 1 cm) in the fundal region. This type of uterine anomaly is rarely associated with any adverse obstetric outcome and does not affect the reproductive outcome.	Diagnosis is usually established on hysterosalpingography, which reveals a single uterine cavity with a saddle-shaped fundal indentation. MRI helps in establishing an accurate diagnosis. Treatment is usually not required. In rare cases with poor reproductive outcome, surgical treatment may be required. Surgical treatment is same as that described for septate uterus.
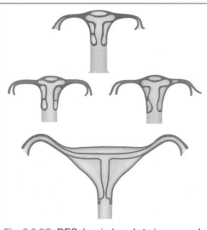 Fig. 9.8.2G: DES drug induced uterine anomaly	Maternal exposure to teratogens such as diethystilbesterol, thalidomide, etc. with a girl child in utero may be associated with Müllerian anomalies such as T-shaped uterus, small hypoplastic uterus, constriction bands, a widened lower uterine segment, a narrowed fundal segment of the endometrial canal, irregular endometrial margins, intraluminal filling defects, etc. in the newborn girl child. Such uterine defects are likely to result in an increased risk of anomalies such as second trimester miscarriages, preterm labor, ectopic pregnancy, cervical incompetence, etc.	Most of these anomalies can be diagnosed using investigations such as HSG, MRI, etc. Presently there is no surgical or medical treatment available for a T-shaped uterus. In order to reduce pregnancy-related complications, close surveillance during early pregnancy associated with frequent clinical and ultrasound examinations is usually sufficient. Proper hormonal support and prophylactic placement of cervical cerclage in the second trimester can be considered. Most patients with a T-shaped uterus who undergo proper surveillance during pregnancy are likely to have an uncomplicated pregnancy and deliver a healthy baby at term. If this does not work, another approach could be to use a gestational carrier along with in vitro fertilization (IVF) treatment.

Picture	Medical/Surgical Description	Management/Clinical Highlights

9.8.3: Vaginal Septum (A and B)

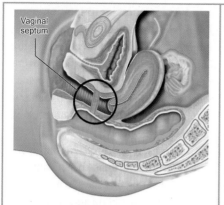

Fig. 9.8.3A: Transverse vaginal septum

Transverse vaginal septum is formed as a result of failure of resorption of tissues between the vaginal plate and caudal aspect of the fused Müllerian ducts. This anomaly causes division of vagina into two segments, thereby reducing its functional length. Incomplete vaginal septum may sometimes result in dyspareunia and obstructed labor. Complete transverse vaginal septum can block the menstrual blood flow, resulting in primary amenorrhea. Accumulation of menstrual debris behind the vaginal septum may result in cryptomenorrhea.

In case of an incomplete vaginal septum, complete surgical excision of the septum may be performed. Ideally, a complete transverse vaginal septum must be incised before menarche to allow for the discharge of menstrual secretions. If there is development of hematometra or hematocolpos, incision and drainage is performed first to relieve obstruction first. Complete excision of the septum is performed after 6–8 weeks, until the tissues have sufficiently healed. Excessive vaginal mucosa must not be removed to prevent shortening of vagina.

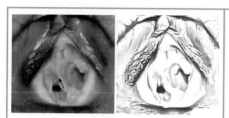

Fig. 9.8.3B: Longitudinal vaginal septum

The longitudinal vaginal septum results due to incomplete fusion of the lower parts of the Müllerian ducts. Presence of a longitudinal vaginal septum results in a double vagina. Sometimes, the defect in fusion may extend toward the upper parts of the Müllerian ducts, resulting in a double cervix and/or uterus didelphys.

The diagnosis of a vaginal septum is usually made on clinical examination. Some patients with a longitudinal vaginal septum may be completely asymptomatic and therefore may not require any treatment. If the longitudinal vaginal septum causes dyspareunia or some other symptom, the vaginal septum can be surgically excised.

9.9: AMENORRHEA

9.9.1: Etiology of Primary Amenorrhea (A to D)

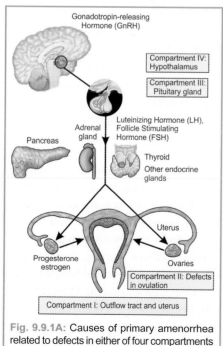

Fig. 9.9.1A: Causes of primary amenorrhea related to defects in either of four compartments

The causes of primary amenorrhea are related to defects in any of the four compartments as described in Figure 9.9.1A. These compartments are:

- *Compartment I*: Defect at the level of outflow tract and the uterus
- *Compartment II*: Defect in ovulation
- *Compartment III*: Defect at the level of pituitary gland
- *Compartment IV*: Defect at the level of hypothalamus and central nervous system

First step in the cases of primary amenorrhea is to determine whether the secondary sexual characteristics are present or not. If the secondary sexual characters are not present, serum gonadotropin levels are determined. If serum gonadotropins are reduced, a diagnosis of hypogonadotropic hypogonadism is made. If serum gonadotropins are raised, a diagnosis of hypergonadotropic hypogonadism is made. Karyotype analysis would reveal premature ovarian failure (46 XX) or Turner's syndrome (45 XO).

If secondary sexual characters are present, pelvic ultrasound is done to see if uterus is present (outflow tract obstruction) or absent (karyotype analysis to differentiate between androgen insensitivity (46 XY) and Müllerian agenesis (46 XX).

Picture	Medical/Surgical Description	Management/Clinical Highlights

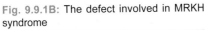

Fig. 9.9.1B: The defect involved in MRKH syndrome

Mayer-Rokitansky-Küster Hauser syndrome may be the probable diagnosis in an individual with primary amenorrhea and no apparent vagina. The syndrome occurs due to defect in fusion of the Müllerian ducts resulting in absence of proximal one-third of vagina with or without the uterus. Since the ovaries are not Müllerian structures, they are normal. Other anomalies including the renal tract anomalies such as ectopic kidney, renal agenesis, horse shoe kidney and abnormal collecting ducts are frequently present.

Treatment of the condition usually involves progressive dilatation using Frank's dilators. By utilizing increasingly larger sized dilators, a functional vagina can be created within a period of several months. Operative treatment (Mc Indoe's vaginoplasty) is used in the patients in whom the Frank's method is unacceptable or fails.

Creating an artificial vagina at the time the patient plans to get married, helps in ensuring that she and her partner would be able to obtain adequate sexual enjoyment following their marriage. Having regular sexual intercourse helps in maintaining the patency of newly created artificial vaginal orifice.

Genetic offsprings can be achieved by collecting oocytes from genetic mother, fertilizing them with sperms obtained from genetic father and their placement in a surrogate carrier.

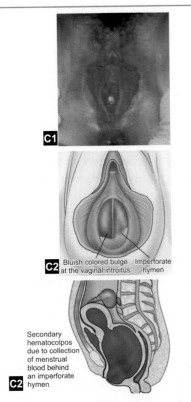

Figs 9.9.1 (C1 to C3): (C1 and C2): Imperforate hymen; (C3) Accumulation of blood in the uterine cavity as a result of imperforate hymen

Imperforate hymen occurs as a result of abnormal or incomplete embryologic development. This condition commonly causes amenorrhea, which is usually associated with cyclical abdominal pain, which tends to worsen over time. If a hematocolpos is present, bluish discoloration is visible behind the translucent membrane.

Prescribing OCPs for suppressing menses can provide symptomatic relief. Use of painkillers such as NSAIDs or narcotic analgesics may be required for providing relief from pain.

An asymptomatic patient having an imperforate hymen without a mucocele during childhood must be treated after the onset of puberty and prior to the development of a hematocolpos or hematometra. In case an adolescent girl presents with hematometra or hematocolpos, the surgical correction (hymenotomy) should be performed as an emergency but with an appropriate preoperative evaluation. The objective of hymenotomy procedure is to open the hymenal membrane in such a way as to form a normally patent vaginal orifice, without scarring. Incision and drainage of the accumulated debris may be also required. During hymenotomy, the hymenal orifice is enlarged by giving either a circular or cruciate incision along the diagonal diameters of hymen.

Picture	Medical/Surgical Description	Management/Clinical Highlights

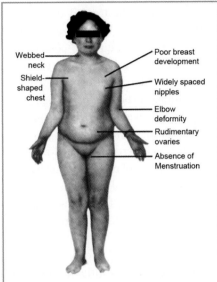

Webbed neck

Shield-shaped chest

Poor breast development

Widely spaced nipples

Elbow deformity

Rudimentary ovaries

Absence of Menstruation

Fig. 9.9.1D: An 18 years old with primary amenorrhea who was diagnosed to be suffering from Turner's syndrome

This is associated with absence of one X chromosome and is characterized by short stature, webbed neck, shield chest, increased carrying angle at the elbow and hypergonadotropic hypoestrogenic amenorrhea. Due to presence of streak gonads, which lack ovarian follicles, no gonadal sex hormones are produced at the time of puberty and the patients present with primary amenorrhea.

The main aims of treatment in the case of a patient with Turner's syndrome are increasing the final height attained and induction of secondary sexual development and menarche. Administration of growth hormone at the age of 4 years or at the time of diagnosis of disorder, (whichever is earlier) may help in increasing the overall height of a child with Turner's syndrome by approximately 8–10 cm (following 3–7 years of treatment).

Estrogen replacement therapy is often started at the time of expected puberty (12 or 13 years) to help trigger the development of secondary sexual characteristics.

Women with Turner's syndrome who wish to become pregnant may consider IVF using a donor egg. Administration of HRT helps in reducing the risk associated with ovarian failure such as osteoporosis and heart failure.

9.9.2: Etiology of Secondary Amenorrhea (A and B)

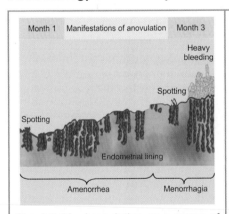

Month 1   Manifestations of anovulation   Month 3

Heavy bleeding

Spotting

Spotting

Endometrial lining

Amenorrhea   Menorrhagia

Fig. 9.9.2A: Anovulation as a cause of amenorrhea

Anovulation is an important cause of secondary amenorrhea. In the absence of ovulation, there is no production of corpus luteum and therefore no progesterone. Due to the absence of progesterone, overgrowth of the endometrium does not occur. Amenorrhea occurs in absence of failed withdrawal. Significant hyperandrogenemia associated with anovulation is another important cause of secondary amenorrhea. Such cases normally give a positive response to the progesterone challenge test.

However, with this unstable, thickened, proliferative phase endometrium, episodic breakdown of the stroma occurs. This kind of endometrial shedding often results in irregular bleeding.

For diagnosis of anovulation as a cause of secondary amenorrhea, the progestational challenge test can be performed by using some progesterone preparation for 3–4 days. Following 2–7 days after cessation of this test, the patient would either bleed or would not bleed.

If the patient bleeds, the diagnosis of anovulation can be established. Presence of bleeding confirms the presence of a functional outflow tract and a uterus, in which endometrium has been prepared by endogenous estrogens.

In cases of anovulation, unopposed exposure of the endometrium to endogenous estrogens in the absence of progesterone can serve as a risk factor for development of endometrial cancer. To prevent this, a progestational agent (for last 15 days of each month) or cyclic OCPs must be prescribed.

Picture	Medical/Surgical Description	Management/Clinical Highlights
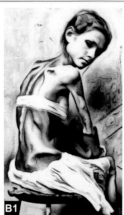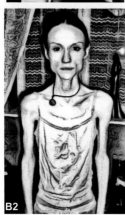 **Figs 9.9.2 (B1 and B2):** Anorexia nervosa as a cause of amenorrhea (*Source*: Computerized generation of images)	Anorexia nervosa is a psychological disorder associated with eating disorders, commonly encountered amongst adolescent women which can sometimes cause secondary amenorrhea. According to American Psychiatric Association (2000), diagnostic criteria for anorexia nervosa are as follows: • The woman is unable to maintain body weight at or above a minimally normal weight for age and height (less than 85% of that expected). • Despite of being extremely underweight, she is extremely fearful of gaining weight or becoming fat. • Women with anorexia tend to show compulsive behaviors, may become obsessed with food, and often show efforts to overly control their food intake and weight. The extreme dieting and weight loss of anorexia can lead to a potentially fatal degree of malnutrition. Besides causing secondary amenorrhea, other possible complications of anorexia include disturbances in heart rate, abnormalities in digestion, loss of bone density, anemia, and hormonal and electrolyte imbalances.	Anorexia may be treated in an outpatient setting, or hospitalization may be sometimes required to correct the malnutrition. A gain of weight between 1 and 3 pounds per week is considered to be a safe and attainable goal. Weight gain may be achieved by devising specific schedules for eating, reducing physical activity, and increasing social activity. Different kinds of psychological therapy such as individual therapy, cognitive behavior therapy, family therapy, etc. have been devised for the treatment of anorexia. While no medications have been identified that can ultimately reduce the urge of starvation in such patients, mood stabilizers such as olanzapine, risperidone, and quetiapine, etc. may prove to be useful. Antidepressants such as SSRI like fluoxetine, sertraline, paroxetine, etc. have also been shown to be helpful.

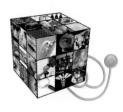

EVIDENCE-BASED BREAKTHROUGH FACTS

1. **ONCOLOGIC AND REPRODUCTIVE OUTCOMES WITH PROGESTIN THERAPY IN WOMEN WITH ATYPICAL ENDOMETRIAL HYPERPLASIA**

Complex atypical endometrial hyperplasia is treated with hysterectomy in most women excepting those desiring future pregnancy. In such women medical treatment with progestins (oral preparations, depot injections, IUD, etc.) have been found to be effective.

Source: Gunderson CC, Fader AN, Carson KA, et al. Oncologic and reproductive outcomes with progestin therapy in women with endometrial hyperplasia and grade 1 adenocarcinoma: a systematic review. Gynecol Oncol. 2012;125:477.

2. **TREATMENT OF PRIMARY DYSMENORRHEA WITH GINGER**

Treatment of primary dysmenorrhea with ginger (500 mg capsules of ginger root powder) for 5 days is able to significantly reduce the intensity and duration of pain.

Source: Rahnama P, Montazeri A, Fallah Huseini H, et al. Effect of Zingiber officinale rhizomes (ginger) on pain relief in primary dysmenorrhea: a placebo randomized trial. BMC Complement Altern Med. 2012;12(1):92.

3. **EFFECTS OF USING HORMONE REPLACEMENT THERAPY**

According to results of the Kronos Early Estrogen Prevention Study (KEEPS), a randomized, double-blind, placebo-controlled clinical trial, use of hormone replacement therapy, containing low-dose oral or transdermal estrogen and cyclic monthly micronized progesterone started soon after the beginning of menopause is likely to cause an improvement in symptoms such as depression, anxiety and cognitive function amongst healthy women. At the same time, use of HRT does not cause an increased risk for cardiovascular disease.

Source: North American Menopause Society (NAMS) 23rd Annual Meeting. Presented October 3, 2012.

The KEEPS preliminary findings presented at NAMS have yet not been peer-reviewed and would be soon submitted for publication in a medical journal.

4. **HOT FLASHES LINKED TO INSULIN RESISTANCE**

According to the data presented at the North American Menopause Society 23rd Annual Meeting, hot flashes and night sweats are likely to be associated with higher serum glucose levels and can be considered as indicators of insulin resistance.

The results of the SWAN study (Study of Women's Health Across the Nation), a large, longitudinal cohort study has indicated that insulin resistance along with the other cardiovascular risk factors such as atherosclerosis, elevated lipids, elevated blood pressure, etc. is likely to be associated with the occurrence of vasomotor symptoms amongst menopausal women. These symptoms may act as a marker of the underlying cardiovascular change amongst women. These results provide a message to the clinician that if a woman in their clinical practice is showing frequent vasomotor symptoms such as hot flashes during the menopause, this might be an indication for the clinician to perform a more intense cardiovascular work-up. Putting these women on HRT is likely to improve their degree of insulin resistance.

Source: North American Menopause Society (NAMS) 23rd Annual Meeting: Abstract S-24. Presented October 5, 2012.

5. GABAPENTIN IMPROVES MENOPAUSAL HOT FLASHES AND INSOMNIA

According to the results of a phase 3 clinical trial known as BREEZE 3, use of extended release gabapentin (*Serada*, Depomed), an investigational nonhormonal drug, is likely to improve sleep and bring about a reduction in hot flashes amongst menopausal women. The drug has yet not gained approval from FDA for use amongst postmenopausal women. Once approved, the drug shall become the first nonhormonal, nonantidepressant treatment for the bothersome symptoms of menopause. Presently FDA has approved use of gabapentin for controlling epileptic seizures and for treatment of restless leg syndrome, and postherpetic neuralgia.

Source: North American Menopause Society (NAMS) 23rd Annual Meeting. Abstract S-8, presented October 5; Abstract S-20, presented October 6, 2012.

6. RELATIONSHIP BETWEEN METABOLIC SYNDROME AND CORONARY EVENTS IN A WOMAN ON HORMONE REPLACEMENT THERAPY

Women receiving HRT who have an underlying metabolic syndrome are likely to be at an increased risk for adverse coronary outcomes. On the other hand, the risk for developing adverse coronary outcomes remains unaffected by the use of HRT amongst women without an underlying metabolic syndrome.

Source: Wild RA, Wu C, Curb JD et al. Women receiving hormone therapy (HT) who have metabolic syndrome (MetS) appear to be at increased risk for adverse coronary outcomes. Menopause. Published online October 25, 2012.

7. EFFECT OF HORMONE REPLACEMENT THERAPY ON CARDIOVASCULAR EVENTS

The results of Women's Health Initiative (WHI) study, 2002 showed that the use of HRT provided no cardiovascular benefits. Moreover, its use may also be associated with an increased the risk of stroke, venous thromboembolism and breast cancer. These conflicting findings have raised speculation regarding the effect of HRT on the woman's cardiovascular risk. Before 2002, prior to the results of this study, use of HRT was characterized as providing significant cardiovascular and skeletal benefits, with minimal or no adverse effects.

However, in contrast to the results of the WHI study (2002), results of the randomized controlled trial (published in the BMJ, 2012) has shown that continued use of HRT amongst the menopausal women for a period of 10 years has been found to be associated with a significant reduction in the risk of myocardial infarction (MI), heart failure, or death with no increased risk of cancer, venous thromboembolism, or stroke.

According to the authors of this study, long-term use of HRT, when started soon after menopause for a prolonged duration of time, does not increase the risk of adverse cardiovascular events. Moreover, in this study, synthetic 17-beta-estradiol was used, while in the WHI study, conjugated equine estrogens were used. This difference in medication, along with variations in patient characteristics, probably was the cause of disparity in the results between this study and the WHI study.

Source: Rossouw JE, Anderson GL, Prentice RL, et al. Risks and benefits of estrogen plus progestin in healthy postmenopausal women: principal results from the Women's Health Initiative randomized controlled trial. JAMA. 2002;288:321-33.

Schierbeck LL, Rejnmark L, Tofteng CL, et al. Effect of hormone replacement therapy on cardiovascular events in recently postmenopausal women: randomised trial. BMJ. 2012;345:e6409.

8. THE FIGO RECOMMENDATIONS ON TERMINOLOGIES AND DEFINITIONS FOR NORMAL AND ABNORMAL UTERINE BLEEDING

Over the past 5 years there has been a major international discussion aimed at reaching agreement on the use of well-defined terminologies to describe the normal limits and range of abnormalities related to patterns of uterine bleeding. One of the main goals of this discussion aimed at discarding the use of long-used, ill-defined and confusing English-language terms of Latin and Greek origin, such as menorrhagia and metrorrhagia, and the term dysfunctional uterine bleeding. The recommendations presented here are the result of an extensive discussion and testing process but should still be regarded as a flexible living document, scheduled for future review through the International Federation of Gynecology and Obstetrics (FIGO) Menstrual Disorders Working Group and sessions at FIGO World Congresses.

Normal menstrual cycle is characterized by normal blood loss occurring at regular intervals and having a normal duration of blood flow.

The abnormalities of blood flow can be classified as follows:

- *Prolonged bleeding*: Greater than or equal to 10 days of bleeding in one episode
- *Frequent bleeding:* Greater than four episodes of bleeding in one 90-day reference period
- *Infrequent bleeding:* Less than two episodes in one 90-day reference period
- *Irregular bleeding*: A range of varying lengths of bleeding free intervals greater than 17 days in one 90-day reference period.
- *Absent Menstrual Bleeding (Amenorrhea)***:** No bleeding in a 90-day period
- *Heavy Menstrual Bleeding (HMB)***:** Most common clinical presentation of AUB, HMB can be defined as excessive menstrual blood loss which interferes with the woman's physical, emotional, social and marital quality of life, and which can occur alone or in combination with other symptoms. Since it is difficult to assess the heaviness of flow with any degree of accuracy in routine clinical practice it was decided the only distinction that could usually be made was between "bleeding" and "spotting", based on whether any sanitary protection is required or not.
- *Heavy and Prolonged Menstrual Bleeding (HPMB)*: This complaint is much less common than HMB on its own. The distinction from HMB is worth making because these two symptomatic components may have different etiologies and may respond differently to therapies.
- *Shortened Menstrual Bleeding*: A very uncommon complaint and is defined as menstrual bleeding, no longer than 2 days in duration. The bleeding is also usually light in volume and is uncommonly associated with serious pathology (such as intrauterine adhesions and endometrial tuberculosis).
- *Irregular Nonmenstrual Bleeding*: Nonmenstrual bleeding is common and usually consists of an occasional episode of intermenstrual or postcoital bleeding associated with minor surface lesions of the genital tract, but such bleeding may herald more serious lesions such as cervical or endometrial cancer. Intermenstrual bleeding is defined as irregular episodes of bleeding, often light and short, occurring between otherwise fairly normal menstrual periods.
- *Bleeding Outside Reproductive Age:* Postmenopausal bleeding (PMB) is common and usually defined as bleeding occurring more than 1 year after the acknowledged menopause.
- *Acute or Chronic Abnormal Uterine Bleeding*: It is proposed that acute AUB is "an episode of bleeding in a woman of reproductive age, who is not pregnant and is of sufficient quantity to require immediate intervention to prevent further blood loss". Chronic AUB is "bleeding from the uterine corpus that is abnormal in duration, volume and/or frequency and has been present for the majority of the last 6 months".

Source: Fraser IS, Critchley HO, Broder M, et al. The FIGO recommendations on terminologies and definitions for normal and abnormal uterine bleeding. Semin Reprod Med. 2011;29(5):383-90.

9. **NEW SYSTEM FOR CLASSIFICATION OF CAUSES OF ABNORMAL UTERINE BLEEDING**

There has been general inconsistency in the nomenclature used for describing AUB in the women of reproductive age group women and there is a plethora of potential causes. The FIGO have approved a new classification system (PALM-COEIN) for causes of AUB in nongravid women of reproductive age. Of the nine categories in the new FIGO classification system (PALM-COEIN), the first four are defined as visually objective structural criteria (PALM: polyp, adenomyosis, leiomyoma, and malignancy and hyperplasia), the pathologies that can be measured visually with imaging techniques, such as sonography and/or histopathology testing. The next four are unrelated to structural abnormalities (COEI: coagulopathy, ovulatory dysfunction, endometrial and iatrogenic), which are the nonstructural entities that are not defined on imaging or histopathology testing. The "iatrogenic" category refers to AUB associated with the use of exogenous gonadal steroids, intrauterine systems or devices, or other systemic or local agents.

The final category stands for the entities that are not yet classified (N). This classification system for the causes of AUB is likely to facilitate clinical care and treatment of such patients. The FIGO classification can be presently regarded as a flexible "living" document, which should undergo review and consideration for modification at regular interval, probably at 3-year intervals, during each FIGO World Congress.

Source: Munro MG, Critchley HOD, Broder MS, et al. FIGO classification system (PALM-COEIN) for causes of abnormal uterine bleeding in nongravid women of reproductive age. Int J Gynaecol Obstet. 2002;113(1):3-13.

Gynecology

Section 10

Benign Tumors of Genital Tract

SECTION OUTLINE

10.1: FIBROIDS

10.1.1: Definition (A and B)

Picture	Medical/Surgical Description	Management/Clinical Highlights
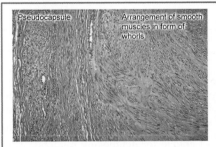 **Fig. 10.1.1A:** Macroscopic appearance of a leiomyoma	Myomas (fibromyomas, leiomyomas or fibroids) are well-circumscribed benign tumors developing from uterine myometrium, most commonly encountered amongst women of reproductive age group (30–45 years), with their prevalence ranging between 20% and 40%.	A typical myoma appears as a pale, firm, rubbery, well-circumscribed mass, which stands out distinctly from the neighboring tissues. Presence of a well-defined outer capsule helps in differentiating it from a malignancy.
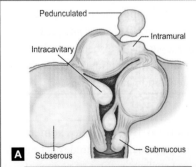 **Fig. 10.1.1B:** Histological appearance of a fibroid	This well-circumscribed mass shows a whorled appearance on histopathological examination due to presence of interlacing fibers of smooth myometrial muscle, separated by varying amount of connective tissue fibers. This type of histopathological arrangement also demonstrates its benign nature.	The fibroid is surrounded by a connective tissue capsule, which helps in fixing the tumor to the myometrium. This connective tissue capsule helps in forming a plane of cleavage along which the tumor can be easily enucleated at the time of surgery. The vessels supplying blood to the tumor lie in the capsule and send radial branches into the tumor. As a result, the central portion of the fibroid receives the least blood supply and is the first to undergo degeneration.

10.1.2: Types of Fibroids (A to C)

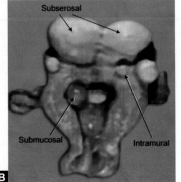 **Figs 10.1.2(A and B):** Different types of leiomyomas	Based on their location inside the uterus, the fibroids can be broadly classified into three types: submucosal, intramural and subserosal. Of the different types of fibroids, the commonest are intramural (interstitial) fibroids, which are present in nearly 75% cases, followed by submucous (15%) and subserous fibroids (10%).	Also known as subendometrial fibroids, the submucosal fibroids grow directly beneath the uterine endometrium. This type of fibroid is thought to be primarily responsible for producing prolonged, heavy menstrual bleeding. Intramural (interstitial) fibroids are the commonest type and are located in the middle of myometrium. Subserosal fibroids are also known as the pedunculated fibroids. These fibroids grow beneath the serosa, the outer uterine covering and are the least common subtype.

Picture	Medical/Surgical Description	Management/Clinical Highlights
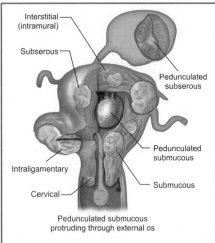 **Fig. 10.1.2C:** Different locations at which fibroids may be present	Though most leiomymas are situated in the body of the uterus, they may be also present at other locations. These include the cervix and broad ligament. Fibroids may be confined to the cervix, specially the supravaginal portion of the cervix in nearly 1–2% cases or they may be sometimes present within the folds of broad ligament.	The fibroids present at extrauterine locations also retain the characteristic histopathological pattern of those present at the uterine locations. The treatment modalities for the fibroids present at the uterine locations are same as those present at extrauterine locations.

10.1.3: Diagnosis of Fibroids Using Ultrasound (A to E)

Picture	Medical/Surgical Description	Management/Clinical Highlights
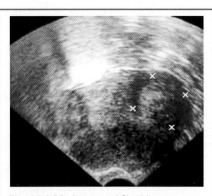 **Fig. 10.1.3A:** Intramural fibroid	In this patient, transvaginal ultrasound examination reveals a well-defined hyperechoic area surrounded by an anechoic capsule located within the myometrium. Ultrasound examination can help in assessing the size, location and number of uterine fibroids. Preoperative finding on sonography can guide the gynecologist while performing surgery, hysteroscopy, laparoscopy, etc.	Nowadays, ultrasound examination (both transvaginal and transabdominal ultrasound) has become the investigation of choice for diagnosing myomas. The advantages of ultrasound imaging include good patient tolerance, noninvasive nature of the investigation, relatively low cost, easy availability and high accuracy rates. Ultrasound examination helps in assessing the overall uterine shape, size and contour; endometrial thickness; adnexal areas and presence of hydronephrosis. It also helps in detection of small, focal, irregular or eccentrically located endometrial lesions.
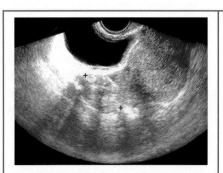 **Fig. 10.1.3B:** Pedunculated fibroid having a diameter of 3.74 cm	Transvaginal ultrasound shows a well-defined mass measuring about 3.74 cm in diameter. The mass is located separately from the uterine fundus and is connected with help of a pedicle.	Subserosal fibroids may sometimes develop a pedicle and extrude out from the serosal surface in form of pedunculated fibroids. Both submucous and subserosal fibroids can be pedunculated. Long pedunculated fibroids may sometimes undergo torsion. The pedunculated subserosal fibroid is best managed through laparoscopic myomectomy.

Picture	Medical/Surgical Description	Management/Clinical Highlights
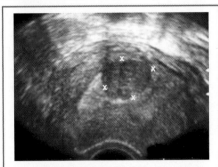 **Fig. 10.1.3C:** Submucous fibroid protruding inside the endometrial cavity	Transvaginal ultrasound in this patient shows a submucous fibroid protruding inside the endometrial cavity. The characteristic symptom of a submucosal leiomymas is menorrhagia. The duration of menstrual period may be normal or prolonged and the blood loss is usually heaviest on 2nd and 3rd day. The nearer the leiomyomas are to the endometrial cavity, the more likely are they to produce menorrhagia.	It may be sometimes very difficult to differentiate between submucous myomas and endometrial polyps on ultrasound examination. In these cases, other investigations such as saline infusion sonography (SIS) and hysteroscopy may help in arriving at the correct diagnosis. Hysteroscopic myomectomy appears to be the best treatment option in these cases.
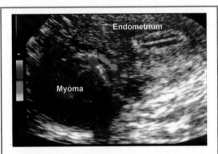 **Fig. 10.1.3D:** Color Doppler shows presence of subserosal fibroids with peripheral vascularization	As previously discussed, the vessels supplying blood to the tumor lie within the capsule and send radial branches into the tumor. This peripheral vascularization can be visualized with the help of color Doppler ultrasound. This pattern of peripheral vascularization helps in differentiating if from a malignancy where low resistance vascularization pattern may be centrally present.	The myoma is subserosal in location and is located far from the endometrial cavity. Laparoscopic myomectomy appears to be the best treatment option in this case.
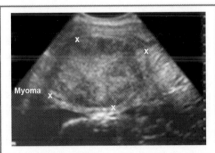 **Fig. 10.1.3E:** Presence of well-circumscribed lesion with homogeneous consistency, which was diagnosed as an intramural fibroid	Fibroids can be single or multiple and may range in size from that of a small seedling to that of bulky masses which can distort and enlarge the uterus. Transvaginal sonography in the adjacent Figure demonstrates presence of a well-circumscribed mass within the uterine myometrium having homogeneous consistency. There was no distortion of uterine cavity or uterine enlargement.	Small fibroids often remain undiagnosed as they rarely produce any symptoms. In this case, initially the myoma was asymptomatic and left as it is. One year later, the woman herself opted for abdominal hysterectomy because she had completed her family and was extremely distressed with the menorrhagia due to fibroids.

10.1.4: Saline Infusion Sonography for Diagnosis of Fibroids (A to D)

Picture		
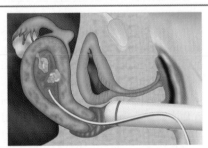 **Fig. 10.1.4A:** Procedure of doing saline infusion sonography	To perform SIS, a small catheter is threaded through internal os into the endometrial cavity. Through this catheter, sterile saline is infused and the uterine cavity distended.	Saline infusion sonography has been demonstrated to cause improved evaluation of the endometrial cavity and assessment of tubal patency. SIS also helps in detection of endometrial pathology such as uterine synechiae, endometrial polyps and submucous leiomyomas.

Picture	Medical/Surgical Description	Management/Clinical Highlights
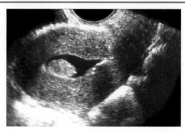**Fig. 10.1.4B:** Saline infusion sonography demonstrating a uterine polyp	Though transvaginal ultrasonography is associated with higher resolution in comparison to transabdominal sonography, it may not always be useful in distinguishing between a submucosal fibroid, endometrial polyp and adenomyosis. A newer technique, called saline infusion sonography or sonohysterography, uses saline infusion into the endometrial cavity to enhance the detection of submucosal fibroids and polyps.	Distension of the uterine cavity with saline revealed a solitary endometrial polyp. This was removed hysteroscopically and sent for biopsy, which revealed a benign growth pattern.
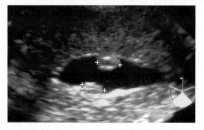**Fig. 10.1.4C:** Multiple submucosal myomas on SIS	Transvaginal ultrasound in this 35-years-old patient showed increased endometrial thickness and suggested presence of a mass. However, no definitive diagnosis could be reached. In this patient, infusion of saline inside the endometrial cavity caused uterine distension, thereby illustrating numerous submucosal myomas.	Hysteroscopic resection was considered as the surgical option of choice because the patient had not completed her family and she wanted to retain her fertility. Moreover, the number of fibroids was countable and were of sufficient size so as to allow their hysteroscopic removal
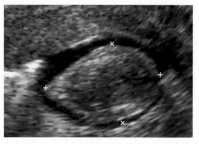**Fig. 10.1.4D:** Visualization of intracavitary fibroid on saline infusion sonography	Transvaginal sonography in this patient was not able to establish any definitive diagnosis. It just demonstrated increased endometrial thickness. Distension of the uterine cavity with saline in this case illustrated a well-defined submucosal fibroid almost completely filling the uterine cavity.	In this 38-years-old patient, the submucosal myoma was causing significant menorrhagia. Hysteroscopic myomectomy was an available option. However, this option was not used because the patient opted for abdominal hysterectomy. The patient's menorrhagia was really troublesome and she wanted to completely get rid of her periods.

10.1.5: Magnetic Resonance Imaging for Diagnosis of Fibroids (A and B)

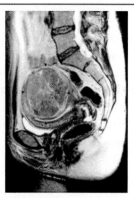**Fig. 10.1.5A:** T1-weighted magnetic resonance image showing an intramural fibroid of size 8 cm	Presently, the ultrasound examination forms the most commonly used investigation modality for initial evaluation. Though magnetic resonance imaging (MRI) is an investigation which helps in accurately establishing the definitive diagnosis of myomas, the high cost associated with its use, prevents its widespread use in clinical practice.	Magnetic resonance imaging was performed in this case because the diagnosis was not clear on ultrasound examination. In this case no definitive diagnosis could be established on transvaginal ultrasound. The likely differential diagnoses in this case were adenomyosis, fibroid uterus and endometrial cancer. MRI established the diagnosis of intramural fibroid.

Picture	Medical/Surgical Description	Management/Clinical Highlights

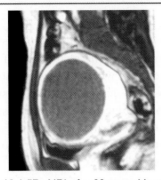

Fig. 10.1.5B: MRI of a 33-year-old woman with large submucosal fibroid. Enhanced T1-weighted magnetic resonance image obtained 4 months after uterine artery embolization show that uterine fibroid decreased to 8 cm in maximum diameter (46% tumor volume reduction) and was not enhancing. Muscular layer of the uterus is enhanced

Though the use of MRI is not routinely recommended, it is useful for mapping the size and location of leiomyomas and in accurately identifying adenomyosis if present. Other pelvic pathology such as ovarian neoplasms can also be identified on MRI.

Though MRI gives images with better resolution, due to its high cost, MRI is usually reserved for only special cases.

Magnetic resonance images are able to clearly delineate the myometrium, junctional zone and endometrium, allowing highly accurate mapping of the size, location and degree of myometrial involvement of uterine leiomyomas. This was very much required in this case because the patient with a large submucosal fibroid about 18 cm in diameter was being treated with uterine artery embolization (UAE). Proper delineation of myometrium, junctional zone and endometrium was essential in this case in order to evaluate tumor regression as a result of UAE.

10.1.6: Hysteroscopy for Diagnosis of Fibroids

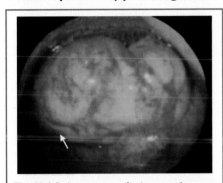

Fig. 10.1.6: Appearance of submucosal myoma on hysteroscopy (indicated by arrow)

Hysteroscope is an instrument which can be inserted inside the uterus through the vaginal orifice. For details regarding the use of hysteroscope, kindly refer to Section 12. Hysteroscopic examination helps in the assessment of endometrial cavity and endometrium.

Hysteroscopic examination helps in diagnosing endometrial masses such as submucosal fibroids and endometrial polyps. In case of suspicion of malignancy, hysteroscopic directed biopsy can be taken to establish the diagnosis. Hysteroscopic myomectomy can also be performed for surgical removal of myoma.

10.1.7: Treatment Option for Symptomatic Fibroids

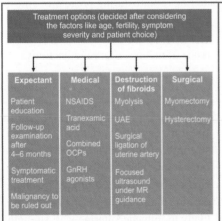

Fig. 10.1.7: Treatment options for a patient diagnosed with fibroid uterus

The following treatment options can be used in the women with fibroids:

Conservative management: Most women with uterine fibroids who are asymptomatic do not require any treatment.

Medical therapy: Though the use of medicines does not help in curing leiomyomas, this may be sometimes used for alleviation of symptoms, improvement of hemoglobin status before surgery, emergency suppression of heavy bleeding, etc.

Surgical therapy: Surgery forms the definite treatment modality for uterine leiomyomas.

The three main surgical options, which can be used in the women with leiomyoma uterus include: myomectomy, hysterectomy and more recently UAE. Hysterectomy, a major surgical operation involving the removal of the woman's uterus helps in providing definitive cure for uterine leiomyomas. Hysterectomy can be performed abdominally, vaginally or through laparoscopic route. Surgical removal of myomas from the uterine cavity is termed as myomectomy and can be performed through hysteroscopic, laparoscopic or abdominal routes. Performing a UAE or myomectomy would potentially allow the women to retain their fertility.

Picture	Medical/Surgical Description	Management/Clinical Highlights

10.1.8: Laparoscopic Myomectomy (A to H)

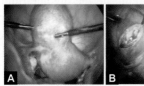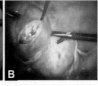

Figs 10.1.8 (A and B): (A) Presence of a subserous fibroid, which is handled laparoscopically; (B) An incision given over the surface of fibroid

The steps for removal of a subserosal myoma are shown in Figures 10.1.8 (A to H). Two or three small, half-inch incisions are made above the pubic hairline and the laparoscopic instruments are passed through these small incisions to perform the surgery. After reaching the uterus, the subserosal fibroid is grasped and freed from its attachments to the normal uterine muscle.

Since in this case, the fibroid was embedded deep in the uterine wall, an incision was given over the surface of the fibroid.

Fibroids can also be removed by laparoscopy. The challenges of this surgery rest with the surgeon's ability to remove the mass through a small abdominal incision and to reconstruct the uterus. Laparoscopic myomectomy is most commonly used for removing subserosal fibroids.

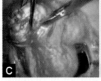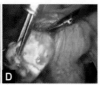

Figs 10.1.8 (C and D): (C) The myoma is gradually shelled out from the underlying myometrium; (D) The myoma has been shelled out completely

After giving an incision over the surface of fibroid, it is gradually shelled out from the uterine musculature. A myoma screw can be used for separating fibroid from the uterine musculature.

Advantages of laparoscopic myomectomy are as follows:
- It is a less invasive procedure, thereby resulting in fewer operative and post-operative complications.
- Surgical morbidity is reduced, resulting in improved postsurgical outcomes.
- There is significantly reduced hospital stay and quick recovery because the procedure may be performed as an outpatient surgery.

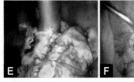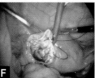

Figs 10.1.8 (E and F): The large fibroid is morcellated and removed from the body; (F) Following the removal of myoma the small raw area left after removal is stitched with Vicryl sutures

After the myoma has been completely freed from the uterine myometrium, it is removed using a morcellator. The uterine wall is repaired using laparoscopically applied sutures. Laparoscopic suturing with small instruments requires considerable amount of surgeon skill, experience and judgment.

Complications of laparoscopic myomectomy are as follows: development of uterine rupture during pregnancy (most commonly third trimester); development of postoperative adhesions and recurrence of myoma after myomectomy.

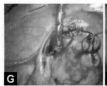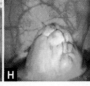

Figs 10.1.8 (G and H): (G) The closure of uterine myometrium is almost complete; (H) The myometrial suture line following the completion of surgery

The uterine incision is completely repaired. The most important complication following myomectomy is the development of adhesions postoperatively. Development of these postoperative adhesions can impair the woman's fertility, resulting in further problems in women desiring future fertility. Development of adhesions postoperatively is less commonly associated with laparoscopic myomectomy in comparison to abdominal myomectomy.

If future fertility is desired, then the strength of the uterine wall repair is important. Thus, before undertaking laparoscopic myomectomy in a woman desiring future fertility, factors which are likely to influence uterine wall strength following repair, need to be taken into consideration. These include size of fibroid and closeness of the myoma to the endometrial cavity.

| Picture | Medical/Surgical Description | Management/Clinical Highlights |

10.1.9: Hysteroscopic Myomectomy (A and B)

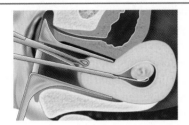

Fig. 10.1.9A: Diagram showing hysteroscopic fibroid resection

Hysteroscopic myomectomy forms the procedure of choice for the removal of completely submucosal myomas or those myomas having less than 50% extension into the myometrium.

Hysteroscopic myomectomy can be performed as a simple outpatient procedure where a hysteroscope is placed inside the uterine cavity and the leiomyomas are resected out.

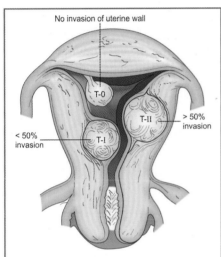

Fig. 10.1.9B: European Society of Hysteroscopy classification of myomas

According to the European Society of Hysteroscopy, submucous leiomyomas have been classified into three categories depending on their degree of myometrial invasion. T-0 corresponds to pedunculated submucous leiomyomas. T-I represents submucous leiomyomas with less than 50% invasion into the myometrial wall and T-II are those with greater than 50% invasion.

Removal of myomas belonging to the categories T-0 and T-1 should be attempted using a hysteroscope.

However, hysteroscopic resection should not normally be attempted in fibromyomas belonging to T-II category because when submucous myomas have intramural extensions greater than 50%, hysteroscopic resection may be associated with a higher rate of complications. These include increased rate of conversion to laparotomy, higher rates of intravascular extravasation of distending media, prolonged operating times and increased requirement for repeat surgery.

10.1.10: Procedure of Hysteroscopic Myomectomy (A to J)

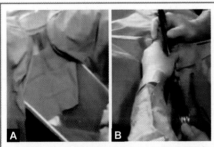

Figs 10.1.10 (A and B): (A) Aseptic preparation of vagina before the introduction of hysteroscope; (B) Introduction of Sim's speculum to retract the posterior vaginal wall.

The steps of hysteroscopic myomectomy have been illustrated in Figures 10.1.10 (A to J). After taking all aseptic precautions, the vulva, vagina, adjacent areas and medial aspect of the thighs must be cleaned with antiseptic solution. Surgical drapes must then be applied. In order to expose the external os, Sim's speculum is applied to retract the posterior vaginal wall. At the same time anterior lip of cervix is grasped with tenaculum forceps.

Asepsis aims at making the operative field free of all pathological organisms, especially the infectious agents before starting the surgery. Besides the step for aseptic preparation of vagina shown in Figure 10.1.10A, another step for asepsis is as follows: all personnel coming in contact with the surgical field must have performed surgical hand scrub with an antiseptic solution and put on sterile surgical cap, gown, mask and gloves.

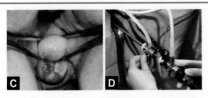

Figs 10.1.10 (C and D): (C) Holding the anterior lip of cervix with tenaculum forceps; (D) Introduction of hysteroscope

Following the exposure of external cervical os, through the use of Sim's speculum and tenaculum, the hysteroscope needs to be inserted. Prior to insertion of hysteroscope, fluid is instilled inside the uterine cavity.

Since the use of hysteroscope requires instillation of fluid inside the uterine cavity, it is important to monitor ongoing fluid balance carefully during hysteroscopic removal of fibroids in order to prevent the fluid overload.

Picture	Medical/Surgical Description	Management/Clinical Highlights
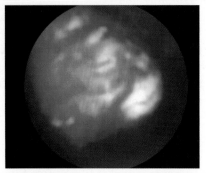 **Fig. 10.1.10E:** Hysteroscopic view of the uterus showing submucous leiomyoma	This figure shows diagnosis of a submucosal fibroid using hysteroscopy. The size of the fibroid and other characteristic features can be visualized.	Hysteroscopic examination of the uterine cavity enables diagnosis of submucosal myomas. Hysteroscopy can also be used for resection of submucous myomas. Hysteroscopic myomectomy enables the woman to retain her fertility, thereby it is preferred in women belonging to reproductive age groups.
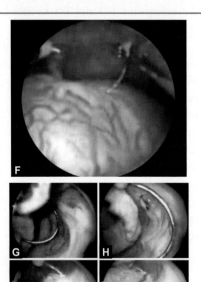 **Figs 10.1.10 (F to J):** (F to I) Progressive resection of successive layers of myomas; (J) Appearance of the uterine endometrium after the resection of uterine myoma is almost complete	The submucosal myoma is progressively resected out in layers using a resectoscope. Sometimes, it may not be possible to perform a complete resection when the tumor invades deeply into the uterine myometrium. All the tissue resected out must be submitted for a histopathological examination.	Resection is carried out with a hysteroresectoscope with a 12° angle lens and a matching electrode.

10.1.11: Abdominal Myomectomy

Picture	Medical/Surgical Description	Management/Clinical Highlights
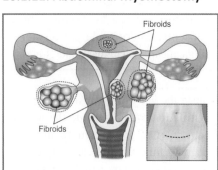 **Fig. 10.1.11:** Abdominal myomectomy	Abdominal myomectomy involves removal of fibroids through an abdominal incision (Pfannenstiel incision is most commonly used). The procedure of abdominal myomectomy has been explained in Figures 10.1.12 (A to I). This procedure enables the surgeon to remove numerous fibroids with varied sizes, present at different locations.	The advantage of abdominal myomectomy is that large fibroids can be quickly removed. The surgeon is able to feel the uterus, which is helpful in locating myomas that may be deep in the uterine wall or are very small in size. The disadvantage of a laparotomy is that it requires an abdominal incision.

Picture	Medical/Surgical Description	Management/Clinical Highlights

10.1.12: Procedure of Abdominal Myomectomy (A to I)

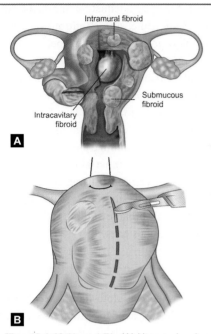

A

B

Figs 10.1.12 (A and B): (A) Uterus showing presence of multiple myomas; (B) A vertical uterine incision given over the anterior surface of the uterus, avoiding a posterior incision wherever possible

Technique of abdominal myomectomy has been explained in Figures 10.1.12 (A to I). Type of abdominal incision to be given at the time of surgery must be decided only after taking into account the size, location and the number of the myomas. Adequate exposure can be usually achieved through a Pfannenstiel incision. After the abdomen has adequately been exposed and the uterus is visualized, the surgeon must plan the uterine incision. This decision is based on the number and location of the myomas. The most preferred incision is a vertical incision on the anterior surface of uterus. The surgeon often can remove multiple myomas from a single incision, whereas at other times, multiple incisions may be required.

A mild Trendelenburg position at the time of surgery helps in ensuring adequate exposure. Planning the appropriate abdominal incision for achieving adequate surgical exposure is of vital importance. In case of small myomas, a transverse Pfannenstiel incision is usually sufficient. However, if more space is required, a modification of the transverse incision, i.e. either a Cherney's or Maylard's incision can be performed. Sometimes a vertical midline incision can also be given if larger space at the time of surgery is required. The operative field must be kept moist and clot-free using a solution of lactated ringer containing heparin. Vertical incision over the anterior surface of uterus helps in minimizing blood loss and preventing the development of adhesions of the ovaries to the posterior uterine walls postoperatively.

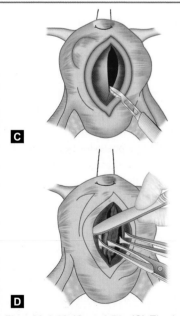

C

D

Figs 10.1.12 (C and D): (C) The incision extended through the pseudocapsule to expose the myoma; (D) The plane of cleavage being developed between the myoma and the myometrium with the help of blunt and sharp dissection

The general strategy employed for removing a myoma involves giving a linear or an elliptical incision through the pseudocapsule of the largest myoma. The myoma is then grasped with a double toothed tenaculum. As the tissue planes are exposed, blunt and sharp dissection is used to enucleate the myoma out of the capsule.

If the dissection can be carried out between the myoma and the pseudocapsule, blood loss can be minimized. As the myoma is completely excised out of the uterine myometrium, an oozing cavitary defect is left in the uterus.

Picture	Medical/Surgical Description	Management/Clinical Highlights

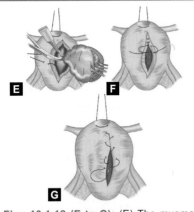

Figs 10.1.12 (E to G): (E) The myoma is enucleated and delivered outside the uterus; (F) The uterine myometrium is being approximated using layered interrupted delayed-absorbable sutures; (G) The uterine serosa is sutured in a running "baseball" fashion

As many myomas as possible are resected out through this incision, following which the uterine defect is closed. Method of closing the resultant uterine defect varies from individual to individual.

Layered interrupted sutures are time consuming but provide the best prospects for tissue coaptation. After the myometrial layers have been adequately reapproximated, excess serosa may be trimmed and the serosal defect repaired with a fine polyglycolic suture in a running "baseball" fashion.

The main aim is to restore normal anatomy and to ensure adequate hemostasis. At the same time, due attention must be paid toward minimizing the dead space. Despite meticulous attempts to reduce the development of uterine defects, many a times, some areas may remain open and fill up with blood. These pockets of blood may serve as the medium for infection. To minimize the development of dead space, most surgeons prefer to close myoma bed using interrupted figure-of-eight sutures or mattress 2-0 delayed absorbable sutures rather than the continuous ones.

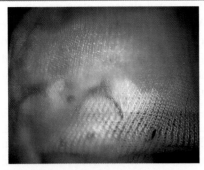

Fig. 10.1.12 H: Use of Interceed® adhesion barrier over the surface of uterine incision in order to prevent the development of adhesions

Following the end of the repair process, an absorbable barrier, such as Interceed® (oxidized regenerated cellulose), can be placed over the uterine corpus to protect the tubes and ovaries from denuded peritoneal surfaces and uterine incision. This technique helps in minimizing the development of uterine adhesions.

Small sheets of cloth-like material can be wrapped around the raw areas created due to surgery and this material prevents nearby tissue from adhering to the site of surgery. After a few weeks, the material dissolves, leaving the newly healed surgery sites fairly free of adhesions. While the use of these barriers may not be completely perfect, they have been shown to help reduce the formation of adhesions.

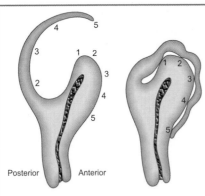

Fig. 10.1.12 I: Bonney's hood approach

In the Bonney's approach, a method for approaching the posterior myoma, an elliptical incision is made transversely across the posterior fundal region, taking care to avoid the interstitial portion of the fallopian tube. After the primary tumor is removed, other leiomyomata can also be removed through the same incision. Excessive myometrium needs to be trimmed away. Interrupted sutures in layers are then used to obliterate the dead space, approximate the myometrium and accomplish satisfactory hemostasis. The posterior flap of myometrium is draped over the fundus and fixed to the anterior surface of the uterus with the help of fine sutures. This is known as the Bonney's hood.

This method helps in creating a functional anterior incision, at the same time avoiding a posterior defect and the various complications, which may be associated with it.

Picture	Medical/Surgical Description	Management/Clinical Highlights

10.1.13: Hysterectomy

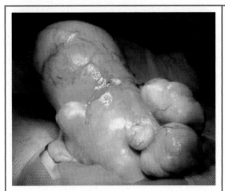

Fig. 10.1.13: Hysterectomy specimen showing presence of multiple subserosal fibroids

A 48-year-old perimenopausal patient presented to the gynecology clinic with the complaints of menorrhagia and severe abdominal pain during periods. Ultrasound examination revealed the presence of multiple large interstitial and subserosal fibroids.

In view of multiple fibroids, patient's age and the fact that she had completed her family, an abdominal hysterectomy was performed. Figure 10.1.13 shows the hysterectomy specimen, showing multiple subserosal fibroids, obtained after the surgery.

10.1.14: Uterine Artery Embolization (A to E)

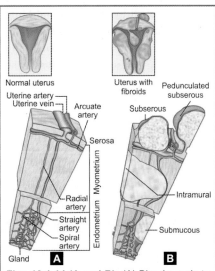

Figs 10.1.14 (A and B): (A) Blood supply to the normal uterine tissue; (B) Blood supply to the fibroids

Uterine artery embolization is a relatively new, novel technique for treatment of uterine fibroids, which was first performed by Ravina, a French Gynecologist in 1995. UAE is a nonhysterectomy surgical technique, which helps in reducing the size of the uterine fibroids by shrinking them, without actually removing them. In this procedure, an embolizing agent is injected into the uterine vessels in order to block the blood supply to the fibroids.

The world-wide success rate of the procedure in producing improvement of symptoms has been considered to be approximately 85%. UAE may be the right treatment choice in women in whom symptomatic relief may be obtained by shrinking the fibroids to a little more than half their present size. However, UAE may not be very helpful for women with extremely large fibroids because they may not shrink enough to make a significant difference in the symptoms.

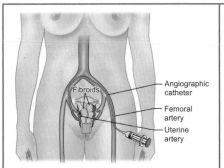

Fig. 10.1.14C: Passing the catheter through femoral artery into the uterine artery

The procedure of UAE itself lasts between 1 hour and 2 hours. Though anesthesia is usually not required, the procedure is commonly performed under sedation. The interventional radiologist introduces and manipulates a catheter through the femoral artery into the internal iliac and uterine arteries. Introduction of an embolizing agent through the catheter inside the femoral vessels helps in reducing blood supply to the fibroids.

Compared to normal uterine cells, fibroid cells are much more sensitive to low oxygen saturation. Thus, due to the lack of sufficient blood supply, the fibroids become avascular and shrink, ultimately resulting in cell death, their degeneration and eventual absorption by the myometrium. The normal myometrium, on the other hand, receives new blood supply from vaginal and ovarian vasculature.

Picture	Medical/Surgical Description	Management/Clinical Highlights

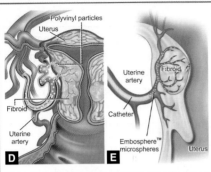

Figs 10.1.14 (D and E): (D) Blocking the blood supply of fibroids through the polyvinyl particles; (E) Magnified view showing UAE blocking the feeding blood vessel

Once the fibroids are visualized on X-ray, an embolizing agent [gelatin microspheres (trisacryl gelatin) or polyvinyl alcohol] is injected, which helps in blocking both the uterine arteries, thereby cutting off the blood supply to the fibroids.

As fibroids begin to undergo necrosis, any active bleeding commonly subsides. The dying cells of the fibroids may release toxins, which may cause irritation of the surrounding tissues, thereby causing pain and inflammation in the first few days following the procedure. Though the rate of recovery usually varies from one woman to the other, it usually takes a few months for the fibroids to fully shrink and the full effect of the procedure to be evident.

10.1.15 : Focused Ultrasound (MRgFUS) for Treatment of Fibroids

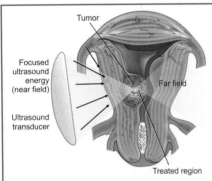

Fig. 10.1.15: Focused ultrasound (MRgFUS) for treatment of fibroids

This is another new technique for destruction of fibroids, which is still under the research stages. In this technique, ultrasound energy, which uses high-frequency energy in the form of sound waves, is used for destroying fibroids. Since the technique uses MRI to focus the ultrasound waves, the term "magnetic resonance guided focused ultrasound (MRgFUS)" is used to describe this technique. The use of focused ultrasound is associated with very low risk and rapid recovery.

This technique is based on the use of ExAblate ® 2000 System, which has been approved by the Food and Drug Administration. The procedure involves repeated targeting and heating of fibroid tissue, using ultrasound energy while the patient is under continuous MRI. The focused ultrasound energy can be used to generate sufficient heat so as to cause protein denaturation and cell death. The procedure can last as long as 3 hours.

While the ExAblate® treatment may succeed in reducing the symptoms by the treatment of fibroids, there may be a recurrence of fibroids in some women.

10.2: BENIGN OVARIAN LESIONS

10.2.1: Definition of a Benign Ovarian Mass (A and B)

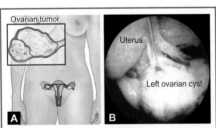

Figs 10.2.1 (A and B): (A) Ovarian tumor in right ovary; (B) Cystic ovarian tumor in left ovary

Ovarian cysts are the most common ovarian masses encountered amongst women belonging to the reproductive age group. Ovarian cysts can be either neoplastic or nonneoplastic in nature. Ovarian neoplasms (tumors) can be benign or malignant in nature. Most ovarian neoplasms (80–85%) are benign and occur in the women between 20 years and 44 years.

Discrimination between benign and malignant lesions of the ovary can usually be made on the basis of ultrasonic patterns. In case, an anechoic unilocular mass is observed on ultrasound and its size is less than 8 cm in premenopausal women, no further action is required. In case of postmenopausal women, follow-up is required after 6 weeks to observe if the resolution of the mass occurs. If there is persistent growth or increase in the size of mass over time, it should be evaluated for ovarian cancer. If size of the mass is greater than 8 cm in any woman, it should be followed-up after 6 weeks.

Picture	Medical/Surgical Description	Management/Clinical Highlights

10.2.2: Histological Pattern of Granulosa Cell Tumor

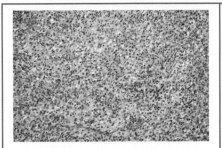

Fig. 10.2.2: Histopathological pattern of granulosa cell tumor. Showing formation of primitive follicles (Call Exner bodies)

Granulosa cell tumor, a type of sex cord stromal tumor comes under the category of neoplastic ovarian growths. It can occur at any age and is composed of cells, which are identical to the granulosa cells of the Graafian follicle.

Functionally active granulosa cell tumors are responsible for producing estrogen. This can cause precocious sexual development in young girls. In adult women, this can cause endometrial hyperplasia, fibrocystic disease of the breast, endometrial carcinoma, etc. In postmenopausal women, this tumor can cause postmenopausal bleeding.

The histopathological examination may show the presence of Call Exner bodies, which can be considered as primitive follicles comprising of granulosa cells arranged haphazardly around a space containing eosinophilic fluid.

Measurement of serum inhibin levels is helpful in the diagnosis of granulosa cell tumors and for monitoring the disease following treatment. Most common treatment modality for these patients is surgery. Chemotherapy and/or radiotherapy may be used for advanced cases of cancer and in cases of cancer recurrence. BEP regimen (bleomycin, etoposide and cisplatin) is the most commonly used chemotherapy regimen.

10.2.3: Histological Picture of a Mature Teratoma

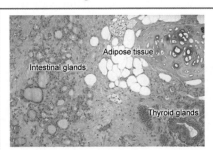

Fig. 10.2.3: Histological picture of a mature teratoma showing adipose tissue and intestinal glands at the right and thyroid tissue on the left

Ovarian teratoma, belonging to the class of germ cell tumors, is a type of neoplastic ovarian growth. They are a complex group of tumors that are subdivided into three major categories: immature, mature, and monodermal and highly specialized. The majority of germ cell tumors are benign cystic teratomas, also known as dermoids. Unlike the immature teratomas, the mature teratomas are exclusively composed of mature tissues. Mature teratomas could be either solid or cystic. In most cases, the tumor contains elements derived from all three germ layers. The dermoid cysts are benign ovarian masses, which may appear as masses having various sonographic appearances ranging from anechoic to echogenic due to a variety of internal contents. The solid areas may be due to the presence of hair follicles in combination with the calcified elements within dermoid. Other types of tissues which may be present include teeth, bone, cartilage, thyroid tissues, bronchial tissues and sebaceous material.

These tumors may be associated with elevated levels of alpha-fetoprotein and βhCG. The diagnosis is made by imaging studies [ultrasonography, computerized tomography (CT) scanning, MRI, etc.]. Fine needle aspiration cytology helps in distinguishing benign from malignant masses. Mature cystic tumor can be removed by simple cystectomy rather than salpingo-oophorectomy. If immature elements are present, surgical staging may be required.

Picture	Medical/Surgical Description	Management/Clinical Highlights

10.2.4: Laparoscopic Appearance of an Ovarian Teratoma (A and B)

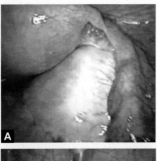
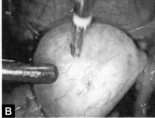

Figs 10.2.4 (A and B): Laparoscopic appearance showing a teratoma arising from the ovary

This picture shows laparoscopic appearance of an ovarian cyst. The ultrasound had shown appearance of an anechoic mass with a few areas of increased echogenicity. Histopathologic examination (HPE) revealed diagnosis of a mature cystic teratoma with clusters of adipose tissue and hair follicles within the mass. No immature elements were identified at the time of HPE.

Since the diagnosis of mature cystic teratoma was established based on the results of HPE, a simple laparoscopic cystectomy was performed for this patient. Bipolar desiccation of the ovarian capsule was done. Simple enucleation of the cyst along with the conservation of maximum possible ovarian tissues was also done. Since these tumors have a tendency to be bilateral, the other ovary must also be checked for presence of any tumor.

10.2.5: Diagnosis with Ultrasound (A to G)

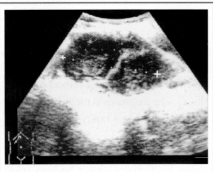

Fig. 10.2.5A: Transabdominal sonography showing a multiloculated mass with presence of cystic areas along with a few brightly echogenic areas

In this case, differential diagnosis of mucinous cystadenoma and dermoid cyst were established based on the findings of sonography. Laparoscopic examination and histopathology confirmed the diagnosis of a mucinous cystadenoma.

Ultrasonography (both transabdominal and transvaginal) is accurate in differentiating tumors of the ovary from other types of tumors of the pelvis, in more than 90% of the patients.

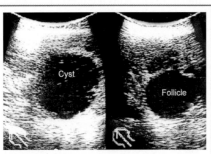

Fig. 10.2.5B: Transvaginal sonography revealing the presence of an ovarian cyst (with multiple internal echoes) on the right side. On the left side the ovary is normal with presence of a dominant follicle

This was a small cyst, which was less than 5 cm in diameter and diagnosed as a functional cyst. Functional cysts usually appear as anechoic, small masses on ultrasound examination. The mass was found to be decreasing in size on repeated sonographic examination. It eventually disappeared on its own within 3–4 months' time.

Discrimination between benign and malignant lesions of the ovary can be made on the basis of ultrasonic patterns. Though sonography cannot definitely rule out malignancy, anechoic or almost anechoic lesions have a high likelihood of being benign. As the percentage of echogenic material in the cysts increases, the likelihood of malignancy also increases.

Picture	Medical/Surgical Description	Management/Clinical Highlights
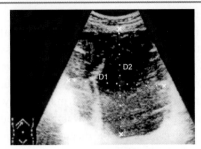 **Fig. 10.2.5C:** Transabdominal sonography showing presence of a large thin-walled cyst of right ovarian origin with multiple septa and numerous internal echoes	The ultrasound features such as presence of a multilocular mass with numerous internal echoes in this mass were indicative of a malignancy. Findings on clinical examination such as presence of solid mass with irregular margins also pointed toward malignancy. The suspicion of malignancy was confirmed on biopsy, which revealed the diagnosis of serous cystadenocarcinoma.	In general, benign lesions are likely to be unilateral, unilocular and thin walled with no papillae or solid areas. Septae, if present in benign masses, are also thin. In contrast, malignant lesions are often multilocular with thick walls, thick septae and mixed echogenicity due to the presence of solid areas. Doppler flow studies of the ovarian artery may also help in differentiating between benign and malignant growths.
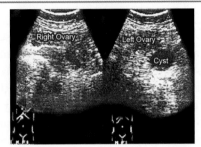 **Fig. 10.2.5D:** Transabdominal sonography revealing presence of a small functional cyst in the left ovary	Ultrasound features in this case such as presence of a small sized, anechoic lesion less than 8 cm pointed toward the diagnosis of a functional cyst. The cyst was asymptomatic and disappeared on its own over time.	Size of tumor may also give clues regarding the nature of the mass. Larger tumors, usually greater than 8 cm in size, have been thought to be associated with higher risk of malignancy in comparison to the smaller ones.
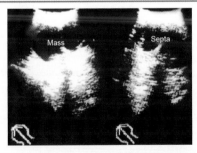 **Fig. 10.2.5E:** Transvaginal sonography showing presence of a single cystic mass with septa arising from left adnexa	In this case, the ultrasound features such as thin-walled, unilocular mass, point toward a benign lesion. Results of HPE revealed a benign serous cystadenoma.	Other signs, which could be suggestive of malignancy include presence of irregular solid parts within the mass, indefinite margins, papillary projections extending from inner wall of the cyst, presence of ascites, hydronephrosis, pleural effusion, matted bowel loops, omental implants, other evidence of peritoneal disseminated disease and lymphadenopathy.
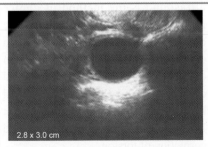 **Fig. 10.2.5F:** Transvaginal sonography showing presence of a small, smooth-walled cystic mass suggestive of functional cyst	Functional cysts develop in the ovary during the normal process of ovulation. Failure to release the egg causes accumulation of fluid within the sac resulting in the development of follicular cysts. Development of a luteal cyst, on the other hand occurs when the egg is released, but the sac gets resealed and filled with fluid.	These cysts are usually asymptomatic and disappear on their own. Usually a follow-up for 2–3 months is sufficient. If the cyst becomes large, there is a risk of torsion, rupture and bleeding. In these cases, its removal may be required. Treatment comprises of using simple pain killer medicines in case the women experiences pain. Treatment with OCPs helps in preventing ovulation and thereby cyst recurrence.

Picture	Medical/Surgical Description	Management/Clinical Highlights
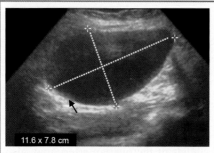 **Fig. 10.2.5G:** Transabdominal sonography showing presence of a large cyst of size 12 × 8 cm in a patient aged 52 years	Transvaginal sonography in this postmenopausal patient showed features of a benign lesion. However, the size of the mass was greater than 8 cm in diameter and the patient was postmenopausal. Both of these serve as risk factors for malignancy.	In view of high risk for malignancy, the patient was called for a repeat ultrasound after 6 weeks. The mass was observed to be increasing in size over serial ultrasound examination. In view of suspicion of malignancy, a staging laparotomy was performed which established the diagnosis of stage I serous cystadenocarcinoma.

10.2.6: Magnetic Resonance Imaging Diagnosis of a Cystadenoma

Picture	Medical/Surgical Description	Management/Clinical Highlights
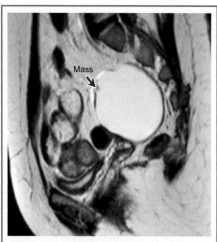 **Fig. 10.2.6:** T1-weighted image on MRI scan showing a benign serous cystadenoma. The mass is smooth walled, having homogenous consistency with no internal septae or lobulations	Sonographic diagnosis of a malignant tumor necessitates further evaluation (e.g. CT or MRI). If these investigations also suggest ovarian cancer, then the best approach is laparotomy for staging and treatment.	Magnetic resonance imaging scans use radio waves and magnetic energy instead of X-ray. MRI scans are not routinely used for diagnosing ovarian cancer. MRI scans help in accurate characterization of ovarian tumors and are also particularly helpful for examining metastatic spread of the cancer to the brain and spinal cord.

10.2.7: Twisted Ovarian Cyst

Picture	Medical/Surgical Description	Management/Clinical Highlights
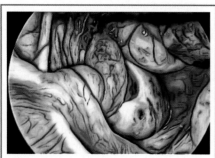 **Fig. 10.2.7:** Twisted ovarian pedicle due to torsion (*Source:* Computerized generation of image)	Ovarian torsion is a condition in which an irregular ovary with a large tumor acts as a point of fulcrum around which the oviduct revolves and subsequently gets twisted. This is likely to result in unilateral, acute lower abdominal pain, accompanied by nausea and vomiting.	The condition is usually diagnosed on ultrasound examination. Color Doppler ultrasound is the method of choice for diagnosis of adnexal torsion. The condition if neglected can result in ovarian necrosis due to the occlusion of blood supply. This is a gynecological emergency and the patient should be admitted in the hospital. Urgent laparoscopy is required for diagnosis and correction of torsion.

Picture	Medical/Surgical Description	Management/Clinical Highlights

10.2.8: Enucleation of a Cystic Ovarian Mass (A to C)

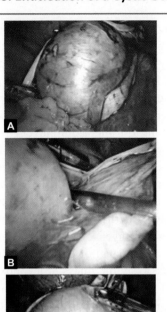

Figs 10.2.8 (A to C): Enucleation of a cystic ovarian mass from the ovary

Removal of an ovarian cyst is usually required in case there is suspicion of malignancy or if it causes some symptoms. Selective cyst removal is usually preferred over the removal of entire ovary because removal of the cyst only helps in preserving the hormonal function and reproductive capacity of the ovaries. During the process of cyst enucleation, the tissues must be handled carefully in order to reduce the formation of postoperative adhesions. Laparotomy is preferred over laparoscopy in case of extensive adhesions or large sized cysts. In general, if a cyst is greater than 10 cm in size, the suspicion of malignancy is sufficiently increased.

During the procedure of cyst removal, the ovarian capsule which overlies the dome of the cyst is incised with help of a scalpel or an electrosurgical needle. The incision is usually given on the antimensentric border surface to prevent excessive bleeding. The incision must be extended into the ovarian stroma up to the level of cyst wall, taking care not to enter or rupture the cyst. The incised edges of the cyst wall must be held with the help of Allis tissues forceps, and blunt dissection must be used to develop a plane of cleavage between the cyst wall and remaining ovarian stroma. Successive traction and counter-traction applied by the surgeon and his assistant respectively, help in gradual enucleation of the cyst. Once the cyst is enucleated out, it is sent for intraoperative frozen section examination. Remainder of the ovarian tissue is used for reconstruction of the ovaries. The ovarian bed is closed using 3-0 or 4-0 delayed absorbable sutures.

10.3: CERVICAL LESIONS

10.3.1: Cervical Polyps (A and B)

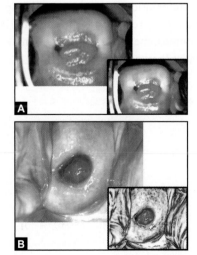

Figs 10.3.1 (A and B): Endocervical polyps
(*Source:* Computerized generation of image)

The hyperplastic projections of endocervical folds in the cervix can result in the development of single, red-colored, smooth, elongated masses known as endocervical polyps. This can be considered as one of the most common benign lesions of the cervix. Endocervical polyps are usually asymptomatic and may sometimes be associated with leukorrhea, menorrhagia or postcoital bleeding. They may be diagnosed during the routine cervical surveillance. They may range in size from several millimeters to a few centimeters.

These polyps are rarely malignant, but must be routinely biopsied to rule out cervical malignancy.

Malignant transformation is likely to occur in less than 1% cases. In case of presence of a slender stalk, the polyp can be removed by using ring forceps after twisting it several times about its base in order to strangulate the feeding vessels. Application of Monsel's solution (ferric subsulfate) along with application of direct pressure can help to achieve hemostasis. In presence of a thick pedicle, surgical excision may be carried out.

10.3.2: Cervicitis

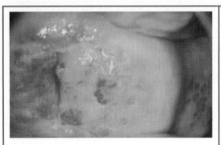

Fig. 10.3.2: Cervicitis

Cervicitis can be defined as inflammation of cervix, which can commonly occur as a result of sexually transmitted diseases. Cervicitis can sometimes be caused as a result of noninfectious causes such as injury due to some birth control device like intrauterine contraceptive device, cervical cap or diaphragm. Cervical cancer can be another noninfectious cause of cervicitis. Cervicitis may frequently cause intermenstrual or postcoital bleeding. Mucopurulent cervicitis may be associated with cervical infection due to organisms such as *Chlamydia trachomatis* and *Neisseria gonorrhoeae*. Cervicitis due to Herpes simplex may result in bleeding.

Microscopic examination of the saline preparation of cervical secretions may show presence of neutrophils and RBCs. Recommended single dose treatment for uncomplicated gonococcal infection is either with ceftriaxone 250 mg IM plus azithromycin 1 g or doxycycline 100 mg twice daily for 7 days. Recommended oral treatment of chlamydial infection is azithromycin 1 g or doxycycline 100 mg twice daily for 7 days. Alternative regimen comprises of erythromycin 500 mg (four times a day for 7 days) or ofloxacin 300 mg twice a day for 7 days or levofloxacin 500 mg daily for 7 days. In order to prevent recurrence, abstinence is recommended until the woman and her partner are treated and become asymptomatic.

10.3.3: Cervical Erosion

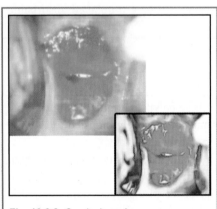

Fig. 10.3.3: Cervical erosion

(*Source:* Computerized generation of image)

Cervical erosion or ectropion is now also known as cervical ectopy. There might be migration of some endocervical tissue onto the vaginal portion of cervix, outward from the endocervical canal resulting in the development of cervical ectopy. The endocervical tissue may then undergo squamous metaplasia and get transformed into stratified squamous epithelium. This is otherwise a benign lesion, but may sometimes mimic early cervical cancer and investigations such as Pap smear and biopsy may need to be performed over it. In prepubertal women, normally the squamocolumnar junction lies at the level of external os. In cases of cervical erosion, the squamocolumnar junction lies external to the os.

The condition may be associated with excessive, but nonpurulent vaginal discharge. It may also be responsible for postcoital bleeding. No treatment is required in asymptomatic cases. In symptomatic cases, hormone therapy may be prescribed. In extremely troublesome cases, it can be ablated under local anesthesia.

Picture	Medical/Surgical Description	Management/Clinical Highlights

10.3.4: Nabothian Cysts (A and B)

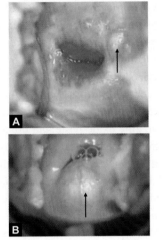

Figs 10.3.4 (A and B): Nabothian cysts (indicated by arrows)

Nabothian cysts develop as a result of a benign process in which squamous metaplasia of ectocervix may cover the invaginations of the glandular columnar cells of the endocervical canal. There may be accumulation of secretions due to blockage of cervical crypts causing the entrapment of the cervical mucus. This might result in the development of smooth, clear, whitish or yellowish-colored rounded elevations which may become visible at the time of per speculum examination.

These are benign lesions for which no treatment is required. They are mostly harmless, but may disappear on their own. If they become large in size, cause discomfort or make Pap testing or cervical examination difficult, they can be opened with help of a biopsy forceps and drained. They can also be removed by electrocautery or cryotherapy. New cysts may sometimes appear even after the procedure.

10.4: VULVAR LESIONS

10.4.1: Lichen Sclerosis

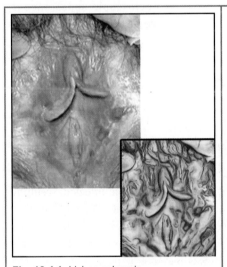

Fig. 10.4.1: Lichen sclerosis
(*Source:* Computerized generation of image)

Lichen sclerosis commonly affects postmenopausal women, though it may be frequently also present in premenopausal women. The etiology, largely, remains unknown, though it can be associated with various causes such as infection, hormones, genetic and autoimmune causes. Most women remain asymptomatic. However, a few may complain of anogenital symptoms such as pruritis and starching, which may worsen during night. Pruritis-induced scratching may result in the development of excoriations and thickening of the vulvar skin. There may be the presence of white atrophic papules, whitish plaques, regression of labia minora, clitoral concealment and introital stenosis. Though this is a non-neoplastic dermatosis, patients may be at an increased risk of malignancy. Malignant transformation can occur in nearly 4-6% cases. Such women would require surveillance every 6–12 months.

No definitive curative therapy is available. Treatment aims at symptom control and prevention of anatomic distortion. Steps for maintaining hygiene for minimizing chemical and mechanical irritation of the skin may be required. Topical corticosteroid ointments such as 0.05% clobetasol propionate or 0.05% halobetasol propionate may be useful due to their anti-inflammatory, antipruritic and vasoconstrictive properties. Topical application of estrogen cream may help in reducing menopausal atrophic changes, labial fusion and dyspareunia. Retinoids may be administered in severe unresponsive cases. Topical calcineurin inhibitors such as tacrolimus and pimecrolimus have anti-inflammatory and immunomodulatory effect.

10.4.2: Vulvar Dystrophy

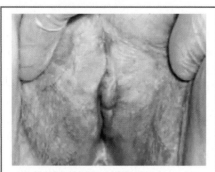

Fig. 10.4.2: Vulvar dystrophy

Vulvar dystrophies comprise of a spectrum of vulvar lesions ranging from atrophic to hypertrophic lesions. This results in development of circumscribed or diffuse white lesions. Histological classification of vulvar dystrophy comprise of the following: hyperplastic dystrophy (squamous cell hyperplasia); lichen sclerosus (atrophic dystrophy) and mixed dystrophy. Lichen sclerosis has been discussed in Figure 10.4.1 (A and B). Hyperplastic dystrophy would be discussed here. The most common etiology for hyperplastic dystrophy is chronic irritation or chronic vulvovaginal infection. There is benign epithelial thickening and hyperkeratosis. In the acute phase, these lesions may appear reddish and moist. As the epithelial thickening develops, there occurs a raised, white lesion, which might be circumscribed or diffuse. This may cause symptoms such as pruritis, soreness, discharge or dyspareunia.

Microscopic examination helps in establishing the diagnosis. Treatment comprises of prescribing estrogens. Conjugated equine estrogens must be prescribed in the dosage of 0.625 mg to help control pruritis. Local application of bland substances such as calamine lotion, zinc oxide paste and crotamine provide a soothing effect. In presence of inflammation, steroid ointments (1% hydrocortisone, betamethasone, etc.) may be helpful. Local application of antimicrobial creams (soframycin, neomycin, etc.) may also be useful. Lignocaine ointment (2%) provides relief from pain.

Biopsy from multiple sites becomes mandatory in case malignancy is suspected because the lesion may show different microscopic appearance at various places in the same lesion.

10.4.3: Lesions Involving Bartholin Glands (A to E)

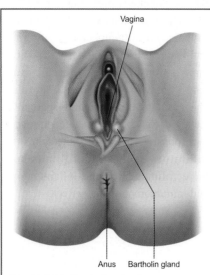

Fig. 10.4.3A: Bartholin glands

Bartholin glands are also known as greater vestibular glands. These are two glands, each of which is located to the left and right of the vaginal introitus, slightly toward the posterior side. These glands secrete mucus, which helps in lubricating the vagina. These glands are homologous to bulbourethral glands in males.

Though the presence of Bartholin glands may remain unnoticed, sometimes, these glands may become infected, resulting in pain and swelling. These glands may develop into a cyst like structure as a result of inflammation. Though the cysts may not be painful, it may result in extreme discomfort and swelling. At times, these cysts may get suppurated resulting in abscess formation.

Picture	Medical/Surgical Description	Management/Clinical Highlights
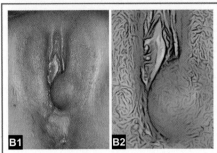 **Figs 10.4.3 (B1 and B2):** Bartholin gland cyst [*Source:* Computerized generation of image (B2)]	Cysts of Bartholin glands are commonly encountered in routine gynecological practice. They typically measure 1–4 cm in size and are frequently asymptomatic. Larger cysts may result in vaginal pressure symptoms and dyspareunia.	Permanent resolution of the cyst is done either using marsupialization or incision, and drainage with Word's catheter placement. Placement of Word's catheter helps in creating a new epithelialized tract for gland drainage after emptying the cyst cavity through the procedure of incision and drainage.
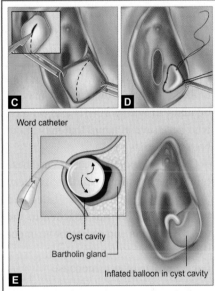 **Figs 10.4.3 (C to E):** (C and D) Marsupialization of Bartholin gland cyst; (E) Placement of Word's catheter	Marsupialization requires greater degree of analgesia, larger incision, placement of sutures and longer procedural time. It may be the preferred procedure in case of recurrence of cysts with previously placed Word's catheter. A vertical incision about 2–3 cm in size is made on the vestibule near the medial edge of labia minora and approximately 1 cm lateral and parallel to the hymenal ring. The cyst wall is then incised with a scalpel and the incision extended with scissors. Allis clamps are then placed on the four edges in order to grasp the edges of the cyst wall. The edges of the cyst wall are then sutured to the adjacent skin edges with interrupted delayed absorbable sutures.	With the introduction of Word's catheter, use of Marsupialization has declined.

10.4.4: Skene's Duct Cysts

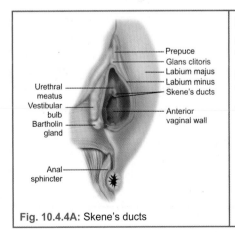 **Fig. 10.4.4A:** Skene's ducts	Skene's ducts are inconsistently present along the side of the female urethra. These ducts drain Skene's glands (periurethral or paraurethral glands). These glands are located on the anterior wall of vagina, adjacent to distal urethra.	Obstruction of these ducts result in the development of Skene's duct cysts. The smaller cysts (< 1 cm in size) are usually asymptomatic. Their management is discussed in Figure 10.4.4B.

Picture	Medical/Surgical Description	Management/Clinical Highlights

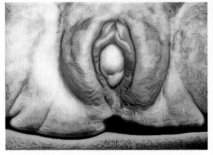

Fig. 10.4.4B: Skene's duct cysts
(*Source:* Computerized generation of image)

The smaller cysts of Skene's ducts (< 1 cm in size) are usually asymptomatic. Larger cysts may result in symptoms such as dyspareunia and outflow tract obstruction (hesitancy, retention, etc.). Suppuration of these cysts may result in abscess formation, which may result in pain and swelling.

Diagnosis is established on clinical examination. Most symptomatic cysts can be palpated adjacent to distal urethra. Surgical excision of these symptomatic cysts may be required. In case of an abscess, broad spectrum antibiotics (cephalexin, 500 mg QID for a week) may be required.

10.5: BENIGN BREAST DISEASE

10.5.1: Fibroadenoma (A to D)

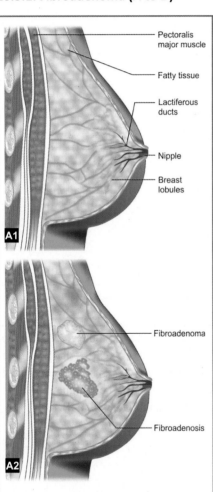

Figs 10.5.1 (A1 and A2): (A1) Normal breast; (A2) Breast showing fibroadenoma

Fibroadenoma is the most common benign tumor of the breast and the most common breast tumor in women under the age of 30 years.

A fibroadenoma is a benign growth composed of glandular and cystic epithelial structures surrounded by a cellular stroma. The etiology behind the development of fibroadenomas is not yet understood.

Fibroadenomas usually present as unilateral lumps. However they may be bilateral in nearly 10–15% of women who have several lumps that may affect both the breasts.

On palpation of the breast tissue, these tumors feel as firm, painless, rubbery lumps having smooth, well-defined borders. They are not attached to the underlying skin and easily move under the skin. Fibroadenomas may often reduce in size after menopause.

Picture	Medical/Surgical Description	Management/Clinical Highlights
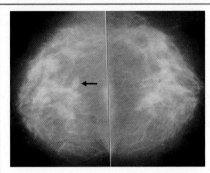 **Fig. 10.5.1B:** In a perimenopausal women aged 45 years, a lesion 1 cm in size was found at the center of right breast on the mammogram (indicated by arrow)	This 45-years-old perimenopausal woman had presented to the clinic with the complaint of feeling a nodular lump in right breast since last 1 month. A small lump (about 2–3 cm in diameter) could be palpated in the right breast on clinical examination. The mass was well-defined, nontender, freely mobile and not attached to the underlying breast tissues. Even though there was a little suspicion of malignancy, a mammogram was performed, which showed a well-defined homogeneous mass about 1 cm in diameter with well-defined margins in the right breast. There were no associated calcifications.	The findings on mammography were suggestive of a benign tumor. Ultrasound as shown in the next figure was also performed to check the diagnosis. Sometimes, an ultrasound (with or without a directed biopsy) and/or a core needle biopsy may be required to confirm the diagnosis in cases of breast lumps.
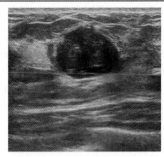 **Fig. 10.5.1C:** Ultrasound examination in the same patient confirmed the diagnosis of fibroadenoma	Ultrasound examination revealed a homogeneous round mass with smooth, well-defined walls.	An ultrasound-guided biopsy was performed taking into account the patient's extreme apprehension for malignancy.
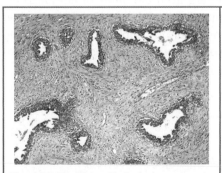 **Fig. 10.5.1D:** Histopathological appearance of the biopsy specimen in the same patient	Microscopic examination of the biopsy specimen revealed proliferation of glandular and stromal elements within the breast tissue in a pericanalicular growth pattern. A well-defined capsule was observed. No features suggestive of atypia, hyperplasia, etc. were observed. The basement membrane was intact.	Most small asymptomatic fibroadenomas can be left in situ as it is and monitored at regular intervals through investigations such as mammography, ultrasound, etc. to exclude malignant conversion. Nearly 10% fibroadenomas may disappear on their own. If the lesions are large, there is a suspicion of malignancy, or if the tumor is symptomatic, it should be removed by surgical excision. Sometimes, the tumor may be destroyed using cryoablation. Some fibroadenomas may respond to treatment with ormeloxifene, a selective estrogen receptor modulator.

SECTION 10 ❖ BENIGN TUMORS OF GENITAL TRACT

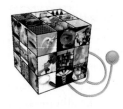

1. ULIPRISTAL ACETATE VERSUS PLACEBO FOR TREATMENT OF FIBROIDS

Ulipristal acetate, a selective progesterone receptor modulator (in the dosage of 5–10 mg per day for 10–12 weeks) has been found to be effective for treatment of symptomatic fibroids prior to surgery. It helps in controlling excessive bleeding as well as in reducing the size of fibroids.

Source: Donnez J, Tatarchuk TF, Bouchard P, et al. Ulipristal acetate versus placebo for fibroid treatment before surgery. N Engl J Med. 2012;366:409.

2. ULIPRISTAL ACETATE VERSUS LEUPROLIDE ACETATE FOR TREATMENT OF FIBROIDS

Ulipristal acetate causes a significantly lower reduction in the size of fibroids as well as the occurrence of hot flashes in comparison to monthly injections of leuprolide acetate, a synthetic GnRH analogue.

Source: Donnez J, Tomaszewski J, Vázquez F, et al. Ulipristal acetate versus leuprolide acetate for uterine fibroids. N Engl J Med. 2012;366:421.)

3. PRETREATMENT WITH GONADOTROPIN-RELEASING HORMONE AGONISTS IN CASES OF UAE

Offering UAE to the women with large fibroids had been a source of concern to the gynecologists due to the risk of infection. However, according to the new study, treatment with GnRH agonists prior to UAE in case of large fibroids (size ≥ 10 cm) is likely to cause a reduction in the size of fibroids. This option therefore serves as a safe and effective nonsurgical method for treatment of fibroids and would help replace hysterectomy.

Source: Kim MD, Lee MS, et al. Uterine artery embolization of large fibroids: comparative study of procedure with and without pretreatment gonadotropin-releasing hormone agonists. Am J Roentgenol. 2012;199:441-6.

4. THE INTERNATIONAL SOCIETY FOR THE STUDY OF VULVOVAGINAL DISEASE (ISSVD, 2011) CLINICAL CLASSIFICATION OF VULVAR DERMATOLOGICAL DISORDERS

ISSVD (2011) appointed a committee comprising of multinational members from the fields of dermatology, gynecology, and pathology in order to formulate a clinically based terminology and classification of vulvar dermatological disorders. The committee identified about 50 of the most commonly encountered disorders along with a few uncommon, but important conditions and categorized them into eight morphological groups, which are described below.

2011 ISSVD Clinical Classification of Vulvar Dermatological Disorders

1. Skin-colored lesions

A. *Skin-colored papules and nodules*
1. Papillomatosis of the vestibule and medial labia minora (a normal finding; not a disease)
2. Molluscum contagiosum
3. Warts (HPV infection)
4. Scar
5. Vulvar intraepithelial neoplasia
6. Skin tag (acrochordon, fibroepithelial polyp)
7. Nevus (intradermal type)
8. Mucinous cysts of the vestibule and medial labia minora (may have yellow hue)
9. Epidermal cyst (syn. epidermoid cyst; epithelial cyst)

Contd...

    10. Mammary-like gland tumor (hidradenoma papilliferum)
    11. Bartholin gland cyst and tumor
    12. Syringoma
    13. Basal cell carcinoma

  B. *Skin-colored plaques*
    1. Lichen simplex chronicus and other lichenified disease
    2. Vulvar intraepithelial neoplasia

2. Red lesions: patches and plaques

  A. *Eczematous and lichenified diseases*
    1. Allergic contact dermatitis
    2. Irritant contact dermatitis
    3. Atopic dermatitis (rarely seen as a vulvar presentation)
    4. Eczematous changes superimposed on other vulvar disorders
    5. Diseases clinically mimicking eczematous disease (candidiasis, Hailey-Hailey disease, and extramammary Paget disease)
    6. Lichen simplex chronicus (lichenification with no preceding skin lesions)
    7. Lichenification superimposed on an underlying preceding pruritic disease.

  B. *Red patches and plaques (no epithelial disruption)*
    1. Candidiasis
    2. Psoriasis
    3. Vulvar intraepithelial neoplasia
    4. Lichen planus
    5. Plasma cell (Zoon) vulvitis
    6. Bacterial soft-tissue infection (cellulitis and early necrotizing fasciitis)
    7. Extramammary Paget disease

3. Red lesions: papules and nodules

  A. *Red papules*
    1. Folliculitis
    2. Wart (HPV infection)
    3. Angiokeratoma
    4. M. contagiosum (inflamed)
    5. Hidradenitis suppurativa (early lesions)
    6. Hailey-Hailey disease

  B. *Red nodules*
    1. Furuncles (boils)
    2. Wart (HPV infection)
    3. Prurigo nodularis
    4. Vulvar intraepithelial neoplasia
    5. M. contagiosum (inflamed)
    6. Urethral caruncle and prolapse
    7. Hidradenitis suppurativa
    8. Mammary-like gland adenoma (hidradenoma papilliferum)
    9. Inflamed epidermal cyst
    10. Bartholin duct abscess
    11. Squamous cell carcinoma
    12. Melanoma (amelanotic type)

4. White lesions

A. *White papules and nodules*
1. Fordyce spots (a normal finding; may sometimes have a yellow hue)
2. M. contagiosum
3. Wart
4. Scar
5. Vulvar intraepithelial neoplasia
6. Squamous cell carcinoma
7. Milium (plural milia)
8. Epidermal cyst
9. Hailey-Hailey disease.

B. *White patches and plaques*
1. Vitiligo
2. Lichen sclerosus
3. Postinflammatory hypopigmentation
4. Lichenified diseases
5. Lichen planus
6. Vulvar intraepithelial neoplasia
7. Squamous cell carcinoma.

5. Dark-colored (brown, blue, gray, or black) lesions

A. *Dark-colored patches*
1. Melanocytic nevus
2. Vulvar melanosis (vulvar lentiginosis)
3. Postinflammatory hyperpigmentation
4. Lichen planus
5. Acanthosis nigricans
6. Melanoma in situ.

B. *Dark-colored papules and nodules*
1. Melanocytic nevus (includes those with clinical and/or histological atypia)
2. Warts (HPV infection)
3. Vulvar intraepithelial neoplasia
4. Seborrheic keratosis
5. Angiokeratoma (capillary angioma, cherry angioma)
6. Mammary-like gland adenoma (hidradenoma papilliferum)
7. Melanoma.

6. Blisters

A. *Vesicles and bullae*
1. Herpes virus infections (herpes simplex, herpes zoster)
2. Acute eczema
3. Bullous lichen sclerosus
4. Lymphangioma circumscriptum (lymphangiectasia)
5. Immune blistering disorders (cicatricial pemphigoid, fixed drug eruption, Steven-Johnson syndrome, pemphigus)

B. *Pustules*
1. Candidiasis (candidosis)
2. Folliculitis.

Contd...

7. Erosions and ulcers

A. *Erosions*

1. Excoriations
2. Erosive lichen planus
3. Fissures arising on normal tissue (idiopathic, intercourse related)
4. Fissures arising on abnormal tissue (candidiasis, lichen simplex chronicus, psoriasis, Crohn disease, etc.)
5. Vulvar intraepithelial neoplasia, eroded variant
6. Ruptured vesicles, bullae and pustules
7. Extramammary Paget disease.

B. *Ulcers*

1. Excoriations (related to eczema, lichen simplex chronicus)
2. Aphthous ulcers (syn. aphthous minor), aphthous major, Lipschütz ulcer (occurring either as an idiopathic process or secondary to other diseases such as Crohn, Behçet, various viral infections)
3. Crohn disease
4. Herpes virus infection (particularly in patients who are immunosuppressed)
5. Ulcerated squamous cell carcinoma
6. Primary syphilis (chancre).

8. Edema (diffuse genital swelling)

A. *Skin-colored edema*

1. Crohn disease
2. Idiopathic lymphatic abnormality (congenital Milroy disease)
3. Postradiation and postsurgical lymphatic obstruction
4. Postinfectious edema (especially staphylococcal and streptococcal cellulitis)
5. Postinflammatory edema (especially hidradenitis suppurativa)

B. *Pink or red edema*

1. Venous obstruction (e.g., pregnancy and parturition)
2. Cellulitis (primary or superimposed on already existing edema)
3. Inflamed Bartholin duct cyst/abscess
4. Crohn disease
5. Mild vulvar edema may occur with any inflammatory vulvar disease.

Syn., synonym

Source: This article was presented at the XXI World Congress of the International Society for the Study of Vulvovaginal Disease, held in Paris, France, on September 3 to 8, 2011. J Low Genit Tract Dis. 2012;16(4):339-44. © 2012 Lippincott Williams & Wilkins

Gynecology

Section 11

Malignancies of Genital Tract

11.1: ENDOMETRIAL CANCER

11.1.1: Definition (A and B)

Picture	Medical/Surgical Description	Management/Clinical Highlights
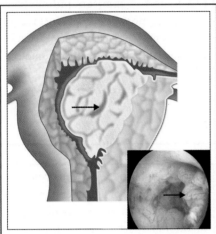 Fig. 11.1.1A: Endometrial cancer. (A) Exophytic growth (indicated by arrow)	Endometrial cancer develops from the lining of the uterus, also known as the endometrium. It may commonly present as exophytic growth or sometimes as an ulcerative lesion. It is the most common gynecologic cancer and the fourth most common cancer amongst women. Approximately, 1 in every 50 women is likely to get affected with the endometrial cancer.	The most common symptom associated with endometrial cancer is abnormal uterine bleeding. Endometrial cancer usually affects women after menopause, commonly in the age groups of 50–65 years. The most important risk factor for endometrial cancer is hyperestrogenism.
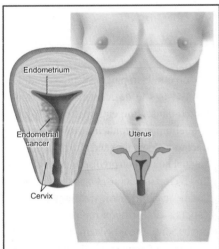 Fig. 11.1.1B: Ulcerative lesion	The endometrial cancer can either appear in form of an exophytic raised lesion or an ulcerative growth of the uterine endometrium. From here the neoplastic cells can grow and invade the surrounding myometrium or may even spread to distant locations. In case of endometrial cancer, an endometrial biopsy may be required to confirm the diagnosis. Most commonly, a hysteroscopic directed biopsy is performed.	An ultrasound (typically a transvaginal ultrasound scan) and a hysteroscopic examination may be performed to further confirm the diagnosis. In case the diagnosis of endometrial cancer has been confirmed, the following investigations are performed to evaluate the spread of cancer: • Blood tests (hematocrit) • Kidney and liver function tests • Chest X-ray • Computed tomography • Magnetic resonance imaging.

11.1.2: Use of Ultrasound and Other Imaging Modalities for the Diagnosis of Endometrial Cancer (A to J)

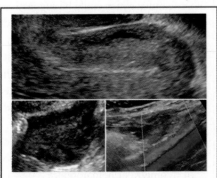 Fig. 11.1.2A: Transvaginal ultrasound in a 58-year-old patient, presenting with postmenopausal bleeding	In this case, the transvaginal sonogram demonstrated normal ultrasound findings in case of a postmenopausal woman. The endometrium appeared to be thin and hyperechogenic, along with the presence of an atrophic uterus and nonfunctioning ovaries, which do not show presence of any growing follicle. Color Doppler demonstrated the presence of iliac vessels adjacent to the ovary with no growing follicle.	Ultrasound (both transabdominal and transvaginal) can be used for evaluating the cancerous growth. Transvaginal ultrasound is especially indicated in the women at high risk for endometrial cancer. If the endometrial stripe on ultrasound examination is greater than 4 mm, endometrial sampling/biopsy should be performed.

Picture	Medical/Surgical Description	Management/Clinical Highlights
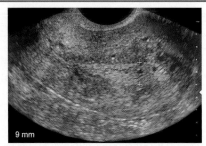 **Fig. 11.1.2B:** TVS in a 48-year-old perimenopausal patient with complaints of postmenopausal bleeding since last 2 months	Measurement of endometrial thickness on transvaginal ultrasound has become a routine investigation in patients with abnormal uterine bleeding, especially those belonging to the perimenopausal age groups. Transvaginal ultrasound in this patient showed an endometrial thickness of 9 mm.	In this case, since the endometrial thickness on transvaginal sonography (TVS) is ≥ 4 mm, an endometrial sampling/biopsy was performed to exclude endometrial hyperplasia. Biopsy revealed the presence of endometrial adenocarcinoma.
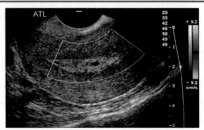 **Fig. 11.1.2C:** Doppler ultrasound in the same patient as described in Figure 11.1.2B	Prior to biopsy, Doppler ultrasound was performed in this patient. It revealed endometrial hyperplasia with prominent peripheral vascular signals.	Increased blood flow and reduced resistance index on Doppler ultrasound is indicative of increased vascularization of the mass, which is a hallmark of malignant growth.
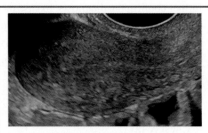 **Fig. 11.1.2D:** Transvaginal sonography in a 50-year-old postmenopausal patient, presenting with irregular bleeding and dyspareunia since 2 months	Transvaginal sonography revealed thin endometrium (thickness = 3 mm) in this patient. Biopsy diagnosed endometrial atrophy. Based on the findings of clinical examination and investigations, a diagnosis of endometrial atrophy was made. Histopathological examination (HPE) is essential because there may be hidden areas of hypertrophic endometrium within the areas of atrophic endometrium.	Endometrial atrophy is a benign condition related to the deficiency of estrogen, which causes the endometrium, vaginal epithelium and epithelium of the urinary tract to become thin and atrophic. Loss of vaginal lubrication predisposes the women to develop infections. Once the diagnosis has been confirmed, treatment usually depends on estrogen replacement. This can be administered systemically or locally (in form of vaginal topical applications).
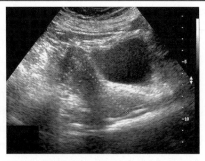 **Fig. 11.1.2E:** Transabdominal ultrasound in a 42-year-old premenopausal patient having irregular bleeding	Transabdominal ultrasound showing an enlarged uterine cavity, measuring 77 × 31 mm, with multiple cystic spaces within. Biopsy confirmed the presence of endometrial cancer.	Besides increased endometrial thickness, other features which could be suggestive of endometrial cancer on ultrasound examination are as follows: • Broad-based polypoid mass present within the endometrial cavity with or without surrounding fluid. The mass is likely to replace the normal endometrial stripe. • Complex fluid collection in the endometrial cavity could be suggestive of pyometra or hematometra • Calcifications may be rarely present in the cases of endometrial cancer.

Picture	Medical/Surgical Description	Management/Clinical Highlights
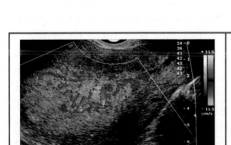 **Fig. 11.1.2F:** Doppler ultrasound in a patient with endometrial carcinoma	There were prominent peripheral and central vascular signals on ultrasound, which revealed presence of an advanced stage III endometrial adenocarcinoma.	Management of stage III endometrial cancer has been discussed in Figure 11.1.4C.
Fig. 11.1.2G: Transvaginal ultrasound in a 52-year-old menopausal patient with the complaints of irregular bleeding and offensive vaginal discharge since 2–3 months	Ultrasound revealed the presence of a heterogeneous mass within the endometrial cavity, which was observed to be replacing the normal endometrial stripe.	Doppler ultrasound was performed (Fig. 11.1.2H), which confirmed the suspicion of malignancy. A hysteroscopic-guided biopsy revealed the diagnosis of endometrial cancer.
Fig. 11.1.2H: Doppler ultrasound in the same patient as described in Figure 11.1.2G	Increased vascular flow was observed on Doppler ultrasound. Hysteroscopic-guided biopsy revealed the diagnosis of advanced stage endometrial cancer.	Evaluation of cases of endometrial cancer using transvaginal color Doppler ultrasound can be considered as a reliable method for reaching the correct diagnosis. Color Doppler examination helps in assessing endometrial angiogenesis and acts as a good predictor factor for tumor progression and metastasis.
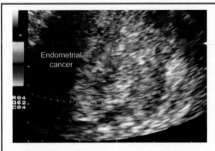 **Fig. 11.1.2I:** Color Doppler examination in a 58-year-old postmenopausal patient presenting with irregular bleeding and abdominal pain since 1 month	Color Doppler ultrasound examination revealed thick heterogeneous endometrium with proliferation of blood vessels. A diagnosis of advanced stage endometrial cancer was made.	In order to further assess the spread of endometrial cancer to distant body organs, an MRI examination as shown in Figure 11.1.2I was performed.

Picture	Medical/Surgical Description	Management/Clinical Highlights

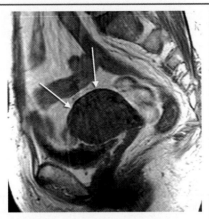

Fig. 11.1.2J: Magnetic resonance imaging scan showing endometrial adenocarcinoma in the same patient as described in Figure 11.1.2I.

T1-weighted images on MRI examination revealed a large tumor of low signal intensity, expanding within the uterine cavity. There was no spread to distant body organs. On the basis of findings of clinical and radiological examination, the disease was classified as stage III endometrial cancer.

Magnetic resonance imaging reveals inconsistent endometrial findings in 80–85% of patients with endometrial carcinoma. The involvement of endometrium can be in variable forms such as focal or diffuse thickening of endometrial lining, widening of endometrial cavity due to the presence of polypoid growth within the cavity, etc. Furthermore, the signal intensity of the tumor can show variable patterns on T1-weighted and T2-weighted images. Treatment of stage III endometrial cancer has been described in Figure 11.1.4C.

11.1.3: Endometrial Biopsy

Kindly refer to Section 9.

11.1.4: Staging of Endometrial Cancer (A to D)

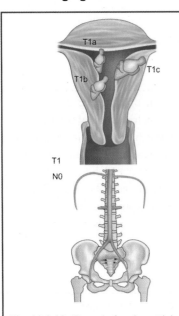

Fig. 11.1.4A: Stage I of endometrial cancer

Stage I endometrial cancers are confined to the uterine corpus. They can be subclassified as follows:
- IA: limited to the endometrium
- IB: invasion of half or less than one half of the myometrium
- IC: invasion of one half or more than one half of the myometrium.

For patients with stage I tumor, the treatment of choice is an extrafascial total abdominal hysterectomy (TAH) and bilateral salpingo-oophorectomy, with lymph node sampling. Removal of a vaginal cuff is usually not required in these cases. The removed tumor specimen is examined for tumor size, depth of myometrial invasion and extension into the cervix. Sampling of the pelvic lymph nodes may be done in selective cases. Surgery alone may serve as an appropriate treatment option for patients with stage I tumors, in whom there is no evidence of invasion of the lymphovascular space, cervix or isthmus; peritoneal cytology is negative and there is no evidence of metastasis. In all the other patients, some form of adjuvant radiotherapy is indicated. In case of lymph node involvement, postoperative radiotherapy in the dosage of 4,000–5,000 cGY is recommended over 5–6 weeks.

Picture	Medical/Surgical Description	Management/Clinical Highlights

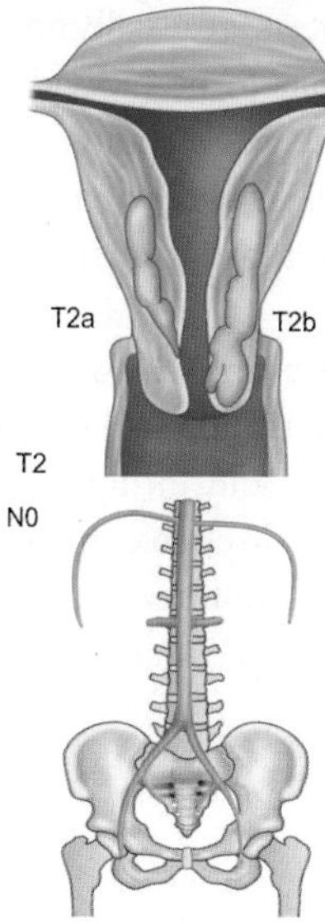

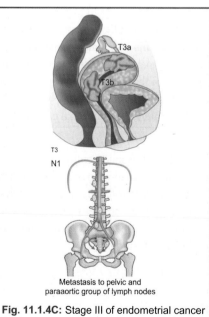

Fig. 11.1.4B: Stage II of endometrial cancer

In stage II endometrial cancer, there is involvement of cervix, but the cancer does not spread beyond the uterus. This can be subclassified as follows:
- IIA: endocervical glandular involvement only
- II B: cervical stromal invasion

Brachytherapy followed by surgery is the treatment of choice for stage II endometrial cancer. External radiotherapy may be administered based on histological findings at the time of surgery. For stage II tumors, radical hysterectomy with bilateral salpingo-oophorectomy and pelvic lymphadenectomy is the most commonly used treatment modality. Alternatively, Wertheim's hysterectomy may also be performed. Pelvic lymphadenectomy is not required in all cases. It is usually based on the results of lymph node sampling. Sampling of the pelvic lymph nodes may be done in selective cases, e.g. presence of stage IIB, size of the tumor is greater than 2 cm or there is an evidence of extrauterine disease.

In stage III endometrial cancer, there is local and/or regional spread. This can be subclassified as follows:
- IIIA: invasion of serosa and/or adnexa and/or positive peritoneal cytology
- IIIB: vaginal metastases
- IIIC: metastases to pelvic and/or para-aortic lymph nodes

For stage IIIA growths, the goal of surgery is TAH and bilateral salpingo-oophorectomy with selective lymphadenectomy, biopsies of suspicious areas, omental biopsy and debulking of tumor followed by radiotherapy or chemotherapy. In stage IIIB and IIIC growths, chemotherapy with doxorubicin in the dosage of 60 mg/m2 with cisplatin and paclitaxel and/or radiotherapy are commonly used following surgery.

Metastasis to pelvic and paraaortic group of lymph nodes

Fig. 11.1.4C: Stage III of endometrial cancer

Picture	Medical/Surgical Description	Management/Clinical Highlights

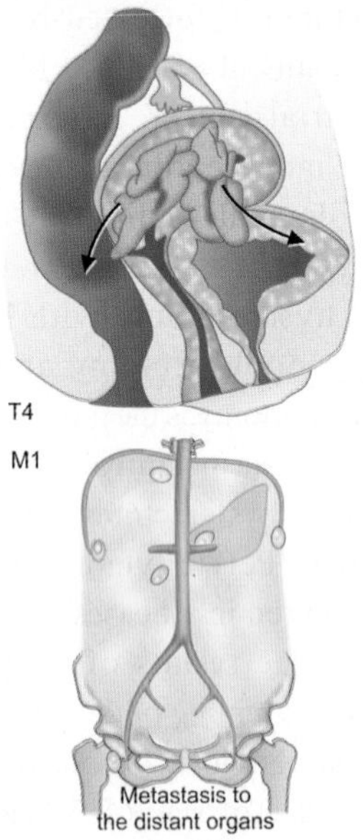

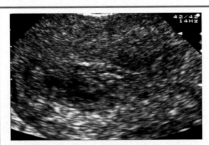

Fig. 11.1.4 D: Stage IV of endometrial cancer

In stage IV, the cancer has become widespread throughout the body. This can be subclassified as follows:
- IVA: invasion of bladder and/or bowel mucosa
- IVB: distant metastases, including intraabdominal metastases and/or inguinal lymph nodes

Stage IV cancers are usually nonoperable. Treatment has to be individualized in those with stage IV tumors. Usually, a combination of surgery, radiotherapy, hormone therapy or chemotherapy is required.

Chemotherapy drugs commonly used in combination include paclitaxel, doxorubicin, and either cisplatin or carboplatin. Medroxyprogesterone acetate administered in the dosage of 1 g weekly, acts as an adjuvant to chemotherapy.

11.2: LEIOMYOSARCOMA (A TO D)

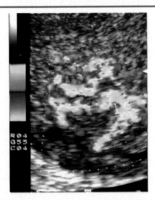

Fig. 11.2A: Ultrasound in a 64-year-old postmenopausal patient presenting with abnormal vaginal bleeding and offensive vaginal discharge since 4 weeks. There was also a history of abdominal pain. The woman had a history of uterine fibroids

Ultrasound examination revealed presence of a hypoechogenic mass. Previous ultrasound examinations done 5 years ago showed presence of small interstitial fibroid about 2 cm in size. Since the patient's fibroids were observed to be increasing in size as observed on the latest transvaginal scans, she was called for a repeat pelvic examination and scan after every 2 months.

The rate of conversion of leiomyoma into a leiomyosarcoma is about 0.5%. Also, the rate of occurrence of uterine leiomyosarcomas is extremely low, with the incidence being about 0.67/1,000 women per year. Since the incidence of sarcomas is so low, it is not clinically justifiable to believe that the growing fibroid in this case indicates malignancy. Since the patient is postmenopausal, any growth in the uterus may be a cause for concern. In this case, efforts were made to first rule out endometrial carcinoma.

Fig. 11.2B: Doppler ultrasound in the same patient as described in Figure 11.2A.

Doppler ultrasound in this patient revealed a highly vascular lesion with low-resistance blood flow.

Doppler ultrasound confirmed the presence of malignancy. In order to establish the exact nature of malignancy, a hysteroscopic-guided biopsy was performed. The findings of HPE confirmed the diagnosis of a leiomyosarcoma.

Picture	Medical/Surgical Description	Management/Clinical Highlights
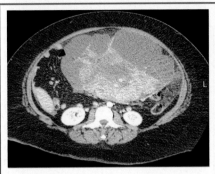 **Fig. 11.2C:** Computed tomography scan in the same patient showed a uterine mass with hemorrhagic and necrotic areas	Computed tomography imaging is useful in evaluating the extent of spread of cancer beyond the uterus into the adjacent structures and organs. CT scan may also be useful in evaluating the patient's response to surgery or presence of any recurrence. Biopsy can be performed using a CT-guided core needle biopsy in order to confirm the diagnosis.	Uterine sarcomas are a rare and aggressive form of uterine cancer, which arise from the smooth muscle fibers of myometrium. Leiomyosarcomas can behave in an unpredictable manner. They can remain dormant for long periods of time and then suddenly recur after many years.
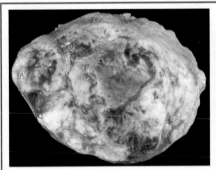 **Fig. 11.2D:** Gross specimen of leiomyosarcoma as obtained upon hysterectomy	Figure 11.2D shows the gross specimen in this patient obtained at the time of surgery. Grossly, the tumor appears soft with areas of hemorrhage and necrosis.	Leiomyosarcomas are usually not responsive to chemotherapy or radiation. The most useful treatment modality is surgical removal with wide excision of the margins. Surgery commonly comprises of extrafascial TAH with bilateral salpingo-oopherectomy and formal surgical staging. While most leiomyosarcomas are usually resistant to radiation and chemotherapy, each case behaves differently and some cases may even respond to radiotherapy or chemotherapy.

11.3: OVARIAN CANCER

11.3.1: Definition

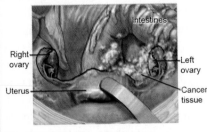 **Fig. 11.3.1:** Ovarian cancer	Ovarian cancer develops most often in women aged 50–70 years. In the United States, it is the second most common gynecologic cancer. However, cancer of the ovaries has the worst prognosis in comparison to any other type of gynecologic cancer. As a result, it is the fifth most common cause of cancer deaths in women. Ovarian cancer usually does not cause symptoms, until it is large or is in an advanced stage.	There are many types of ovarian cancer. Nearly 80% of the cancers are epithelial cell cancers, which begin from the surface epithelium of the ovaries. Other types of ovarian cancers include the germ cell tumors or the stromal cell tumors. The ovarian cancer is one of the most aggressive types of cancers, which can spread directly to the surrounding tissues and through the lymphatic system to other parts of the pelvis and abdomen. It can also spread through the bloodstream to the distant body organs, mainly the liver and lungs.

| Picture | Medical/Surgical Description | Management/Clinical Highlights |

11.3.2: Diagnosis (A and B)

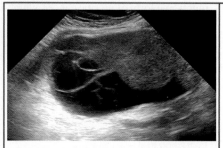

Fig. 11.3.2A: Transvaginal scan in a 52-year-old patient with complaints of anorexia, bloating sensation, vague pain in the left iliac fossa, fatigue, weakness, increased frequency of micturition and history of severe weight loss since 1 month

Transvaginal scan in this patient, shown in Figure 11.3.2A, demonstrated presence of a multiseptated complex adnexal mass having heterogeneous solid areas. These features were highly suggestive of a malignancy. Discrimination between benign and malignant lesions of the ovary on imaging studies has been discussed in Section 10.

For establishing the diagnosis of ovarian cancer, the investigations which are most commonly performed include ultrasonography, CT and MRI. Biopsy of the tumor tissue and examination of the ascitic fluid may also be performed to reach a definitive diagnosis. In addition, blood tests to measure levels of ovarian cancer markers, such as cancer antigen 125 (CA 125) may also be performed.

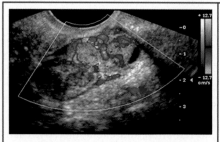

Fig. 11.3.2B: Transvaginal sonography color Doppler in the same patient

Color Doppler ultrasound in the patient described in Figure 11.3.2A showed increased blood flow. Biopsy revealed presence of an ovarian cystadenocarcinoma.

Presence of low pulsatile index (< 1) and low resistance index (< 0.4) on Doppler ultrasound is suggestive of high blood flow within the mass. This is indicative of a malignant growth.

11.3.3: Clinical Staging

11.3.3.1: Spread of Ovarian Cancer (A and B)

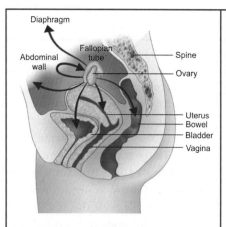

Fig 11.3.3.1A: Spread of ovarian cancer via transcelomic implantation

Figure 11.3.3.1A demonstrates the spread of ovarian cancer to the peritoneal cells via transcelomic implantation. The cancer can also spread to the epithelial lining of bowel or bladder.

The ovarian cancer has a propensity to spread in the early stages. The epithelial tumors arising from the epithelial lining of the ovaries are the most common ovarian tumors. Since the ovaries are located in the pelvic cavity and therefore have a direct access to it, the cancer cells can easily get disseminated to the cells lining the peritoneal cavity and spread directly from there via transcelomic implantation.

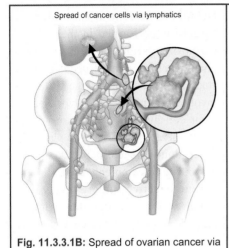

Fig. 11.3.3.1B: Spread of ovarian cancer via lymphatics

Figure 11.3.3.1B demonstrates the spread of ovarian cancer via lymphatics.

The initial spread of ovarian cancer is via transcelomic implantation and in later stages via lymphatics and blood vessels. The tumor can spread to distant organs such as lungs and liver through blood vessels.

11.3.3.2: Staging of Ovarian Cancer (A to D)

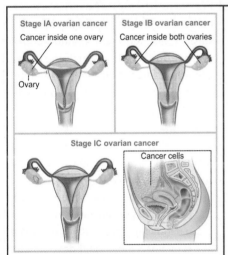

Fig. 11.3.3.2A: Stage I of ovarian cancer

In stage I ovarian cancer, cancer growth is limited to the ovaries. This stage is divided into three subgroups:

Stage IA: The growth is limited to one ovary. There is no ascites containing malignant cells, no tumor is present on the external surface and capsule is intact.

Stage IB: The growth is limited to both the ovaries. There is no ascites containing malignant cells, no tumor is present on the external surface and capsule is intact.

Stage IC: The cancer is either at stage IA or IB, but with tumor on the surface of one or both the ovaries or with capsule ruptured or with ascites present, containing malignant cells or with positive peritoneal washings.

Primary treatment for stage IA (grade I) epithelial ovarian cancer is surgical, i.e. a TAH and a bilateral salpingo-oophorectomy and surgical staging. The uterus and contralateral ovary can be preserved in woman with stage IA, grade I disease, who desire to preserve their fertility.

However, such women must be periodically monitored with routine pelvic examinations and determination of serum CA 125 levels.

For stage IA and IB (grade II and grade III), and IC disease, treatment options include additional chemotherapy or radiotherapy besides surgery as described above. Chemotherapy is the more commonly used option. According to the current treatment recommendations, the treatment must be in form of either cisplatin or carboplatin or combination therapy of either of these drugs with paclitaxel for three to four cycles. Short course of melphalan (four to six cycles) may be preferable in the older women.

Radiotherapy could be administered either in the form of intraperitoneal radiocolloids (P-32) or whole abdominal radiation.

Picture	Medical/Surgical Description	Management/Clinical Highlights

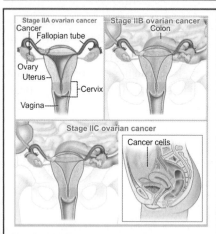

Fig. 11.3.3.2B: Stage II ovarian cancer

Stage II cancer growth involves one or both ovaries with pelvic extension. There are three subgroups:

Stage IIA: The cancer has spread to the uterus and/or fallopian tubes.

Stage IIB: There is extension to other pelvic tissues such as the rectum or bladder.

Stage IIC: The cancer is either at stage IIA or IIB, with tumor on the surface of one or both ovaries or with capsule ruptured or with ascites present containing malignant cells or with positive peritoneal washings.

Debulking surgery or cytoreductive surgery is performed in the stage II cases of ovarian cancer. Adjuvant chemotherapy can be used in some stage II cases such as stage II disease involving the pelvis, high grade disease, clear cell histology, etc. Intravenous chemotherapy comprising of platinum-based doublet such as paclitaxel and carboplatin is commonly used.

Cytoreductive surgery involves an initial exploratory procedure with the removal of as much disease as possible (both tumor and the associated metastatic disease).

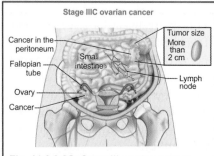

Fig. 11.3.3.2C: Stage III ovarian cancer

Stage III tumor involves one or both the ovaries, with peritoneal implants outside the pelvis and/or positive retroperitoneal or inguinal nodes. Superficial liver metastasis equals stage III. Tumor is limited to the true pelvis, but with histologically proven extension to small bowel or omentum. It can be divided into the following subtypes:

Stage IIIA: Tumor is grossly limited to true pelvis with negative nodes, but with histologically confirmed seeding of abdominal/peritoneal surfaces.

Stage IIIB: Tumor of one or both ovaries with histologically confirmed implants of abdominal peritoneal surfaces, none exceeding 2 cm in diameter. Nodes are negative.

Stage IIIC: Abdominal implants > 2 cm in diameter and/or positive retroperitoneal or inguinal lymph nodes.

For stage III cases of ovarian cancer, treatment comprises of cytoreductive surgery and adjuvant chemotherapy. Cytoreductive surgery includes abdominal hysterectomy and bilateral salpingo-oophorectomy, complete omentectomy and resection of metastatic lesions from the peritoneal surface. The surgeon also takes the biopsies or removes some of the lymph nodes in the abdomen and pelvis. They may also have to remove the omentum, the appendix and part of the peritoneum.

Chemotherapy previously comprised of cyclophosphamide and doxorubicin. Nowadays, most surgeons prefer platinum and taxane-based chemotherapy such as intravenous carboplatin and paclitaxel for six cycles. For patients with no clinical evidence of disease and negative tumor markers at the completion of chemotherapy, the woman must be evaluated again for residual disease. Second-look laparotomy as done in the past is no longer recommended due to poor prognosis. If there is an evidence of residual disease, the woman must be considered as being platinum resistant. For women with platinum-resistant cancer after a platinum and taxane-based combination, the preferred first line agent is pegylated liposomal doxorubicin.

Picture	Medical/Surgical Description	Management/Clinical Highlights

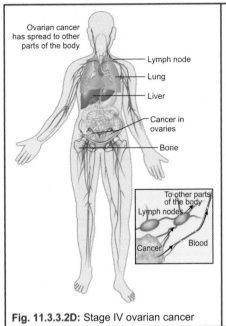

Fig. 11.3.3.2D: Stage IV ovarian cancer

Stage IV growth involves one or both ovaries with distant metastasis. If pleural effusion is present, there must be positive cytological test results to allot a case to stage IV. Parenchymal liver metastasis equals stage IV. The above mentioned categories are based on the findings of clinical examination and/or surgical exploration.

For stage IV cases of ovarian cancer, palliative treatment comprises of cytoreductive surgery and adjuvant chemotherapy. The goal of cytoreductive surgery is resection of the primary tumor and all the metastatic disease. If this is not possible, the goal must be to reduce the tumor burden by resection of the tumor to an "optimal status". The study by the Gynecologic Oncology Group (2004) has defined optimum debulking as residual tumor diameter of < 1 cm. Many patients are given a few cycles of chemotherapy following the surgery. For some patients with completely resected disease, whole abdominal radiation therapy may be used.

11.4: CERVICAL INTRAEPITHELIAL NEOPLASIA

11.4.1: Definition (A to C)

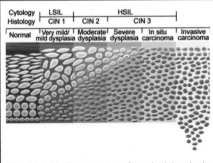

Fig. 11.4.1A: Progression of cervical dysplasia

Figure 11.4.1A shows diagrammatic progression of cervical dysplasia. Dysplasia is the process, which is associated with an abnormal maturation of cells within a tissue. This process differs from metaplasia in the sense that normal differentiated cells are replaced by abnormal undifferentiated cells unlike metaplasia in which one type of differentiated epithelial cells are replaced by another type of normal differentiated epithelial cells. Dysplasia is often indicative of an early neoplastic process and is characterized by presence of nuclear changes such as anisocytosis (abnormality in size), poikilocytosis (abnormality in shape), hyperchromatism and presence of mitotic figures.

Dysplasias can be graded as follows:

Mild dysplasia (CIN-I): The undifferentiated cells are confined to the lower one-third of the epithelium. The cells are more differentiated toward the surface. According to Bethesda classification, CIN-I has been lately described as low-grade squamous intraepithelial lesion (LSIL).

Moderate dysplasia (CIN-II): Undifferentiated cells occupy the lower 50–75% of the epithelial thickness.

Severe dysplasia and carcinoma in situ (CIN-III): In this grade of dysplasia, the entire thickness of epithelium is replaced by abnormal cells. The basement membrane, however, remains intact and there is no stromal infiltration. According to latest Bethesda classification CIN-II and CIN-III are described as high-grade squamous intraepithelial lesions (HSIL). The presence of HSIL is significant because these lesions have a high-degree potential to progress to invasive cancer that needs to be treated.

Picture	Medical/Surgical Description	Management/Clinical Highlights
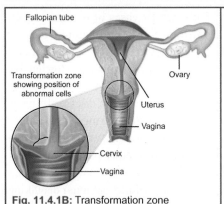 **Fig. 11.4.1B:** Transformation zone	The cervix is anatomically composed of two parts: ectocervix and endocervix. The part of the cervix projecting into the vagina is known as the portio vaginalis or ectocervix, whereas the region of the cervix opening into the uterine cavity is known as the endocervix. The ectocervix is lined by squamous cells, while endocervical cells are mainly of the columnar type. The transformation zone lies at the junction of ectocervix and endocervix.	Columnar cells are constantly changing into squamous cells in the transformation zone. Since the cells in the squamocolumnar zone are constantly changing, this is the most common place for rapid cell turnover, squamous metaplasia and the site of oncogenic transformation or development of cervical malignancy.
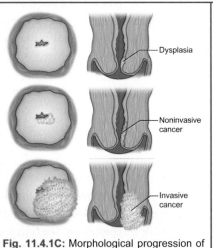 **Fig. 11.4.1C:** Morphological progression of cervical cancer	Figure 11.4.1C shows morphological progression of cervical cancer. Though cervical cancer may be sometimes visible on clinical examination, changes such as dysplasia and carcinoma are usually not visible on clinical examination. These changes may be diagnosed using a Pap smear or colposcopic examination.	Cancer of cervix is usually the end stage of the spectrum of disorders progressing from mild through moderate to severe dysplasia and carcinoma in situ. The peak incidence of occurrence of dysplasias appears to be 10 years earlier than that of frank invasive cancer. Presence of dysplasia may be associated with minimal findings on clinical examination.

11.4.2: Histopathological Examination (A to C)

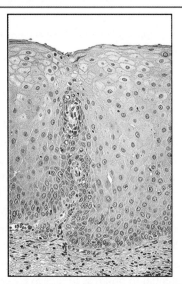 **Fig. 11.4.2A:** Normal cervical epithelium (HPE)	Figure 11.4.2A shows histopathological appearance of normal cervical epithelium.	In the normal cervix, the ectocervix is composed of nonkeratinized squamous epithelium, whereas the endocervix is composed of columnar epithelium. The columnar epithelium of cervix is thrown into longitudinal folds and invaginations, which form the endocervical glands. Presence of these crypts and channels may create problems in detection of carcinoma.

Picture	Medical/Surgical Description	Management/Clinical Highlights
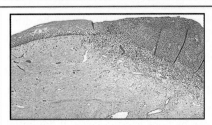 **Fig. 11.4.2B:** Histopathological picture showing the transformation of the normal cervical squamous epithelium (at the left) into dysplasia (at the right)	Figure 11.4.2B shows transformation zone of the normal cervical squamous epithelium at the left hand side, which gets transformed into dysplastic changes at the right hand side.	Treatment of dysplasia at early stages prevents conversion into invasive cancer at a later date. Treatment of CIN I lesions is given to the adolescents only if the lesion persists beyond 2 years. For CIN II in adult women and CIN III lesions at any age, treatment in form of excision or ablation is recommended. "See and treat" approach involving loop excision at the time of colposcopic examination is also an acceptable option. Treatment of CIN is presently limited to ablative or excisional procedures.
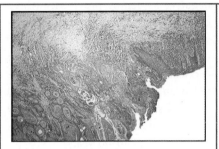 **Fig. 11.4.2C:** Histopathology of invasive squamous cell carcinoma	Histopathological examination in case of invasive carcinoma as presented in Figure 11.4.2C shows nests of squamous cancer cells, which have invaded the underlying stroma in the center and left side of the figure.	Presence of abnormal results on Pap test or symptoms of cervical cancer may mandate further testing in form of colposcopy, colposcopic directed biopsy and endocervical curettage, which can help in confirming if abnormal cells are dysplastic or cancerous.

11.4.3: Pap Smear for Diagnosis (A to E)

Picture		
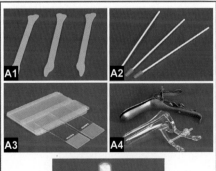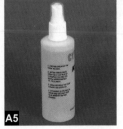 **Figs 11.4.3A (A1 to A5):** Equipment for taking Pap smear: (A1) Ayre's spatula; (A2) Endocervical brush; (A3) Slides; (A4) Per vaginal speculum; (A5) Fixative	Since its introduction in the 1940s, cytological screening in form of Pap smear has become the investigation of choice for detection of precancerous lesions of the cervix. The widespread introduction of the Papanicolaou test for cervical cancer screening has resulted in significantly reducing the incidence and mortality of cervical cancer in developed countries.	According to the latest recommendations by the "Screening for cervical cancer; US Preventive Services Task Force" (USPSTF, 2012) recommendations statement, screening for cervical cancer must be done within the age groups of 21–29 years with Pap smear testing to be done every 3 years and in the age group within 30–65 years, a combination of cytology and human papillomavirus (HPV) testing to be done every 5 years. Screening for cervical cancer in women must not be initiated before the age of 21 years, regardless of the age of initiation of sexual activity.

Picture	Medical/Surgical Description	Management/Clinical Highlights

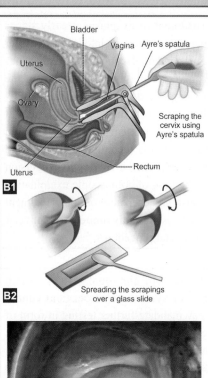

B1

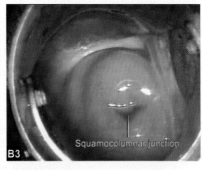

Spreading the scrapings over a glass slide

B2

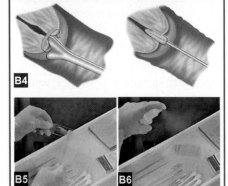

Squamocolumnar junction

B3

The procedure of performing a Pap smear comprises of the following steps:

- The patient is made to lie in a dorsal position and adequate light must be used to visualize the cervix and vagina properly.
- After exposing the cervix with a Cusco's speculum, an endocervical brush or a cotton-tipped swab must be placed inside the endocervix and rotated firmly against the canal in order to take an endocervical sample, which is then placed on the glass slide.
- Next, the Ayre's spatula must be placed against the cervix with the longer protrusion in the cervical canal.
- The spatula must be rotated clockwise for 360° against the cervix. This would help in scraping the entire transformation zone.
- The sample from the spatula is placed onto the glass slide by rotating the spatula against the slide in a clockwise manner.
- The slide must be immediately fixed with the help of a spray fixative, which is held at a distance of about 9–12 inches.

Pap smear screening should be done every 3 years in an average-risk women aged 21–29 years. For an average-risk women aged 30–65 years, Pap smear testing must be done every 3 years or a combination of Pap and HPV testing can be done every 5 years, if the initial results are negative. Women with an increased risk of cancer (history of exposure to DES, CIN II, CIN III or cervical cancer, HIV infection or immunosuppression) require more frequent screening. Women aged 65 years or older who have had adequate negative screening previously (three consecutive negative cytology tests within the previous 10 years) may not be required to undergo further screening for cervical cancer. Older women who have not been adequately screened should undergo screening (either by cytology every 3 years or co-testing every 5 years until the age of 70–75 years).

Figs 11.4.3B (B1 to B6): Procedure of taking a Pap smear: (B1) Diagrammatic representation of the procedure; (B2) Normal squamocolumnar junction; (B3) Ayre's spatula inserted for taking ectocervical scrapings; (B4) Endocervical brush inserted inside to take endocervical scrapings; (B5) Scrapings spread on the slide; (B6) Spraying of fixative to fix the slide

Picture	Medical/Surgical Description	Management/Clinical Highlights

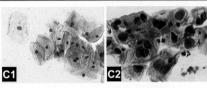

Figs 11.4.3C (C1 and C2): Histopathological appearance: (C1) Normal Pap smear result; (C2) Abnormal Pap smear result

As previously mentioned, the normal ectocervix is composed of nonkeratinized squamous epithelium. Abnormal Pap smear (Figure 11.4.3C2) is associated with atypical cells having features of atypia and dysplasia such as anisocytosis (abnormality in size), poikilocytosis (abnormality in shape), increased nuclear-cytoplasmic ratio, polymorphism, hyperchromatism of the nuclei, loss of nuclear polarity, presence of mitotic figures, etc.

Pap smear is an outpatient technique of screening for premalignant cervical changes. This enables early intervention in order to prevent conversion of premalignant changes into invasive malignant lesions.

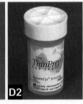

Figs 11.4.3D (D1 and D2): Equipment for liquid-based cytology: (D1) Cervex-Brush®; (D2) ThinPrep vial

Figures 11.4.3 (D1 and D2) demonstrate the equipment used for performing sampling using liquid-based cytology methods. The sample is taken using a plastic spatula with either an endocervical brush or a cervical broom, also known as the cervex. The figure also shows the vial containing the preservative solution into which the endocervical brush is rinsed. After collection of the sample, the vial is capped, labeled and sent to the laboratory, where it is processed.

Liquid-based cytology is a new way of sampling and preparing cervical cells. While the conventional "Pap smear" involves direct preparation of the slide from the cervical scrape obtained, the procedure of "ThinPrep" involves making a suspension of cells from the sample, which is then used to produce a thin layer of cells on a slide. Advantage of liquid-based Pap smear is that it is associated with fewer drying artifacts. Since the cells are spread more evenly on the surface of a glass slide, the chances of unsatisfactory smears are reduced.

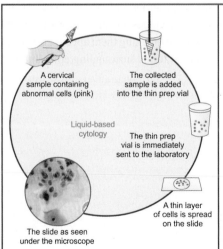

Fig. 11.4.3E: Procedure of performing a liquid-based cytology

Using this technique, the cells collected from the cervix are placed in a preservative fluid, which is then sent to the laboratory rather than being directly spread onto a slide. At the laboratory, the sample is mixed and treated to disperse the cells and remove unwanted material (blood, mucus and inflammatory material). The sample is then centrifuged to form a cell pellet, which is then fixed on a glass slide and stained by the Papanicolaou staining method and then examined under a microscope.

According to the latest recommendations by the "Screening for cervical cancer; US Preventive Services Task Force" (USPSTF, 2012) recommendations statement liquid-based testing has not been shown to significantly improve the accuracy of Pap test in comparison to the conventional cytology testing using a Pap smear.

11.4.4: Diagnosis by Colposcopy (A to D)

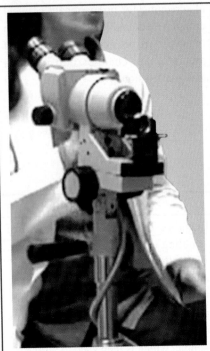

Fig 11.4.4A: Colposcope

A colposcope is like a small microscope with a light and enables the gynecologist to perform a thorough examination of the cervix. Colposcopy is an office-based procedure during which the cervix is examined under illumination and magnification before and after application of dilute acetic acid and Lugol's iodine.

If abnormal cells are found in a Pap smear test or liquid-based cytology, the patient may be referred for a colposcopic examination and/or a colposcopic directed biopsy. While the Pap smear detects abnormal cells, colposcopy helps in locating the abnormal lesions.

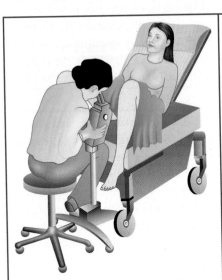

Fig. 11.4.4B: Colposcopic examination

Colposcopic examination comprises of the following steps:
- The patient is placed in the lithotomy position.
- Under all aseptic precautions, a speculum is inserted into the vagina.
- The colposcope is brought into the position. The perineum, vulva, vagina and cervix must be examined for presence of lesions using the colposcope's white light and then green light.
- The entire cervix must be viewed both under the low and high power magnification. Higher-power magnification helps in visualization of small details and features.
- Cervix is visualized after the application of both dilute 5% acetic acid and Lugol's iodine in order to enhance any abnormal epithelial findings.
- A scoring system such as "the Reid Colposcopic Index" may be used to help the colposcopist in classifying the colposcopic appearance.

Satisfactory colposcopy requires visualization of the entire squamocolumnar junction and transformation zone for the presence of any visible lesions. Both a regular white light and a green light are used during colposcopy. The green filter enhances visualization of blood vessels by making them appear darker in contrast to the surrounding epithelium.

Picture	Medical/Surgical Description	Management/Clinical Highlights

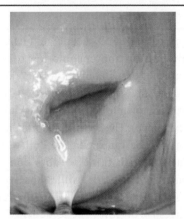

Fig. 11.4.4C: Normal appearance of cervix

The normal appearance of cervix on colposcopic examination is shown in Figure 11.4.4C. On colposcopic examination, the squamous epithelium of cervix appears pale and transparent in color, having a pinkish hue. The columnar epithelium of endocervix appears dark red in color. Usually no apparent vascular pattern can be visualized over the original squamous epithelium.

The indications for colposcopic examination are as follows:
- Presence of abnormal cells on the Pap smear: In these cases colposcopy helps in assessing the location and extent of abnormal lesions on the cervix.
- Biopsy can be taken from the areas of abnormality.
- Conservative surgery (e.g. conization) can be performed under colposcopic guidance.
- Follow-up examination of cases that have undergone conservative therapy.

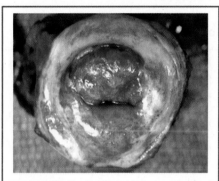

Fig. 11.4.4D: Cervix with carcinoma as observed on colposcopic examination

Squamous cell carcinoma of cervix in early stages may appear as acetowhite lesions or areas of leukoplakia with uneven density of the surface epithelium. There may be areas of coarse punctuation or mosaicism in the periphery of these lesions. Presence of atypical vessels having abnormal caliber and form are the hallmarks of invasive vascularization. There may be presence of hemorrhagic changes or bleeding on touch.

The characteristic features of malignancy and premalignancy on colposcopic examination include changes such as acetowhite areas, abnormal vascular patterns, mosaic pattern, punctuation and failure to uptake iodine stain.

Later stages of cancer may not require colposcopic examination for diagnosis because in these cases there is presence of ulcerated lesions, which may be visible even without the use of magnification. In these cases punch biopsy of the periphery of the lesion rather than the center of ulcerated lesion helps in establishing the diagnosis.

11.4.5: Visual Inspection under Lugol's Iodine or VILI (A and B)

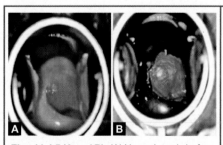

Figs 11.4.5 (A and B): (A) Normal cervix before the application of Lugol's iodine; (B) Normal cervix after the application of Lugol's iodine

VILI or visual inspection under Lugol's iodine, also known as Schiller's test involves application of Lugol's iodine solution onto the cervix with the help of a cotton swab and is allowed to remain there for at least 30 seconds. The cervix is then visualized with the naked eye to identify any changes in color.

This test is based on the fact that normal squamous epithelial cells contain glycogen, whereas precancerous or invasive cells and normal columnar cells contain little or no glycogen. Therefore, on performing the VILI test, iodine is taken up by the glycogen in normal squamous cells, turning them to mahogany brown or black. This is known as VILI negative test.

Precancerous or invasive cancer cells will not take up iodine and would appear as well-defined thick yellow-saffron areas. This is known as VILI positive test.

11.4.6: Visual Inspection under Acetic Acid or VIA (A and B)

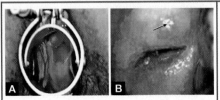

Figs 11.4.6 (A and B): (A) Normal cervix after the application of acetic acid; (B) Abnormal cervix following the application of acetic acid (area of abnormality is indicated by an arrow)

In areas where facilities for Pap smear screening do not exist, visual inspection with 5% acetic acid (VIA) can be done.

Application of 5% acetic acid causes dehydration and coagulation of the abnormal areas containing increased nuclear material and protein, which turns acetowhite (opaque and white in appearance). The areas of abnormalities can then be biopsied. The dull white plaques with faint borders can be considered as LSIL, while those with sharp borders and thick plaque are suggestive of HSIL. The acetic acid does not affect the mature glycogen producing epithelium.

11.4.7: Cone Biopsy for Treatment of Cervical Intraepithelial Neoplasia (A to D)

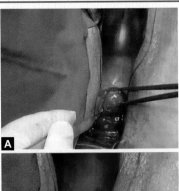
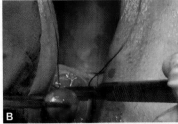
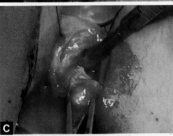
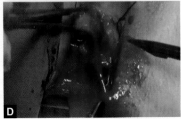

Figs 11.4.7 (A to D): Procedure of cone biopsy

Cone biopsy serves as both a diagnostic and therapeutic procedure. The procedure involves the removal of entire area of abnormality [Figures 11.4.7 (A to D)]. It is capable of providing tissue for HPE. The cone biopsy may be performed under general or local anesthesia. This method involves obtaining a wide cone of excision including the entire outer margin of the lesion and the entire endocervical lining.

Indications for cone biopsy are as follows:
- The area of the abnormality is large, or its inner margin has receded into the cervical canal.
- The squamocolumnar junction is not completely visible on colposcopy.
- There is discrepancy between the findings of cytology and colposcopy.
- There is a suspicion of microinvasion based on the results of biopsy, colposcopy or cytology.
- The findings of endocervical curettage are positive for CIN II or CIN III.

Picture	Medical/Surgical Description	Management/Clinical Highlights

11.4.8: Loop Excision (A to C)

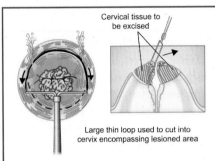

Cervical tissue to be excised

Large thin loop used to cut into cervix encompassing lesioned area

Fig. 11.4.8A: Large loop excision of the transformation zone

In the procedure of large loop excision of the transformation zone, the loop of wire is advanced into the cervix lateral to the lesion until the required depth is reached. The loop is then taken across to the opposite side and a cone of tissue is removed. The area of abnormal cells is removed completely using a loop of wire and electrosurgery.

LLETZ stands for "large loop excision of the transformation zone" and is commonly the name used in the UK. In the USA, this procedure is called LEEP—loop electrosurgical excision procedure. This method basically uses low voltage diathermy and may be done at the same time as colposcopy. It is an outpatient treatment and is usually performed under local anesthesia. If a large area of tissue needs to be removed, or if the patient is very anxious about the treatment, the surgery may also be performed under general anesthesia.

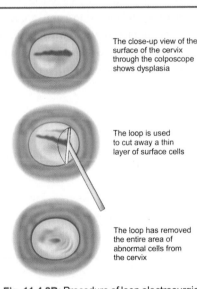

The close-up view of the surface of the cervix through the colposcope shows dysplasia

The loop is used to cut away a thin layer of surface cells

The loop has removed the entire area of abnormal cells from the cervix

Fig. 11.4.8B: Procedure of loop electrosurgical excision procedure

In this procedure, a thin wire loop that carries an electric current is used to remove abnormal areas of the cervix. The excised area of the cervix removed is sent to the laboratory for HPE. This electric energy is also used to coagulate the blood vessels on the surface of the cervix.

The procedure of LEEP is one of the most commonly used treatment modalities for management of CIN II and CIN III lesions observed on colposcopy and/or cone biopsy. It is an easy-to-use, cost-effective method associated with high success rates.

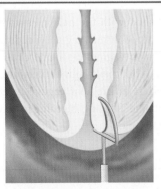

Fig. 11.4.8C: Magnified view showing the procedure of loop electrosurgical excision

The LEEP equipment comprises of a thin wire loop electrode attached to an electrosurgical generator, which generates current to cut away the cervical tissue that comes in the vicinity of the wire loop. LEEP is even simpler than LLETZ and is applicable anywhere in the lower genital tract whereas LLETZ is applicable only to the cervix.

Loops of various shapes and sizes can be used during the procedure depending on the size of the lesion. The excision is usually performed to a depth of 8 mm and extends 4–5 mm beyond the region of the lesion.

11.5: INVASIVE CANCER OF THE CERVIX

11.5.1: Definition

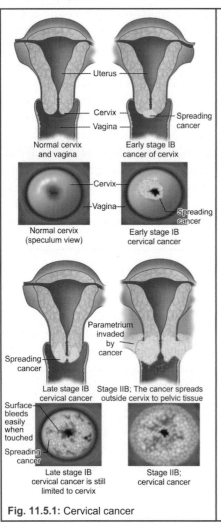

Uterus

Cervix

Vagina

Spreading cancer

Normal cervix and vagina

Early stage IB cancer of cervix

Cervix

Vagina

Spreading cancer

Normal cervix (speculum view)

Early stage IB cervical cancer

Parametrium invaded by cancer

Spreading cancer

Late stage IB cervical cancer

Stage IIB; The cancer spreads outside cervix to pelvic tissue

Surface bleeds easily when touched

Spreading cancer

Late stage IB cervical cancer is still limited to cervix

Stage IIB; cervical cancer

Fig. 11.5.1: Cervical cancer

Cervical cancer develops from the cervix. Cervical cancer usually results from infection with the HPV transmitted at the time of sexual intercourse. This cancer may result in abnormal bleeding such as irregular vaginal bleeding, postcoital bleeding, bleeding in between periods, etc. This cancer usually affects women aged 35–55 years, but it can also affect women as young as 20 years.

Pap smear is able to accurately detect cervical cancers in up to 90% of the cases in the early stages, even before the symptoms have developed. In case an abnormality is detected on Pap smear, a colposcopic examination and biopsy may be performed to further confirm the diagnosis. Different types of biopsies, which can be performed are punch biopsy, endocervical curettage, cone biopsy, etc. Once the cervical cancer has been diagnosed, its exact size and stage are determined. Staging begins with a physical examination of the pelvis. Various investigations, which help in the staging include cystoscopy, a chest X-ray, sigmoidoscopy, CT, MRI, barium enema, bone and liver scans and positron emission tomography.

11.5.2: Imaging Studies for Diagnosis (A to E)

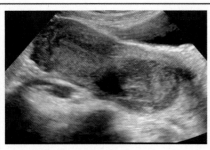

Fig. 11.5.2A: Transabdominal sonography showing solid heterogeneous cervical mass

Transabdominal sonography in a 52-year-old postmenopausal patient with the history of abnormal vaginal bleeding revealed presence of a heterogeneous cervical mass.

Diagnosis of cervical cancer is established with the help of symptoms such as abnormal vaginal bleeding and offensive vaginal discharge or leukorrhea. Abnormal vaginal bleeding may manifest as irregular vaginal bleeding, postcoital bleeding, bleeding in between periods, etc.

PART II ❖ GYNECOLOGY

Picture	Medical/Surgical Description	Management/Clinical Highlights
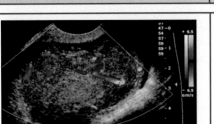 **Fig. 11.5.2B:** Color Doppler of the same patient	In the same patient as described in Figure 11.5.2A, a color Doppler examination was performed, which showed presence of randomly distributed irregular vessels in the mass arising from the posterior aspect of the cervix. This was highly suggestive of a malignancy. CT examination as shown in the next figure was performed, which revealed the diagnosis of stage I cervical malignancy. The tumor was limited to the cervix. No lymph node involvement or spread to adjacent organs was observed on the CT examination.	Pelvic examination shows the following findings in a patient with cervical cancer: • A growth may be present on the cervix, which bleeds upon touching. • The growth may be cauliflower-like-proliferative growth or an ulcerative lesion. • Uterus may be bulky due to pyometra. • Involvement of uterosacral ligaments may present as an area of thickened induration on pelvic and rectal examination.
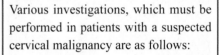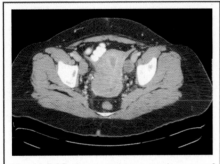 **Fig. 11.5.2C:** Computed tomography scan of the same patient as shown in Figure 11.5.2B	In the same patient as described in Figure 11.5.2A, a CT scan was performed. It showed a large lobulated cervical mass with central hypoattenuation.	Various investigations, which must be performed in patients with a suspected cervical malignancy are as follows: *PAP smear*: Pap smear is able to accurately detect cervical cancers in up to 90% of the cases in the early stages, even before the symptoms have developed. *Colposcopic examination and biopsy*: In case an abnormality is detected on Pap smear, a colposcopic examination and biopsy may be performed to further confirm the diagnosis. *Tissue biopsy*: HPE helps in establishing the accurate diagnosis. Different types of biopsies, which can be performed, are punch biopsy, endocervical curettage, cone biopsy, etc. *Imaging studies*: These include ultrasound (transabdominal, transvaginal and color Doppler) and CT examination [Figs 11.5.2 (A to E)]. *Investigations for staging*: Various investigations, which help in the staging the cancer include cystoscopy, chest X-ray, sigmoidoscopy, CT, MRI, barium enema, bone and liver scans, and positron emission tomography.

Picture	Medical/Surgical Description	Management/Clinical Highlights
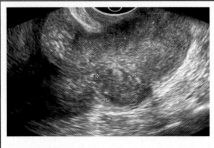 **Fig. 11.5.2D:** Transvaginal sonography of cervix of a 47-year-old patient with severe suprapubic pain	Figure 11.5.2D shows TVS of cervix in another patient, 47 years old, who presented with severe suprapubic pain. Transvaginal sonography showed presence of a solid cervical mass measuring 3 × 2 × 2.5 cm.	Biopsy of the cervical lesion helps in establishing the diagnosis in most of the cases.
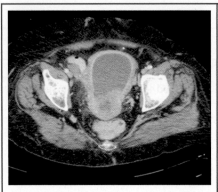 **Fig. 11.5.2E:** CT scan of the same patient as shown in Figure 11.5.2D	Figure 11.5.2E shows CT scan of the same patient as in Figure 11.5.2D, showing spread of the cancer. CT scan, however, is not accurate for assessment of subtle parametrial invasion or deep invasion of cervical stroma. Moreover, it may be sometimes difficult to differentiate between reactive nodal hyperplasia and lymph node enlargement due to true metastatic disease.	CT scan is one of the most commonly used imaging modalities for evaluation of metastasis and lymph node involvement in cases of cervical carcinoma. CT scan also provides a high resolution image of the pelvic anatomy, especially when used with a contrast medium. Though CT scanning is not a component of FIGO (International Federation of Gynecology and Obstetrics) staging, it does give a fairly accurate idea about the tumor size and extension, and presence of enlarged lymph nodes or distant metastasis.

11.5.3: Cervical Punch Biopsy for Diagnosis

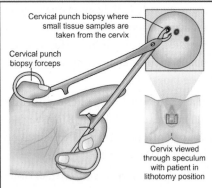 Cervical punch biopsy where small tissue samples are taken from the cervix Cervical punch biopsy forceps Cervix viewed through speculum with patient in lithotomy position **Fig. 11.5.3:** Cervical punch biopsy	Cervical punch biopsy is performed as an outpatient department procedure, in which small pieces of tissue are removed from the affected areas using punch biopsy forceps. More than one punch may be taken from the areas at the time of performing biopsy. Biopsy specimen is then sent for HPE. It is purely for the diagnostic and not for curative purposes.	In presence of HSIL (CIN II and III), cervical punch biopsy is required in order to confirm the presence of any invasive lesion. Following the identification of biopsy site, the cervical punch biopsy forceps are used to obtain the specimen under colposcopic visualization. Specimens are firstly obtained from the most inferior aspect of the cervix to avoid bleeding from the biopsy site and obscuring other biopsy sites. Monsel's paste or silver nitrate can be used to achieve hemostasis after cervical punch biopsy.

Picture	Medical/Surgical Description	Management/Clinical Highlights

11.5.4: Staging of Cervical Cancer as Devised by International Federation of Gynecologists and Obstetricians (A to D)

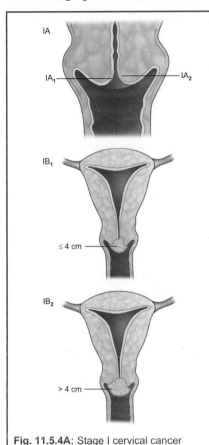

Fig. 11.5.4A: Stage I cervical cancer

Stage I cervical carcinoma is confined to uterus (extension to corpus should be disregarded). It can be subclassified as follows:

IA: This includes invasive carcinoma diagnosed only by microscopy. All other macroscopically visible lesions—even with superficial invasion—are classified as IB. Stage IA tumors can be further subclassified as:
- IA1: Measured stromal invasion is 3 mm or less in depth and 7 mm or less in lateral spread
- IA2: Measured stromal invasion is more than 3 mm, but not more than 5 mm with a horizontal spread of 7 mm or less

IB: Clinically visible lesion confined to the cervix or microscopic lesion greater than IA2. This can be further subclassified as:
- IB1: Clinically visible lesion 4 cm or less in greatest dimension
- IB2: Clinically visible lesion more than 4 cm.

For stage IA cervical cancer, simple hysterectomy without pelvic node dissection proves useful in most cases. Conization with clear margins may be considered adequate in young patients with stage IA disease, who want to conserve their uterus. However, these patients require close follow-up including cytology, colposcopy and endocervical curettage.

For stage IB cancers, radical hysterectomy with pelvic lymph node dissection, or external beam and intracavitary radiotherapy proves useful.

Lymph node dissection is not required, if the depth of invasion is less than 3 mm and no lymphovascular invasion is noted on microscopic examination. Patients with lymphatic or the vascular channel infiltration require treatment as in stage IB.

Postoperative radiotherapy may be administered in cases where the nodes are positive.

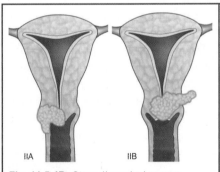

Fig. 11.5.4B: Stage II cervical cancer

Stage II cervical carcinoma invades beyond uterus but not to pelvic wall or to the lower third of vagina. This can be subclassified as follows:

IIA: Tumor without parametrial invasion

IIB: Tumor with parametrial invasion

The treatment options for stage IIA are surgical treatment or radiotherapy or both combined surgery and radiotherapy. Radiotherapy can be either in the form of external beam and intracavitary radiotherapy.

Surgery includes a radical hysterectomy (Wertheim's hysterectomy or Schauta's vaginal hysterectomy, known as Mitra operation in India or extended vaginal hysterectomy). Wertheim's hysterectomy involves removal of the entire uterus, both adnexa, medial one-third of parametrium, uterosacral ligaments, upper 2–3 cm cuff of the vagina and dissection of pelvic lymph nodes. Oophorectomy is usually not necessary in premenopausal women.

Picture	Medical/Surgical Description	Management/Clinical Highlights
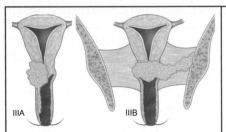 **Fig. 11.5.4C:** Stage III cervical cancer	Stage III cervical cancer extends to the pelvic wall and/or involves the lower third of the vagina and/or causes hydronephrosis or nonfunctioning kidney. This can be subclassified as follows: *IIIA*: Tumor involves lower third of vagina; no extension to pelvic wall. *IIIB*: Tumor extends to pelvic wall and/or causes hydronephrosis or nonfunctioning kidney.	In stage III cancer, as the tumor invades local organs, radiation therapy becomes the mainstay of treatment. However, in some cases combination of chemotherapy and radiotherapy is employed. Recently, the chemotherapy comprises of administering cisplatin (40 mg/m²) on weekly basis.
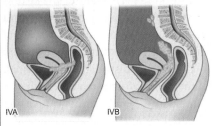 **Fig 11.5.4D:** Stage IV cervical cancer	Stage IV cervical carcinoma extends beyond the true pelvis or involves (biopsy proven) the bladder mucosa or rectal mucosa. Bullous edema does not qualify as criteria for stage IV disease. Stage IV disease is further subclassified as follows: IVA: Spread to adjacent organs (bladder, rectum or both) IVB: Distant metastasis	In stage IV cancer, due to invasion of local organs, radiation therapy has become the mainstay of treatment. Patients with distant metastases (stage IVB) also require chemotherapy with or without radiotherapy to control systemic disease. In advanced cases of cervical cancer, the most extreme surgery called pelvic exenteration in which all of the organs of the pelvis, including the bladder and rectum, are removed may be employed.

11.6: VULVAR CANCER

11.6.1: Definition (A and B)

Picture	Medical/Surgical Description	Management/Clinical Highlights
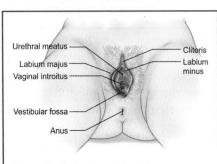 **Fig. 11.6.1A:** Anatomy of vulva	Vulvar cancer affects the vulva, an area of external female genitalia. Vulva refers to the region of female external genitalia and includes various anatomical structures such as labia majora, mons pubis, labia minora, clitoris, vestibule and the vaginal introitus.	In the United States, cancer of the vulva is the fourth most common gynecologic cancer, accounting for 3–4% of these cancers. Vulvar cancer usually occurs after menopause. The average age at diagnosis is 70 years. The main risk factor for developing vulvar cancer is the presence of precancerous/dysplastic changes, lichen sclerosus, etc. in the vulvar tissues.
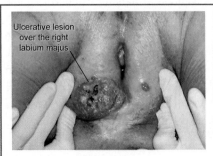 **Fig. 11.6.1B:** Vulvar cancer	In 50% of cases of vulvar cancer, presentation is in the form of a lump or a mass along with a long-standing history of pruritus. In majority of the cases, the lesion is in labia majora. The vulvar cancer can spread by direct extension to the adjacent structures; by lymphatic route to adjacent lymph nodes (inguinal group) and via hematogeneous route to distant organs such as lungs, liver and bone.	Diagnosis of vulvar cancer is done by carrying out biopsy of the abnormal skin over the vulva. Pap smear is obtained from the cervix. Colposcopic examination of the cervix and vagina must be performed due to common association with other squamous epithelial cell neoplasms of the lower genital tract. Wedge biopsy of the lesions is commonly performed. In case the lesion is < 1 cm in diameter, an excisional biopsy may be performed.

11.6.2: Staging of Vulvar Carcinoma (A to D)

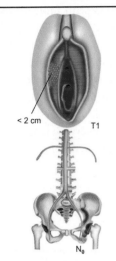

Fig. 11.6.2A: Stage I vulvar cancer

Stage I vulvar cancer is confined to the vulva or perineum, is less than 2 cm in greatest dimension and nodes are negative. It can be further subclassified as:

IA: Stromal invasion < 1 mm

IB: Stromal invasion > 1 mm

In the patients, where the stromal invasion by the tumor is < 1 mm, there is no risk of lymph node metastasis.

Groin dissection is usually required for the cases of vulvar cancer having more than 1 mm of stromal invasion. Groin dissection in the patients with early vulvar cancer should be in the form of a thorough inguinal-femoral lymphadenopathy and the dissected lymph nodes are then submitted for the HPE. If one microscopically positive groin lymph node is found, no additional treatment is required. In case of two or more positive groin nodes, there is an increased risk of groin and pelvic recurrence. In these cases, postoperative groin and pelvic radiation must be administered.

The management of patients with T1 cancer of the vulva is individualized. Radical local excision, rather than a radical vulvectomy is advocated for the primary lesions for patients with T1 tumors. If the lesions are present on the posterior lateral aspect of the vulva, where the preservation of clitoris is feasible, radical local excision appears to be the most appropriate form of therapy. In young patients with preclitoral lesions, small field of radiation therapy can be considered. Small vulvar lesions may respond to about 5,000 CGy of external radiation. After this radiation therapy, biopsy can be performed to rule out the presence of any residual disease. Some type of vulvar reconstruction is usually required after radical local excision.

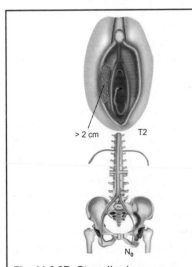

Fig. 11.6.2B: Stage II vulvar cancer

Stage II vulvar cancer is confined to vulva and/or perineum, is greater than 2 cm in greatest dimension and nodes are negative.

Management of patients with T2 and early T3 tumors comprises of radical vulvectomy with bilateral inguinal-femoral lymphadenectomy. Two types of surgical approaches, which can be used are:

1. En bloc approach using a single trapezoid or a butterfly incision.
2. The second approach comprises of groin dissection using three separate incisions.

Picture	Medical/Surgical Description	Management/Clinical Highlights
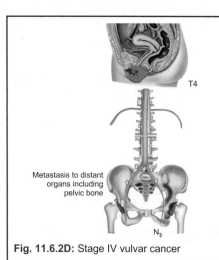 **Fig. 11.6.2C:** Stage III vulvar cancer	Stage III vulvar cancer include tumor of any size with: • Adjacent spread to the lower urethra or the anus • Unilateral regional lymph node metastasis.	In these cases, pelvic exenteration in combination with radical vulvectomy and bilateral groin dissection may be required. Nowadays, preoperative radiation with or without concurrent chemotherapy is regarded as the treatment of choice for patients with advanced vulvar cancer, who would otherwise require some form of pelvic exenteration.
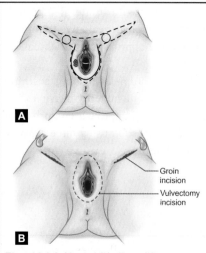 **Fig. 11.6.2D:** Stage IV vulvar cancer	Stage IV tumor invades the distant organs. It can be subclassified as follows: *IVA*: Invasion of upper urethra, bladder mucosa, rectal mucosa, pelvic bone or bilateral lymph node metastasis. *IVB*: Any distant metastasis including the pelvic lymph nodes.	In the cases of stage IV vulvar cancer, pelvic exenteration in combination with radical vulvectomy and bilateral groin dissection may be required. Bornow's combination therapy comprising of combined radiosurgical approach has been suggested in patients with advanced vulvar cancer, as an alternative to pelvic exenteration. In this approach, intracavitary radium with or without external irradiation is administered prior to the surgery, which usually comprises of radical vulvectomy and bilateral groin dissection for the treatment of external genital disease.

11.6.3: Treatment (A and B)

Picture	Medical/Surgical Description	Management/Clinical Highlights
Figs 11.6.3 (A and B): Two different types of surgical approaches: (A) Single butterfly incision; (B) Three separate skin incisions	Depending on the extent and type of the cancer, vulvectomy is performed. Lymphadenectomy may be also done depending upon the involvement of lymph nodes. For early stage cancers such treatment is usually all that is required. However for more advanced cancers, radiation therapy along with cisplatin is usually required. After the removal of the cancerous tissues, surgical reconstruction of the vulva and vagina may be performed.	Management of patients with T2 and early T3 vulvar cancers comprises of radical vulvectomy with bilateral inguinal-femoral lymphadenectomy. Two types of surgical approaches, which can be used are an en bloc approach using a single trapezoid or butterfly incision, and groin dissection. Groin dissection by three separate groin incisions is a recent modification and involves three separate incisions. This is associated with improved healing and comparatively less chances of wound separation (15%).

Picture	Medical/Surgical Description	Management/Clinical Highlights

11.7: CANCER OF THE FALLOPIAN TUBES

11.7.1: Diagnosis (A and B)

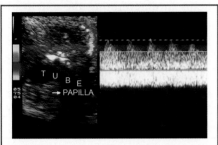

Fig. 11.7.1A: Patient with fallopian tube cancer having sausage shaped adnexal mass with presence of papillomatous protrusions and solid parts

Fallopian tube cancer, also known as tubal cancer, develops in the fallopian tubes that connect the ovaries and the uterus. It is very rare and accounts for only 1–2% of all cases of gynecologic cancers. The most common type of tumor is an adenocarcinoma and typically affects women between the ages of 50 years and 60 years. It is bilateral in nearly one-third cases. Women who have inherited the BRCA1 gene (linked with the development of ovarian and breast cancer) are also at an increased risk of developing fallopian tube cancer. This cancer is more common in nulliparous menopausal women.

Investigations comprise of Pap smear, which can be considered as an unreliable test for the diagnosis of fallopian tube cancer, and endometrial biopsy. Negative findings on the biopsy of the uterine curettings and a negative hysteroscopic examination in a patient with postmenopausal bleeding should raise the suspicion of fallopian tube cancer.

Imaging studies have an important role in the diagnosis of cancer of fallopian tubes. Transvaginal ultrasound may show presence of an adnexal mass as is seen in this case.

CA 125 test: An estimated 85% of women with gynecological disease have increased levels of CA 125.

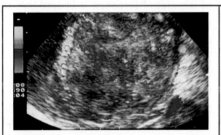

Fig. 11.7.1B: Color Doppler shows increased venous blood flow signals

Doppler flow velocimetry also plays an important role in the diagnosis of fallopian tube cancer and may show low resistance blood flow in the mass.

Treatment for fallopian tube cancer usually involves surgery and comprises of total abdominal hysterectomy with bilateral salpingo-oophorectomy, pelvic lymph node sampling and omentectomy. Postoperative radiotherapy, chemotherapy and hormonal therapy with progestogens may be required depending upon the spread of cancer.

11.8: BREAST CANCER

11.8.1: Definition (A and B)

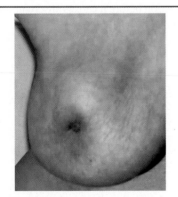

Fig. 11.8.1A: Nipple retraction

The most common sign of breast cancer is appearance of a new lump or mass in the breast. The mass may not be freely mobile, may have irregular margins and be fixed to the underlying tissues. Other possible signs of breast cancer include nipple discharge or redness, breast or nipple pain, swelling of part of the breast or dimpling or retraction of nipple, etc. Figure 11.8.1A shows nipple retraction in a patient who was later diagnosed as stage II invasive ductal carcinoma.

Breast cancer is a malignant growth, arising from the breast tissues, (ducts and/or lobules). Although breast cancer primarily occurs in women it can also affect men. Various types of breast cancers are as follows: ductal carcinoma in situ (DCIS) (commonest type of noninvasive breast cancer); invasive ductal carcinoma (commonest invasive lesion); invasive lobular carcinoma and a few less common ones such as mucinous carcinoma, mixed tumors, medullary carcinoma, inflammatory breast cancer, etc.

Picture	Medical/Surgical Description	Management/Clinical Highlights

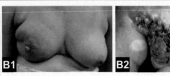

Figs 11.8.1(B1 and B2): (B1) Ulcerative-nodular growth in the breast; (B2) Growth involving the axillary lymph nodes of ipsilateral side

Figures 11.8.1 (B1 and B2) shows an ulcerative-nodular growth of the right breast in a 50-years-old postmenopausal patient, which has involved the skin of breast, chest wall and axilla. The axillary lymph nodes of ipsilateral side were involved. There was no distant metastasis. According to the tumor, node, metastases (TNM) staging system, this tumor was classified as $T_4 N_3 M_0$.

Following the diagnosis of cancer, staging is usually performed. This helps in determining the extent of the cancer and its spread in the body. Staging also helps in determining the appropriate therapy and in predicting chances for survival. The most widely used system in the United States is the TNM system as devised by the American Joint Committee on Cancer.

11.8.2: Fine Needle Aspiration Cytology for Diagnosis

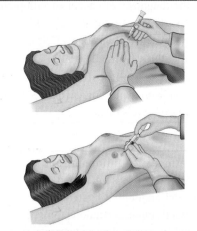

Fig. 11.8.2: Fine needle aspiration cytology for diagnosis of breast lesion

Figure 11.8.2 illustrates the procedure of fine needle aspiration cytology (FNAC) for detection of malignant changes in a breast lesion.

FNAC is a simple, rapid procedure commonly performed for assessment of a breast lesion in which there is suspicion of a malignancy. It is usually performed as an OPD procedure without requirement of any anesthesia. It provides rapid results, which can be immediately correlated with the findings of imaging. Moreover, it is associated with minimal complications and is easily repeatable for multiple lesions. The limitations of this method are that it is operator dependent and may result in high failure rates in unskilled hands. It also cannot differentiate between in-situ lesions and invasive cancer.

11.8.3: Mammography (A to G)

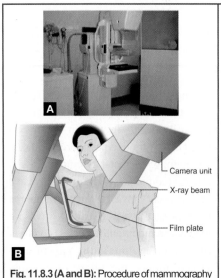

Camera unit
X-ray beam
Film plate

Fig. 11.8.3 (A and B): Procedure of mammography

Mammography is performed after removing all jewelry and clothing in the chest and breast area, following which the breasts are placed on a flat panel. Gentle, but firm pressure is then applied with the help of another panel. This helps in the compression of breast tissue between the two panels.

Screening mammography is commonly performed in women above the age of 40 years in order to facilitate early cancer detection before it causes any symptoms and can be easily treated.

Picture	Medical/Surgical Description	Management/Clinical Highlights

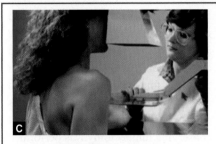

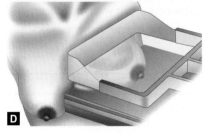

Figs 11.8.3 (C and D): Correct placement of the breasts within the mammography machine

Figures 11.8.3 (C and D) illustrate the correct placement of breasts within the mammography machine. During mammography, two X-ray images must be obtained for each breast [craniocaudal (CC) and mediolateral oblique (MLO) views]. In order to obtain good quality, high resolution clear images of the breasts, proper compression of the breast tissues is essential. The breasts are first compressed horizontally and then obliquely in order to take images in CC and MLO views respectively. The patient should be advised not to wear any perfume, deodorants or talcum powder prior to the procedure because it may create difficulty in interpretation of results due to blurring and fogging of images or production of areas of microcalcifications.

According to the latest recommendations by USPTF (2009), there is no requirement for routine screening of women between 40 years and 50 years of age. After 50 years of age, 2-yearly mammograms are recommended. Screening mammography is usually not required after the age of 75 years. The decision to start regular, screening mammography, every 2 years before the age of 50 years should be individualized and taken by the clinician after taking into account the patient's risk as well as patient context including the patient's values regarding specific benefits and harms for developing breast cancer.

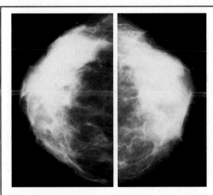

Fig. 11.8.3E: Normal breast mammogram

Figure 11.8.3E shows a normal breast mammogram. Mammograms can be considered as modified X-ray image of the breast tissues. In a normal mammogram, the areas of fatty tissue usually appear dark because the adipose tissue is normally radiolucent. The denser tissues such as breast ducts, lobes (glandular structures) and fibrous connective tissues appear relatively lighter.

Treatment of breast cancer is usually based on the type of cancer and the cancer staging. Various treatment options are as follows:

Surgery: Surgeries for breast cancer can be broadly categorized as breast conserving surgery (partial mastectomy, lumpectomy) and mastectomy (simple, radical, and modified radical mastectomy).

Radiation therapy: This comprises of external beam radiation and brachy-therapy.

Chemotherapy: Various chemotherapy drugs which can be used for treatment of breast cancer include cyclophosphamide, methotrexate, 5-fluorouracil, doxorubicin, etc. Chemotherapy can be administered either as adjuvant chemotherapy (chemotherapy is administered after surgery has removed all the visible cancer) or as neoadjuvant chemotherapy (chemotherapy is administered prior to surgery). Hormone therapy (tamoxifen, fulvestrant, etc.) is used to help reduce the risk of cancer reoccurrence after surgery, but it can also be used as adjunct treatment.

Picture	Medical/Surgical Description	Management/Clinical Highlights
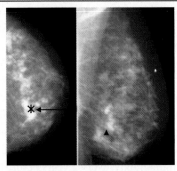 **Fig. 11.8.3F:** Invasive ductal carcinoma (arrow and the asterisk mark show the location of carcinoma)	A 52-years-old woman presented with a lump in breast and bloody discharge from nipples since last 6 months. Mammogram in this patient (Figure 11.8.3F) revealed a small mass (about 1 cm in size) with fine spikes radiating from the mass. Suspicion of an abnormal growth/cancer on a mammogram was confirmed by biopsy. In this case, the biopsy revealed the presence of an invasive ductal carcinoma.	In order to assess metastatic spread in this case, other tests which were performed included an ultrasound examination, CT scan, MRI, positron emission tomography scan, bone scan and chest X-ray. No metastasis was detected on these investigations. Breast conserving lumpectomy was performed in this case along with radiotherapy.
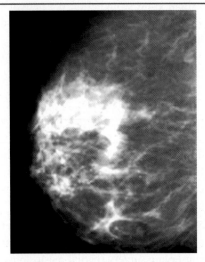 **Fig. 11.8.3 G:** Benign deposits of calcium on mammogram	Areas of calcifications are usually detected on the mammogram and are produced due to the deposits of calcium. Microdeposits of calcium usually develop in the necrotic calcium cells. Therefore presence of microcalcifications on a mammogram could sometimes be suggestive of a malignancy, however not always. Presence of irregular deposits of calcium in form of tight clusters or patterns (circles or lines) may be indicative of DCIS. However, scattered microcalcifications or macrocalcifications are usually nonmalignant (Figure 11.8.3G).	No specific follow-up or treatment is required for benign calcifications. If the microcalcifications appear to be probably benign, a follow-up mammogram is required after 6 months. In case of suspicious calcification, likely to be malignant, follow-up is usually required with investigations such as ultrasound, repeat mammograms, biopsy (stereotactic core biopsy), etc. Benign calcifications could be related to the presence of mastitis, benign breast cysts, use of ointments, powder or deodorants by the patient, calcifications in a fibroadenoma, calcifications in the blood vessels of the breast tissues, and previous history of injury or trauma to the breasts.

11.8.4: Ultrasound for Detection of Breast Lesions (A and B)

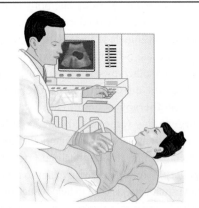 **Fig. 11.8.4A:** Performing an ultrasound of the breast	Figure 11.8.4A shows the method of performing an ultrasound of the breast. While performing an ultrasound, the transducer is moved back and forth over the surface of breast.	Breast ultrasound makes use of sound waves to study the lesions found to be suspicious of malignancy on mammography.

Picture	Medical/Surgical Description	Management/Clinical Highlights
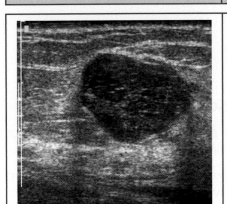 **Fig. 11.8.4B:** Breast ultrasound showing a malignant mass	Breast ultrasound does not replace a mammogram, rather it acts as supplement to it. Breast ultrasound usually makes use of sound waves to further evaluate the lesions found to be suspicious of malignancy on mammography. Figure 11.8.4B shows a malignant mass on ultrasound examination. The diagnosis of malignancy was confirmed by performing an ultrasound-directed biopsy.	A cystic fluid-filled, well defined lesion with regular margins is usually suggestive of a benign lesion. On the other hand, presence of a complex or a solid mass is usually suggestive of malignancy.

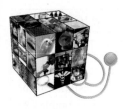

EVIDENCE-BASED BREAKTHROUGH FACTS

1. AGE AT LAST BIRTH IN RELATION TO RISK OF ENDOMETRIAL CANCER

Childbearing at an older age irrespective of parity can be considered as a factor associated with reduced risk for development of endometrial cancer, which persist over many years following the last childbirth.

Source: Setiawan VW, Pike MC, Karageorgi S, et al. Age at last birth in relation to risk of endometrial cancer: pooled analysis in the Epidemiology of Endometrial Cancer Consortium. Am J Epidemiol. 2012;176(4):269-78.

2. PACLITAXEL PLUS CARBOPLATIN VERSUS PACLITAXEL PLUS CISPLATIN IN STAGE IVB, PERSISTENT OR RECURRENT CERVICAL CANCER

Carboplatin rather than cisplatin in combination with paclitaxel is more beneficial and is associated with fewer side effects in women with metastatic or persistent cervical cancer.

Source: Kitagawa R, Katsumata N, Shibata T, et al. A randomized, phase III trial of paclitaxel plus carboplatin (TC) versus paclitaxel plus cisplatin (TP) in stage IVB, persistent or recurrent cervical cancer: Japan Clinical Oncology Group study (JCOG0505). J Clin Oncol. 2012;30(15):5006.

3. ASSOCIATION BETWEEN BRCA1 AND BRCA2 MUTATIONS AND SURVIVAL IN WOMEN WITH INVASIVE EPITHELIAL OVARIAN CANCER

Presence of mutations on the BCRA 1 and BCRA 2 gene in cases of ovarian cancer is associated with a better prognosis in comparison to those who do not carry this mutation. Amongst the carriers of these mutations, the carriers of BCRA 2 gene mutation had a better prognosis in comparison to those with BCRA1 gene mutation.

Source: Bolton KL, Chenevix-Trench G, Goh C, et al. Association between BRCA1 and BRCA2 mutations and survival in women with invasive epithelial ovarian cancer. JAMA. 2012;307:382-90.

4. RELATIONSHIP BETWEEN FATTY ACIDS AND ENDOMETRIAL CANCER

Intake of long chain polyunsaturated fatty acids, eicosapentaenoic and docosahexaenoic acid, in food or in form of supplements is likely to provide protection against endometrial cancer.

Source: Arem H, Neuhouser ML, Irwin ML, et al. Omega-3 and omega-6 fatty acid intakes and endometrial cancer risk in a population-based case-control study. Eur J Nutr. 2012 Aug 23. [Epub ahead of print]

5. RELATIONSHIP BETWEEN LEEP AND PRETERM BIRTH

The treatment for CIN with LEEP and other similar modalities is unlikely to cause an increase in the risk for subsequent preterm birth.

Source: Castanon A, Brocklehurst P, Evans H, et al. Risk of preterm birth after treatment for cervical intraepithelial neoplasia among women attending colposcopy in England: retrospective-prospective cohort study. BMJ. 2012;345:e5174.

6. HUMAN PAPILLOMAVIRUS VACCINE

Quadrivalent, recombinant HPV vaccine, (*Gardasil*, Merck and Co. Inc), has gained FDA approval in 2006. It is likely to provide protection against a range of diseases attributed by multiple types of HPV (types 6, 11, 16, and 18). The vaccine is indicated for females aged 9–26 years and provides protection against genital warts and gynecologic cancer for females and for providing protection against anal cancer in both males and females. No major adverse effects were found to be associated with this vaccine, though first day syncope and skin infections (after 2 weeks) were observed in some patients.

Source: Klein NP, Hansen J, Chao C, et al. Safety of Quadrivalent Human Papillomavirus Vaccine Administered Routinely to Females. Arch Pediatr Adolesc Med. 2012 Oct 1:1-9. doi:10.1001/archpediatrics.2012.1451. [Epub ahead of print]

7. NEW CERVICAL CANCER SCREENING RECOMMENDATIONS

The American Society for Colposcopy and Cervical Pathology (ASCCP), and the American Society for Clinical Pathology (ASCP) have recently updated their joint guidelines for cervical cancer screening. An update to the U.S. Preventive Services Task Force recommendations also has been issued. The biggest change in the guideline is aimed at women between the ages of 30 years and 65 years. In such women, co-testing with cervical cytology (either the conventional pap or liquid-based method) in combination with human papilloma virus testing is indicated after every five years in cases where the initial testing on pap smear was negative. If HPV testing is not available, women can get a Pap test by itself (without HPV co-testing) every 3 years.

Population	Recommended Screening Method	Comments
Aged less than 21 years	No screening	
Aged 21 to 29 years	Cytology alone every 3 years	
Aged 30 to 65 years	*Preferred screening method*: HPV and cytology co-testing every 5 years. In case of non-availability of HPV testing, cytology alone is indicated every 3 years	Screening by HPV testing alone is not recommended
Aged more than 65 years	No screening necessary after adequate negative prior screening results	Routine age-based screening must be continued for at least 20 years in women with a history of CIN II, CIN III, or adenocarcinoma in situ
After total hysterectomy	No screening necessary in women without a history of CIN II, CIN III, adenocarcinoma in situ, or cancer in the past 20 years	
After HPV vaccination	Follow the same age-specific recommendations as unvaccinated women	

Source: Saslow D, Solomon D, Lawson HW, et al. American Cancer Society, American Society for Colposcopy and Cervical Pathology, and American Society for Clinical Pathology screening guidelines for the prevention and early detection of cervical cancer. CA Cancer J Clin. 2012;62:147-72.

8. RISK FACTORS FOR ENDOMETRIAL CANCER AFTER BENIGN RESULTS OF ENDOMETRIAL BIOPSY

Personal history of colorectal cancer, presence of endometrial polyps, and morbid obesity are the strongest risk factors for having endometrial cancer even after having a benign endometrial biopsy or D&C result. On the other hand, use of OCPs appears to be the strongest protective factor against the development of endometrial cancer.

Source: Torres ML, Weaver AL, Kumar S, et al. Risk factors for developing endometrial cancer after benign endometrial sampling. Obstet Gynecol. 2012;120(5):998-1004.

9. USE OF NEOADJUVANT CHEMOTHERAPY

According to a new Cochrane review, neoadjuvant chemotherapy is a reasonable alternative to primary debulking surgery in women with stage IIIc/IV ovarian cancer. Treatment with neoadjuvant chemotherapy before surgery in women with stage IIIc/IV ovarian cancer is associated with fewer serious adverse events related to surgery and serves as a reasonable treatment option, especially for women with bulky tumors. The rates of overall survival and disease-free survival are similar for women with stage IIIc/IV ovarian epithelial cancer, regardless of treatment order (chemotherapy first then surgery or surgery first then chemotherapy).

Source: Morrison J, Halder K, Kehoe S, et al. Chemotherapy versus surgery for initial treatment in advanced ovarian epithelial cancer. Cochrane Database Syst Rev. 2012;8:CD005343.

10. HUMAN PAPILLOMAVIRUS TEST VS PAP SMEAR: WHICH IS MORE SENSITIVE?

While both HPV testing and pap smear are quite useful for a short term (2 year) follow-up period, a study has demonstrated that a baseline negative HPV test provides the greatest guarantee against the future development of grade III CIN during a very long-term follow-up (10–18 years) period, in comparison with normal Pap smears.

Source: Castle PE, Glass AG, Rush BB, et al. Clinical human papillomavirus detection forecasts cervical cancer risk in women over 18 years of follow-up. J Clin Oncol. 2012;30:3044-50.

11. SCREENING FOR OVARIAN CANCER BY USPSTF

The US Preventive Services Task Force has recommended against routine preventive screening of asymptomatic women with no risk factors for ovarian cancer. While this recommendation applies to asymptomatic women, those with known genetic mutations which increase their risk for ovarian cancer (e.g. BRCA mutations) are not included in this recommendation.

Source: Virginia A Moyer, MD, MPH; and on behalf of the U.S. Preventive Services Task Force. Screening for Ovarian Cancer: U.S. Preventive Services Task Force Reaffirmation Recommendation Statement. *Ann Intern Med.* 11 September 2012

12. TALCUM POWDER USE AND RISK OF ENDOMETRIAL CANCER

Use of talcum powder in the perineal area has been associated with an increased risk of ovarian cancer, and a recent cohort study also found positive association between the use of talc and endometrial cancer. The data from the Australian National Endometrial Cancer Study (ANECS), however, does not confirm any positive association between the use of talc in the perineal area and endometrial cancer as observed in the previous study.

Source: Neill AS, Nagle CM, Spurdle AB, et al. Use of talcum powder and endometrial cancer risk. Cancer Causes Control. 2012;23(3):513-9.

Section 12

Uterus

Gynecology

SECTION OUTLINE

12.1: UTERINE PROLAPSE

12.1.1: Definition (A to F)

Picture	Medical/Surgical Description	Management/Clinical Highlights
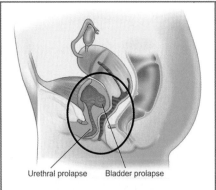**Fig. 12.1.1A:** Different pelvic compartments	Anatomically, the vaginal vault has three compartments: an anterior compartment (consisting of the anterior vaginal wall), a middle compartment (cervix) and a posterior compartment (posterior vaginal wall). Different pelvic compartments are shown in Figure 12.1.1A.	Weakness of the anterior compartment results in cystocele (weakness of upper two-thirds) and urethrocele (weakness of lower one-thirds of anterior vaginal wall), whereas that of the middle compartment in the descent of uterine vault. The weakness of the posterior compartment results in development of enterocele (weakness of upper one-third of posterior vaginal wall) and rectocele (weakness of lower two-thirds of posterior vaginal wall).
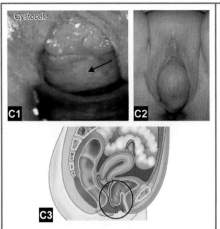**Fig. 12.1.1B:** Urethrocele with moderate cystocele	Cystocele and urethrocele can be defined as the protrusion of bladder/urethra respectively into the anterior vaginal wall, thereby causing its descent. Cystocele produces a bulge in the upper two-thirds of anterior vaginal wall, whereas urethrocele produces a bulge in lower one-third of anterior vaginal wall. Along with the descent of the vaginal wall, there also occurs prolapse of bladder and/or urethra.	Urethrocele and cystocele occur as a result of weakness of anterior pelvic compartment and may be associated with difficulty in emptying the bladder. Prolapse of the urethral tissues is likely to result in stress urinary incontinence. The tissues around the urethra and bladder can be strengthened with the help of Kegel exercises. Surgery for repair of cystocele (anterior colporrhaphy) has been discussed later in this Section.
Figs 12.1.1C (C1 to C3): (C1) Photograph of grade I cystocele; (C2) Photograph of grade III cystocele; (C3) Diagrammatic representation of cystocele (demonstrated by the circle)	Cystocele can be classified as follows: Mild (grade I): The bladder descends halfway up to the vaginal introitus. Severe (grade II): Bladder descends up to the vaginal introitus. Advanced (grade III): Bladder bulges out through the vaginal introitus.	Management of cystocele has been discussed later in this Section.

Picture	Medical/Surgical Description	Management/Clinical Highlights

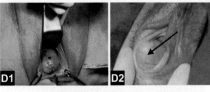
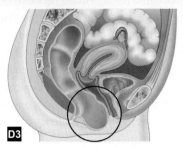
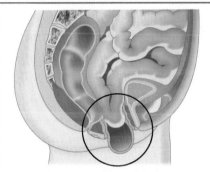

Figs 12.1.1D (D1 to D3): (D1 and D2) Photographic appearance of rectocele; (D3) Diagram showing rectocele (demonstrated by the circle)

Rectocele occurs due to the weakness of posterior pelvic compartment. Bulging of anterior rectal wall into the vagina can produce vaginal symptoms such as vaginal bulging, the sensation of a mass in the vagina, etc., and rectal symptoms such as constipation, and difficult evacuation with straining. Rectocele is associated with the weakness of lower two-thirds of posterior vaginal wall.

The woman should be advised to avoid constipation by eating a high fiber diet, drinking plenty of fluids (at least 6–8 glasses of water) and avoiding prolonged straining. If this conservative management is not successful, surgical therapy is indicated. Surgical repair of rectocele has been discussed later in this Section.

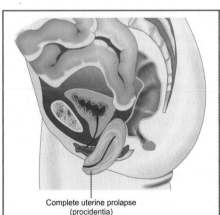

Fig. 12.1.1E: Enterocele (demonstrated by the circle)

Enterocele can be defined as protrusion of small intestines and peritoneum into upper one-third of the posterior vaginal wall.

Surgical treatment is required to replace the prolapsed bowel in its proper place and to strengthen the muscles of pelvic floor.

Complete uterine prolapse (procidentia)

Fig. 12.1.1 F: Complete uterine prolapse

Uterine descent can be defined as follows:
First degree: There is descent of cervix into the vagina.
Second degree: There is descent of cervix up to the vaginal introitus.
Third degree: There is descent of cervix outside the vaginal introitus.
Procidentia can be defined as the descent of whole of the uterus outside the vaginal introitus.

There is no medical treatment available, which can cure prolapse. Though nonsurgical methods (pessary use) and conservative management may provide symptomatic relief, surgery provides the definitive cure. In women who desire future child bearing, conservative surgical repair options are indicated. In perimenopausal and postmenopausal patients, vaginal hysterectomy with repair of pelvic floor is the surgical treatment of choice.

12.1.2: Etiology: Damage Caused by Childbirth to the Muscles of Pelvic Floor

Picture	Medical/Surgical Description	Management/Clinical Highlights
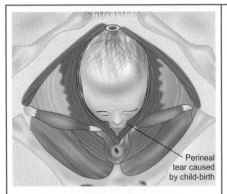 Fig. 12.1.2: Damage caused by the child-birth to the muscles of pelvic floor	Uterine prolapse usually occurs in postmenopausal and multiparous women, in whom the pelvic floor muscles and the ligaments that support the female genital tract have become slack and atonic. Injury to the pelvic floor muscles during repeated child-births, causing excessive stretching of the pelvic floor muscles and ligaments, acts as a major risk factor for causing reduced tone of pelvic floor muscles.	Perineal tears occurring at the time of delivery and parturition tend to either divide the decussating fibers of levator ani or cause damage to the perineal body. Both these factors can cause the hiatus urogenitalis to become patulous and result in the development of prolapse. Conditions which result in reduced tone of levator muscles tend to increase the dimensions of hiatus urogenitalis, thereby increasing the tendency of pelvic organs to prolapse.

12.1.3: Stages of Uterine Prolapse (A to C)

Picture	Medical/Surgical Description	Management/Clinical Highlights
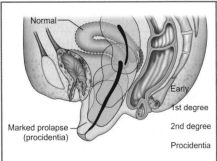 Fig. 12.1.3A: Stages of uterine prolapse	This figure describes the stages in which the descent of pelvic organs occurs stage by stage.	The Baden-Walker Halfway system for evaluation of pelvic organ prolapse is shown in Figure 12.1.3B and the POP-Q System for quantification of pelvic prolapse is described in Figure 12.1.3C.
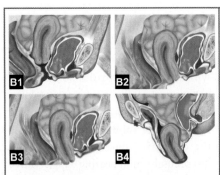 Figs 12.1.3B (B1 to B4): Baden-Walker Halfway system for evaluation of pelvic organ prolapse: (B1) Stage I uterine prolapse; (B2) Stage II uterine prolapse; (B3) Stage III uterine prolapse; (B4) Uterine procidentia	Baden-Walker Halfway system for evaluation of pelvic organ prolapse is as follows: • Stage 0: Normal position for each respective site • Stage I: Descent of the cervix to any point in the vagina above the introitus • Stage II: Descent of the cervix until the introitus • Stage III: Descent of the cervix halfway past the hymen • Stage IV: Total eversion or procidentia	Diagnosis of pelvic organ prolapse is usually based on the findings of clinical examination. Surgery forms the definitive cure and comprises of replacing the prolapsed organ and strengthening the weakened pelvic compartment. Routine investigations must be performed before undertaking a major gynecological surgery. Cervical cytology must be obtained in all cases to rule out the possibility of malignant changes in the cervix.

Picture	Medical/Surgical Description	Management/Clinical Highlights

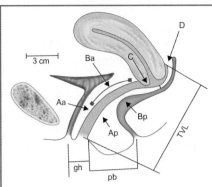

Fig. 12.1.3C: POP-Q system for quantification of pelvic prolapse (gh, genital hiatus; pb, perineal body; TVL, total vaginal length)
(*Source:* Bump RC, Mattiasson A, Bo K, et al. The standardization of terminology of female pelvic organ prolapse and pelvic floor dysfunction. Am J Obstet Gynecol. 1996;175(1):10-7)

In 1966, the international continence society defined a system for quantification of pelvic organ prolapse (POP-Q system). This system is based on a series of site-specific measurements of the woman's pelvic organ support system in relation to the hymen in each of the segments. This system is based on the measurement of six points, which are located with the reference to the plane of the hymen: two on the anterior vaginal wall (Aa and Ba); two in the apical vagina (C and D) and two on the posterior vaginal wall (Ap and Bp). All these six points are measured with the patient engaged in maximum protrusion.

Stages of POP-Q system for measurement of pelvic organ prolapse are as follows:
Stage 0: No prolapse is demonstrated
Stage 1: The most distal portion of the prolapse is more than 1 cm above the level of hymen
Stage 2: The most distal portion of the prolapse is 1 cm or less proximal or distal to the hymenal plate
Stage 3: The most distal portion of the prolapse protrudes more than 1 cm below the hymen, but protrudes no further than 2 cm less than the total vaginal length
Stage 4: Complete vaginal eversion
Management of cases of pelvic prolapse has been discussed in forthcoming topics.

12.1.4: Pessary Use for Correction of Prolapse (A and B)

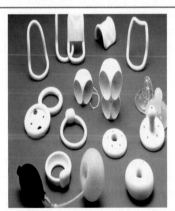

Fig. 12.1.4A: Different types of pessaries used for treatment of uterine prolapse

Pessaries are a nonsurgical method for supporting the uterine and vaginal structures. A small pessary may help in maintaining normal uterine position. Figure 12.1.4A shows different types of pessaries which can be used for treatment of uterine prolapse.

Pessaries are usually used for attaining temporary relief in cases with symptomatic prolapse. Pessaries work as a first-line option for women with pelvic organ prolapse who want nonsurgical management or have desire for future childbearing. Pessaries also prove useful in patients who have early-stage prolapse or are too weak for surgery. One of the important indications for using pessary is in young women following child birth. Additionally, pessaries are a valid option for patients with stress incontinence worsened by strenuous physical activity.

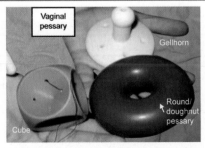

Fig. 12.1.4B: Some commonly used pessaries for treatment of uterine prolapse

Figure 12.1.4B highlights some of the commonly used pessaries for the treatment of uterine prolapse. Some of these include the Gellhorn pessary, cube pessary and round/donut pessary. All these three types of pessaries can be used in patients with rectoceles and enterocele.

The Gellhorn pessary is most often used for patients with significant uterine prolapse and a large introital diameter who have not obtained relief with other pessaries because this pessary provides strong pelvic support. Both Gellhorn and donut pessaries can be used for patients with third degree uterine prolapse. Additionally, the cube can be used in patients with large cystocele.

12.1.5: Anterior Repair: Anterior Colporrhaphy (A to F)

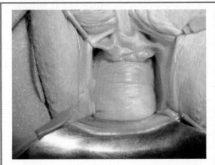

Fig. 12.1.5A: Appearance of cystocele just before giving the incision

Anterior colporrhaphy operation is one of the most commonly performed surgeries to repair a cystocele and cystourethrocele. The steps of surgery have been illustrated in Figures 12.1.5 (A to F). This surgery is usually performed under general or regional anesthesia. A speculum is inserted into the vagina to expose it during the procedure. Traction is applied on the cervix using Allis forceps, in order to expose the anterior vaginal wall. Figure 12.1.5A shows appearance of cystocele just before giving the incision.

Anterior colporrhaphy comprises of the following steps: (i) excision of a portion of relaxed anterior vaginal wall; (ii) mobilization of bladder; (iii) pushing the bladder upward after cutting the vesicocervical ligament and (iv) permanently supporting the bladder, by tightening the pubocervical fascia.

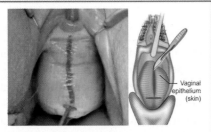

Fig. 12.1.5B: Skin incision is given over the skin overlying the cystocele

Figure 12.1.5B shows the way a T-shaped incision is given over the skin overlying the cystocele.

Firstly an inverted T-shaped incision is made on the anterior vaginal wall, starting with a transverse incision on the bladder sulcus. Through the midpoint of this transverse incision, a vertical incision is given, which extends up to the urethral opening.

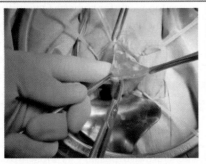

Fig. 12.1.5C: Dissection of the underlying fascia

Figure 12.1.5C shows dissection of the underlying fascia in order to expose the bladder and vesicovaginal fascia.

The vaginal walls are reflected to either side to expose the bladder and vesicovaginal fascia. Bladder is pushed upward and the vaginal skin is separated from the underlying fascia.

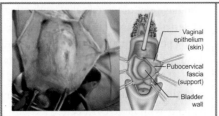

Fig. 12.1.5D: Dissection of the underlying fascia is continued until the midline defect in pubocervical fascia is visualized

Figure 12.1.5D shows that the continued dissection of underlying fascia reveals that the patient has a cystocele due to weakness of the pubocervical fascia in the midline.

Dissection until the visualization of midline defect in pubocervical fascia facilitates the repair of cystocele.

Picture	Medical/Surgical Description	Management/Clinical Highlights
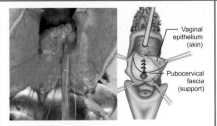 **Fig. 12.1.5 E:** The tissue under the bladder is plicated and pulled together in the midline, thus reducing the bulge	In order to strengthen the weakened pubocervical fascia, the tissue under the bladder is pulled together in the midline and plicated (Figure 12.1.5E). Following the reduction, excess vaginal skin is then cut off, which can create a shortened or constricted vagina.	The overlying vesicovaginal and pubocervical fascia is plicated with interrupted 0 catgut sutures, to correct the vaginal wall laxity and to close the hiatus through which the bladder herniates. Following the reduction, excess vaginal skin is then cut off, which can create a shortened or constricted vagina.
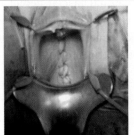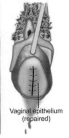 **Fig. 12.1.5 F:** Closure of the vaginal epithelium	Figure 12.1.5 F shows final step of surgical repair by anterior colporrhaphy.	Cut margins of vagina are apposed together. In women suffering from stress incontinence, a Kelly's suture to plicate the bladder neck, just prior to closure, helps in correcting stress incontinence.

12.1.6: Posterior Colporrhaphy and Colpoperineorrhaphy (A to F)

Picture	Medical/Surgical Description	Management/Clinical Highlights
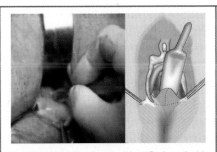 **Fig. 12.1.6A:** Rectocele identified and skin incised: a bulge is apparent on the bottom (posterior) floor of the vagina. The dotted line represents the skin incision, performed in this posterior repair procedure	The surgical procedure for rectocele repair is illustrated in Figures 12.1.6 (A to F). While repairing the rectocele, most surgeons also perform a posterior colporrhaphy. This process involves nonspecific midline plication of the rectovaginal fascia, after reducing the rectocele.	In this surgery, the lax vaginal tissue over the rectocele is excised. The medial fibers of the levator ani are then pulled together, approximated and sutured over the top of rectum.
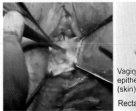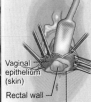 **Fig. 12.1.6 B:** Identification of the fascia break: the defect is readily identified and the rectal wall is found to be protruding through this break in the rectovaginal fascia	With the dissection of vaginal epithelium (skin), the area of weakness in the rectovaginal fascia is identified. Rectocele exists because of a break in the supportive layer known as the rectovaginal fascia.	Identification of the area of weakness is essential because this allows the surgeon to repair the defect, at the same time strengthening the posterior vaginal wall.

Picture	Medical/Surgical Description	Management/Clinical Highlights
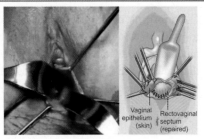 **Fig. 12.1.6C:** The distal defect is repaired	The rectovaginal fascia is reattached to the perineal body, where the distal defect was located.	Following the excision of lax vaginal skin over the rectocele and reduction of rectocele, the rectovaginal fascia is repaired by approximation of the medial fibers of levator ani.
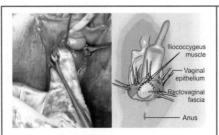 **Fig. 12.1.6D:** The rectovaginal fascial defect has been repaired	Figure 12.1.6D shows the appearance of posterior vaginal wall following closure of rectovaginal fascia prior to closure of vaginal epithelium.	As the rectovaginal fascial defect is repaired, the caliber of hiatus urogenitalis is restored, the perineal body is repaired and an adequate perineum is created.
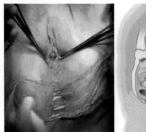 **Fig. 12.1.6E:** The rectovaginal fascia is reattached to the iliococcygeal muscles bilaterally with permanent sutures	In order to further strengthen the posterior vaginal wall, the rectovaginal fascia is reattached to the iliococcygeal muscles bilaterally with help of permanent sutures	In order to prevent recurrence of prolapse and to reinforce the weakened fascia, mesh such as mersilene, prolene or gore-tex can be used.
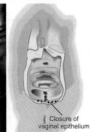 **Fig. 12.1.6F:** Closure of the vaginal epithelium (skin) completes the operation	Figure 12.1.6F shows the appearance of posterior vaginal wall following closure of vaginal epithelium.	Though the surgery for rectocele repair is quite effective in the treatment of rectocele, these patients often suffer from dyspareunia following surgery.

12.1.7: Manchester Repair (A to E)

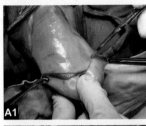

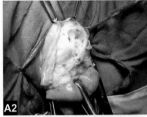

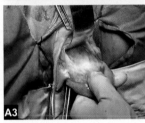

Figs 12.1.7A (A1 to A3): Anterior colporrhaphy: (A1) The anterior vaginal wall is separated from bladder; (A2 and A3) Paravesical fascia is dissected out so that bladder is separated from vagina and can be pushed up

Manchester repair (also called Fothergill operation) is performed in those cases of prolapse where removal of the uterus is not required. The procedure for Manchester repair is described in Figures 12.1.7 (A to E). Anterior colporrhaphy is firstly performed [Figures 12.1.7 (A1 to A3)]. The bladder is dissected from the cervix. Dissection of paravesical fascia is done so as to separate the bladder and push it up.

Indications of Manchester operation are as follows:
- Presence of a small cystocele with only first or second degree prolapse
- Absence of an enterocele
- Symptoms of prolapse are largely due to cervical elongation.
- Patient requires preservation of the menstrual function.
- Child bearing function is not required.
- Malignancy of the endometrium has been ruled out by performing a D&C.
- There is absence of urinary tract infection.

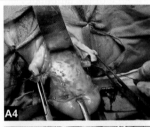

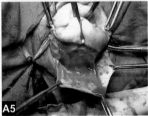

Figs 12.1.7A (A4 and A5): (A4) The base of cardinal ligament is exposed, clamped and cut; (A5) Posterior vaginal wall is similarly separated from the cervix

The attachment of Mackenrodt's ligaments to the cervix on each side are exposed, clamped and cut. The vaginal incision is then extended posteriorly round the cervix.

The principles of Manchester repair are as follows:
- Dilatation and curettage is done prior to the procedure in order to rule out endometrial malignancy
- Anterior colporrhaphy
- Shortening of the Mackenrodt's ligaments and anchoring them to the anterior surface of cervix in order to antevert the retroverted uterus.
- Amputation of cervix
- Formation of lip of cervix using Sturmdorf's suture.

Picture	Medical/Surgical Description	Management/Clinical Highlights
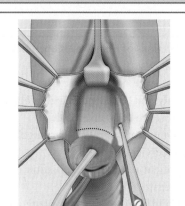 **Fig. 12.1.7 A6:** Steps A1 to A5 are summarized in this Figure	The adjacent figure shows the following: • The bladder is dissected from the cervix. • A circular incision is given over the cervix. • The base of cardinal ligament is exposed, clamped and cut.	Ligation and transfixation of Mackenrodt's ligaments is done with the help of No. 1 delayed absorbable vicryl sutures. Vicryl is used because it has a great tensile strength and easy knotability.
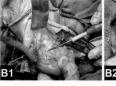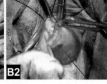 **Fig. 12.1.7B (B1 and B2):** (B1) The cervix is amputated; (B2) Posterior lip of cervix is covered with a flap of mucosa	The cervix is amputated and posterior lip of cervix is covered with a flap of mucosa.	Cervix can be amputated using a cautery. The advantage of using cautery is that the blood vessels can be coagulated simultaneously. Some surgeons prefer to ligate the descending cervical vessels prior to cervical amputation.
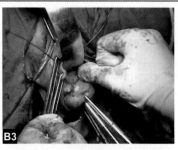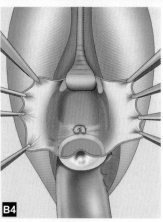 **Figs 12.1.7B (B3 and B4):** (B3) The base of cardinal ligament is sutured over the anterior surface of cervix; (B4) This diagram summarizes steps B1 to B3	The base of cardinal ligament is sutured over the anterior surface of cervix. The raw area of the amputated cervix is then covered.	The suturing of cardinal ligaments over the anterior surface of cervix helps in strengthening the supports of uterus. The raw area of the amputated cervix is covered using the vaginal mucosa with the help of Sturmdorf's suture.

Picture	Medical/Surgical Description	Management/Clinical Highlights
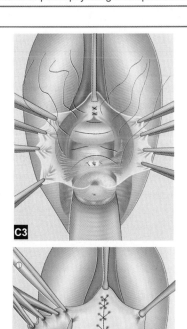**Figs 12.1.7C (C1 and C2):** (C1) Application of bladder buttressing sutures; (C2) Completion of anterior colporrhaphy using interrupted sutures	Anterior colporrhaphy is completed by the application of bladder buttressing sutures.	Approximately 25% of patients who undergo Manchester repair may experience recurrence of prolapse in future and eventually require a hysterectomy.
Figs 12.1.7C (C3 and C4): (C3) Diagram showing approximation of pubovesicocervical fascia in the midline; (C4) The fascial approximation has been completed and excessive vaginal mucosa has been excised	Following the completion of bladder buttressing sutures, the pubovesicocervical fascia is approximated in the midline.	This step helps in repairing cystocele, if present. However care must be taken not to excessively tighten the tissue under the bladder neck as it can result in voiding dysfunction.

SECTION 12 ❖ UTERUS

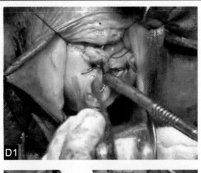

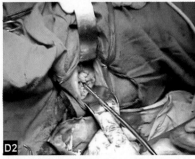

Figs 12.1.7D (D1 and D2): (D1) Formation of anterior lip of cervix; (D2) Newly formed cervix at the end of surgery

The new anterior lip of cervix is formed. While application of Sturmdorf's sutures, a dilator (8 mm to 10 mm) must be placed inside the cervical canal.

Both the anterior and posterior lips of cervix are fashioned with the help of Sturmdorf's suture. Sturmdorf's suture begins from the posterior vaginal wall and the stitch is brought in an "outside-in" direction into the posterior vaginal wall. The needle is then taken through the cervical canal (from "outside-in" direction) and emerges out through the cervical opening. From here the suture is taken in an "inside-out" direction (reverse direction) from the tip of vagina into the cervical canal and then outside (again in an inside-out direction). Once the stitch is tied, the posterior lip of cervix is formed. The same procedure is then repeated anteriorly to form the anterior lip of cervix.

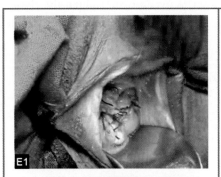

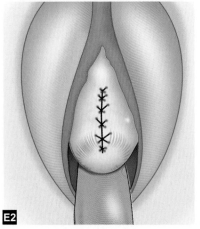

Figs 12.1.7E (E1 and E2): Appearance of vagina at the end of surgery

This figure shows appearance of vagina at the end of the surgery.

Immediately after the surgery the lips of cervix may appear slightly ugly due to the presence of numerous stitches.

Following 6 months of surgery, new lips of cervix are completely healed up and it appears normal looking. The end result of surgery is formation of a shorter cervix which is more strongly supported.

12.1.8: Le fort Colpocleisis (A to E)

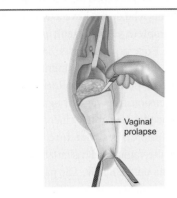

Fig. 12.1.8A: Incision over the mucosa of anterior vaginal wall

In the Le Fort colpocleisis, a patch of anterior and posterior vaginal mucosa is removed. The cut edge of the anterior vaginal wall is sewn to its counterpart on the posterior side. As the approximation is continued on each side, the most dependent portion of the mass is progressively inverted. A tight perineorrhaphy is also performed to help support the inverted vagina and prevent recurrence of the prolapse.

For patients who cannot undergo long surgical procedures and who are not contemplating sexual activity, obliterative procedures, such as the Le Fort colpocleisis or colpectomy and colpocleisis, are viable options.

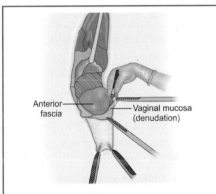

Fig. 12.1.8B: Incision and removal of skin: mucosa is removed from the prolapse to expose the anterior fascia (pubocervical fascia) and posterior fascia (rectovaginal fascia)

The procedure involves excision of rectangular strips of mucosa from the upper portions of anterior and posterior vaginal walls.

The main problem specific to this obliterative operation is that it limits coital function. Also, it does not correct an enterocele because they are both extraperitoneal procedures. Moreover, there is a 25% incidence of postoperative urinary stress incontinence caused by induced fusion of the anterior and posterior vaginal walls and flattening of the posterior urethrovesical angle. In addition, if the uterus is retained, the patient can later bleed from many causes including carcinoma.

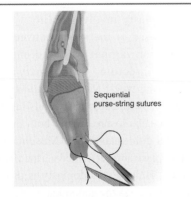

Fig. 12.1.8C: Suturing: The exposed submucosal fascia is then closed together

Once the mucosa has been removed and the underlying strong tissues (pubocervical and rectovaginal fascia) have been identified, the tissue is sewn together in a circular fashion (like the drawstrings on a purse).

Colpocleisis is an excellent surgery for the treatment of uterine prolapse or complete vaginal vault prolapse for patients who are:
- not sexually active,
- have no future plans for sexual activity,
- medically fragile and
- elderly patients who do not require preservation of their sexual functioning.

Picture	Medical/Surgical Description	Management/Clinical Highlights
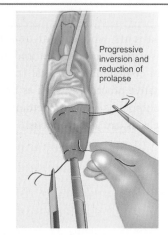 **Fig. 12.1.8D:** Reducing the prolapse	The most protruding portion of the vagina is inverted (pushed in upon itself) and the last suture placed is tied. The suture holds the rest of the vagina from coming back out or prolapsing.	The procedure is called total colpocleisis for patients who do not have a uterus and have complete vaginal vault prolapse, and Le Fort colpocleisis for those patients who still have a uterus. Total colpocleisis procedure is often coupled with a tension free vaginal tape (TVT) sling procedure for urinary incontinence. The colpocleisis procedure is done through the vagina and essentially closes the vagina on the inside. The patient can no longer engage in sexual intercourse due to the closing up of the vagina. The completed procedure usually leaves the patients with a much shortened vagina. As a result, the patient becomes incapable of engaging in sexual intercourse.
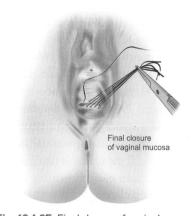 **Fig. 12.1.8E:** Final closure of vaginal mucosa	Figure 12.1.8E shows the appearance of vagina after multiple circular sutures have been placed and the prolapse has been completely reduced back into the patient's vagina and pelvis. The skin edges from the original incision are closed using sutures.	Colpocleisis is associated with the following advantages: • Closes the vagina together • Inhibits the patient from future sexual intercourse • Is associated with 90–95% cure rate • Can be performed using local, epidural, or spinal anesthesia. There is no requirement for general anesthesia • It is a quick procedure which takes only 45 minutes to perform. • There is minimal pain or complications. • Can be coupled with TVT sling (incontinence) operation

12.1.9: Halban's Culdoplasty (A to C)

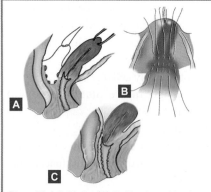 **Figs 12.1.9 (A to C):** Halban's culdoplasty with uterus in situ	Figures 12.1.9 (A to C) demonstrate the procedure of Halban's Culdoplasty. In Halban's procedure, vertical closure of the peritoneum is performed with help of interrupted long acting, absorbable or monofilament/permanent sutures. Figure 12.1.9A is lateral view of uterus showing the attachment of the suture to anterior rectal wall, upper vagina and lower uterine segment. Figure 12.1.9B is superior view of the cul-de-sac, while Figure 12.1.9C is lateral view showing completed closure.	Culdoplasty involves obliteration of cul-de-sac or the space between the posterior vaginal wall and anterior wall of rectum. Culdoplasty is of following types: Mc Call's culdoplasty, Moschcowitz culdoplasty and Halban's cul-de-sac closure. While both the Mc Call's culdoplasty and Moschcowitz culdoplasty are performed via the vaginal route, Halban's culdoplasty is usually performed via the abdominal route.

Picture	Medical/Surgical Description	Management/Clinical Highlights

12.1.10: Transvaginal Sacrospinous Ligament Fixation for Uterine Suspension

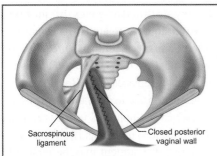

Fig. 12.1.10: Transvaginal sacrospinous ligament fixation

In this method, the vaginal apex is attached, using permanent sutures, to the sacrospinous ligament.

The posterior vaginal wall is opened vertically, following which a window space is created between the vagina and the rectum toward the right sacrospinous ligament. Using Deschamps ligature carrier, a synthetic ligature is used for fixing the vaginal vault to the sacrospinous ligament, 3–5 cm away from the ischial spine. The suture must be placed through the ligament, rather than around it.

Vault prolapse is a delayed complication of both abdominal and vaginal hysterectomy when the supporting structures, i.e. paravaginal fascia and levator ani muscles become weak and deficient. It may also result from failure to identify and repair an enterocele during hysterectomy. Uterine suspension procedures involve putting the uterus back into its normal position. Various types of uterine suspensions can be performed either via the abdominal or vaginal route.

12.1.11: Abdominal Sacral Colpopexy for Uterine Suspension

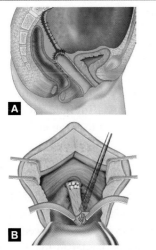

Figs 12.1.11 (A and B): Abdominal sacral colpopexy: (A) Lateral view; (B) Surgery as visualized from the abdominal incision (superior view)

This procedure comprises of suspending the vaginal vault to the sacral promontory extraperitoneally using various grafts, such as harvested fascia lata, abdominal fascia, dura mater, marlex, prolene, goretex, mersilene or cadaveric fascia lata, via a low transverse or vertical incision over the abdominal wall. Injury to the ureter, bladder, sigmoid colon, middle sacral artery and presacral venous plexus should be avoided at the time of surgery.

The aim of surgery is to restore the normal pelvic anatomy as far as possible. At the end of the surgery, normal vaginal length should be maintained with its axis directed toward S3-S4 vertebra. Abdominal sacral colpopexy has the highest cure rate for vault prolapse, probably because of the use of graft tissue with high strength and not relying on the patient's own tissue, which may not be strong enough to hold up the vaginal vault.

12.2: UTERINE RETROVERSION

12.2.1: Definition

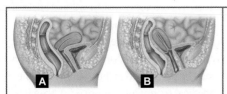

Figs 12.2.1 (A and B): Uterine positions: (A) Uterus in position of anteversion and anteflexion; (B) Retroverted uterus where the long axis of uterus is directed backward

Normal uterine position is that of anteversion and anteflexion, i.e. the uterine body is bent forward at the uterocervical junction over the bladder. Anteflexion refers to forward inclination of the body of the uterus on cervix. Retroversion is a type of uterine displacement in which the uterine body is displaced backward at the uterocervical junction.

Retroversion could be either fixed or mobile. The two main symptoms of retroversion are dyspareunia and dysmenorrhea. Other symptoms may include: menorrhagia, pressure symptoms, infertility, etc.

Picture	Medical/Surgical Description	Management/Clinical Highlights

12.2.2: Management (A and B)

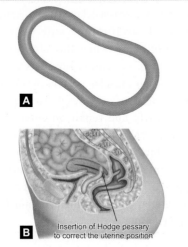

Figs 12.2.2 (A and B): (A) Hodge pessary; (B) Hodge pessary being used to correct retroversion for correction of uterine retroversion

Diagnosis of retroversion is mainly established on the basis of findings of pelvic examination.

Bimanual examination: On bimanual examination, a mass is felt in the Pouch of Douglas. Since this mass moves with the cervix, it can be considered to be a part of the uterus. Uterus may be tender to touch.

Hodge pessary test: If application of Hodge pessary helps in providing relief against the symptoms related to retroversion, the clinician can assume that surgery undertaken to correct the uterine position would be useful.

In asymptomatic cases of mobile retroversion, no treatment is required. Insertion of a pessary may be required in symptomatic cases, where the uterus is bimanually replaced and a Hodge pessary is inserted inside to keep the uterus in an anteverted position. It is usually retained in position for 3 months and then removed.

Surgical treatment may be required in the cases of fixed retroversion and comprises of the following options:
- *Modified Gilliam's ventrosuspension*: This is the most commonly used surgical option in which the round ligaments are anchored to the anterior rectus sheath.
- *Plication of the round ligaments*
- *Baldy-Webster's operation*

12.3: ADENOMYOSIS

12.3.1: Definition

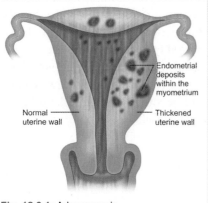

Fig. 12.3.1: Adenomyosis

Adenomyosis is a condition in which there is a growth of endometrial cells inside the uterine myometrium (usually > 2.5 mm beneath the basal endometrium). It is associated with myometrial hypertrophy and may be either diffuse or localized (adenomyoma). The exact cause of adenomyosis is unknown. Some likely causes include the following: uterine trauma (as a result of surgery, pregnancy and pregnancy termination), conditions associated with the production of excessive estrogens and abnormal level of various inflammatory substances in the blood.

Commonly occurring symptoms of adenomyosis include menorrhagia (unresponsive to hormonal therapy or uterine curettage) and progressively increasing dysmenorrhea. Other symptoms may include pelvic pain, backache, dyspareunia and subfertility.

On pelvic examination, the uterus is enlarged to about 12–14 weeks in size, and may be tender to touch, soft and boggy. Adenomyosis is associated with uterine fibroids in about 6–20% cases.

12.3.2: Diagnosis (A to C)

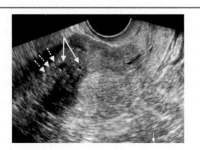

Fig. 12.3.2A: Ultrasound showing features suggestive of adenomyosis

Upon ultrasound examination, adenomyosis may present with heterogeneous myometrial echotexture, ill-defined, anechoic areas of thickened myometrium consisting of blood-filled, irregular cystic spaces, or as an area of hyperechoic myometrium with several cysts (hypoechoic lacunae). Other features suggestive of adenomyosis include asymmetrical uterine enlargement, indistinct endometrial-myometrial border and subendometrial halo thickening.

Total hysterectomy with or without bilateral salpingo-oophorectomy is the treatment of choice in elderly patients who are past their childbearing age. Conservative resection may be performed in the younger patients. Medical treatment comprises of NSAIDs, hormone therapy, danazol, GnRH agonists and Mirena IUCD. Recently, uterine artery embolization is emerging as an effective and safe method in the treatment of adenomyosis.

Picture	Medical/Surgical Description	Management/Clinical Highlights
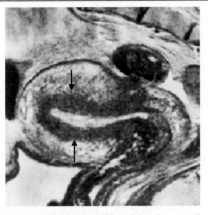 Fig. 12.3.2B: Sagittal T2-weighted magnetic resonance (MR) image showing diffuse, even thickening of the junctional zone (as depicted by arrows), which is consistent with the diagnosis of diffuse adenomyosis	Magnetic resonance imaging is superior to ultrasound for diagnosis of adenomyosis. The presence of heterotopic endometrial glands and stroma in the myometrium appear as bright foci within the myometrium on T2-weighted MR images. Adjacent smooth muscle hyperplasia may present as areas of reduced signal intensity on MRI.	Magnetic resonance imaging had a higher specificity than transvaginal sonography, but similar sensitivity regarding the diagnosis of adenomyosis. Though MRI is superior to ultrasound for the diagnosis of adenomyosis, the diagnosis of adenomyosis can only be confirmed by pathological examination.
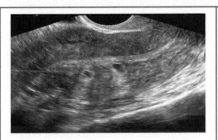 Fig. 12.3.2C: Transvaginal ultrasound in longitudinal plane suggestive of adenomyosis	On ultrasound examination, the uterus was enlarged and myometrium was heterogeneous. Presence of cystic structures just adjacent to the myometrium was suggestive of superficial adenomyosis.	Management of cases of adenomyosis has been described in 12.3.2A.

12.4: UTERINE MALFORMATIONS

12.4.1: Definition

For obtaining further information regarding the classification of the uterine anomalies, kindly refer to 9.8.1 (Section 9).

12.4.2 Management of Vaginal Agenesis

12.4.2.1: Use of Vaginal Dilators

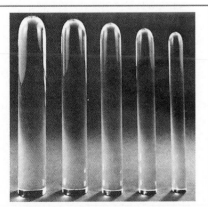 Fig. 12.4.2.1: Vaginal dilators with progressively increasing size	Though surgery remains one of the most effective methods for management of vaginal agenesis, the nonsurgical approach is also sometimes employed. The nonsurgical approach relies on the use of graduated dilators with progressively increasing size that help to create a neovagina. Two methods of nonsurgical treatment are practiced: active dilatation (Frank's method) and passive dilatation (Ingram's method).	In Frank's method, the woman is asked to apply manual pressure to the fourchette with a vaginal dilator, twice a day for 15–20 minutes. In this method, dilators are placed against the fourchette and firm pressure is applied for up to 15 minutes twice a day or more often. Size of the dilators is gradually increased till a full length of vagina can be achieved. This method may take several months or a few years before a functional vagina is formed.

12.4.2.2: Vaginoplasty (A to L)

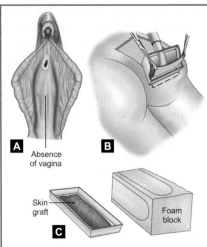

Figs 12.4.2.2 (A to C): (A) Congenital absence of vagina; (B) Obtaining split-thickness skin grafts from the buttock region using a Padgett electrodermatome; (C) Cutting out a vaginal form from a rubber block; skin graft is placed in a sterile pan filled with saline solution

One of the most important steps in performing the modified Mc Indoe's procedure is obtaining a split-thickness skin graft. The graft harvested from each buttock should measure about 8–9 cm wide, and be excised to a depth of approximately 0.045 cm (0.018 inches). The length of the graft should be double the vaginal width, which is about 16–20 cm. The graft is usually taken from the buttocks. The alternative sites are the thighs and hips. After preparing the graft site with antiseptic solution, a single layer is removed. Many surgeons support the use of the pneumatic Padgett electrodermatome for obtaining the skin graft. Following retrieval, the graft is placed between the two layers of the saline-moistened gauze and reserved for later use.

Skin graft remains the most popular material used in vaginoplasties; however, scar formation at the graft site has been a major concern. In the United States, full-thickness skin grafts are often used. These are associated with reduced incidence of graft contracture and stenosis in comparison to that associated with the use of split-thickness grafts. A graft that is slightly thicker is better than a thin graft. The vaginal mold cut from the rubber block should be of sufficient length and width to fit snugly into the new cavity without causing extra pressure onto the rectum, bladder and urethra. A foam-rubber form measuring $10 \times 10 \times 20$ cm works well as a mold. The mold is sterilized and the size is customized to fit the patient's vagina.

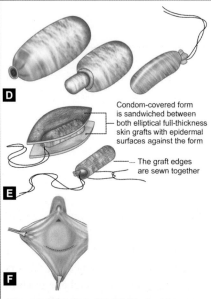

Figs 12.4.2.2 (D to F): (D) Vaginal forms are covered with a condom; (E) The skin grafts are placed over a condom-covered vaginal form and the margins are sutured with synthetic absorbable sutures; (F) Dimple on the introital area is identified, labia are retracted with Allis clamp and a transverse incision is made in the epithelium

The skin graft is draped around the vaginal form after covering it with a condom in such a way that its epithelial surface faces outward before insertion. The margins of the graft are sutured with synthetic absorbable sutures. The patient is then placed in the dorsal lithotomy position and a transurethral catheter is placed inside the bladder. A transverse incision is made in the mucosa at the apex of the vaginal dimple after identifying the dimple on the introital area and retracting the labia.

The prosthetic material used as a vaginal mold is cut to twice the desired size of the vagina, folded in half and compressed by the placement of two condoms over the surface. The condoms are tied at the open end.

Picture	Medical/Surgical Description	Management/Clinical Highlights

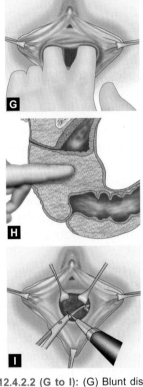

Figs 12.4.2.2 (G to I): (G) Blunt dissection performed with fingers to open the space between the bladder and rectum; (H) Sagittal section showing the dissection being carried out 2 cm from the peritoneum; (I) Hemostasis to be maintained throughout the cavity

Vaginal space is created between the rectum and the bladder by performing blunt dissection through a 0.5 cm incision made across the region of fourchette. Blunt dissection with a finger is carried out until an optimal vaginal length of 10–12 cm has been achieved. The dissection is continued up to the peritoneum. The dissection should be carried as high as possible without entering the peritoneal cavity and without cleaning away all the tissue beneath the peritoneum.

The graft is placed over the mold with the epidermis approximating the surface of the mold and the dermis facing out. The graft-covered prosthesis is carefully inserted into the vaginal canal.

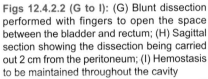

Figs 12.4.2.2 (J to L): (J) Graft-covered mold inserted inside the newly formed vaginal cavity; (K) Sagittal view of pelvis showing skin covered form inserted in the newly created vaginal cavity; (L) Labia are sutured in the midline to hold the vaginal form in space

The graft-covered mold is then inserted in the newly created space and the labia minora are sutured in the midline so that the vaginal mold can remain in position and is then left as such.

After 1 week following insertion, the mold is removed and the cavity irrigated with warm saline solution to reveal a newly formed vaginal cavity lined with the skin graft. The clinician also needs to inspect the vaginal cavity to assess if the graft has been taken up properly or not. At the time of discharge, the patient is instructed to remove the form daily and douche the vagina with warm water. She is advised to continue wearing the form for 6 weeks. Following this, she is instructed to wear it in the night for next 12 months. There remains a risk of contracture of the newly formed vaginal orifice. Regular coital activity helps in solving this problem.

12.4.3: Management of Bicornuate Uterus

12.4.3.1: Strassman's Metroplasty (A to E)

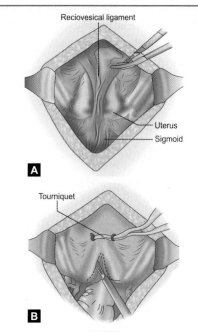

Figs 12.4.3.1 (A and B): (A) If a rectovesical ligament is present, it should be removed; (B) Incision is made on the medial side of each hemicorpora. The incision should be deep enough so as to enter the uterine cavity

In Strassman's metroplasty, a Pfannenstiel incision is made over the abdomen following which the pelvic organs, vessels and ureters are examined.

The rectovesical ligament or a broad peritoneal band, which is frequently present, should be completely excised before performing the uterine wedge resection. Before performing the wedge resection of the uterine horns, tourniquets are applied over the uterine vessels at the level of lower uterine segment and cervix in order to promote hemostasis. A penrose drain or a rubber catheter is inserted through the avascular space in the broad ligament just lateral to the uterine vessels on the each side. A wedge-shaped incision, deep enough to enter the endometrial cavity, is made on the medial aspect of each hemicorpora, along their longitudinal axis.

Strassman's metroplasty is the most commonly used surgery for the unification of two horns of bicornuate uterus. However, bicornuate uterus rarely requires surgical reconstruction. Surgery in cases of bicornuate uterus is recommended only for those women who have experienced more than three recurrent spontaneous abortions, midtrimester loss or premature births, and in whom no other etiologic factor for recurrent miscarriages has been identified.

The wedge-shaped incision, which is made, should not be too close to the interstitial portions of the fallopian tubes in the superior direction. In the inferior direction, the incision must be extended so as to achieve a single endocervical canal. If duplex cervices are present, no attempts are made to join the cervix.

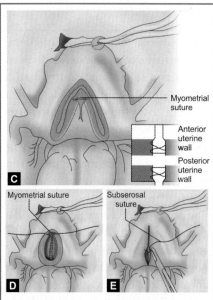

Figs 12.4.3.1 (C to E): (C and D) Approximating the myometrium using the interrupted vertical figure-of-eight polyglycolic acid sutures; (E) Serosa is stitched using continuous polyglycolic acid subserosal sutures

The uterus is closed in three layers with interrupted figure-of-eight polyglycolic acid sutures. The inner layer must include one-third of thickness of myometrium along with the endometrium. The middle layer must include most of the myometrium (nearly two-thirds of the myometrium, which is left). Final layer must mainly includes the serosa and part of myometrium, if any is left. The stitches of the innermost layers must be placed in such a way that the knots are tied in the endometrial cavity. While tying these sutures, the two uterine hemicorpora must be manually pressed together to avoid tension on the suture line. After placing a few stitches and before the first layer is completed, stitches of the second layer can be put in order to avoid tension. Serosa is stitched using continuous polyglycolic acid subserosal sutures.

After resecting the wedge, the myometrial edges naturally evert. Therefore the everted edges are sutured together. The suture line must be then examined for hemostasis. When suturing the fundal region, the surgeon must be careful, not to place the sutures too close to the tubal ostia.

Following the uterine repair and removal of the tourniquets, dilatation of the cervix is performed in order to ensure proper drainage of the endometrial cavity. The patient should be advised to wait for 4–6 months before attempting pregnancy.

12.4.3.2: Jones Metroplasty (A to G)

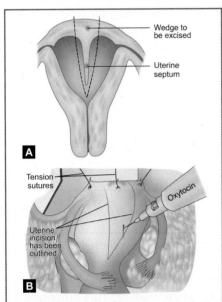

Figs 12.4.3.2 (A and B): Jones metroplasty: (A) Diagram outlining the wedge-shape incision to be made on the uterine serosal surface; (B) Injection of vasopressin to ensure hemostasis

The procedure of Jones metroplasty is illustrated in Figures 12.4.3.2 (A to G). In this procedure, the abdomen is opened through a transverse incision. The uterine septum is surgically excised in the form of a wedge. The uterine incision should begin at the fundus of the uterus. The incision at the top of the fundus is usually within 1 cm or less of the insertion of the fallopian tubes. Two methods to control the bleeding can be used during the procedure. In the first, a tourniquet is applied at the junction of the lower uterine segment and the cervix, and tied anterior to the uterus (as described previously with Strassman's metroplasty. The second method of hemostasis (as shown in this Figure) involves the use of vasopressin diluted in saline into the anterior and posterior walls of the uterus.

Jones procedure is used for surgical repair in case of a septate uterus. It involves wedge resection of the portion of uterine fundus containing the uterine septum after making a triangular wedge-like incision in the anterior-posterior plane of the uterus.

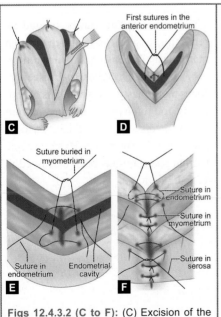

Figs 12.4.3.2 (C to F): (C) Excision of the uterine wedge containing most of the septum; (D to F) Closure of the uterine cavity

Figure 12.4.3.2 C demonstrates the excision of uterine wedge containing most of the septum. Figures 12.4.3.2 (D to F) demonstrate the method closure of uterine incision.

The method of closure of the uterine incision is in form of three layers, same way as that described with Strassman's metroplasty Figure 12.4.3.1 (C to E).

Picture	Medical/Surgical Description	Management/Clinical Highlights
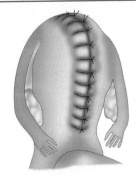 **Fig. 12.4.3.2G:** Appearance of the uterine surface following the closure	After the uterine wedge has been removed, the uterus is closed in three layers with interrupted stitches. The innermost layer of stitches includes about one third of the thickness of myometrium and must also include the endometrium. Figure 12.4.3.2G shows appearance of the uterine surface following the closure.	If a double cervix is present, the surgeon must not try to unify the cervix because this may result in the development of an incompetent os.

12.4.3.3: Tompkin's Metroplasty

Picture	Medical/Surgical Description	Management/Clinical Highlights
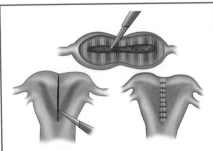 **Fig. 12.4.3.3:** Median bivalving technique of Tompkins metroplasty	In Tompkins procedure, the uterine corpus and the septum is divided with the help of a single median incision. The incision is carried inferiorly, until the endometrial cavity is reached. Each lateral septal half is then incised to within 1 cm of the tubes. No septal tissue is removed. The myometrial tissue is then reapproximated taking care not to place the sutures too close to the interstitial portion.	The procedure is believed to be simpler than the Jones procedure mainly because nearly all myometrial tissue is conserved by this procedure. This procedure is supposed to provide better results, a comparatively normal looking uterotubal junction and better pregnancy outcomes in comparison to Jones metroplasty.

12.4.4: Management of Uterine Septum

12.4.4.1: Diagnosis of Uterine Septum (A to D)

Picture	Medical/Surgical Description	Management/Clinical Highlights
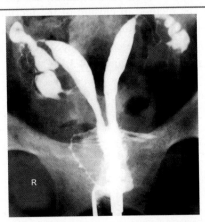 **Fig. 12.4.4.1A:** Hysterosalpingography showing presence of uterine septum which was confirmed on hysteroscopy	Initial investigations for diagnosis of uterine septum include hysterosalpingography (HSG) and two-dimensional ultrasound examination. HSG shows presence of an elongated fibrous structure arising from the uterine fundus, which is observed to be dividing the uterine cavity and is observed as a filling defect on HSG. Since HSG is not able to reveal the outer uterine contour, the diagnosis needs to be confirmed with the help of combined hysteroscopy, laparoscopy, three-dimensional ultrasound examination and/or MRI examination. Both HSG and two-dimensional ultrasound act as first line tools for diagnosis of uterine septum. Moreover, HSG helps in establishing tubal patency, while ultrasound also helps in detecting co-existing renal anomalies.	The uterine septum can be treated by removing it surgically, either through metroplasty (reconstructive uterine surgery) or through hysteroscopic resection. Jones metroplasty and Tompkins metroplasty for removal of uterine septum have been discussed in 12.4.3.2 (A to G) and 12.4.3.3 respectively. Hysteroscopic uterine resection has been discussed in 12.4.4.2 (A to C).

Picture	Medical/Surgical Description	Management/Clinical Highlights
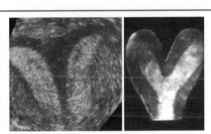Figs 12.4.4.1 (B and C): Three-dimensional reconstruction of a uterine septum: (B) Partial; (C) Complete	Three-dimensional ultrasound imaging and MRI are the best noninvasive techniques for confirming the diagnosis of uterine septum.	Both three-dimensional ultrasound and MRI examination help in determining the fundal contour. While the fundal contour is round in shape in case of septate uterus, the fundus is intended (> 1 cm) in cases of bicornuate uterus.
Fig. 12.4.4.1D: Visualization of outer uterine contour with three-dimensional ultrasound showing complete bicornuate uterus	On three-dimensional ultrasound, the central myometrial tissue extends up to internal cervical os and there are two endometrial cavities. The outer fundal contour was not round, but instead showed an indentation (> 1 cm), which confirmed the diagnosis of bicornuate uterus.	Other investigations, which help in confirming the diagnosis of bicornuate uterus and differentiating it from septate uterus include laparoscopic (invasive) and MRI (noninvasive) examination. MRI examination not only helps in confirming diagnosis of bicornuate uterus by determining the fundal contour, but an intercornual diameter (> 4 cm) is also diagnostic of bicornuate uterus.

12.4.4.2: Hysteroscopic Resection of the Uterine Septum (A to C)

Picture	Medical/Surgical Description	Management/Clinical Highlights
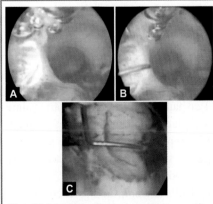Figs 12.4.4.2 (A to C): Hysteroscopic resection of the uterine septum: (A) Hysteroscopic appearance of the uterine septum; (B and C) Resectoscope loop transecting the uterine septum	The surgical procedure of choice for cases of septate uterus is hysteroscopic metroplasty under general endotracheal anesthesia and comprises of the following steps: • The uterus is first distended using dextran 70 or Hyskon® via a hysteroscope, which is inserted inside the cervix. • Using microscissors, electrosurgery or a laser, the surgeon can cut the uterine septum. • The inferior aspect of the septum is identified, and the septum is progressively dissected until a cavity with a normal-appearing contour is attained.	The hysteroscopic resection of septum is often accompanied with concurrent laparoscopic guidance. Concomitant laparoscopy at the time of hysteroscopic resection helps in reducing the risk of uterine perforation at the time of septal incision. When electrosurgical resectoscope is used for cutting the uterine septum, the septum is incised electrosurgically by advancing the cutting loupe and using the trigger mechanism of the resectoscope. When microscissors are used, flexible microscissors are passed through the operating channel of the hysteroscope.

12.5: HYSTERECTOMY

12.5.1: Abdominal Hysterectomy (A to O)

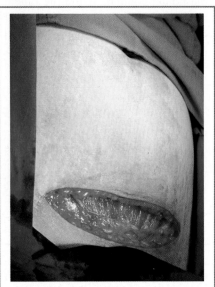

Fig. 12.5.1A: Pfannenstiel transverse abdominal incision

Due to good cosmetic results, better incision strength and reduced postoperative pain, transverse incisions in the abdomen (Pfannenstiel incision) versus vertical incisions are usually preferred for abdominal hysterectomy.

Once the uterus is reached, self-retaining retractors are placed in the abdominal incision, and the bowel is packed off with warm, moist gauze packs. Some surgeons prefer placing a No. 0 synthetic absorbable suture in the fundus of the uterus in order to provide adequate uterine traction.

Since the transverse incisions may not provide adequate exposure, they are usually reserved for benign uterine pathology, when the uterus is not very large in size. In general, cases where an increased exposure is required (e.g. presence of a malignant disease), either a midline subumbilical incision or modifications of transverse incision (Maylard's or Cherney's incision) may be performed. These types of incisions would result in an increased exposure. Moreover, with the midline subumbilical incision there is a possibility for extension of the abdominal incision around and above the umbilicus for provision of appropriate exposure in cases where required.

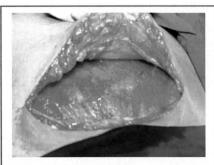

Fig. 12.5.1B: Opening of the rectus sheath

Following the dissection of skin and subcutaneous fat, rectus sheath is encountered which is visible as a glistening white structure and is composed of the aponeurosis of three abdominal muscles: external oblique, internal oblique and transversus abdominis. For details related to the anatomy of rectus sheath, kindly refer to Section 8.

A transverse incision is given with a scalpel in the midline of rectus sheath. It is then extended laterally on both sides with help of a scissors, following the direction of the fibers of aponeurosis in each of the layers. The rectus muscles are separated from the sheath superiorly and inferiorly. The pyramidalis muscles may be left attached to the undersurface of the fascia or left on the rectus muscles.

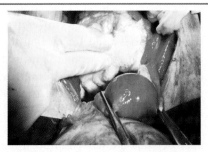

Fig. 12.5.1C: Intestines pushed back by packing the abdomen

After the rectus sheath has been cut and the rectus muscles separated, the parietal peritoneum becomes visible. A vertical incision is given over the parietal peritoneum in order to enter the peritoneal cavity. Once the peritoneal cavity is entered, intestines must be pushed back by packing the abdomen.

Two gauze packs soaked in warm saline are placed on the two sides to push the loops of intestines in the paracolic gutters so that the uterine surface is fully exposed and comes into view. Placement of Kelly's clamp across each uterine cornu, running down along the sides of uterus help in the elevation of the uterus.

Picture	Medical/Surgical Description	Management/Clinical Highlights

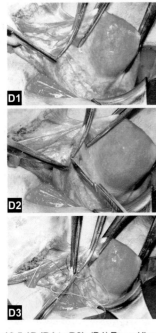

Figs 12.5.1D (D1 to D3): (D1) Round ligaments clamped; (D2) Round ligaments are cut; (D3) Round ligaments are ligated

The uterus is manually deviated to the left side, thereby stretching the round ligament. Following this, the round ligaments are clamped, cut and ligated.

Once the round ligaments are transected, the anterior leaf of broad ligament is cut out and opened.

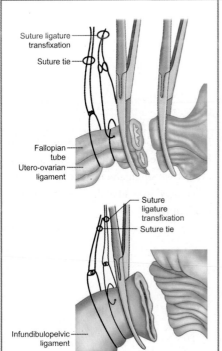

Fig. 12.5.1E: Diagrammatic representation of transection of utero-ovarian and infundibulopelvic ligaments

The next step depends on whether the tubes and ovaries have to be preserved or removed. If the fallopian tubes and ovaries are to be removed, then the infundibulopelvic ligaments are clamped, cut and ligated. Three Oschner's clamps are placed across the infundibulopelvic ligament, using a window in the broad ligament. After the ureter is located, the lateral most clamp is placed first. The ligament is then incised between the medial and middle clamp. The pedicle is then doubly ligated with No. 0 delayed absorbable suture.

If the tubes and ovaries have to be conserved, the fallopian tube and the utero-ovarian ligament are clamped, cut and ligated close to the uterus.

Ovaries are usually preserved if they appear normal and the patient is below 50 years of age. After the age of 50 years, the ovaries are removed after taking the woman's consent in order to prevent the occurrence of ovarian carcinoma at a later date.

Picture	Medical/Surgical Description	Management/Clinical Highlights

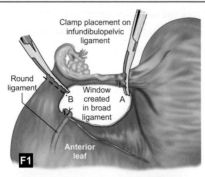

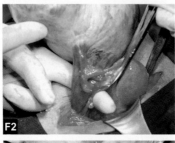

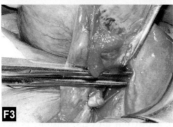

Figs 12.5.1F (F1 to F3): (F1) Diagrammatic representation of ligation of the infundibulopelvic ligament; (F2) Identifying the infundibulopelvic ligament; (F3) Infundibulopelvic ligament clamped and later cut and ligated

Figures 12.5.1 (F1 to F3) illustrates the method of identifying, clamping, cutting and ligation of infundibulopelvic ligaments.

As discussed previously, infundibulopelvic ligaments are cut in case the tubes and ovaries are to be removed.

Ovaries are left behind in case they appear healthy on direct examination; there is no family history of ovarian cancer and the patient's age is less than 50 years. Direct inspection of the ovaries at the time of hysterectomy serves as the best screening method for ovarian cancer. If ovaries appear unhealthy or suspicious of malignancy (enlarged or appears to have solid areas), they must be removed.

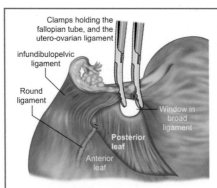

Fig. 12.5.1G: Transection of the utero-ovarian ligament and fallopian tube

The uterus is retracted toward the pubic symphysis and deviated to one side with the infundibulopelvic ligament, tube and ovary on tension. A finger should be inserted through the peritoneum of the posterior leaf of broad ligament under the suspensory ligament of the ovary and fallopian tube. Three Ochsner's clamps are placed across the tube and utero-ovarian ligaments as close to the uterus as possible. An incision is made between the middle and medial clamp. As a free tie is placed lateral to the lateral most clamp, the pedicle is completely surrounded and the vessels are occluded. The middle clamp is replaced by a transfixation suture ligature that is tied securely around both sides of the pedicle.

In case, the tubes and ovaries have to be conserved, the fallopian tube and the utero-ovarian ligament are clamped, cut and ligated instead of the infundibulopelvic ligaments.

Picture	Medical/Surgical Description	Management/Clinical Highlights

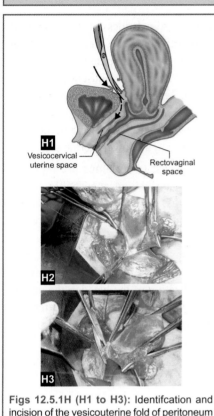

Figs 12.5.1H (H1 to H3): Identifcation and incision of the vesicouterine fold of peritoneum

Figure 12.5.1H illustrates the procedure of identifying and incising the vesicouterine fold of peritoneum.

A curvilinear incision is given over the vesicouterine fold of peritoneum.

After separating the bladder peritoneum from the lower uterine segment, the incision along the vesicouterine fold is extended over the anterior leaf of broad ligament.

Figure 12.5.1H1 shows dissection of the vesicouterine plane to mobilize the bladder. Figure 12.5.1H2 shows identification of loose uterovesical (UV) fold. Figure 12.5.1H3 shows cutting of UV fold.

The vesicouterine fold of peritoneum is identified by its loose nature. The bladder can be dissected off the lower uterine segment of the uterus and cervix by either blunt or sharp dissection. If there has been extensive lower segment disease, previous cesarean sections or pelvic irradiation, blunt dissection of the bladder off the cervix is dangerous, and a sharp dissection technique should be performed.

Both blunt and sharp dissection helps in removing the loose connective tissues overlying the external iliac artery.

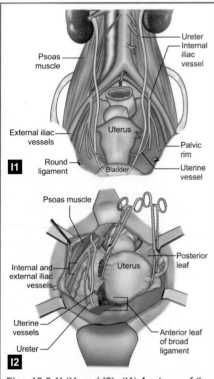

Figs 12.5.1I (I1 and I2): (I1) Anatomy of the pelvic retroperitoneum; (I2) Identification of the ureter in the retroperitoneal space

The retroperitoneum is then entered by extending the incision on the posterior leaf of broad ligament cephalad, remaining lateral to both the infundibulopelvic ligaments and the iliac vessels. The ureter is identified as it crosses the common iliac vessels by following the external iliac artery cephalad to the bifurcation.

Ureter is left attached to the medial or posterior leaf of the broad ligament so as not to disrupt its blood supply.

The left ureter is usually more medial than the right one. If the surgeon encounters extensive pelvic disease, he/she may need to dissect the ureter down toward the bladder as far as is necessary.

Picture	Medical/Surgical Description	Management/Clinical Highlights

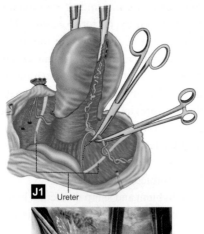

J1 Ureter

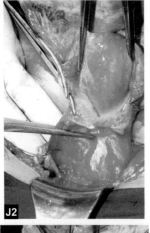

J2

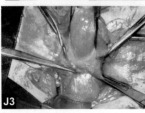

J3

Figs 12.5.1J (J1 to J3): (J1) Diagram showing ligation of uterine vessels; (J2) Uterine artery ligation; (J3) Uterine arteries of both the sides have been clamped

Figure 12.5.1J shows clamping, cutting and ligation of the uterine vessels. Bladder is sharply dissected off the lower uterine segment and the cervix. The uterus is then retracted cephalad to one side of the pelvis, placing the ligaments in the lower uterine segment on a stretch. Any loose connective tissue overlying the uterine vessels is sharply removed in order to skeletonize the vessels.

After the uterine vessels are skeletonized, they are triply clamped and cut.

Three cardinal rules must be followed while clamping the uterine vessels in order to avoid clamping the ureters:
- The lowest clamp must be placed first
- The lowest clamp must be placed at the level of internal os
- The lowest clamp must be at right angles to the lower uterine segment.

The lowest two clamps are replaced by No. 0 delayed absorbable suture ligatures. Following these principles help in avoiding injury to the ureters. The ureters lie close to the cervix as they travel through the pelvis. By gentle upward uterine traction and downward mobilization of the bladder, the ureters that lie approximately 2 cm lateral to the cervix are further displaced from the uterine vessels.

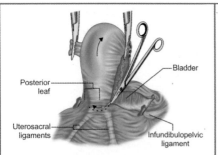

Bladder

Posterior leaf

Uterosacral ligaments

Infundibulopelvic ligament

Fig. 12.5.1K: Incision of the rectouterine peritoneum and mobilization of the rectum from the posterior cervix

Figure 12.5.1 K illustrates the dissection of the rectum and incision of the rectouterine peritoneum inferiorly toward uterosacral ligaments to help mobilize the uterus and reflect sigmoid colon.

The posterior leaf of broad ligament is then incised to the point where the uterosacral ligaments join the cervix and across the posterior lower uterine segment between the rectum and cervix.

Picture	Medical/Surgical Description	Management/Clinical Highlights

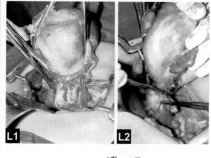

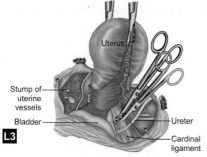

The uterosacral ligaments and the Mackenrodt's ligament are identified and then clamped, cut and ligated.

Mackenrodt's ligaments, also known as cardinal or transverse cervical ligaments, are found at the base of broad ligament and help in attaching the cervix and lower uterine segment to the lateral pelvic wall. Since ureters are present in close vicinity to the cardinal ligaments, care must be taken at the time of clamping and ligating these ligaments so as not to damage the ureters. The uterosacral ligaments help in attaching the cervix and the lower uterine segment to the sacrum and posterior pelvic wall.

Figs 12.5.1L (L1 to L3): (L1) Mackenrodt's ligament are identified; (L2) Mackenrodt's ligaments are clamped; (L3) Diagrammatic representation of clamping and cutting the cardinal ligaments

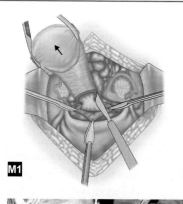

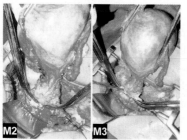

Figures 12.5.1M (M1 to M3) shows identification, clamping and cutting of the vaginal angles. After the surgeon has determined with certainty that the bladder and rectum have been completely dissected away from the vagina, curved Ochsner's clamps are placed across the vaginal angles. The vagina is entered by a stab wound with a scalpel and is cut across with either a scalpel or scissors. First the anterior vaginal fornix is opened and the incision is extended circumferentially close to the cervix in order to maintain the length of the vagina. The uterus is removed.

After removing the uterus, the edges of the vagina are picked up with straight Ochsner's clamps in a 3 O'clock, 6 O'clock, 9 O'clock and 12 O'clock positions.

Figs 12.5.1M (M1 to M3): (M1) Diagrammatic representation of cutting the cervix from the vaginal vault; (M2) Vaginal angles are clamped; (M3) Vaginal angles are cut

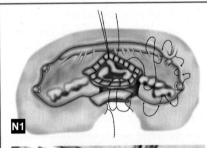

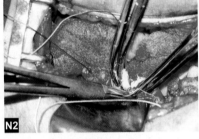

Figs 12.5.1N (N1 and N2): (N1) Vaginal cuff is left open with running locking stitch sutures placed along the cut edge of the vaginal mucosa; (N2) Closure and support of the vaginal vault

The vaginal cuff may be left open and the edges of the vaginal mucosa are sutured with a running locking no. 0 synthetic absorbable suture starting at the midpoint of the vagina underneath the bladder and carried around to the stumps of the cardinal and uterosacral ligaments, which are sutured into the angle of the vagina.

The cardinal and uterosacral ligaments of the opposite side are included in the running locking no. 0 synthetic absorbable suture, and the reefing process is then completed to the midpoint of the anterior vaginal wall.

At this point, meticulous care should be taken to ensure that the lateral angle of the vagina is adequately secured and that hemostasis is complete between the lateral angle of the vagina and the stumps of the cardinal and uterosacral ligaments because this can be a site of hemorrhage. When tied, this suture approximates the uterosacral ligaments behind the upper posterior vagina and pulls the posterior vaginal fornix in a posterior direction. This helps in supporting the vaginal vault, thereby preventing the possibility of development of vaginal vault prolapse or enterocele in subsequent years following total abdominal hysterectomy.

The next step for the surgeon to decide is whether to or not to close the vaginal vault. Some surgeons prefer to close the vaginal vault using interrupted No. 0 chromic catgut sutures. However, in our setup, the vaginal cuff usually is not closed. If additional support of the posterior vagina is required, obliteration of the cul-de-sac by Moskowitz or Halban's technique can be considered.

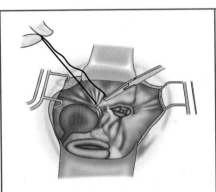

Fig. 12.5.1O: Reperitonization of the pelvis

The pelvis is reperitonized with running 2-0 synthetic absorbable suture from the anterior to the posterior leaf of the broad ligament. The stumps of the tubo-ovarian, round, suspensory ligament of the ovary, and the cardinal and uterosacral ligaments are buried retroperitoneally. In order to avoid leaving the ovaries above the vaginal vault, the utero-ovarian ligament should be extraperitonized as separate sutures. Retroperitonization is completed by suturing the bladder peritoneum to the cul-de-sac peritoneum with 3-0 delayed absorbable sutures.

Reperitonization of pelvis is followed by abdominal closure, which completes the procedure of abdominal hysterectomy. Prior to closing the abdomen, all the stumps must be inspected for hemostasis. The pelvis is thoroughly washed with sterile saline solution. Meticulous care is taken to ensure that hemostasis is present throughout the dissected area.

Picture	Medical/Surgical Description	Management/Clinical Highlights

12.5.2: Vaginal Hysterectomy (A to N)

Picture	Medical/Surgical Description	Management/Clinical Highlights
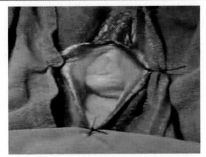 **Fig. 12.5.2A:** Application of labial sutures	After cleaning and draping the patient under all aseptic precautions and induction of anesthesia, the labial sutures are applied to facilitate the exposure of cervix. The anterior and posterior lips of the cervix are grasped with a single or double-toothed tenaculum.	Figures 12.5.2 (A to M) demonstrate the procedure of vaginal hysterectomy. In vaginal hysterectomy, the steps of surgery are based on the same principle as that in abdominal hysterectomy described previously, it is just that the uterus is removed through the vaginal route rather than the abdominal route and the various steps as described previously with abdominal route are now performed vaginally.
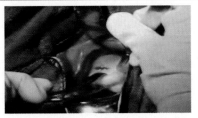 **Fig. 12.5.2B:** Transverse incision is made over the anterior vaginal wall just below the bladder reflection	Figure 12.5.2 shows the procedure for grasping and circumscribing the cervix.	Traction in downward direction is applied on the cervix after grasping its anterior and posterior lips. A circumferential incision is made in the vaginal epithelium at the junction of the cervix just below the bladder sulcus.
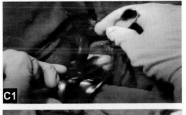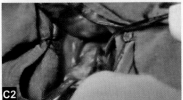 **Figs 12.5.2C (C1 and C2):** The incision is deepened to cut the pubovesicocervical ligament	After making the incision below the bladder sulcus, the vaginal epithelium may be dissected sharply from the underlying tissues or pushed bluntly with an open sponge. The vesicouterine fascia is dissected away. Uterovesical fold of peritoneum is visualized and incised.	Cutting of the pubovesicocervical ligament helps in visualizing the uterovesical fold of peritoneum, which is then cut.
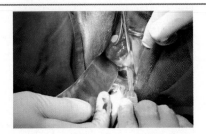 **Fig. 12.5.2D:** The circular vaginal incision is extended posteriorly and laterally and the bladder is retracted anteriorly	Figure 12.5.2D shows that the circular incision over the vagina is extended posteriorly and laterally and the bladder is retracted anteriorly.	After the initial incision is made, the vaginal epithelium may be sharply dissected from the underlying tissues or pushed bluntly with an open sponge.

Picture	Medical/Surgical Description	Management/Clinical Highlights
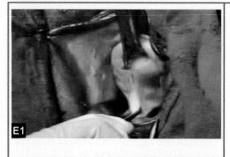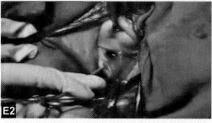**Figs 12.5.2E (E1 and E2):** (E1) Loose fold of posterior vaginal wall at cervico-vaginal junction is lifted with Allis; (E2) An incision is given to open the vagina and Pouch of Douglas at the same time	Figure 12.5.2E shows the opening of vagina and Pouch of Douglas. The peritoneal reflection of the posterior cul-de-sac can be identified by stretching the vaginal mucosa and underlying connective tissues with forceps.	To open the posterior peritoneum, the uterus is pulled up. The peritoneum is grasped with surgical forceps and opened with scissors. The posterior vaginal wall is separated from the Pouch of Douglas.
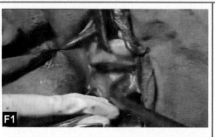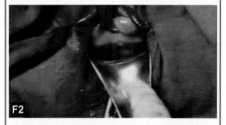**Figs 12.5.2F (F1 and F2):** Peritoneum is dissected and incised; rectum and Pouch of Douglas are retracted with Sims speculum	As the peritoneum is dissected and incised, rectum and the Pouch of Douglas are retracted with the help of Sims speculum.	In order to gain entry into the posterior cul-de-sac, the peritoneal reflection of the posterior cul-de-sac can be identified by stretching the vaginal mucosa and underlying connective tissues with forceps. To open the posterior peritoneum, the uterus is pulled up. The peritoneum is grasped with surgical forceps and opened with scissors. The posterior vaginal wall is separated from the Pouch of Douglas.

Picture	Medical/Surgical Description	Management/Clinical Highlights

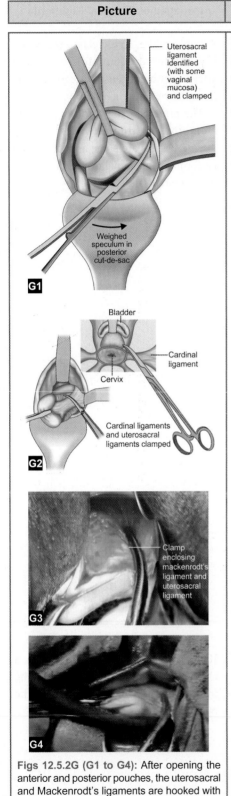

Uterosacral ligament identified (with some vaginal mucosa) and clamped

Weighed speculum in posterior cut-de-sac

G1

Bladder

Cardinal ligament

Cervix

Cardinal ligaments and uterosacral ligaments clamped

G2

Clamp enclosing mackenrodt's ligament and uterosacral ligament

G3

G4

Figs 12.5.2G (G1 to G4): After opening the anterior and posterior pouches, the uterosacral and Mackenrodt's ligaments are hooked with help of a finger, following which they are clamped, cut and ligated with Heaney's clamp

Figures 12.5.2G (G1 to G4) shows ligation of uterosacral ligaments. With the retraction of lateral vaginal wall and counter traction on the cervix, the uterosacral ligaments are clamped with the tip of clamp incorporating the lower portion of the uterosacral ligaments, following which it is cut and ligated.

The clamp is placed perpendicular to the uterine axis, and the pedicle is cut close to the clamp and sutured. Following the cutting of uterosacral ligaments, the cardinal ligaments are identified, clamped, cut and suture ligated.

Picture	Medical/Surgical Description	Management/Clinical Highlights
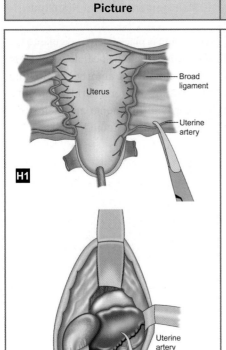 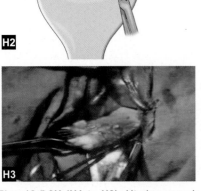 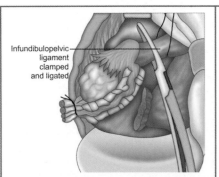 **Figs 12.5.2H (H1 to H3):** Uterine vessels are then clamped, cut and ligated without transfixation	Figures 12.5.2H shows ligation of the uterine vessels. Contralateral and downward traction is applied on the cervix with an effort to incorporate the anterior and posterior leaves of the visceral peritoneum. The uterine vessels are identified, clamped, cut and suture ligated. This is usually done without transfixation.	A single suture, single clamp technique is considered adequate for uterine artery ligation because it decreases the potential risk of ureteral injury. The principles to be followed while clamping, cutting and ligating the uterine vessels are same as those while performing abdominal hysterectomy and have been discussed before.
Fig. 12.5.2I: Removal of the fallopian tubes and ovaries by clamping across the infundibulopelvic ligament	As the anterior and posterior peritoneum are opened, the remainder of broad ligament, utero-ovarian ligaments and round ligament are clamped, cut and ligated.	If the ovaries have to be removed, a Heaney's clamp is placed across the infundibulopelvic ligaments, and the ovaries and tubes are excised.

Picture	Medical/Surgical Description	Management/Clinical Highlights
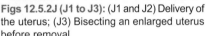 **Figs 12.5.2J (J1 to J3):** (J1 and J2) Delivery of the uterus; (J3) Bisecting an enlarged uterus before removal	Figures 12.5.2J (J1 to J3) shows delivery of the entire uterus once the various uterine support structures have been successfully released.	Sometimes when the uterus is big in size to be delivered outside, it may be partially divided starting from the fundal region to facilitate its delivery outside through the vagina.
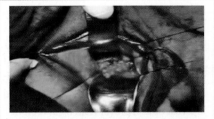 **Fig. 12.5.2K:** Following the removal of uterus, pedicles are inspected for any bleeding	Before the uterus is removed, the pedicles must be inspected for presence of any bleeding.	In case any bleeding points are visualized, steps must be taken to suture ligate the bleeding points.
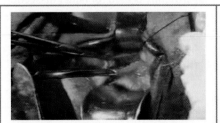 **Fig. 12.5.2L:** Uterovesical fold of peritoneum is identified and sutured transversely using monocryl 2-0 sutures	Figure 12.5.2L shows the method of peritoneal closure. Peritoneal closure may not be always performed. If the peritoneal closure is performed, the anterior edge of peritoneum is identified and grasped with forceps. The peritoneum is reapproximated in a purse-string fashion using continuous absorbable sutures.	Since the pelvic peritoneum does not provide support and usually reforms within 24 hours after surgery, many surgeons do not reapproximate the peritoneum as a routine procedure. If the peritoneum is reapproximated, high posterior reperitonealization is performed because it shortens the cul-de-sac and prevents the formation of enterocele in the future.

Picture	Medical/Surgical Description	Management/Clinical Highlights
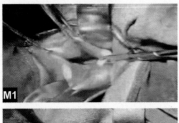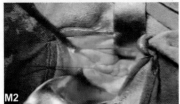 **Figs 12.5.2M (M1 and M2):** Vaginal walls identified and sutured with 1-0 vicryl sutures	Figures 12.5.2M (M1 and M2) shows the method of closing the vaginal mucosa.	The vaginal mucosa can be reapproximated in a vertical or horizontal manner using either interrupted or continuous sutures.
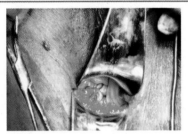 **Fig. 12.5.2N:** Final appearance of vagina following closure	After the uterus and cervix have been removed from the top of the vagina, the upper part of the vagina where the surgical incision was made is closed with suture material.	The final appearance of vagina following the closure of vaginal mucosa is shown in Figure 12.5.2N.

12.5.3: Laparoscopic Assisted Vaginal Hysterectomy (A to L)

Picture		
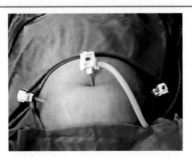 **Fig. 12.5.3A:** Insertion of laparoscope and others surgical tools	The procedure of laparoscopic assisted hysterectomy is illustrated in Figures 12.5.3 (A to F). Patients are placed in a dorsal lithotomy position with pneumoboots. Laparoscopic assisted vaginal hysterectomy (LAVH) begins with several small abdominal subumbilical incisions to allow the insertion of the laparoscope and other surgical tools. Pneumoperitoneum is created by inserting a Veress needle into the peritoneal cavity. Once intraperitoneal pressure has reached 15 mm Hg, an optical trocar is inserted through the umbilicus under direct vision. The lower quadrant trocar sleeves are placed under direct vision. These trocars are placed lateral to the rectus abdominis muscles, 2 cm above and 2 cm medial to the anterior superior iliac spine.	Three approaches can be taken by the surgeons toward use of minimally invasive surgery at the time of hysterectomy. These include LAVH, laparoscopic hysterectomy and laparoscopic supracervical hysterectomy. The procedure of LAVH is quite similar to the procedure of vaginal hysterectomy described above, but in this case laparoscopy is used for better dissection of the abdominal tissues. The procedure is performed under general anesthesia.

Picture	Medical/Surgical Description	Management/Clinical Highlights
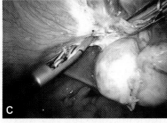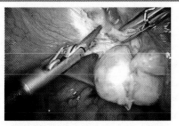**Figs 12.5.3 (B and C):** (B) Ovarian ligament is held taut, (C) following which they are desiccated and cut	The infundibulopelvic, or utero-ovarian ligaments and fallopian tubes are occluded and divided, depending on whether the ovaries would be removed or not respectively.	Laparoscopic assisted vaginal hysterectomy enables performance of a difficult vaginal hysterectomy and also serves as an alternative to abdominal hysterectomy. Thus the mortality and morbidity associated with LAVH is similar to that associated with vaginal hysterectomy and is much less in comparison with abdominal hysterectomy.
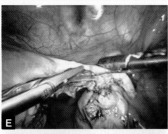**Fig. 12.5.3 D:** Laparoscopic clamping, desiccation and cutting of the fallopian tube, adnexa and round ligaments in succession	The fallopian tube, adnexa and round ligament are then clamped, cut and desiccated in a similar fashion.	At the time of LAVH, if any concomitant pathology is encountered such as presence of adhesions, simple ovarian cysts, etc., they are dealt with simultaneously.
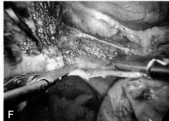**Figs 12.5.3 (E and F):** (E) The broad ligament is opened to separate the anterior and posterior sheath; (F) Anterior and posterior leaves of the broad ligament are cut	The anterior and posterior leaves of the broad ligament are separated with the help of a Harmonic scalpel.	As the anterior and posterior leaves of broad ligament are separated and a proper plane of cleavage formed between the two, the anterior and posterior leaves of broad ligament are cut separately.

Picture	Medical/Surgical Description	Management/Clinical Highlights
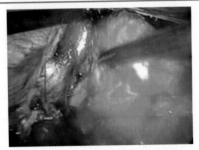 **Fig. 12.5.3G:** Uterovesical fold of peritoneum is lifted and opened up by giving a small nick	The vesicouterine peritoneal fold is identified, following which it is lifted and then incised with help of a small nick. The bladder is then mobilized off the lower uterine segment and pushed down.	As a small nick is given in the vesicouterine fold, it opens up on its own immediately under the pressure of pneumoperitoneum. The physician may also choose to laparoscopically incise the posterior cul-de-sac.
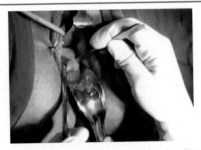 **Fig. 12.5.3 H:** The bladder is separated from cervix	As the bladder is separated from the cervix, rest of the procedure of hysterectomy is carried out vaginally.	At the time of laparoscopic surgery, uterus is lifted with help of a uterine manipulator, moving the uterus in various directions. This helps in keeping the various structures taut so that they can be properly cut and/or dissected.
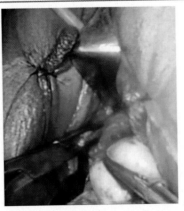 **Fig. 12.5.3I:** A semilunar incision is given over cervix	A semilunar incision is given over the cervix to separate the lower uterine segment and cervix from the vaginal apex.	The bladder has already been separated from cervix at the time of laparoscopy.
Fig. 12.5.3J: Uterosacral ligaments are clamped and cut through vaginal route	The remaining pedicles, i.e. the uterosacral ligaments and cardinal ligments are clamped, desiccated and cut through the vaginal route.	The Pouch of Douglas between the two uterosacral ligaments had already been cut at the time of laparoscopy.

Picture	Medical/Surgical Description	Management/Clinical Highlights
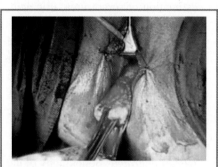 **Fig. 12.5.3K:**Uterine vessels are doubly clamped and cut through vaginal route	Uterine vessels are then doubly clamped, occluded and cut.	At the time of clamping, occluding and cutting the uterine vessels, care must be taken not to injure the ureter due to its close proximity with the uterine vessels.
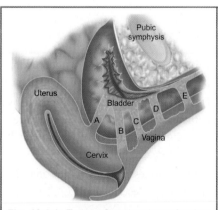 **Fig. 12.5.3L:** Uterus is delivered out vaginally	Since all attachments of the uterus with the pelvic side walls have now been cut, the uterus and cervix can be easily removed through the vagina, following which the top of the vaginal cuff is sutured. The closure of the vaginal cuff is also performed vaginally. Following the closure of vaginal cuff, a re-look laparoscopy is performed during which the pelvis can be irrigated and hemostasis at all sites assured. The port sites are then closed.	If the uterus is too large to come out through the vagina, it can be carefully morcellated transvaginally prior to the removal.

12.6: GENITOURINARY FISTULAE

12.6.1: Types

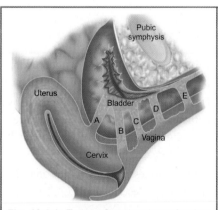

Fig. 12.6.1: Types of genitourinary fistulas: (A) uterovesical fistula; (B) cervicovesical fistula; (C) midvaginal vesicovaginal fistula (VVF); (D) VVF involving the bladder neck; (E) urethrovaginal fistula

Urogenital fistulas (UGFs) can be defined as abnormal communication tracts (lined with epithelium) between the genital tract and the urinary tract or the alimentary tract or both. UGFs can be classified as follows:
Urethrovaginal fistula
- Vesical fistula (VVF or vesicocervical)
- Ureterovaginal fistula
- Rectovaginal fistula

Vesicovaginal fistula is an abnormal fistulous tract extending between the bladder and the vagina that allows the continuous involuntary discharge of urine into the vaginal vault. The uncontrolled continuous leakage of urine into the vagina is the hallmark symptom of patients with UGFs.
- Patients may complain of urinary incontinence or an increase in vaginal discharge.
- Constant wetness in the genital areas can lead to the excoriation of the vagina, vulva, perineum and thighs.
- Presence of recurrent cystitis or pyelonephritis, abnormal urinary stream and hematuria following surgery may point toward an underlying UGF.

12.6.2: Surgical Management

12.6.2.1: Latzko's Partial Colpocleisis (A to C)

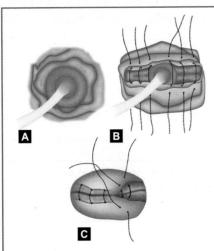

Figs 12.6.2.1 (A to C): Steps of Latzko's partial colpocleisis

Latzko's partial colpocleisis involves denuding the vaginal epithelium all around the edge of the fistula and then approximating the wide raw surfaces with rows of absorbable sutures. The vesical edges of the fistula are not denuded. The posterior vaginal wall becomes the posterior bladder wall and re-epithelializes with transitional epithelium.

Methylene blue three-swab test is diagnostic of VVF and is performed prior to surgery to identify the fistula. In this test, with the vaginal cavity packed with three sterile swabs, a catheter is introduced into the bladder through the urethra. Approximately 50–100 mL of methylene blue dye is injected into the bladder via the catheter. In case of VVF, dye stains the uppermost swab. The lowermost swab gets stained if the leakage is from urethra. If none of the swabs get stained, but get wet from urine, leakage is from the ureter.

Other investigations, which need to be done prior to surgery are as follows:
- *Blood investigations*: This includes complete blood count, hemoglobin, etc.
- *Urine investigations*: This includes urine routine, microscopy, and urine culture and sensitivity.
- *Renal function tests*: This includes estimation of serum urea, uric acid, creatinine and electrolytes.
- *Cystoscopy*: With the vagina filled with water or isotonic sodium chloride solution, the infusion of gas through the urethra through a cystoscope produces air bubbles in the vaginal fluid at the site of a UGF (Flat tire sign).
- *Methylene blue three-swab test Ultrasonography*: Sonography of the kidney, ureter and bladder must be performed.
- *Methylene blue dye test*: The bladder can be filled with sterile milk or methylene blue in retrograde fashion using a small transurethral catheter to identify the site of leakage.

12.6.2.2: Chassar Moir Flap-splitting Technique (A to E)

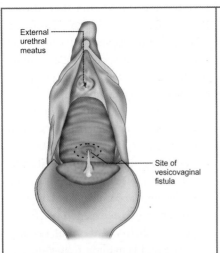

Fig. 12.6.2.2A: Vesicovaginal fistula located on the posterior wall of the bladder

Figures 12.6.2.2 (A to E) illustrate the flap-splitting technique for repair of VVF. Figure 12.6.2.2A shows a VVF located on the posterior wall of the bladder. Sometimes a Foley's catheter may be inserted through the fistula and its bulb inflated with 5 cc of saline. This helps in better delineation of the fistula margins.

Preoperative steps: Before undertaking surgery, the following need to be done:

Urine sample must be collected by catheterization and must be submitted for culture and sensitivity. Any infection must be treated prior to surgery.

Other investigations which may be required are described in 12.6.2.1.

Picture	Medical/Surgical Description	Management/Clinical Highlights
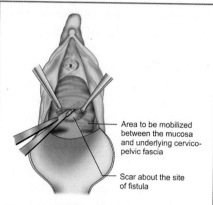 **Fig. 12.6.2.2B:** An incision is made about the fistula opening, which is extended into a transverse vaginal incision	After making an incision around the fistula, the vagina is dissected from the bladder to allow mobilization of tissues and subsequently reduced tension on the suture lines.	In case, the patient has extensive fibrosis, application of omental grafts or interpositioning of maritus or gracilis muscle graft between the bladder and vaginal muscles promotes healing. If the first attempt at the fistula repair fails, the second must be undertaken only after a period of 3 months. Urinary diversion procedures (e.g. implantation of ureters into the sigmoid colon, creating an ileal loop bladder or a rectal bladder) can be considered in cases where there is extensive loss of bladder tissue, previous failed attempts at fistula closure or fistula formation due to radiation injury.
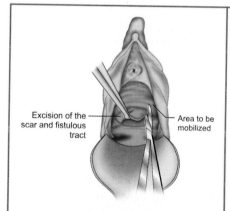 **Fig. 12.6.2.2C:** The fistula scar is excised converting the opening into fresh injury	As the scarred area around the fistulous tract is excised, it gets converted into a fresh wound.	At the time of surgery, routine excision of the fistula tract is not mandatory.
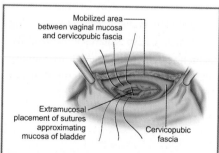 **Fig. 12.6.2.2D:** Closure performed with the initial suture layer of 4-0 delayed absorbable sutures placed in an extramucosal fashion	The bladder and vaginal mucosa are sutured in two layers with delayed absorbable sutures in order to obtain water-tight seal.	Successful fistula repair requires adequate dissection and mobilization of tissues, meticulous hemostasis and reapproximation under minimal tension.

Picture	Medical/Surgical Description	Management/Clinical Highlights
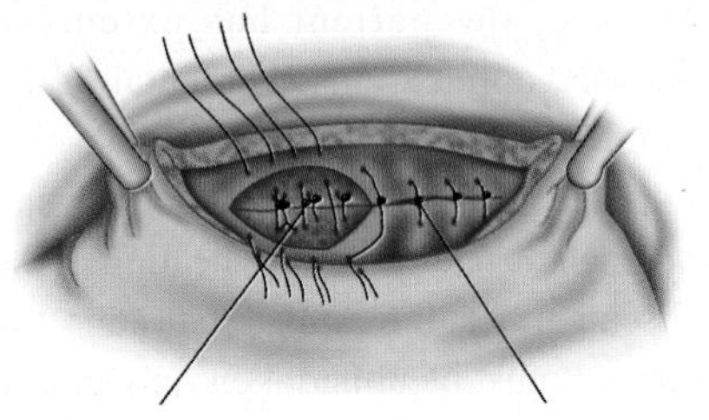 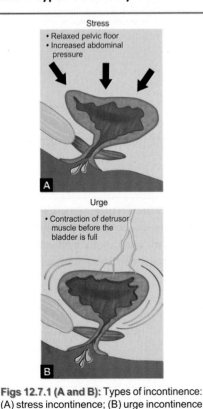 **Fig. 12.6.2.2E:** The initial suture line is inverted with similar suture	Each suture line inverting the previous suture line is placed 3–4 mm lateral to the initially closed suture line.	Postoperative management in these patients comprises of the following steps: • *Bladder drainage*: Continuous bladder drainage postoperatively is vital for successful UGF repair. • *Antibiotics*: Treatment with antibiotics helps in eradication of infection. • *Acidification of urine*: This helps in reducing the risk of complications such as cystitis, mucus production and formation of bladder calculi. Vitamin C in the dosage of 500 mg orally three times per day may be used to acidify urine. • *Pelvic rest*: Pelvic and speculum examinations of the vagina must be avoided during the first 4–6 weeks postoperatively because during this time, the tissue is fragile and delicate. Sexual intercourse and tampon use must also be prohibited.

12.7: URINARY INCONTINENCE

12.7.1: Types of Urinary Incontinence (A and B)

Stress
- Relaxed pelvic floor
- Increased abdominal pressure

A

Urge
- Contraction of detrusor muscle before the bladder is full

B

Figs 12.7.1 (A and B): Types of incontinence: (A) stress incontinence; (B) urge incontinence

Urinary incontinence can be defined as an involuntary loss of urine which is a social or hygienic problem and can be demonstrated with objective means. There are two main types of urinary incontinence: stress incontinence and urge incontinence.

Stress urinary incontinence can be defined as involuntary leakage of urine during conditions causing an increase in intra-abdominal pressure (exertion, sneezing, etc.) which causes the intravesical pressure to rise higher than that which the urethral closure mechanisms can withstand (in the absence of detrusor contractions). Urge urinary incontinence can be defined as involuntary leakage of urine accompanied by or immediately preceded by urgency. The corresponding urodynamic term is detrusor overactivity, which is evident in form of involuntary detrusor contractions at the time of filling cystometry.

Picture	Medical/Surgical Description	Management/Clinical Highlights

12.7.2: Diagnosis of Urinary Incontinence

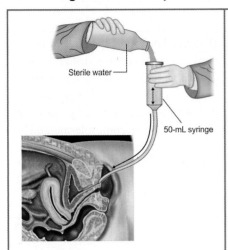

Sterile water

50-mL syringe

Fig. 12.7.2: Cystometry for diagnosis of urinary incontinence

Cystometrogram requires a 50 cc syringe and a No. 16 Foley's catheter. After the patient has emptied her bladder, a Foley's catheter is inserted inside the urethra, through which a premeasured amount of fluid is injected inside the bladder. This catheter may be connected to a cystometer which measures the pressure when fluid is inserted inside the catheter. When the patient gets a feeling to micturate, the pressure is recorded again. In the adjacent picture, the special catheter performs both the functions, transfering the liquid as well as acting as a manometer (pressure sensor).

Cystometry is a diagnostic procedure used for evaluating the bladder function (ability of the bladder to contract and expel urine). The bladder function is evaluated in terms of a cystometrogram generated, which plots the volume of liquid emptied by the bladder against the pressure generated in the bladder at that time. This test helps in evaluating the functioning of the bladder and its ability to hold or release the urine. The chart generated from cystometric analysis is known as cystometrogram.

12.7.3: Retropubic Bladder Neck Suspension Procedures for Surgical Management

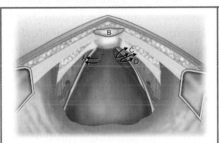

Fig. 12.7.3: Point of attachment of endopelvic fascia during bladder neck suspension procedures: (A) arcus tendineus; (B) periosteum of the pubic symphysis; (C) iliopectineal ligaments (Cooper's ligaments); (D) obturator internus fascia

Various retropubic bladder neck suspension procedures are performed through lower abdominal incision and involve the attachment of periurethral and perivesical endopelvic fascia to some other supporting structure in the anterior pelvis. The various supporting structures which can be used are shown in Figure 12.7.3.

Supporting structure in the anterior pelvis for various bladder neck suspension procedures are as follows:
- Paravaginal procedure: Arcus tendineus
- Modified Marshall-Marchetti- Krantz procedure: Back of pubic symphysis
- Burch colposuspension: Iliopectineal ligament (Cooper's ligament)
- Turner-Warwick vaginal obturator shelf procedure: Fascia over obturator internus

12.7.4: Transvaginal Urethropexy/Needle Suspension Procedure

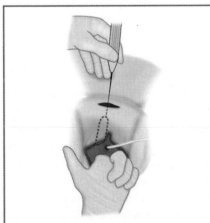

Fig. 12.7.4: Guiding a long needle through the Retzius space using the index finger

This procedure involves passage of sutures between the vagina and anterior abdominal wall using an especially designed long needle carrier, which is inserted through the vaginal incision made at the level of bladder neck. The endopelvic fascia is perforated and the Retzius space is entered from below. A permanent suture is passed down through a small abchominal incision to the Retzius space where it is fixed to the endopelvic fascia at the level of bladder nuck. The needle is then passed back up through the retropubic space to the abdominal incision where the suture is tied.

Postoperative care involves the following steps:
- Bladder drainage is an essential aspect of postoperative care. Most patients are able to void spontaneously in 3–7 days.
- Measures must be taken to control chronic cough and to avoid or treat constipation.
- The patient should avoid lifting anything heavier than 10 pounds for 12 weeks.

12.8: HYSTEROSCOPY

12.8.1: Definition

Picture	Medical/Surgical Description	Management/Clinical Highlights
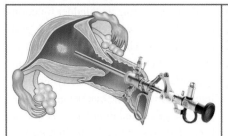 **Fig. 12.8.1:** Diagrammatic view of a hysteroscope inside the uterine cavity (© 2010 Karl Storz GmbH & Co. KG)	Hysteroscopy is a minimally invasive procedure, involving the direct inspection of the cervical canal and endometrial cavity through a rigid, flexible or a contact hysteroscope.	Both diagnostic and operative hysteroscopy has now become a standard part of routine gynecological practice. Besides diagnosing certain uterine pathologies and aiding in the biopsy, hysteroscopy has now also become the method of choice for treatment of intrauterine pathology.

12.8.2: Equipment (A to I)

Picture	Medical/Surgical Description	Management/Clinical Highlights
  Fig. 12.8.2A: Telescope (© 2010 Karl Storz GmbH & Co. KG)	The hysteroscopic system comprises of a rigid telescope that is used together with an outer sheath for instillation of the distension media. Telescopes of different diameters (2–4 mm) and a variety of viewing capabilities are available (0°, 12°, 30°, 70°). The most popular hysteroscope is a 4 mm, 30° telescope with a 5.5 mm outer sheath for diagnostic as well as operative hysteroscopy. The telescopes are available with a 0° straight-on or a 30° fore-oblique view. The major advantage of the 0° lens is that it allows the operator to see the operative devices as a relatively distant panorama, whereas this view is lost when 30° lens is used. The telescope has three parts: (1) the eyepiece; (2) the barrel and (3) the objective lens.	Hysteroscopy not only allows for the diagnosis of intrauterine pathology, it also serves as a method for surgical intervention (operative hysteroscopy). Hysteroscopy has the benefit of allowing direct visualization of the uterine cavity, thereby avoiding or reducing iatrogenic trauma to delicate reproductive tissues. Not only does hysteroscopy allow direct observation of the intrauterine/endometrial pathology (presence of submucous fibroids, endometrial cancer, etc.), it also acts as a way of sampling the endometrium under direct visualization.
  Fig. 12.8.2B: Continuous flow diagnostic sheath (© 2010 Karl Storz GmbH & Co. KG)	The diagnostic sheath helps in the delivery of the distension media inside the uterine cavity. A 6.5 mm double channel continuous flow sheath is available and is useful when the uterine cavity is bleeding. The telescope fits into the sheath and is secured by means of a watertight seal that locks into place. Improper coupling between the telescope and sheath is likely to result in leakage of the medium at that interface.	The diagnostic sheath, commonly used is 5 mm and allows 1 mm clearance space between its inner wall and the telescope, through which the distending medium is delivered. The hysteroscope must be inserted under direct vision and the axis of the cervical and uterine canal must be carefully followed until the uterine corpus has been reached. This helps in minimizing the chances of uterine perforation.

Picture	Medical/Surgical Description	Management/Clinical Highlights
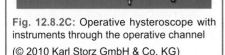 **Fig. 12.8.2C:** Operative hysteroscope with instruments through the operative channel (© 2010 Karl Storz GmbH & Co. KG)	The diameter of the operative sheath is usually greater than that of the diagnostic sheath and ranges from 7 mm to 10 mm.	The operative sheath has space for instillation of the distension medium, for the 4 mm telescope and for the insertion of operating devices.
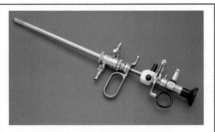 **Fig. 12.8.2D:** Resectoscope (Karl Storz) (© 2010 Karl Storz GmbH & Co. KG)	The resectoscope is a specialized electrosurgical endoscope comprising of an inner and outer sheath. In the inner sheath, there is a common channel for the telescope, medium and electrode. There is a trigger device, which pushes the electrode out beyond the sheath and pulls it back within the sheath. The operating tool comprises of two basic electrodes: (1) a 4 mm ball and (2) a 5 mm cutting loop.	The internal lumen of the sheath must be of adequate size to allow the passage of telescope and operative instruments, e.g. scissors, biopsy forceps, catheters and coagulation electrodes.
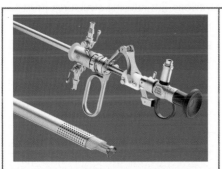 **Fig. 12.8.2E:** Resectoscope sheath including connecting channels for inflow and outflow for continuous irrigation and suction with bipolar electrode (© 2010 Karl Storz GmbH & Co. KG)	The external sheath of resectoscope has diameter ranging from 3.7 mm to 7 mm to allow the passage of telescope, operative instruments and liquid distension medium.	Resectoscope has been used by gynecologists to perform operative procedures such as excision of submucous myomas, polypectomy, division of uterine septa and endometrial ablation or resection.
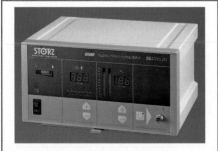 **Fig. 12.8.2F:** Hysteromat of Hamou (© 2010 Karl Storz GmbH & Co. KG)	This is a hysteroscopic insufflator device, which helps in distending the uterine cavity with the distension medium. It is applicable for both surgical and diagnostic hysteroscopy.	Hysteromat of Hamou helps in providing a constant flow of low-viscosity fluid, which helps in maintaining sufficient pressure to keep the uterine walls distended, thereby facilitating its visualization during hysteroscopic examination.

Picture	Medical/Surgical Description	Management/Clinical Highlights
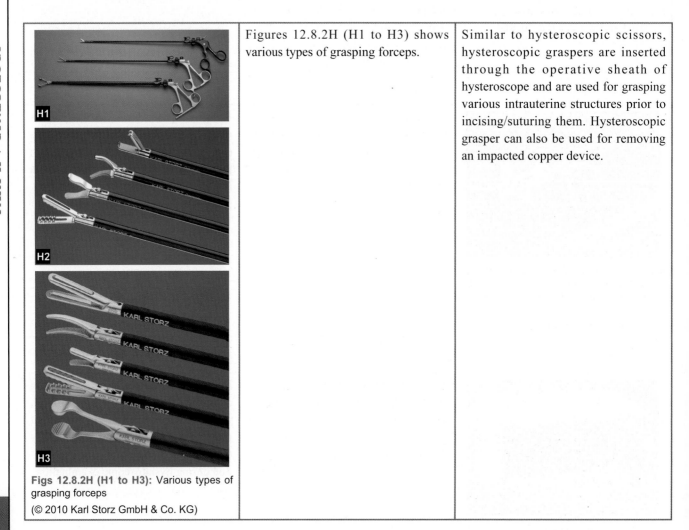 **Figs 12.8.2G (G1 and G2):** Various types of scissors (© 2010 Karl Storz GmbH & Co. KG)	Various types of hysteroscopic scissors are shown in Figures 12.8.2G (G1 and G2). Hysteroscopic scissors are commonly used for procedures such as resection of small polyps, lysis of intrauterine adhesions, incision of uterine septa, etc.	A variety of rigid, semirigid and flexible instruments have been developed for use during hysteroscopic surgery. Scissors are a type of rigid instruments, which are inserted through the operative sheath of hysteroscope.
Figs 12.8.2H (H1 to H3): Various types of grasping forceps (© 2010 Karl Storz GmbH & Co. KG)	Figures 12.8.2H (H1 to H3) shows various types of grasping forceps.	Similar to hysteroscopic scissors, hysteroscopic graspers are inserted through the operative sheath of hysteroscope and are used for grasping various intrauterine structures prior to incising/suturing them. Hysteroscopic grasper can also be used for removing an impacted copper device.

Picture	Medical/Surgical Description	Management/Clinical Highlights
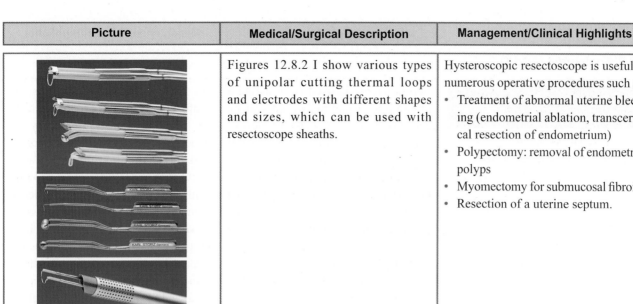 **Fig. 12.8.2 I:** Unipolar cutting loops and electrodes (for use with resectoscope sheaths) (© 2010 Karl Storz GmbH & Co. KG)	Figures 12.8.2 I show various types of unipolar cutting thermal loops and electrodes with different shapes and sizes, which can be used with resectoscope sheaths.	Hysteroscopic resectoscope is useful in numerous operative procedures such as: • Treatment of abnormal uterine bleeding (endometrial ablation, transcervical resection of endometrium) • Polypectomy: removal of endometrial polyps • Myomectomy for submucosal fibroids • Resection of a uterine septum.

12.9: LAPAROSCOPY

12.9.1: Definition

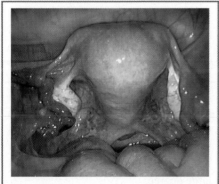 **Fig. 12.9.1:** Normal laparoscopic view of the pelvis	Laparoscopy is a type of endoscopy, which helps in visualization of the peritoneal cavity. During the last 35 years, gynecologic laparoscopy has evolved from a limited surgical procedure used only for diagnosis and tubal ligations to a major surgical tool used for the treatment of a large number of gynecological indications such as treatment of ectopic pregnancy, and endometriosis or removal of a benign ovarian cyst.	Laparoscopy is a hybrid surgical approach that shares characteristics of both minor and major surgery. Compared with laparotomy, laparoscopy is a form of minimal invasive surgery which is associated with a low complication rate, reduced pain, better cosmetic result, reduced rate of adhesion formation, shorter recovery time and reduced duration of hospital stay. However, it may be associated with various intraoperative complications such as injury to abdominal structures.

Picture	Medical/Surgical Description	Management/Clinical Highlights

12.9.2: Equipment (A to K)

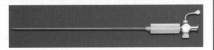 **Fig. 12.9.2A:** Veress needle (© 2010 Karl Storz GmbH & Co. KG)	Veress needle is used for creating a pneumoperitoneum, which can be considered as the first step of most of the laparoscopic surgeries. This helps in separating the internal organs and tissues from the abdominal wall so that the trocar can be inserted safely without causing any injury to the surrounding structures. The Veress needle is available in three sizes depending upon its length: 80 mm, 100 mm and 120 mm. It has an inner blunt tip, which springs out when the needle enters the peritoneal cavity.	The most commonly used gas for insufflation is CO_2. It is a noncombustible gas, which is rapidly absorbed by the blood where it gets converted to carbonic acid after combination with water. A CO_2 gas insufflator must provide continuous flow rate of gas in order to maintain the intra-abdominal pressure between 10 mm and 15 mm Hg. A high intra-abdominal pressure facilitates the introduction of the trocar as well as helps in increasing the distance between the trocar and the retroperitoneal vessels.
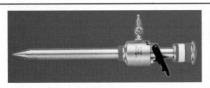 **Fig. 12.9.2B:** Primary trocar and cannula (© 2010 Karl Storz GmbH & Co. KG)	First generation laparoscopic instruments consist of two parts: a removable central trocar and an encasing outer cannula. Once this access instrument is placed inside the body's cavity, the central trocar is removed in order to place the laparoscope and other operating instruments. The most commonly used trocars vary between the size of 5 mm and 10 mm. Trocars usually have two types of valves to prevent the escape of gas. These include the flap valve and trumpet valve.	There are two types of laparoscopic access equipment: first generation equipment (with a central trocar and an encasing outer sheath or cannula) and the second generation equipment (based on visual access method). The proximal end of the primary trocar is designed to accommodate the palm of surgeon's dominant hand. The distal end of the trocar could have a pointed, sharp, conical or beveled pyramidal cutting blade tip. Conical first generation trocars have pointed nonbladed sharp tips with no cutting edges.
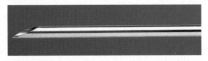 **Fig. 12.9.2C:** Cannula tip shown separately without the trocar (© 2010 Karl Storz GmbH & Co. KG)	Figure 12.9.2 shows the hollow cannula tip without the accompanying trocar.	The cannula allows the insertion of laparoscopic instruments inside the abdominal cavity.
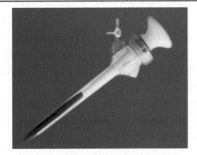 **Fig. 12.9.2D:** Disposable trocar (© 2010 Karl Storz GmbH & Co. KG)	Disposable trocars are also available, which have the advantage of being sharp. However, the sharp edges of the trocars may sometimes cause damage to the small blood vessels and other organs.	With the blunt trocar tips, the chances of injury are relatively low in comparison to the sharp trocar tips because the blood vessels are pushed aside at the time of insertion and are thereby protected to a large degree.

Picture	Medical/Surgical Description	Management/Clinical Highlights

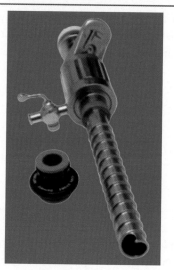

Fig. 12.9.2E: EndoTIP reusable visual access cannula

(© 2010 Karl Storz GmbH & Co. KG)

Second generation laparoscopic access instruments with visual access method are also sometimes used. These include the optical access trocars, which helps in visualizing the layers of abdominal wall during placement.

The EndoTIP, a sheath with screw threading is a new second generation instrument, which allows safe peritoneal entry under direct vision. In this method, the sheath which has screw thread tip is inserted with the telescope inside so that as the sheath is screwed in, the tissue layers can be visualized and therefore inadvertent injury to the internal organs may be avoided. This technique may especially prove to be safe in cases where dense adhesions are expected, especially in cases where the patient had a previous laparotomy. The screwed EndoTIP prevents it from slipping out of the intraperitoneal space.

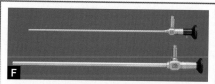

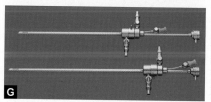

Figs 12.9.2 (F and G): (F) Laparoscopic telescope; (G) Operative telescope

(© 2010 Karl Storz GmbH & Co. KG)

Following the removal of the primary trocar, the laparoscopic/operative telescope are inserted through the cannula in order to visualize the abdominal cavity.

Laparoscopic telescopes can vary in size from 2 mm to 13 mm with visualization angle varying from 0° to 45°. At the end of the telescope is a lens system, which helps in creating an inverted and real image of the object. This image is finally transported to the eye piece containing the magnifying lens, which produces an uninverted, magnified image.

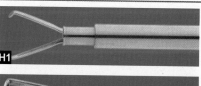

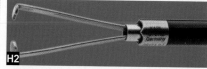

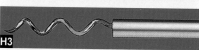

Figs 12.9.2H (H1 to H3): Grasping and holding equipment

(© 2010 Karl Storz GmbH & Co. KG)

Graspers with different sizes and designs (claw forceps, Allis type forceps, spoon forceps, atraumatic forceps, etc.) are important for any laparoscopic procedure.

The grasping and holding instruments are essential for holding and grasping various pelvic structures while performing laparoscopic surgery.

A myoma screw like holding instrument can be used for grasping a myoma at the time of laparoscopic myomectomy.

Picture	Medical/Surgical Description	Management/Clinical Highlights
Fig. 12.9.2I: Straight and curved blade scissors (© 2010 Karl Storz GmbH & Co. KG)	Scissors are essential for dissection and cutting of various structures, adhesions, etc. They can be either straight or curved types. Besides these two types, other types of laparoscopic scissors include serrated scissors, hook scissors, microtip scissors, etc.	At the time of laparoscopic surgery, scissors can be used for cutting variety of tissues, sutures, structures, etc.
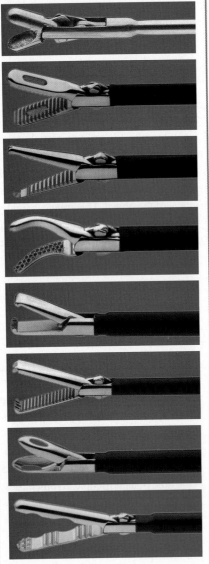 Fig. 12.9.2J: Various types of laparoscopic bipolar forceps (© 2010 Karl Storz GmbH & Co. KG)	Figure 12.9.2J demonstrate various types of laparoscopic bipolar forceps. Some of these forceps include Maryland forceps, atraumatic and fenestrated forceps, biopsy forceps, bipolar tong forceps, bipolar rippled bar forceps, ruby forceps, etc.	These instruments are connected to bipolar electrosurgical units. The tips of these instruments combine grasping of tissues and precise dissection with coagulation of blood vessels for obtaining hemostasis.

Picture	Medical/Surgical Description	Management/Clinical Highlights

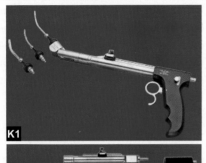

Figs 12.9.2K (K1 and K2): Uterine manipulator (© 2010 Karl Storz GmbH & Co. KG)

This is one of the simplest instruments and is used for stabilizing or manipulating the organs, especially the uterus. This helps in providing good view of the surgical field at the time of laparoscopic surgery and for creating tension on the tissues, which may facilitate cutting and incision of various structures.

Some of these manipulators also facilitate the instillation of an inert colored solution (such as sterile saline with indigo carmine dye) into the uterine cavity to determine the patency of the fallopian tubes.

12.10: ROBOTIC SURGERY

12.10.1: Incisions of Robotic Surgery

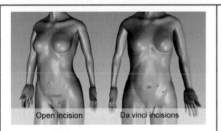

Fig. 12.10.1: Incision given in traditional open surgery compared to the minimal small incisions given in the robotic surgery

Robotic surgery is a type of minimally invasive procedure, in which several small incisions (0.25–0.75 inch) are made along the abdomen and the surgical equipment are inserted through these incisions. In traditional abdominal surgery a 7–8 inches long vertical or horizontal incision is usually given over the anterior abdominal wall.

Due to its minimal invasive nature, robotic system can offer numerous benefits over traditional open surgery such as shorter duration of hospital stay, reduced pain, faster recovery, reduced amount of blood loss, requirement for fewer transfusions and reduced risk of infection, risk of scar formation and overall improved quality of life.

12.10.2: Robotic Equipment (A to L)

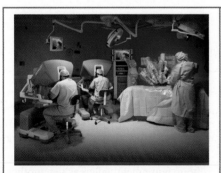

Fig. 12.10.2A: Robotic Da Vinci® operating system. (A) An operating room featuring Da Vinci® Si HD robotic operating system along with the operating console where the surgeon sits; a nurse can be seen attending the patient (© 2012 Intuitive Surgical, Inc.)

Da Vinci® apparatus is the most advanced surgical platform, which has three integrated components: an operating console where the surgeon sits; the second component of the machine is the patient side cart with four interactive robotic arms. Seated at the Da Vinci® counsel, the surgeon sees a high resolution three-dimensional image of the operative site powered by robotic and computerized technology. Surgeon's hand movements are transferred into precise movements of the EndoWrist instruments, resulting in unparalleled precision, dexterity and controlled surgery. Third component is the video tower housing. This has dedicated system processors and high precision three-dimensional vision system.

Robotic surgery has seen enormous growth over the past decade in the field of gynecology. Key features of the robotic surgical platform are as follows:
- Complex surgeries can be performed with minimally invasive approach.
- Motions are scaled to micromovements of robotic EndoWrist equipment; moreover the hand tremors are filtered out.
- This system also provides high definition three-dimensional view of surgery and enables accurate perception of depth.
- Digital zoom allows tissue magnification, which provides superior vision of the tissue planes and critical anatomy.

Picture	Medical/Surgical Description	Management/Clinical Highlights
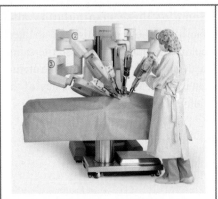 **Fig. 12.10.2B:** Patient cart with instruments (Da Vinci® Surgical S System) (© 2012 Intuitive Surgical, Inc.)	The patient side cart with four interactive robotic arms is one of the three components of the machine.	Of the four arms, the first arm helps in holding and positioning the high resolution stereo endoscope. The remaining arms help in controlling the high precision fully articulated EndoWrist instruments.
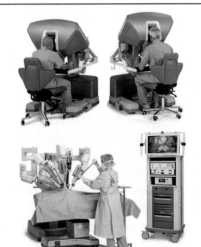 **Fig. 12.10.2C:** Full Da Vinci® Si HD surgical system with two surgical consoles both with surgeons seated; one patient cart; one female nurse attending vision cart (© 2012 Intuitive Surgical, Inc.)	As shown in the adjacent Figure, surgical robotic system is composed of three parts: a patient-side robot, a vision cart and the robotic master console.	The current version of the Da Vinci® robotic surgical system, the Da Vinci® S (with or without high definition) allows for telestration. Through this feature, surgeon sitting on the console is able to give instructions to other surgeons using touch screen, thereby guiding the dissection, and supervising the direction in which a particular robotic instrument would be moved in order to accomplish a particular surgical task, e.g. tying a suture.
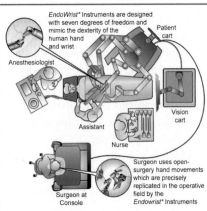 **Fig. 12.10.2D:** Set up of the operating room (© 2012 Intuitive Surgical, Inc.)	Figure 12.10.2D illustrates set-up in an operating room utilizing the Da Vinci® robotic equipment. The robotic surgeon operates from the remote master console and uses a combination of hand controls and foot pedals. The patient-side cart is positioned in between the patient's legs, and the robotic arms are attached to stainless steel robotic trocars through a process termed as docking.	One of the foot pedal controls the movements of camera; another one may control the focus; another pedal helps in providing a range of motions to the robotic equipment, whereas yet another one controls both monopolar and bipolar energy sources. The hand controls of the surgeon sitting on the side console help in the movements of the camera as well as the various robotic instruments. There are about three operative robotic arms. Despite all of these advancements, a bedside assistant is still required.

Picture	Medical/Surgical Description	Management/Clinical Highlights
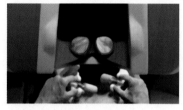 **Fig. 12.10.2E:** Robotic operating equipment after being inserted into the patient's abdomen (© 2012 Intuitive Surgical, Inc.)	A new minimally invasive surgical procedure for gynecologic patients, which has nowadays been commonly employed, is robotic surgery using Da Vinci® robotic system. The robotic equipment can be used for performing surgeries such as hysterectomy, myomectomy (for removal of submucosal fibroids), sacrocolpopexy (treatment for pelvic organ prolapse), removal of ovarian cysts and masses, treatment of cervical and endometrial cancer, lymph node dissections, etc.	The movement of each instrument and each surgical maneuver is controlled by the surgeon, who sits on a console slightly away from the site of surgery. While robotic system is used for performing various gynecological surgeries, robotic surgery is yet not used for the treatment of ovarian cancer.
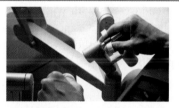 **Fig. 12.10.2 F:** Cameras of the robotic system (© 2012 Intuitive Surgical, Inc.)	Figure 12.10.2F shows cameras of the robotic system.	These cameras help in providing magnified, three-dimensional, high definition view of the operating field. This helps in facilitating depth perception by the patient.
Fig. 12.10.2G: Surgeon's hand movements over the surgical console (© 2012 Intuitive Surgical, Inc.)	The robotic master console also provides the surgeon with three-dimensional imaging through a stereoscopic viewer.	Seated at the Da Vinci® counsel, the surgeon sees a high resolution three-dimensional image of the operative site powered by the robotic computerized technology.
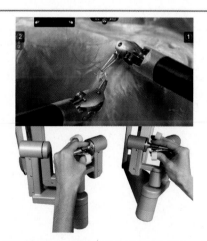 **Fig. 12.10.2H:** Movement of surgeon's hand controls the movement of robotic equipment (© 2012 Intuitive Surgical, Inc.)	Figure 12.10.2H illustrates translation of surgeon's hand movements into precise movements of the EndoWrist instruments.	This results in unparalleled precision, dexterity and controlled surgery by robotic equipment.

Picture	Medical/Surgical Description	Management/Clinical Highlights
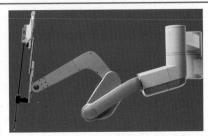 **Fig. 12.10.2I:** Instrument arm of Da Vinci® Surgical S system (© 2012 Intuitive Surgical, Inc.)	Figure 12.10.2I shows the instrument arm of Da Vinci® Surgical S system. The surgeon sitting on the nearby console controls the movements of the robotic equipment.	By controlling the movements of these arms, the robotic operative instruments can be manipulated, thereby facilitating the repositioning, grasping, retraction, cutting, dissection, coagulation and suturing of various structures required during surgery.
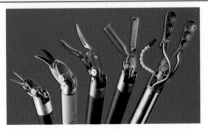 **Fig. 12.10.2J:** Array of robotic equipment (© 2012 Intuitive Surgical, Inc.)	Figure 12.10.2 illustrates an assortment of equipment used for performing robotic surgery. These may include various types of scissors, forceps and graspers.	These instruments can be used for grasping, stabilizing and incising various pelvic structures.
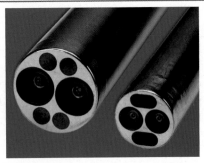 **Fig. 12.10.2K:** Da Vinci® 12 mm and 8.5 mm endoscope (© 2012 Intuitive Surgical, Inc.)	Figure 12.10.2K demonstrates Da Vinci® endoscopes having diameters of 8 mm and 12 mm respectively.	Robotic endoscopes have space for insertion of various robotic equipment. The endoscopes with wider diameter facilitate the entry of more instruments in comparison to those with narrower diameter.
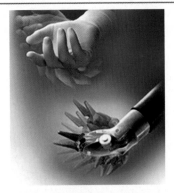 **Fig. 12.10.2L:** Comparison of hand movements with that of Da Vinci® robot (© 2012 Intuitive Surgical, Inc.)	Figure 12.10.2L shows a comparison between the ranges of movements possible with robotic equipment in comparison with the hand movements.	The robotic equipment in comparison to laparoscopic and hysteroscopic equipment shows much greater dexterity and versatility of movements.

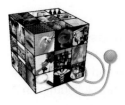

EVIDENCE-BASED BREAKTHROUGH FACTS

1. USE OF SILS IN GYNECOLOGY

Single incision laparoscopic surgery can be considered as a safe and feasible technique for surgical management of various gynecological conditions, such as endometriosis, divisions of adhesions, ovarian cystectomies and performance of surgical procedures such as hysterectomies and mesh sacrohysteropexies. SILS is associated with a high rate of patient satisfaction due to improved cosmesis and reduced requirement for analgesia postoperatively.

Source: Behnia-Willison T, Foroughinia L, Sina M, et al. Single incision laparoscopic surgery (SILS) in gynaecology: Feasibility and operative outcomes. Aust N Z J Obstet Gynaecol. 2012;52(4):366-70.

2. NEW CLINICAL GUIDELINES ON THE DIAGNOSIS AND TREATMENT OF NON-NEUROGENIC OVERACTIVE BLADDER

The American Urological Association (AUA) and the Society of Urodynamics, Female Pelvic Medicine and Urogenital Reconstruction (SUFU) have released a new clinical guideline on the diagnosis and treatment of non-neurogenic overactive bladder (OAB) in adults and include the following recommendations:

Approach to Diagnosis

A thorough history, physical examination and urinalysis should be performed initially. If required, a urine culture and/or postvoid residual assessment can be done. The patient can be asked to maintain a bladder diary or fill up symptom questionnaire. Investigations such as urodynamic studies, cystoscopy, and diagnostic renal and bladder ultrasound are not required in the initial workup in most cases.

Treatment

Some patients may choose to receive no treatment at all. Behavioral therapies (e.g. bladder training, bladder control strategies, pelvic floor muscle training, and fluid management) and education should be offered as first line therapy.

Second Line Treatment

Antimuscarinics should be offered as second line therapy. Extended-release preparations should be preferred over immediate-release preparations to reduce incidence of side effects such as dry mouth, etc.

Third-Line Treatments

- Sacral neuromodulation (FDA approved) can be offered as third-line treatment to carefully selected patients with severe refractory OAB symptoms or "patients who are not candidates for second line therapy and are willing to undergo a surgical procedure."
- Another FDA approved treatment which the panel offers as third-line treatment, is peripheral tibial nerve stimulation using an acupuncture needle.
- Intradetrusor injection of onabotulinumtoxinA (non FDA approved) may be offered as "third-line treatment in the carefully selected patients who had been refractory to first-and-second-line OAB treatments.

Source: Gormley EA, Lightner DJ, Burgio KL, et al. Diagnosis and Treatment of Overactive Bladder (Non-Neurogenic) in Adults: AUA/SUFU Guideline. Published online in the journal of urology 23 October 2012.

3. OVERACTIVE BLADDER SYMPTOMS IMPROVED WITH BOTOX INJECTIONS

Oral anticholinergic therapy and intradetrusor onabotulinumtoxinA (Botox) injection are associated with similar reductions in the frequency of daily episodes of urgency urinary incontinence. The patients receiving onabotulinumtoxinA are less likely to experience anticholinergic symptoms such as dry mouth and are also more likely to have complete resolution of urgency urinary incontinence. However, injection of onabotulinumtoxin A may be associated with a higher rate of transient urinary retention and urinary tract infections.

Source: Visco AG, Brubaker L, Richter HE, et al. for the Pelvic Floor Disorders Network. Anticholinergic Therapy vs. Onabotulinumtoxin A for Urgency Urinary Incontinence. N Engl J Med. 2012;367:1803-13.

4. UTERINE TRANSPLANTATION—A REAL POSSIBILITY?

Uterine transplantation has been proposed as a potential solution to absolute uterine factor infertility (AUFI).

Causes of AUFI include the following:

- Congenital causes (absence/ hypoplasia of uterus or other uterine malformation) and
- Acquired uterine factors (e.g. hysterectomy for uncontrollable hemorrhage)

Source: Del Priore G, Saso S, Meslin EM, et al. Uterine transplantation—a real possibility? The Indianapolis consensus. Hum Reprod. 2012. (Epub ahead of print).

Section 13

Abnormalities in Conception

13.1.1: Female Causes of Infertility (A and B)

Picture	Medical/Surgical Description	Management/Clinical Highlights
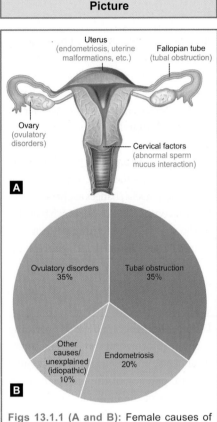 **Figs 13.1.1 (A and B):** Female causes of infertility	Infertility is defined as the inability to conceive even after trying with unprotected intercourse for a period of 1 year for couples in which the woman is under 35 years and 6 months of trying for couples in which the woman is over 35 years of age. Infertility commonly results due to the disease of the reproductive system, in either a male or a female, which inhibits the ability to conceive and deliver a child. Nearly one-third of the cases of infertility are related to male causes; one-third are related to female causes and remaining one-third of the cases are related to both male and female causes. Among the female causes of infertility, ovulatory dysfunction and tubal obstruction are each responsible for 35% cases of infertility. Endometriosis may be responsible for nearly 20% cases whereas idiopathic causes may be responsible for the remainder 10% cases.	Management of both male and female infertility is different from one another and is largely based on the treatment of the underlying cause. Nevertheless, the evaluation for infertility must focus on the couple as a whole and not on one or the other partner. Both the partners must be encouraged to attend the clinic at the time of each appointment. Tests for ovulatory dysfunction include determination of serum midluteal progesterone levels (day 21 levels suggestive of ovulation are 4–6 ng/mL in a 28-day cycle), basal body temperature (BBT) and endometrial biopsy (for diagnosis of luteal phase defects). Tests for assessment of tubal/pelvic disease include hysterosalpingography and laparoscopy with chromotubation. Tests for uterine factors include hysterosalpingography, transvaginal sonography, saline infusion sonography, magnetic resonance imaging, hysteroscopy, laparoscopy, etc. Postcoital test is used for the evaluation of cervical factors.

13.1.2: Male Causes of Infertility

Picture	Medical/Surgical Description	Management/Clinical Highlights
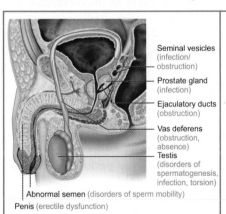 **Fig. 13.1.2:** Male causes of infertility	Amongst the various causes of male infertility, nearly 50% cases are due to disorders of spermatogenesis. Factors which raise scrotal temperature (e.g. workers in a blast furnace), presence of varicocele, etc. can adversely affect spermatogenesis. Nearly 30% cases could be due to obstruction of ductus deferens. This could be due to damaged sperm ducts, testicular torsion, testicular infection (mumps, gonorrhea and tuberculosis), etc. Disorders of sperm motility may be responsible for another 15% cases. Approximately 5% of male causes of infertility include psychological or behavioral problems such as erectile dysfunction, premature ejaculation, ejaculatory incompetence, etc.	Male infertility is evaluated by performing a comprehensive semen analysis in a certified andrology laboratory. The primary values that are evaluated at the time of semen analysis include the volume of the ejaculate, sperm motility, total sperm concentration, sperm morphology, motility and viability. The next step in the management of male infertility is the correction of underlying abnormality, e.g. surgical correction of varicocele, administration of antibiotics for treatment of infection and administration of hormones such as testosterone and gonadotropin-releasing hormone (GnRH) for improvement of spermatogenesis, etc.

13.2: DIAGNOSIS OF INFERTILITY

13.2.1: Evaluation of Cervical Factors for Infertility

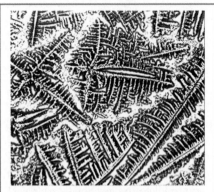

Fig. 13.2.1: Ferning pattern of the cervical mucus

The most important method for evaluating the cervical factor involves assessment of the quality of cervical mucus. Just prior to ovulation, the cervical mucus becomes thin, watery, alkaline, stretchable, acellular, and elastic in appearance due to increase in the concentration of salt and water in the mucus under the influence of estrogen. Also, during this phase, the mucus assumes a fern-like pattern (as shown in the adjacent Figure) when allowed to dry on a slide under the microscope.

In normal women, at the beginning of the menstrual cycle, cervical mucus is scanty, viscous, and very cellular. This mucus does not allow the sperms to pass into the uterine cavity. Mucus secretion from the cervix increases during the mid follicular phase and reaches its maximum approximately 24–48 hours before ovulation. Following ovulation, under the effect of progesterone, the cervical mucus changes its character and becomes opaque and viscid, which is hostile to the sperms. The ferning pattern also cannot be demonstrated during this phase.

13.2.2: Tests of Tubal Patency

13.2.2.1: Hysterosalpingography

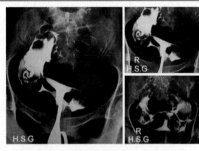

Fig. 13.2.2.1: Normal hysterosalpingogram showing bilateral spillage of dye

The hysterosalpingogram (HSG) is the most frequently used diagnostic tool for evaluation of the endometrial cavity as well as the tubal pathology. Tubal patency is indicated by bilateral spillage of dye into the peritoneum. A normal HSG depicts a smooth triangular uterine outline with opacification of both fallopian tubes. HSG is best performed during the 2–5 days interval period immediately following the end of menses. During hysterosalpingography, diluted, water soluble, hyperosmolar iodinated contrast agent is injected into the uterine cavity via the Foley's catheter.

Hysterosalpingogram helps in providing accurate information about the endocervical canal, endometrial cavity, cornual ostium, patency of the fallopian tubes and status of the fimbriae. HSG is able to accurately define the shape and size of the uterine cavity. It can help in diagnosing uterine developmental anomalies, (e.g., unicornuate uterus, septate uterus, bicornuate uterus and uterus didelphys), submucous myomas, intrauterine adhesions and endometrial polyps. Normal uterine cavity is symmetrical and triangular in shape. It is widest at the level of cornual orifices near the fundus.

13.2.2.2: Hysterosalpingography for Diagnosis of Hydrosalpinx (A and B)

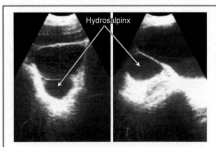

Fig. 13.2.2.2A: Transabdominal sonography revealing the presence of bilateral masses with multiple internal echoes suggestive of hydrosalpinx

In this 28-year-old patient presenting with infertility, ultrasound revealed presence of bilateral tubular, cystic mass with multiple internal echoes. This mass was suggestive of hydrosalpinx.

In order to establish a definitive diagnosis, a HSG was performed (Figure 13.2.2.2B).

Picture	Medical/Surgical Description	Management/Clinical Highlights
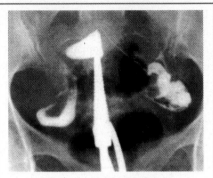 Fig. 13.2.2.2B: Hysterosalpingogram in the same patient showing the presence of mass bilaterally	Figure 13.2.2.2B shows the findings of HSG in the patient in whom ultrasound revealed the presence of hydrosalpinx. In this case HSG shows presence of tubular convoluted structures on both sides of the uterus, representing bilateral hydrosalpinges. No intraperitoneal spillage of contrast was demonstrated.	During HSG, the contrast material is inserted through the catheter into the uterine cavity, fallopian tubes and peritoneal cavity, following which the fluoroscopic images are taken. X-ray pictures are taken as the uterine cavity begins filling. Following this, additional contrast material is injected inside the uterine cavity so that the tubes fill up and the dye begins to spill into the abdominal cavity. More X-ray pictures are taken as the spillage of dye occurs.

13.2.2.3: Bilateral Cornual Block on Hysterosalpingogram

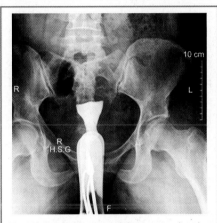 Fig. 13.2.2.3: Hysterosalpingogram showing bilateral cornual block	Hysterosalpingogram in Figure 13.2.2.3 shows a triangular-shaped uterine cavity. However, there is no movement of dye beyond the tubal cornu on both sides. Bilateral cornual blockage was therefore demonstrated.	The X-ray images taken during hysterosalpingography can help in determining whether the fallopian tubes are patent or blocked and whether the blockage is located at the proximal or at the distal end of the fallopian tube.

13.2.2.4: Laparoscopic Test for Tubal Patency (A to C)

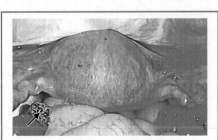 Fig. 13.2.2.4A: Slight spillage of dye from right-sided tube (indicated by the arrow)	Laparoscopic chromotubation involves injection of the methylene blue dye through the cervix to visualize free spill or absence of spillage to diagnose patent or blocked tubes respectively. Laparoscopic examination also allows visualization of fallopian tubes, ovary and the pelvis. Figure 13.2.2.4A shows slight spillage of methylene blue dye (in form of bubbles) from the right-sided fallopian tube. The laparoscopic examination also reveals a normal looking uterus, fallopian tubes and the peritoneal cavity.	During this procedure, under all aseptic precautions, a blue colored dye (methylene blue) is injected into the uterine cavity with the help of a plastic or metal cannula placed in the cervical canal. If both the fallopian tubes are patent, they first become slightly distended as they fill with the dye. As the injection of dye is continued, it spills out through the tubal ostia into the a peritoneal cavity. In the beginning, the spillage may be in form of bubbles.

Picture	Medical/Surgical Description	Management/Clinical Highlights
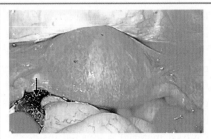 Fig. 13.2.2.4B: Spillage of dye more pronounced on right side (indicated by the arrow)	Figure 13.2.2.4B shows that as the injection of dye is continued, the spillage of dye on the right side becomes more pronounced.	Laparoscopic chromotubation is normally being regarded as the gold standard for the assessment of fallopian tubes, especially in women with infertility suspected to be suffering from tubal pathology. This test has now become part of the routine assessment for infertility.
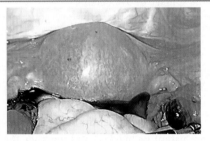 Fig. 13.2.2.4C: Bilateral spillage of dye on both the sides	Figure 13.2.2.4C shows bilateral spillage of dye on both sides. As the spillage of dye continues, it can also be observed in the peritoneal cavity. Bilateral free spillage of dye is indicative of patent tubes. If the spillage of dye is not observed either on one or both the sides, this could indicate an obstruction, which could be due to infection, inflammation or muscle spasm (temporary obstruction).	Hysterosalpingography and laparoscopic chromotubation are usually complementary to each other. HSG is able to outline the shape of uterine cavity and is also able to show presence of the filling defects, (which could be due to the presence of polyps, fibroids, etc.). Laparoscopy, on the other hand, is able to visualize the uterus and peritoneal cavity externally and also diagnose the presence of adhesions.

13.2.2.5: Diagnosis of Hydrosalpinx (A and B)

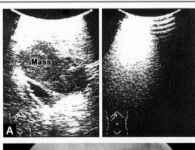 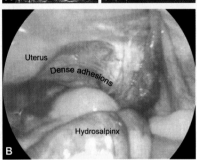 Figs 13.2.2.5 (A and B): Diagnosis of a hydrosalpinx: (A) Ultrasonogram showing a mass of variable echogenicity arising from left adnexa suggestive of a tubo-ovarian mass; (B) Laparoscopic appearance of hydrosalpinx arising from left tube	Figure 13.2.2.5A shows an anechoic elongated, cystic, tubal mass on ultrasonography. Laparoscopic examination (as shown in Figure 13.2.2.5B) helps in confirming the diagnosis of a left-sided hydrosalpinx.	Hydrosalpinx is formed due to distal occlusion of the fallopian tubes (commonly due to pelvic inflammatory disease). As the blocked fallopian tube gets distended with fluid, it develops into a retort-shaped structure called hydrosalpinx. When there is no tubal blockage, this fluid normally gets discharged into the peritoneal cavity. Women with bilateral hydrosalpinx may be infertile. In these cases, either tubal surgery in form of neosalpingostomy or in vitro fertilization (IVF) may be required to achieve pregnancy.

13.2.2.6: Hysteroscopic Assessment of Tubal Ostia

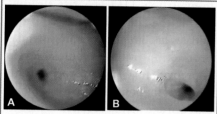

Figs 13.2.2.6 (A and B): Hysteroscopic evaluation of tubal ostium: (A) Right sided; (B) Left sided

Figures 13.2.2.6 (A and B) show left and right tubal ostia as visualized on hysteroscopic examination. Tubal ostia refer to the opening where fallopian tube enters the uterine cavity. Evaluation of both the tubal ostia is important because presence of membrane or any other blockage over the tubal ostia (especially if bilateral) may be responsible for producing infertility.

Diagnostic hysteroscopy is a commonly performed procedure, which can help evaluate the endocervical canal, endometrial cavity and tubal ostia. In case of suspected endometrial pathology, endometrial biopsy can be performed.

13.2.3: Tests for Ovulation (A to C)

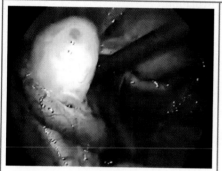

Fig. 13.2.3A: Laparoscopic view showing an ovary with a developing follicle

Laparoscopic examination can help visualize the ovary. Figure 13.2.3A shows presence of a single dominant follicle protruding from the surface of ovary, just a few hours prior to ovulation.

The maturing ovarian follicle is also known as the preovulatory follicle. It has an ovum surrounded by cumulus oophorus, composed of granulosa cells. This is surrounded by a large antrum composed of follicular fluid. Since this preovulatory follicle can increase in size to about a few millimeters, it may be visible from the surface of ovary on laparoscopic examination.

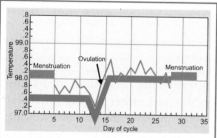

Fig. 13.2.3B: Basal body temperature method

Basal body temperature charts can be used for predicting ovulation. In this method, the woman is asked to measure her oral temperature with an oral glass or mercury thermometer, the first thing when she wakes up in the morning or after at least 3 hours of uninterrupted sleep. She should measure her temperature throughout the entire duration of her menstrual cycle for at least three menstrual cycles. The temperatures are then plotted on a graph paper. BBT serves as a useful method for evaluation of ovulation in couples who are reluctant or unable to pursue more formal and costly investigations.

Basal body temperature varies between 97.0°F and 98.0°F during the follicular phase of the cycle and rises by 0.4–0.8°F over the average preovulatory temperature during the luteal phase. The thermogenic shift in BBT occurs when serum progesterone levels rise above 5 ng/mL, usually occurring for up to 4 days following ovulation. In a normal ovulating woman, there occurs a rise in body temperature by 0.5–1.0°C immediately following ovulation under the thermogenic effect of progesterone. This increase in temperature remains sustained throughout the luteal phase. The temperature again falls to baseline just before or after the onset of menses. This biphasic pattern is evident in ovulatory women.

Picture	Medical/Surgical Description	Management/Clinical Highlights

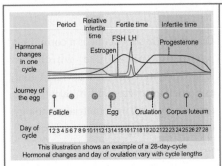

Fig. 13.2.3C: Hormonal changes suggestive of ovulation in a 28 days cycle

The events preceding ovulation are as follows: estrogen production peaks (must be greater than 200 pg/mL for more than 24 hours) and is responsible for triggering the follicle stimulating hormone (FSH) and luteinizing hormone (LH) surge. Rupture of the ovarian follicle follows, resulting in ovulation.

A surge of LH takes place just prior to ovulation. LH levels rise steadily during the late follicular phase. LH initiates luteinization and progesterone production in the granulosa layer. A preovulatory rise in progesterone facilitates the positive feedback action of estrogen and may be required to induce the midcycle FSH peak.

Ovulation occurs about 10–12 hours after the LH peak and 24–36 hours after the peak of estradiol levels have been attained. The onset of LH surge is the most reliable indicator of impending ovulation.

13.3: ASSISTED REPRODUCTIVE TECHNIQUES FOR TREATMENT OF INFERTILITY

13.3.1: Artificial Insemination (A and B)

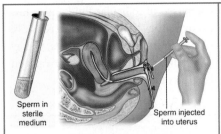

Fig. 13.3.1A: Diagrammatic representation of intrauterine insemination

Artificial insemination can be performed by depositing the sperms at the level of internal cervical os (cervical insemination) or inside the endometrial cavity [intrauterine insemination (IUI)].

The underlying principle of IUI is that increasing the density of both eggs and sperm near the site of fertilization helps increase the chances of pregnancy.

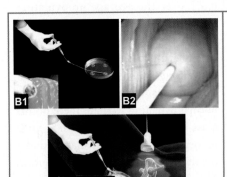

Figs 13.3.1 (B1 to B3): Procedure of intrauterine insemination

As shown in the adjacent Figure, the procedure of IUI comprises of the following steps:
- Using a "no touch" technique, IUI catheter is introduced through the cervix up to the uterine fundus under ultrasound guidance.
- An amount of 0.3–05 mL of processed semen is then slowly injected through the catheter.
- The catheter is then slowly withdrawn out.

Intrauterine insemination may be performed either during a natural cycle (unstimulated IUI) or following ovulation induction with clomiphene citrate (CC) or gonadotropins (stimulated IUI). The average pregnancy rate achieved after a natural-cycle IUI is 8%. This rate increases by 5–10% in the stimulated cycles. The procedure is performed 30–34 hours after the spontaneous LH surge or 36 hours after the administration of 10,000 U of human chorionic gonadotropin. The procedure is repeated within 12 hours, if the oocyte is not released till then.

Picture	Medical/Surgical Description	Management/Clinical Highlights

13.3.2: In Vitro Fertilization

13.3.2.1: Diagrammatic Representation of In Vitro Fertilization

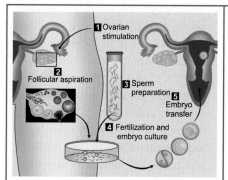

Fig. 13.3.2.1: Diagrammatic representation of the procedure of in vitro fertilization

In vitro fertilization is one of the most commonly used assisted reproductive technique (ART). It consists of retrieving a preovulatory oocyte from the ovary; fertilizing it with sperm in the laboratory and subsequently transferring the embryo within the endometrial cavity.

In vitro fertilization is now being recognized as an established treatment for infertility. Indications for IVF include the following:
- Uterine malformations (e.g. unicornuate uterus)
- Damage/absence of fallopian tubes
- Severe pelvic adhesions and/or endometriosis
- Severe oligospermia or a history of obstructive azoospermia in the male partner
- Premature ovarian failure.

13.3.2.2: Procedure of In Vitro Fertilization (A to G)

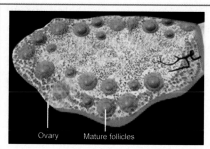

Fig. 13.3.2.2A: Follicular stimulation

The success of IVF is related to the patient's age and the number of embryos transferred into the endometrial cavity. Therefore, in order to increase the number of ovarian follicles, which are recruited, selected and finally get transformed into dominant follicle, several protocols may be used. Some such protocols include long and short protocols. GnRH agonists are usually preferred over GnRH antagonists for the long protocol. The agents used for pituitary down-regulation can be used in a "step-up" or "step-down" approach. In a "step-down" protocol, the starting dose of gonadotropin is high and this is followed by gradual reductions in dose during the cycle depending on the response. In a "step-up" protocol, the starting dose of gonadotropin is low and is then gradually increased during the cycle depending on the response.

Another type of protocol, which is commonly used is flare protocol. GnRH agonist flare protocol is used in patients who are poor responders to stimulation. In this protocol, GnRH agonists are administered in conjunction with ovarian stimulation, so that the agonistic response of the pituitary can be used for ovarian stimulation.

"Long protocols" involve administration of either a GnRH agonist (Lupron) or antagonist or oral contraceptive pills (OCPs) 7 days before the next expected cycles. This helps in pituitary down-regulation, thereby inhibiting the production of gonadotropins by the pituitary. Pituitary suppression of LH secretion is important because it helps in preventing a surge of endogenous LH before there is full maturation of the cohort of ovarian follicles. In "short protocols", GnRH agonists are started at the time of the natural menstrual cycle. Following pituitary suppression, in order to stimulate follicular growth and ovulation (there are two or more follicles with a mean diameter of 18 mm or more and a serum estradiol level of 200 pg/mL), hMG or FSH or both are administered in a dose of 225–300 IU/day subcutaneously on day 2–7 of the menstrual cycle. Treatment with CC is also sometimes used for ovulation induction. Simultaneously, GnRH agonists (or antagonists) are continued at a lower dose to prevent a premature surge of LH secretion.

Picture	Medical/Surgical Description	Management/Clinical Highlights
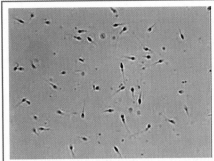 Fig. 13.3.2.2B: Follicular aspiration	Oocytes are aspirated from the ovary 35–36 hours following administration of hCG. Initially all aspirations were performed under laparoscopic guidance. However, now, follicular aspirations are commonly performed under ultrasonographic guidance. The transvaginal route for follicular aspiration has presently become the preferred procedure in most IVF programs.	The procedure of follicular aspiration comprises of the following steps: • The oocyte aspiration is usually performed under heavy sedation, while the patient has been placed in the dorsal lithotomy position. • Under ultrasound guidance, a 17-gauge needle is passed via the needle guide through the vaginal fornix into the ovaries in order to aspirate the follicular fluid, which is sent to the IVF laboratory as soon as possible.
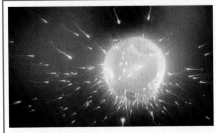 Fig. 13.3.2.2C: Preparation of sperm concentrate	The procedure of preparing sperm concentrate involves the removal of certain components of the ejaculate (i.e. seminal fluid, excess cellular debris, leukocytes, morphologically abnormal sperms, etc.) along with the retention of the motile fraction of sperms.	A semen sample is obtained after a 3- to 5-day period of sexual abstinence immediately prior to the oocyte retrieval. The sperms are incubated for 60 minutes in an atmosphere of 5% carbon dioxide in air. The motile portion of the sperms is separated via the process of centrifugation through a discontinuous density gradient system.
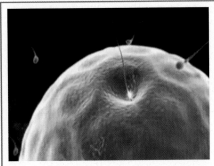 Fig. 13.3.2.2D: Oocyte insemination with multiple sperms	In order to achieve fertilization between a sperm and ovum, a single ovum is incubated with multiple sperms. Fertilization usually occurs within 12–24 hours.	Approximately 200,000 motile sperms, placed in a small volume of media with a layer of mineral oil on top, are added to the oocytes. This usually helps in fertilizing the ovum by atleast one sperm.
Fig. 13.3.2.2E: Fertilization of the ovum with a single sperm	Once an ovum has been fertilized by a sperm, the fertilized egg is monitored to ensure that further cell division occurs. At the time of fertilization, there occurs fusion between the male and female pronuclei.	In cases where there is low probability of fertilization due to abnormalities such as azoospermia, etc., the procedure of intracytoplasmic sperm injection (ICSI) may be used to ensure fertilization.

Picture	Medical/Surgical Description	Management/Clinical Highlights
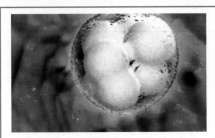 Fig. 13.3.2.2F: Embryo culture	The inseminated oocytes are incubated in an atmosphere of 5% carbon dioxide in air with 98% humidity. Presence of two pronuclei and the extrusion of a second polar body are the criteria which ascertain fertilization, and should occur approximately 18 hours following insemination. The fertilized embryos are transferred into growth media and placed in the incubator. No further evaluation is performed over the next 24 hours. A 4- to 8-cell stage, pre-embryo is observed approximately 36–48 hours after insemination.	Embryos can be cultured in an artificial culture medium or autologous endometrial cell culture. Embryos can be graded based on morphological characteristics. In order to achieve optimal pregnancy rate, the embryos with the highest grading characteristics are selected for transferring into the uterine cavity.
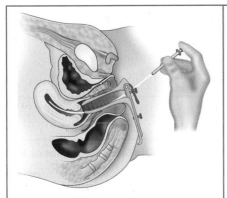 Fig. 13.3.2.2G: Transfer of the embryo inside the uterine cavity	The procedure of embryo transfer is performed within 72 hours after oocyte insemination, when the embryo has become approximately 8–16 cells in size. The transfer is usually performed transcervically under guidance of transabdominal ultrasound.	The embryos should be loaded with 15–20 µL of culture media at the time of transfer. The catheter is advanced up to the fundus of the endometrial cavity, and then withdrawn slightly. The embryos are ejected into the miduterine cavity, approximately 1–2 cm away from the fundus. In the UK and Australia, no more than two embryos must be transferred during any one cycle. In the USA, many embryos can be transferred in younger women based on individual fertility diagnosis.

13.3.3: Intracytoplasmic Sperm Injection

13.3.3.1: Artist's Demonstration of Intracytoplasmic Sperm Injection (A to C)

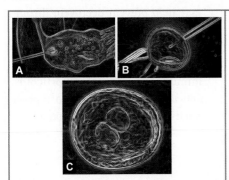

Figs 13.3.3.1 (A to C): (A) Retrieval of a mature ovum from the surface of ovary; (B) Injection of spermatozoan inside the ovum; (C) Fertilization occurring from the fusion of male and female pronuclei
(*Source*: Computerized generation of image)

Intracytoplasmic sperm injection has revolutionized the treatment of severe male factor infertility because this procedure requires only a single live sperm, which is injected directly into the ovum, thereby improving the rate of fertilization. The woman has to undergo the process of follicular stimulation and follicular aspiration prior to the infection of sperm. ICSI is commonly used in cases of male factor infertility such as obstructive azoospermia (due to congenital absence of the vas deferens), severe deficit of semen quality, etc.

Indications for ICSI are as follows:
- Severe deficits in semen quality
- Obstructive azoospermia
- Nonobstructive azoospermia
- Low sperm motility
- Couple desiring pregnancy, where male partner has undergone vasectomy, and reversal of vasectomy is unsuccessful.
- Failure of previous IVF treatment cycles.

Couples should be informed that ICSI improves fertilization rates compared to IVF alone, but once fertilization is achieved, the pregnancy rate is no better than with IVF.

13.3.3.2: Procedure of Intracytoplasmic Sperm Injection (A to E)

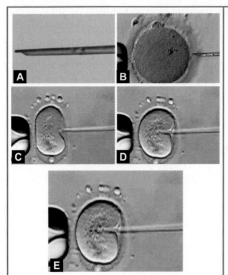

Figs 13.3.3.2 (A to E): (A) Microneedle is loaded with a sperm; (B) The microneedle approaches the oocyte; (C) The microneedle pierces the oocyte membrane; (D) The microneedle is advanced deeper inside the cytoplasm; (E) The spermatozoon is released inside the oocyte

Figures 13.3.3.2 (A to E) illustrate the procedure of ICSI. The oocyte membrane is pierced with the microneedle and the oolemma is entered. The spermatozoon is released inside the oolemma, and the microinjected oocyte is kept in the incubator.

The sperm can be obtained through masturbation, epididymal aspiration, testicular biopsy or needle puncture of the testes. The sperm is paralyzed by stroking the distal portion of its tail.

The oocyte is stripped from the cumulus using a solution of hyaluronidase. To inject the sperm, first the oocyte is stabilized with a micropipette, then the sperm is loaded, tail first, into a microneedle. As the microneedle is advanced deeper inside the cytoplasm, the spermatozoan is eventually released inside the oocyte.

13.3.4: Complications of Assisted Reproductive Techniques

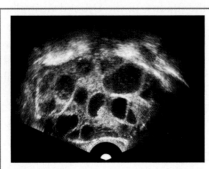

Fig. 13.3.4: Ovarian hyperstimulation syndrome showing "wheel-spoke appearance" on transvaginal examination

Ovarian hyperstimulation syndrome (OHSS) is the commonest iatrogenic complication occurring due to ovarian stimulation during ART and other infertility treatments. Various risk factors for OHSS include raised levels of LH (cases of polycystic ovarian disease), administration of hCG, administration of high doses of stimulation-causing drugs, and the size and number of ovarian follicles. The condition is diagnosed on the basis of clinical presentation and ultrasound findings. Ultrasound shows bilateral symmetric enlargement of ovaries (often > 12 cm in size). There may be the presence of multiple cysts, having varying sizes. This is often termed as the "wheel-spoke appearance". Associated ascites and pleural with or without pericardial effusion (which is due to capillary leak) may also be present.

According to Galen's classification, OHSS has been classified into three classes: mild, moderate and severe.

Treatment of OHSS comprises of the following steps:

- Infusion of intravenous fluids (colloids, plasma, human albumin infusion) for correction of hypovolemia.
- Continuous autotransfusion of ascitic fluid may be required in cases of ascites.
- Thigh high venous support stockings may help prevent deep vein thrombosis.
- Other medicines, which may prove to be helpful include intravenous immunoglobulins, glucocorticoids, anticoagulants, dopamine (to improve renal blood flow and oliguria), etc.

13.4: SURGERY FOR TREATMENT OF INFERTILITY

13.4.1: Fimbrioplasty for Fimbrial Agglutination (A to C)

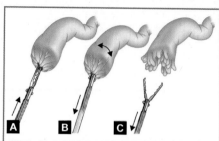

Figs 13.4.1 (A to C): Deagglutination of agglutinated fimbriae: (A) Introduction of an alligator-jawed forceps through the stenosed opening; (B) Opening of the jaws of forceps within the tube; (C) Withdrawing the forceps gently while keeping the jaws open

The procedure comprises of the following steps:
- A fine forceps with jaws closed is introduced through phimotic fimbrial opening. This opening is usually covered by fibrous tissues.
- The tube must be distended prior to the fimbrioplasty by transcervical chromopertubation. This step helps in defining the exact area of pathology especially the presence of fibrous tissue.
- Deagglutination is achieved by opening the jaws of the forceps within the tubal lumen and then gently withdrawing the forceps. This movement is repeated several times.

Fimbrioplasty involves reconstruction of fimbriae in cases of fimbrial agglutination. This surgery aims at opening the blocked tubes and salvaging enough function of the fimbriae so as to be able to successfully entrap and transport the oocyte. Meticulous hemostasis is essential for the success of this surgery.

13.4.2: Fimbrioplasty for Prefimbrial Phimosis (A to C)

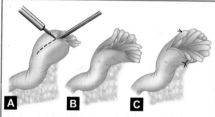

Figs 13.4.2 (A to C): Correction of prefimbrial phimosis: (A) Placing an incision along the antimesosalpingeal border of the tube; (B) Extending the incision; (C) Everting the flaps

Figures 13.4.2 (A to C) demonstrate steps of fimbrioplasty for correction of prefimbrial phimosis. In this case, fimbrioplasty refers to the tubal reconstructive surgery involving broadening of the phimotic tubal opening.

Inflammatory damage may cause stenosis of the apex of tubal infundibulum, resulting in prefimbrial phimosis. The opening in this case is created with the help of sharp dissection or incision either with laser or electrosurgical microelectrode. The incised flaps are then everted in order to create a proper opening.

13.4.3: Salpingostomy (A to E)

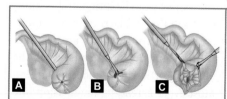

Figs 13.4.3 (A to C): Salpingostomy: (A) Distal end of the tube showing the area of occlusion in form of a centrally avascular area with scarred lines extending in a cart-wheel manner; (B and C) Incision being made along the avascular lines toward the ovary

The procedure of salpingostomy involves the following steps:
The occluded terminal end of tube is inspected under magnification, which helps in the identification of the relatively avascular zones radiating from a central punctum. Using a microelectrode or a microsurgical scissors, an incision is made over this central point and then extended toward the ovary in accordance with the avascular line until a satisfactory stoma is created.

This involves creation of a new stoma in a tube with a completely occluded distal end. Often, presence of adhesions in these cases may require the performance of a salpingo-ovariolysis first. While performing salpingostomy, the occluded distal end is distended by hydrochromopertubation. Not only this confirms the diagnosis, it also helps in improving the visualization of tubes.

Picture	Medical/Surgical Description	Management/Clinical Highlights

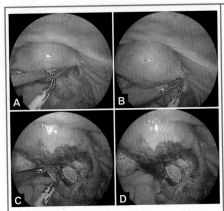

Figs 13.4.3 (D and E): The flaps of the stoma are everted by placing a few sutures

Following the creation of stoma, the flaps which have been created are then everted by securing them to the ampullary seromuscularis using interrupted No. 8-0 vicryl sutures.

The eversion of the newly created flaps is essential to prevent reclosure of the tube.

13.4.4: Laparoscopic Salpingo-ovariolysis (A to D)

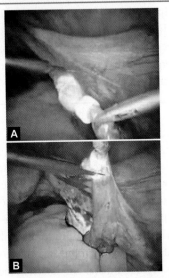

Figs 13.4.4 (A to D): Laparoscopic salpingo-ovariolysis

Presence of periadnexal adhesions is an important cause of infertility. Figures 13.4.4 (A to D) show how the periadnexal adhesions are lysed with the help of laparoscopic salpingo-ovariolysis. This can be considered as a low-risk procedure, which is associated with a high success rate. This procedure helps in avoiding major abdominal surgery.

Salpingo-ovariolysis refers to the lysis of adhesions surrounding the fallopian tubes and ovary, which may be interfering with the pick-up of ovum, resulting in infertility. This procedure is commonly performed prior to fimbrioplasty or salpingostomy.

13.4.5: Tubotubal Anastomosis (A to F)

Figs 13.4.5 (A and B): Steps of tubotubal anastomosis: (A) Grasping the portion of the tube in which tubal ligation had been performed; (B) Transecting the blocked portion of the tube

The tubotubal anastomosis is performed under general anesthesia.
- Bladder is catheterized by inserting a No. 13 Foley's catheter inside the uterine cavity and inflating its bulb.
- The proximal tubal segment is distended by transcervical chromopertubation to help identify the site of occlusion.
- The occluded end of the tube is then grasped with the help of a toothed forceps.
- Tubal transection is performed adjacent to the site of occlusion with a straight scissors or a microblade. Successive transection of the tube at 1–2 mm intervals help in identifying the normal segments, which lie distal and proximal to the site of occlusion.

Tubotubal anastomosis is usually performed to reverse the previous tubal sterilization or for reconstruction of tubes after removal of lesions, which are occlusive and affect the tube at sites other than the fimbriated end.

Depending upon the tubal segments that are approximated, tubotubal anastomosis can be intramural-isthmic, intramural-ampullary, isthmic-isthmic, isthmic-ampullary or ampullary-infundibular. While transecting the blocked portion of the tube, the surgeon must avoid extending the incision into the mesosalpinx in order to avoid damage to the adjacent vascular arcade.

Picture	Medical/Surgical Description	Management/Clinical Highlights

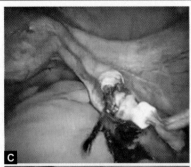
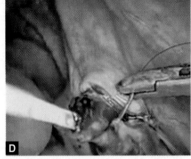

Figs 13.4.5 (C and D): Steps of tubotubal anastomosis: (C) Chromopertubation performed to check the patency of the proximal segment; (D) Stitching the cut segments

The dye (methylene blue) is injected through the intrauterine catheter until it is seen coming out through the medial cut segment of the tube.

- The cut surface of the tubes must be examined under magnification to ensure that the tube is normal, exhibiting normal muscular and vascular architecture with intact mucosal folds.
- If there is no significant luminal disparity between the two tubal segments, the distal portion of the tubes is prepared in a similar manner. Before transecting this segment, it is distended by performing descending chromopertubation, which is performed through the fimbriated end of the tube in order to identify the distal limit of the occluded portion.
- The two prepared tubal segments are then approximated in two layers using 8-0 vicryl sutures, with the first layer joining the epithelium and muscularis, and the second layer joining the serosa.

Once the tube has been cut in the region of obstruction, chromotubation is performed to see if the tube has been adequately transected. If the tubes have been properly transected in the region of obstruction, dye solution would be observed to be escaping freely from the transected tubal lumen. After preparation, the two cut ends of the tube are stitched together in two layers, the inner being continuous and outer being interrupted.

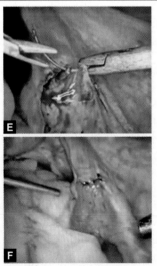

Figs 13.4.5 (E and F): Steps of tubotubal anastomosis: (E) Stitching the cut at the ends of the tube; (F) Appearance of tube following the completion of recanalization procedure

After the approximation of the inner layer, chromopertubation is performed again to demonstrate the tubal patency and a water tight anastomotic site. Once this is demonstrated, the serosa is joined either with interrupted sutures or with two continuous sutures, one running anteriorly and the other posteriorly, starting at the 12'O clock position (antimesosalpingeal border). Finally, the defect in the mesosalpinx is repaired. After checking the patency of the tubes by injecting the dye through the intrauterine Foley's catheter and seeing the dye oozing out through the fimbriated end, the uterus and tubes are gently pushed back into the pelvis.

During the surgical procedure, continuous intraoperative irrigation is provided by heparinized lactated ringer solution. This helps in providing periodic irrigation of the exposed peritoneal surfaces and ovaries, and preventing desiccation. It also helps in the visualization of the individual bleeders. At the time of closure, the operative site is properly inspected to ensure that the complete hemostasis has been achieved. A thorough pelvic lavage is performed with the help of an irrigation solution until the irrigated fluid remains clear. This helps in removing blood clots or debris from the peritoneal cavity.

Picture	Medical/Surgical Description	Management/Clinical Highlights
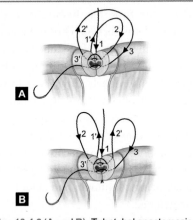 **Figs 13.4.6 (A and B):** Tubotubal anastomosis: placement of sutures using a single strand of sutures as a continuous series of loops	Figures 13.4.6 (A and B) demonstrate the technique of placement of sutures using a single strand of sutures with continuous series of loops. These sutures include the epithelium and muscularis layer.	The approximation of tubal segment is performed in two layers: first one involving the epithelium and muscularis, and second one involving the serosa. The first suture of the inner musculoepithelial layer is placed at the mesosalpingeal border (6'O clock position). This helps in ensuring proper alignment of the two segments. After tying the sutures at 6'O clock position, additional sutures are placed in order to appose the inner layers as shown in the figure.

13.5: POLYCYSTIC OVARIAN DISEASE

13.5.1: Definition (A to D)

Picture	Medical/Surgical Description	Management/Clinical Highlights
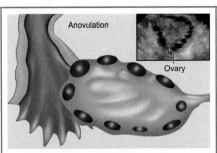 **Fig. 13.5.1A:** Comparison of polycystic ovary (gross and ultrasound appearance)	Polycystic ovarian syndrome (PCOS) was first described by Stein and Leventhal (1935) who reported dramatic effect of ovarian wedge resection in women with secondary amenorrhea, secondary infertility, obesity, hirsutism and cystic ovaries. PCOS is frequently associated with weight gain, excessive hair growth on the face and body, oligomenorrhea or amenorrhea, infrequent or absent ovulation, miscarriage and infertility.	In PCOS, the ovaries are characterized by the presence of numerous small cysts (about size of a pearl). These cysts contain oocytes, which have yet not been released as a result of hormonal imbalance. Therefore, instead of follicle rupturing and releasing ovum, it gets converted into a cyst-like structure. Such structures gradually built up in the ovary, resulting in irregular or absent ovulation. Built up of these cystic structures give a polycystic appearance to the ovaries.
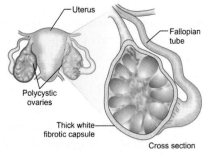 **Fig. 13.5.1B:** Macroscopic appearance of polycystic ovary	The condition, PCOS is a relatively common endocrine disorder amongst women of reproductive age group. It is associated with anovulation, features of androgen excess, obesity, infertility and hypersecretion of LH. This condition is characterized by the presence of many minute cysts in the ovaries and excessive production of androgens.	The Rotterdam criteria for the diagnosis of PCOS is as follows: 1. Infrequent or absent ovulation. 2. Clinical or biochemical features of hyperandrogenism such as excessive hair growth, acne, raised LH and raised androgen levels. 3. Morphologically there is bilateral ovarian enlargement, thickened ovarian capsule, multiple follicular cysts (usually ranging between 2 mm and 8 mm in diameter) and an increased amount of stroma. Any two of the above-mentioned three manifestations must be fulfilled in order to establish the diagnosis of PCOS.

Picture	Medical/Surgical Description	Management/Clinical Highlights
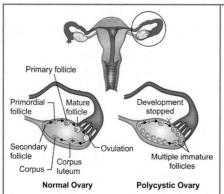 **Fig. 13.5.1C:** Formation of multiple follicles in case of polycystic ovarian disease	Diagnosis of PCOS is made through ultrasound examination or diagnostic laparoscopy. Blood levels of hormones, such as LH, FSH, androgens and serum hormone binding globulins must also be measured in these patients. FSH levels are low or normal, and LH levels are often raised, resulting in a raised LH/FSH ratio. The levels of androgens and testosterone may also be raised.	Under normal circumstances, the ovarian follicles grow, mature and eventually ovulate during each menstrual cycle. If these eggs mature, but cannot be released from the ovary, they develop into fluid-filled cystic structures. These cyst-like structures are either observed on ultrasound examination or on diagnostic laparoscopy.
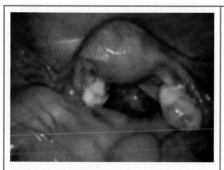 **Fig. 13.5.1D:** Bilateral polycystic ovaries as observed on laparoscopic examination	When observed on laparoscopic examination, the polycystic ovaries are nearly 1.5 to 3 times larger than the normal ovaries. The ovaries appear large and round in shape, and are surrounded by a thick, white capsule. Though the small cysts may not be as clearly visible as observed on ultrasound examination, some bluish colored cystic structures may be visible sometimes through the ovarian capsule.	Inside the ovary, multiple cysts are present giving it an appearance of string of pearls or a pearl necklace appearance. However, this may not be visible on laparoscopic examination. This is only observed on ultrasound examination. Therefore, diagnosis of PCOS cannot be just established on the basis of laparoscopic examination. An ultrasound examination and evaluation of blood levels of various hormones is also essential before arriving at a particular diagnosis.

13.5.2: Diagnosis

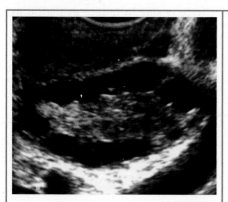 **Fig. 13.5.2:** Ultrasound features of polycystic ovarian morphology	Ultrasound examination is essential before establishing the diagnosis of PCOS. Ultrasound gives an internal picture of the ovary, demonstrating the presence of numerous cystic structures. It is not possible to see this picture of the ovary on laparoscopic examination.	Features of polycystic ovarian morphology on ultrasound scan are as follows: • Greater than 12 follicles measuring between 2 mm and 9 mm in diameter, located peripherally, resulting in a pearl necklace appearance. • Increased echogenicity of ovarian stroma and/or ovarian volume > 10 mL. The distribution of the follicles is not required, with one ovary being sufficient for the diagnosis.

| Picture | Medical/Surgical Description | Management/Clinical Highlights |

13.5.3: Pathophysiology

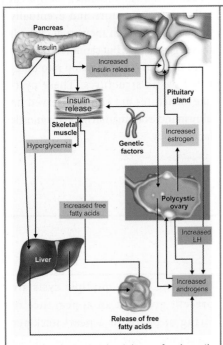

Fig. 13.5.3: Pathophysiology of polycystic ovarian syndrome
(*Source*: Nestler JE. Metformin for the treatment of the polycystic ovary syndrome. N Engl J Med. 2008;358:47-54.)

Despite of many years of research, the pathophysiology of PCOS has not been completely understood. Common endocrine abnormalities in PCOS include chronically high levels of LH, thereby resulting in an elevated LH/FSH ratio (usually 2.5 or greater), hyperandrogenism, hyperinsulinemia, insulin resistance and dyslipidemia. These endocrine disturbances interfere with ovarian folliculogenesis and result in anovulation. Two important biochemical features associated with PCOS include insulin resistance to a standard glucose challenge, and compensatory hyperinsulinemia and obesity.

Elevated LH levels in patients with PCOS result in the hyperplasia of stromal and thecal cells in the ovarian follicles. This ultimately results in an increased androgen production by the adrenal glands (DHEA and DHEAS) and ovarian stroma (androstenedione). High intraovarian androgen levels may further contribute to follicular atresia. This also results in an increased peripheral availability of ovarian testosterone (androstenedione), which gets converted in the skin to dihydrotestosterone, with the help of the enzyme 5-reductase, thereby accounting for acne and hirsutism in these women. Moreover, increased androstenedione secretion results in an increased production of estrone.

Low levels of FSH in the follicle prevent induction of aromatase activity and result in the lack of ovarian estrogen production. As granulosa cell mitosis and follicular growth requires an estrogenic follicular microenvironment, follicular maturation gets arrested. This is responsible for producing anovulation.

13.5.4: Treatment

13.5.4.1: Treatment of Patients Desiring Fertility

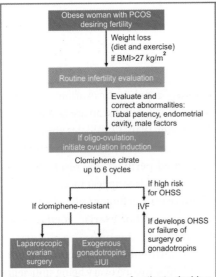

Fig. 13.5.4.1: Treatment of patients desiring fertility

Stepwise approach for women with PCOS who want to conceive is as follows:
1. Weight loss: Weight loss is especially required, if BMI is greater than 30 kg/m².
2. Use of ovulation inducing agent such as CC.
3. Combination of CC with corticosteroids (if DHES > 2 µg/mL)
4. Combination of CC with insulin sensitizing agents (such as glucophage and metformin) in case of insulin resistance
5. Low dose FSH injection
6. Combination of low dose FSH injection with metformin
7. Laparoscopic ovarian drilling (LOD)
8. IVF

For the woman with PCOS who wants to conceive, CC is used initially because of its high success rate, and relative simplicity and inexpensiveness. Clomiphene citrate is able to induce ovulation in nearly 50–80% of the individuals and of these approximately 40–50% are able to conceive. Other possible therapeutic approaches for ovulation induction include the use of insulin-sensitizing agents, gonadotropins, FSH alone, pulsatile GnRH and LOD.

Picture	Medical/Surgical Description	Management/Clinical Highlights

13.5.4.2: Treatment of Patients not Desiring Fertility

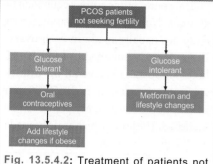

Fig. 13.5.4.2: Treatment of patients not desiring fertility

In women with PCOS, not desiring fertility, treatment primarily aims at prevention of long-term health problems such as hirsutism, endometrial hyperplasia, dysfunctional uterine bleeding, insulin resistance, etc.

The treatment must be individualized according to the needs and desires of each patient. The aims of treatment in women with PCOS, who do not desire fertility, are to control hirsutism, to prevent endometrial hyperplasia from unopposed acyclic estrogen secretion and to prevent the long-term consequences of insulin resistance.

Use of OCPs or cyclic progestational agents can help to maintain a normal endometrium, and also reduce the increased risk of endometrial hyperplasia and carcinoma.

13.5.4.3: Laparoscopic Ovarian Drilling (A to D)

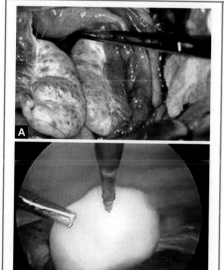

Figs 13.5.4.3 (A and B): (A) Laparoscopic visualization of the pelvis in an effort to locate the ovaries; (B) Lifting the ovaries out of the ovarian fossa and placing them over the cervicouterine junction

The steps of LOD, as described in Figures 13.5.4.3 (A to D), are as follows:

- Immediately after the insertion of laparoscope, the entire pelvis is inspected to rule out other causes of infertility.
- Chromotubation is done by transcervical injection of the methylene blue dye. The under-surface of the ovaries is inspected for any evidence of endometriosis.
- A good uterine manipulator is used to stretch the ovarian ligament and move the uterus to the contralateral side.
- The ovary is then lifted out of the ovarian fossa using a blunt instrument.
- The monopolar needle for drilling holes in the ovary is inserted from the contralateral lower abdominal port and is introduced at right angles to the ovary, at the same time, avoiding injury to the hilum.
- A thorough suction irrigation and lavage should be now done, in order to clear the pelvis of any smoke, blood, clot, debris, etc. In order to minimize the formation of adhesions, it is important to achieve proper hemostasis and minimize bleeding.

The main advantages associated with the procedure of LOD are enumerated below:

- There is no additional risk of multiple gestation or ovarian hyperstimulation syndrome, as reported with the use of gonadotropins for ovulation induction.
- The procedure is considered to be associated with fewer postoperative adhesions in comparison to laparotomy.
- It is associated with minimum morbidity and no requirement for cyclic monitoring, as required with the ovulation-inducing drugs.
- LOD yields a better ovulation and pregnancy rate in comparison to other surgical modalities for ovulation induction.
- LOD is associated with a low miscarriage rate (14%) in comparison to that associated with ovulation induction, using gonadotropins (50%).

Picture	Medical/Surgical Description	Management/Clinical Highlights

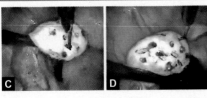

Figs 13.5.4.3 (C and D): (C)The procedure of laparoscopic ovarian drilling using electrocauterization; (D) Appearance of the ovary following the procedure

The number of holes to be made during LOD is usually decided on the basis of ovarian size and volume, and preoperative ultrasound appearance of the ovaries. Usually all bluish subcapsular follicles, which are visible, must be cauterized. Though treatment of both ovaries is usually preformed, reports in which treatment with drilling of only one ovary proved to be successful have also been published.

Laparoscopic ovarian drilling is performed utilizing pure cutting current equivalent to 40 watts. Number of holes varying from 4–20 are usually made in each ovary. In moderately enlarged ovaries, 10–12 holes are made. However, if the ovaries are extremely voluminous, i.e. 50–60 mm in size, number of cautery points can be increased. The holes, which are to be made are usually 3 mm wide and 3–4 mm deep.

13.5.5: Long-term Consequences

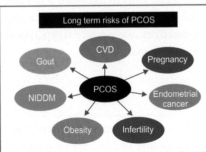

Fig. 13.5.5: Long-term consequences of polycystic ovarian syndrome (CVD, Cardiovascular disease, NIDDM, non-insulin dependent diabetes mellitus)

Polycystic ovarian syndrome has been found to be associated with insulin resistance, which in the long run may result in the development of impaired glucose tolerance and type 2 diabetes. PCOS has also been found to be associated with obstructive sleep apnea, which itself acts as an independent risk factor for the development of cardiovascular disease.

These women are also at an increased risk of cardiovascular diseases and cardiometabolic syndrome due to a higher incidence of hypertension, dyslipidemia, visceral obesity, insulin resistance and hyperinsulinemia. Gestational diabetes may be observed in women with PCOS. Oligomenorrhea or amenorrhea in women with PCOS may predispose to endometrial hyperplasia and later carcinoma.

Lifestyle changes through diet and exercise remain the first line for treatment in cases of PCOS.

In order to prevent the risk for development of endometrial cancer as a result of exposure to unopposed estrogens, progestogens must be prescribed for last 10–15 days in order to induce a withdrawal bleed at least every 3–4 months.

Both metformin and thiazolidinediones (troglitazone) have been shown to have beneficial short-term effects on insulin resistance in women with PCOS who are not diabetic. Antiobesity drugs such as orlistat and sibutramine have been shown to significantly reduce body weight and hyperandrogenism in women with PCOS.

13.6: HIRSUTISM

13.6.1: Definition (A to C)

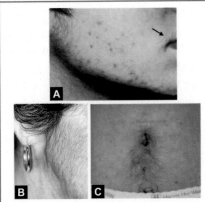

Figs 13.6.1 (A to C): Excessive hair: (A) Over the upper lip; (B) Over the sideburn area; (C) Abdominal hair

Hirsutism is defined as the presence of coarse, dark, terminal hair in a male pattern in a woman. This is in contrast with virilization, which reflects very high levels of androgens and manifests in form of increased muscle mass, reduced breast size, deepening of voice, clitoromegaly, etc. The most common areas, where increased hair growth is apparent are upper lips, chin, side burns, chest and linea alba of abdomen [Figures 13.6.1 (A to C)].

The mainstay of treatment of hirsutism is removal of excessive hair using mechanical methods such as plucking, shaving, waxing, using depilatory creams, bleaching, etc. and clinic-based treatments such as clinic-based waxing, electrolysis, laser hair removal, etc. These methods can also be combined with drug therapy. The drugs most commonly used for treatment of hirsutism include OCPs, containing low-androgenic progestins; antiandrogenic drugs such as spironolactone, cyproterone, flutamide, etc.; insulin sensitizers, such as metformin (glucophage), GnRH analogues, etc.

Picture	Medical/Surgical Description	Management/Clinical Highlights

13.6.2: Original Ferriman and Gallwey Scoring System

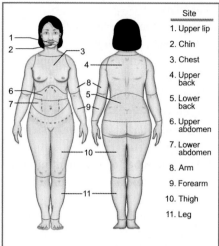

Site
1. Upper lip
2. Chin
3. Chest
4. Upper back
5. Lower back
6. Upper abdomen
7. Lower abdomen
8. Arm
9. Forearm
10. Thigh
11. Leg

Fig. 13.6.2: Ferriman and Gallwey scoring system

The Ferriman-Gallwey scoring system was developed in 1961 by Dr D Ferriman and Dr JD Gallwey to quantify the degree of hirsutism, and it was later modified in 1981. In the modified system, the abnormal distribution of hair is assessed in nine areas of the body [Figures 13.6.3 (A to D)] and given a score ranging from 0 to 4. The score increases with the increasing hair density and include the following areas: upper lip, chin, chest, upper abdomen, lower abdomen, upper arms, thighs, buttocks and back. Therefore total score can vary from a minimum of 0 to a maximum of 36. In the original method, eleven areas of the body were assessed (two extra regions being forearm and legs).

Polycystic ovary syndrome clinically presents with menstrual irregularities such as oligomenorrhea or amenorrhea, infertility and signs of hyperandrogenism such as hirsutism, acne, etc. Using a Ferriman-Gallwey scoring system can help evaluate hirsutism. A Ferriman-Gallwey score of 8 or higher is considered to be hirsutism.

13.6.3: Scoring the Extent of Hirsutism Using the Modified Method (A to D)

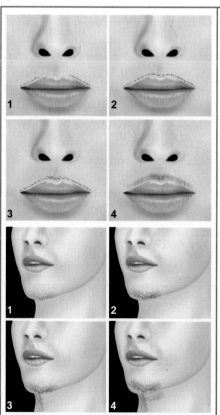

Fig. 13.6.3A: Hair growth on upper lip and chin

Scoring over the chin region is as follows:
1. Sparse terminal hair on chin
2. Sparse terminal hair with small thickened areas
3. Entire chin covered with light growth
4. Entire chin covered with a heavy growth

Scoring over the upper lip region is as follows:
1. Small number of terminal hair over the upper lip and outer lip border
2. The moustache covering less than 50% of the upper lip or at the outer border
3. Moustache covering 50% from the outer margin of the lip or 50% of the lip height
4. Moustache covering most of the upper lip and crossing the midline up

The physical examination in cases of hirsutism involves use of the Ferriman-Gallwey hirsutism scoring system, which helps categorize the severity and distribution of excess hair growth.

Picture	Medical/Surgical Description	Management/Clinical Highlights
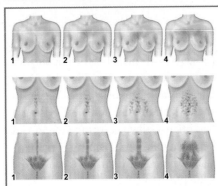 **Fig. 13.6.3B:** Hair growth on chest, upper abdomen and lower abdomen	For a modified Ferriman-Gallwey scoring system, total score can vary from a minimum of 0 to a maximum of 36. A Ferriman-Gallwey score of 8 to 15 indicates moderate hirsutism, whereas a score above 15 indicates severe hirsutism. *Scoring over the chest region is as follows:* 1. Circumareolar or midline terminal hair 2. Circumareolar and midline terminal hair 3. About 75% of the chest region is covered with terminal hair 4. Entire chest is covered with terminal hair growth.	*Scoring over the upper abdominal region is as follows:* 1. Scattered midline terminal hair 2. More hair, still midline 3. Fifty percent of upper abdomen is covered 4. Entire area covered with terminal hair growth. *Scoring over the lower abdominal region is as follows:* 1. Small number of scattered midline terminal hair in the length of linea alba 2. Midline concentration of terminal hair along the length of linea alba 3. A midline thickened band of terminal hair less than half width of the pubic hair at the base 4. An inverted V-shaped coverage of half width of pubic hair at the base.
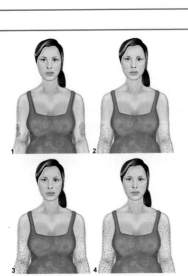 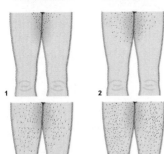 **Fig. 13.6.3C:** Hair growth over arms and thighs	*Scoring over the arms is as follows:* 1. Scattered terminal hair over less than 25% of the upper arm 2. Increased but incomplete coverage 3. Entire area covered with a light growth 4. Entire area covered with a heavy growth. *Scoring over the thighs is as follows:* 1. Scattered terminal hair over less than 25% of thighs 2. Increased but incomplete coverage 3. Entire area covered with a light growth 4. Entire area covered with a heavy growth.	During physical examination of cases with hirsutism, the clinician must also look for other cutaneous signs of hyperandrogenism such as acne, seborrhea, etc. Acanthosis nigricans may be also observed in cases of PCOS and is a sign of insulin resistance. It is a skin disorder characterized by skin, which becomes thicker, hyperpigmented and acquires a velvety texture. Height and weight should be measured in these cases to calculate the body mass index.

Picture	Medical/Surgical Description	Management/Clinical Highlights

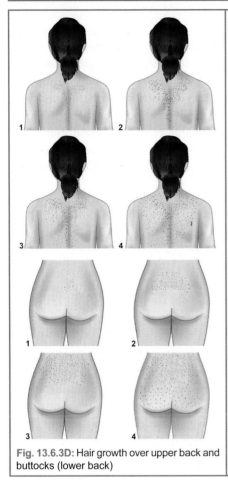

Fig. 13.6.3D: Hair growth over upper back and buttocks (lower back)

Scoring over the upper back is as follows:
1. Sparse terminal hairs over the upper back
2. Increased number of spread terminal hairs
3. Entire area is covered with a light growth
4. Entire area is covered with a heavy growth

Scoring over the buttocks (lower back) is as follows:
1. Sacral area with the hair coverage less than 4 cm wide
2. Increased coverage on the sides
3. Approximately 75% of the lower back is covered with terminal hair
4. Entire area is covered with heavy growth.

Tests suggested for the work up of hirsutism in cases of PCOS include:

Hormone levels: Measurement of androgens such as early-morning total or free testosterone levels, and levels of sex hormone binding globulins, DHEAS, and androstenedione needs to be done. Ratio of LH:FSH greater than 2 has been considered indicative but is not diagnostic of PCOS.

Ultrasound: Transvaginal ultrasound examination must be performed for assessment of polycystic ovaries.

Metabolic profile: A fasting lipid profile and fasting serum glucose are usually recommended. If the fasting serum glucose is normal, an oral glucose tolerance test is recommended.

13.7: ENDOMETRIOSIS

13.7.1: Definition

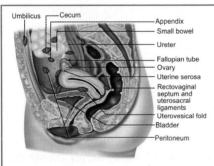

Fig. 13.7.1: Common sites of endometriotic lesions

Endometriosis, which is an important cause of infertility is a clinical entity characterized by the presence of ectopic endometrial glands and stroma, outside the uterine cavity. The common sites of endometrial implants include the pelvic cavity, ovaries, uterine ligaments, rectovaginal septum, parietal peritoneum, intestinal serosa, etc.

Endometriosis is one of the most common causes of chronic pelvic pain in women belonging to the reproductive age groups and may be associated with infertility in nearly 30–40% cases. This disease can be associated with a varied clinical presentation. There can be pelvic symptoms (e.g. dysmenorrhea, dyspareunia, chronic pelvic pain, sciatica, premenstrual spotting); gastrointestinal symptoms (e.g. constipation, diarrhea, dyschezia, tenesmus, hematochezia); urinary symptoms (e.g. flank, abdominal and back pain, urinary urgency, frequency and hematuria); infertility and pulmonary symptoms (e.g. hemoptysis, chest pain, pneumothorax, etc.).

13.7.2: Pathophysiology of Endometriosis

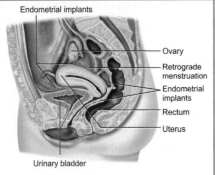

Fig. 13.7.2: Basic anatomy of retrograde menstruation

Though the pathophysiology of endometriosis is not yet understood, the most widely accepted theory for pathogenesis of endometriosis involves retrograde menstruation. According to this theory, reflux of degenerated menstrual endometrium through the fallopian tubes occurs during menstrual cycles. This tissue subsequently gets implanted on the pelvic peritoneum and the surrounding structures and starts growing. These refluxed cells implant in the pelvis, bleed in response to cyclic hormonal stimulation and increase in size along with progression of symptoms at the time of menses.

Although retrograde menstruation seems to be the most likely cause involved in the pathogenesis of endometriosis, this theory does not explain the full spectrum of the disease. For example, this theory is unable to explain the presence of endometrial implants at remote sites such as the lung, pleura, endocardium, etc.

13.7.3: Diagnosis (A to E)

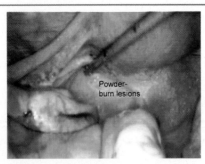

Fig. 13.7.3A: Powder-burn lesions

Laparoscopy can help in establishing the diagnosis of endometriosis by identifying various lesions. Laparoscopic findings are variable and may include discrete endometriotic lesions, endometriomas and adhesion formation. Endometriotic lesions are typically located over the pelvic organs and pelvic peritoneum, and may acquire variable colors such as red, white, reddish-pink, yellow, yellowish-brown, black or blackish-blue. Endometrial lesions may appear as smooth blebs on peritoneal surface, as holes or defects in the peritoneum or as flat stellate lesions surrounded by scar tissue.

Powder-burn lesions, also known as the gunshot lesions can be considered as the classical pigmented endometriotic lesion. These lesions may acquire dark brown, dark blue or black color, and may become cystic in appearance due to the accumulation of menstrual blood within the endometriotic deposits. These implants may attain a size of 5–10 mm. As the disease progresses, these lesions may increase in size and number, and there may be development of extensive adhesions.

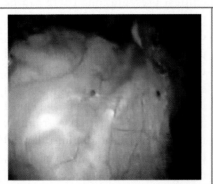

Fig. 13.7.3B: Nodular endometrial lesions

Small fluid-filled nodular lesions represent early stage of the disease and they result due to implantation of endometriotic cells on the peritoneal surface.

Endometrial lesions may be either superficial, or may deeply invade the peritoneum or pelvic organs. Presently, biopsy and histological evaluation are not recommended for the diagnosis of endometriosis. Diagnosis is presently established on the basis of laparoscopic findings only (ASRM, 1997).

Picture	Medical/Surgical Description	Management/Clinical Highlights
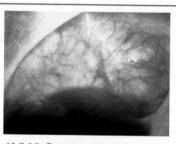 Fig. 13.7.3C: Presence of blood in cul-de-sac	Laparoscopy can also detect presence of blood or endometriotic deposits or blood in the cul-de-sac and its obliteration as shown in Figure 13.7.3C.	Treatment of endometriosis depends upon on the woman's specific presenting symptoms, symptom severity, location of endometriotic lesions, goal of treatment and desire to conserve future fertility. If the woman's presenting symptom is infertility, fertility-preserving treatment for ovulation suppression would be required.
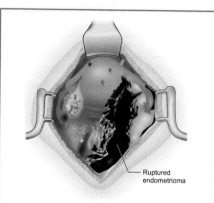 Fig. 13.7.3D: Ruptured chocolate cyst of ovary	In the ovary, endometrial cysts may get enlarged to several centimeters resulting in the development of endometriomas or chocolate cysts. Once intracystic pressure inside the chocolate cyst rises, the cyst perforates, spilling its contents within the peritoneal cavity. This can cause severe abdominal pain typically associated with endometriosis exacerbations. The inflammatory response may result in the development of adhesions, which may further increase the disease related morbidity.	The classic lesion of endometriosis is a chocolate cyst of the ovary that contains old blood that has undergone hemolysis. On gross microscopic examination, the tunica albuginea appears to be thickened. Red vascular lesions may be well marked on the under surface of the ovary.
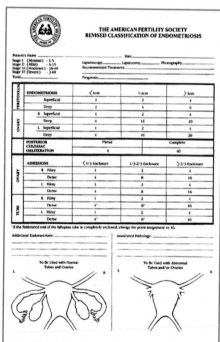 Fig. 13.7.3E: Classification of endometriosis *If the fimbriated end of the fallopian tube is completely enclosed, the point assignment is changed to 16. (*Source:* Revised American Society for Reproductive Medicine classification of endometriosis: 1996. Fertil Steril. 1997; 67:817-21)	Before initiating treatment for endometriosis, it is important to classify the disease as minimal, mild, moderate or severe. The American Fertility Society's revised staging for endometriosis is currently the most widely used staging system. In this scoring system, point scores are assigned based on the number of lesions, their bilaterality, size of the lesions, depth of endometrial implants, presence and extent of adnexal adhesions, and degree of obliteration of the Pouch of Douglas. If the total number of points is scored between 1 and 5, the disease is classified as minimal (stage I); if the total number of points are between 6 and 15, the disease is classified as mild (stage II); if the total number of points are between 16 and 40, the disease is classified as moderate (stage III) and it is classified as severe (stage IV) if the number of points is more than 40. Minimal invasive surgery is often employed in mild to moderate cases of endometriosis.	For patients with mild disease, hormonal treatment (e.g. GnRH analogs, danazol and medroxyprogesterone) has been shown to be effective in reducing pain, but has no impact on fertility. For severe endometriosis, the efficacy of hormonal treatment has not yet been established. Medical treatment should be reserved for use in patients with pain or dyspareunia, and comprises of oral analgesic agents such as NSAIDs, progesterone therapy, oral contraceptive agents, GnRH agonists, danazol and Mirena intrauterine contraceptive device. If the medical therapy does not prove to be successful, the gynecologist may have to resort to surgical treatment, which is the preferred approach for treatment of infertile patients with advanced endometriosis. Surgical care can be broadly classified as conservative when reproductive potential is retained, semiconservative when reproductive ability is eliminated but ovarian function is retained, and radical when both the uterus and ovaries are removed.

Picture	Medical/Surgical Description	Management/Clinical Highlights

13.7.4: Treatment of Endometriosis (A to F)

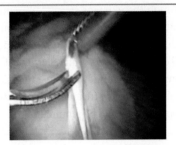

Fig. 13.7.4A: Laparoscopic excision of nodular endometrial lesions overlying the round ligament

Figure 13.7.4A shows laparoscopic excision of nodular endometrial lesions overlying the round ligament. Besides removing the endometriotic lesions, the minimal invasive surgery is also useful in restoration of patient's fertility.

Age, desire for future childbearing and deterioration of quality of life are the main considerations when deciding on the type of surgery to be employed in cases of endometriosis. Surgical treatment improves pregnancy rates and is the preferred initial treatment for infertility caused by endometriosis. Surgery also appears to provide better long-term pain relief than medical treatment.

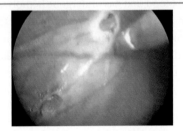

Fig. 13.7.4B: Laser ablation of endometriotic lesions

Figure 13.7.4B demonstrates laser ablation of endometriotic lesions at the time of laparoscopy.

Besides diagnosis of endometriotic lesions at various locations, laparoscopy can also help in treating the patient. Powder-burn lesions over the uterine surface may be amenable to laser obliteration. Some of the cystic or nodular endometrial lesions can also be excised at the time of laparoscopy.

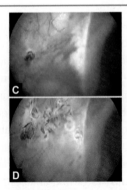

Figs 13.7.4 (C and D): Appearance of the uterine surface after the ablation of endometriotic lesions

Figures 13.7.4 (C and D) show appearance of the uterine surface following ablation of endometriotic lesions.

Until recently, surgery in infertile patients with limited disease was thought to be no better than expectant management. However, according to the recent evidence, surgery (especially minimal invasive surgery) has been found to significantly improve the fertility rates among infertile women with minimal or mild endometriosis. Infertile patients with documented endometriosis can also benefit from the ARTs such as superovulation, IVF, etc.

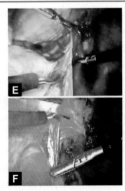

Figs 13.7.4 (E and F): Laparoscopic excision of endometrial adhesions

Laparoscopic surgery can also be used for excision of endometrial adhesions. The benefit of surgery in these patients may be entirely due to the mechanical clearance of adhesions and obstructive lesions.

When the diagnosis of endometriosis is made at laparoscopy, laparoscopic modalities of treatment such as surgical ablation of the lesions, laparoscopic excision of adhesions, etc. are frequently performed. Definitive surgery, which includes hysterectomy and oophorectomy, is reserved for use in women with intractable pain who no longer desire pregnancy.

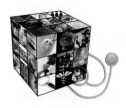

EVIDENCE-BASED BREAKTHROUGH FACTS

1. POSTPERATIVE LEVONORGESTREL-RELEASING INTRAUTERINE SYSTEM FOR PELVIC ENDOMETRIOSIS-RELATED PAIN

In patients with endometriosis treated through conservative laparoscopic surgery, hormonal suppression using progestin therapy (levonorgestrel-releasing intrauterine system) postoperatively has been found to be associated with reduced rate of dysmenorrhea and pelvic pain after 1 year of surgery in comparison with expectant management following surgery for endometriosis. However, its beneficial effect on the future pregnancy rate remains unknown.

Source: Tanmahasamut P, Rattanachaiyanont M, Angsuwathana S, et al. Postoperative levonorgestrel-releasing intrauterine system for pelvic endometriosis-related pain: a randomized controlled trial. Obstet Gynecol. 2012;119:519.

2. MODIFIED FERRIMAN-GALLWEY SCORING SYSTEM

A modified Ferriman-Gallwey scoring of greater than 4 can be used to diagnose hirsutism amongst women. Also, hair growth involving the upper lip, thighs, and lower abdomen with scores greater than 2 can be used to diagnose hirsutism in women.

Source: Li R, Qiao J, Yang D, et al. Epidemiology of hirsutism among women of reproductive age in the community: a simplified scoring system. Eur J Obstet Gynecol Reprod Biol. 2012;163(2):165-9.

3. BREAST CANCER AND IN VITRO FERTILIZATION

There was no overall increase in the rate of breast cancer in women who had IVF but there was an increased rate amongst women who commenced IVF at a young age (< 24 years). Therefore, commencing IVF treatment at a young age is associated with an increased rate of breast cancer.

Source: Stewart LM, Holman CD, Hart R, et al. School of Population Health, In vitro fertilization and breast cancer: is there cause for concern? Fertil Steril. 2012;98(2):334-40

4. REVISED REFERENCE LIMITS FOR SEMEN ANALYSIS

The World Health Organization (WHO, 2010) has published revised lower reference limits for semen analyses as described below:

Parameter	Older WHO criteria for being normal	Newer WHO criteria (2010) for being normal
Volume	2–5 mL	1.5 mL
Sperm concentration	20 million spermatozoa/mL	15 million spermatozoa/mL
Total sperm number	40 million spermatozoa per ejaculate	39 million spermatozoa per ejaculate
Morphology	≥ 4%	≥4 % normal forms (using "strict" Tygerberg method)
Vitality	75% or more live	58% or more live
Progressive motility	50%, forward progression	32%

Source: Cooper TG, Noonan E, von Eckardstein S, et al. World Health Organization reference values for human semen characteristics. Hum Reprod Update. 2010;16(3):231.

5. INFLUENCE OF VITAMIN D LEVELS ON IVF OUTCOMES

Levels of vitamin D are likely to play a role in the woman's reproductive capacity. Higher IVF pregnancy rates have been demonstrated in woman with optimal levels of vitamin D. Vitamin D deficiency has been found to be associated with lower pregnancy rate in non-Hispanic whites, but not in Asians. This could be related to low rate of IVF success in these women. Vitamin D deficiency could not be correlated with ovarian stimulation parameters or with markers of embryo quality. This implies that its effect may be mediated through the endometrium.

Source: Rudick B, Ingles S, Chung K, et al. Characterizing the influence of vitamin D levels on IVF outcomes. Hum Reprod. 2012;27(11):3321-7.

Section 14

Infections of the Genital Tract

14.1: Vaginal Discharge
14.2: Sexually Transmitted Diseases
14.3: Pelvic Inflammatory Diseases

14.1: VAGINAL DISCHARGE

14.1.1: Discharge in Candidal Vaginitis

Picture	Medical/Surgical Description	Management/Clinical Highlights
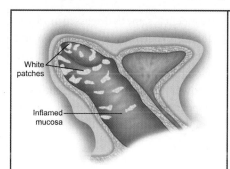 **Fig. 14.1.1:** Type of vaginal discharge in cases of candidal vaginitis	Vulvovaginal candidiasis (VVC) is the second most common cause of vaginitis in the United States and the most common cause of vulvovaginitis in Europe. In most of the cases, the infecting agent is the yeast *Candida albicans*. In this condition, the discharge is usually white and thick (curd-like), with no odor and a normal pH. Pruritus vulva is a cardinal feature of this condition.	Imidazoles and triazoles are presently the most extensively used antifungal drugs for treatment of VVC. Imidazole antifungal agents, which can be used in form of creams and pessaries for treatment of VVC, include butoconazole, clotrimazole and miconazole. Some of these agents are freely available over the counter. Triazole agents include systemically acting agents such as fluconazole. A single dose of triazole antifungals (e.g. 150 mg of fluconazole orally) has also been shown to be effective in most cases.

14.1.2: Appearance of Vulva and Vagina in Cases of Vulvovaginal Candidiasis

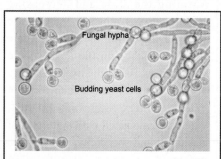 **Fig. 14.1.2:** Appearance of vulva and vagina in cases of vulvovaginal candidiasis	Women with VVC frequently complain of pruritus, vaginal irritation, dysuria, vulvar and vaginal erythema and occasionally, scaling and fissures of vulvar tissue.	Management of VVC has been discussed in Figure 14.1.1. In case of recurrent vulvovaginitis, oral fluconazole in the dosage of 140 mg every 72 hours for three doses serves as an effective therapy. This should be then followed by weekly doses for a few weeks. Ideally, both the partners should be treated and the underlying predisposing factors be corrected to provide long-term relief.

14.1.3: Diagnosis of Candidal Infection

Fig. 14.1.3: Appearance of wet-mount preparation of *Candida albicans*	Microscopic examinations of wet mount and potassium hydroxide (KOH) preparations are positive in 50–70% of patients with candidal infections. In candidal infections, KOH preparation may reveal budding filaments, mycelia, or pseudohyphae. A fungal culture may be used if the diagnosis is uncertain. Microscopy for candidal disease has an estimated sensitivity of 65%.	Positive findings on microscopic examination are likely to confirm the diagnosis. In patients whose symptoms are strongly suggestive of candidal vaginitis, but the microscopic examination is negative, gram staining or culture using Nickerson's medium or Sabouraud's dextrose agar may prove to be helpful. Though candidiasis is not considered to be a sexually transmitted disease, VVC may be sometimes associated with sexual activity. However, treatment of male partner may not be always required.

14.1.4: Type of Vaginal Discharge in Cases of Trichomonal Vaginitis

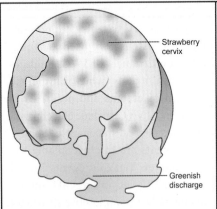

Fig. 14.1.4: Type of vaginal discharge in cases of trichomonal vaginitis

Trichomonal vaginitis is caused by the protozoa *Trichomonas vaginalis*, a motile organism currently accounting for 10–25% of vaginal infections. Trichomonads are usually transmitted sexually and may be identified in 30–80% of the male sexual partners of infected women. Classic manifestations of vaginal trichomoniasis include a purulent, frothy, yellow discharge with an abnormal odor, pruritus and dysuria. The typical discharge associated with this infection is profuse, thin, creamy or slightly green in color, irritating and frothy.

Metronidazole in the dose of 200 mg TDS or 375 mg BID must be prescribed to both the partners for a period of 7 days. The Centers for Disease Control and Prevention (CDC), however, recommends a single dose of 2 g of metronidazole. Since tricomoniasis is largely believed to be a sexually transmitted disease, both the partners should be advised to avoid intercourse or use a condom during the course of therapy. An alternative to metronidazole could be to prescribe tinidazole in the dose of 300 mg BID for 7 days or secnidazole in a single dose of 1,000 mg daily for 2 days.

14.1.5: Appearance of Vulva and Vagina in Trichomoniasis

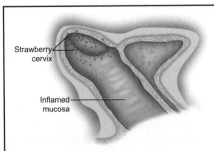

Fig. 14.1.5: Appearance of vulva and vagina in trichomoniasis

Since the discharge commonly causes pruritus and inflammation of the vulva and vagina, the vaginal walls are often tender and appear angry looking. There may be presence of multiple, small, punctate, strawberry spots on the vaginal vault and portio vaginalis of the cervix resulting in a "strawberry vagina".

Treatment is same as discussed in 15.1.4. During pregnancy and lactation use of metronidazole is contraindicated. During early pregnancy, vinegar douches to lower the vaginal pH, trichofuran suppositories and betadine gel may be useful.

14.1.6: Histopathological Appearance of *Trichomonas vaginalis*

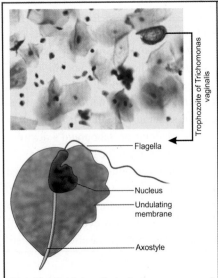

Fig. 14.1.6: Histopathological appearance of *Trichomonas vaginalis*

Motile trichomonads are usually observed on microscopic examination of wet mounts. If the index of suspicion for trichomoniasis is high and microscopic examination of the wet-mount preparation reveals negative results, the microorganism may be cultured using Diamond's medium.

Warming the slide and decreasing the intensity of substage lighting are ways for increasing the detection rate of trichomonads on the microscopic examination. Additionally, tests using DNA probes, polymerase chain reaction tests and latex agglutination test, which are associated with high rates of sensitivity and specificity, may also be performed.

Picture	Medical/Surgical Description	Management/Clinical Highlights

14.1.7: Transmission of *Trichomonas vaginalis*

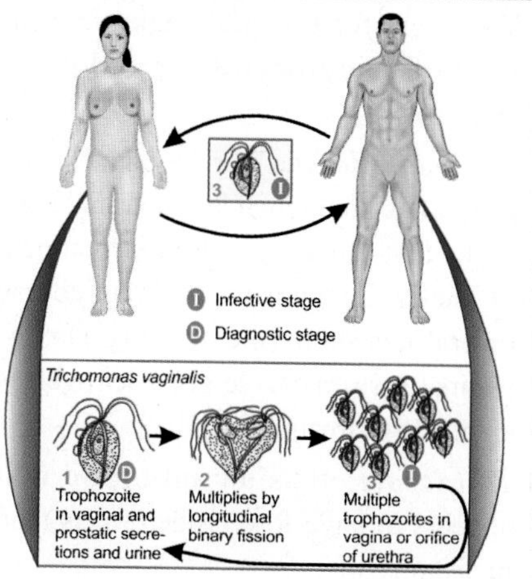

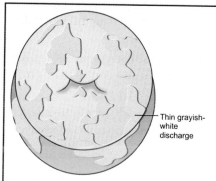

Fig. 14.1.7: Transmission of *Trichomonas vaginalis*

Trichomonads are usually transmitted sexually and may be identified in 30–80% of the male sexual partners of infected women. Trichomoniasis may commonly act as a vector for other sexually transmitted diseases, including the human immunodeficiency virus.

Risk factors for trichomoniasis include use of an intrauterine device (IUD), cigarette smoking and having multiple sexual partners. Since trichomoniasis is a sexually transmitted disorder, both the sexual partners must be treated and instructed to avoid sexual intercourse until both of them have been cured.

14.1.8: Type of Vaginal Discharge in Cases of Bacterial Vaginosis

Thin grayish-white discharge

Fig. 14.1.8: Type of vaginal discharge in cases of bacterial vaginosis

Bacterial vaginosis, initially also known as bacterial vaginitis, is one of the most important causes of vulvo-vaginitis. This condition is primarily caused due to the alteration of normal vaginal flora, rather than due to any specific infection. The classic presentation is a vaginal discharge with its characteristic fishy odor and a clinical examination that is otherwise normal. There is presence of white milky, non-viscous discharge which is adherent to the vaginal wall. pH of the discharge is more than 4.5.

Bacterial vaginosis typically is associated with a reduction in the number of the normal hydrogen peroxide-producing *Lactobacilli* in the vagina (which is toxic to other aerobic and anaerobic bacteria). The resultant change in pH allows proliferation of organisms that are normally suppressed such as *Hemophilus vaginalis, Gardnerella mobiluncus, Mycoplasma hominis, Gardnerella vaginalis, Peptostreptococcus* species, etc.

14.1.9: Clue Cells in Case of Bacterial Vaginosis

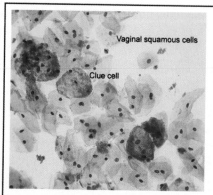

Fig. 14.1.9: Clue cells

A typical sign of bacterial vaginosis on microscopic examination is presence of an unusual vaginal cell known as "clue cell". Clue cells are believed to be the most reliable diagnostic sign of bacterial vaginosis.

Clue cells are vaginal epithelial cells, which are studded with bacteria on their surface. This results in the obscuration of their borders. In addition to the presence of clue cells, a vaginal pH greater than 4.5 is also suggestive of bacterial vaginosis.

14.1.10: Amsel's Diagnostic Criteria for Bacterial Vaginosis

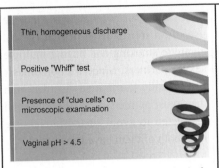

Fig. 14.1.10: Amsel's diagnostic criteria for bacterial vaginosis

- Thin, homogeneous discharge
- Positive "Whiff" test
- Presence of "clue cells" on microscopic examination
- Vaginal pH > 4.5

Bacterial vaginosis is mainly diagnosed using Amsel's criteria, with three of the four findings required to establish its diagnosis. Amsel's criteria as shown in Figure 14.1.10 helps in establishing the diagnosis of bacterial vaginosis in nearly 90% of affected women. Of the various criteria mentioned, presence of clue cells on microscopic examination is a highly significant criterion for diagnosis of bacterial vaginosis.

Treatment for bacterial vaginosis consists of using one of the following antibiotics:

Metronidazole: The World Health Organization has recommended metronidazole as the first-line therapy for the treatment of bacterial vaginosis. A 7-day course of oral metronidazole, 400 mg TDS or vaginal metronidazole gel (metrogel) is an effective treatment.

Tinidazole: It is an antibiotic that appears to have fewer side effects than metronidazole.

Ornidazole: Ornidazole, 500 mg vaginal tablet daily for 7 days is another effective option. Use of vaginal tablets help in avoiding first pass metabolism.

Ampicillin: Ampicillin 500 mg TDS or cephalosporins 500 mg BID for 7 days are also effective.

Tetracyclines: Tetracycline 500 mg, four times a day or doxycycline 100 mg twice daily for 7 days is effective.

Lincosamides: Vaginal clindamycin cream, 2% (cleocin) or oral clindamycin, 300 mg daily for 7 days is also effective.

14.1.11: Whiff Test

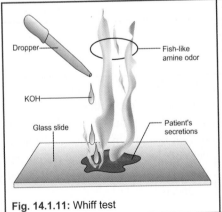

Fig. 14.1.11: Whiff test

- Dropper
- Fish-like amine odor
- KOH
- Glass slide
- Patient's secretions

Whiff test is diagnostic of bacterial vaginosis and is performed using 10% KOH solution. The test is said to be positive if a fishy odor is produced when the discharge of a woman with bacterial vaginosis is mixed with 10% KOH solution.

The fishy odor is produced due to production of amino metabolites from various organisms. As a result, Whiff's test is also known as the amine test.

Picture	Medical/Surgical Description	Management/Clinical Highlights

14.2: SEXUALLY TRANSMITTED DISEASES

14.2.1: Life Cycle of *Chlamydia trachomatis*

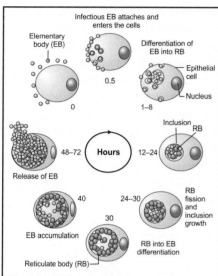

Fig. 14.2.1: Life cycle of *Chlamydia trachomatis*

Chlamydia trachomatis is a Gram-negative, aerobic, intracellular pathogen and can be considered as one of the most common causes for STD, worldwide in association with blindness and infertility. *Chlamydia* has a very unique life cycle, which alternates between a nonreplicating, infectious elementary body (EB) and a replicating, noninfectious reticulate body (RB). The EB, which is metabolically inactive can be considered equivalent to the spore and helps in transmitting the disease. The infectious EB attaches to the host cells. Following the entry into the cell, it gets differentiated into a RB. Once inside a cell, the EB germinates as the result of interaction with glycogen and gets converted into its reticulate form. The reticulate form divides by binary fission every 2–3 hours and has an incubation period of about 7–21 days in its host. Within 40–48 hours, the RBs transform back into infective EBs, which are subsequently released from the infected cell through the process of exocytosis and infect the neighboring cells.

The majority of women with chlamydial infection remain asymptomatic. However, some women may develop vaginal discharge, dysuria, abdominal pain, increased urinary frequency, urgency, urethritis and cervicitis. Chlamydia is very destructive to the fallopian tubes. If left untreated, nearly 30% of women with chlamydia may develop pelvic inflammatory disease. Pelvic infection often results in symptoms such as fever, pelvic cramping, abdominal pain or dyspareunia. Pelvic infection can often lead to infertility or even absolute sterility and ectopic pregnancy.

Diagnosis can be established with the help of following tests:
- *Direct immunoflorescence test*: Fluorescein-conjugated monoclonal antibodies can be used on smears prepared from urethral and cervical swabs for detecting chlamydial antigens.
- *Enzyme-linked immunosorbent assay (ELISA)*: Can help in detecting the chlamydial antigen.
- *Polymerase and ligase chain reactions*: For routine diagnostic use, newer and inexpensive diagnostic tests such as polymerase and ligase chain, which depend upon identification and amplification of the genetic material of the organism, have replaced the older, time-consuming culture methods.

Treatment of *Chlamydia* involves the use of broad spectrum antibiotics. A convenient single-dose therapy for chlamydia is 1 g of azithromycin per orally. Alternatively, doxycycline can be used orally in the dosage of 100 mg BID for 7 days. The combination of cefoxitin and ceftriaxone with doxycycline or tetracycline also proves to be useful. Erythromycin or amoxicillin in TID or QID dosage may also be given during pregnancy. Use of protective barrier such as condoms often helps prevent the spread of the infection. *Chlamydia* is observed to frequently occur with gonorrhea, another bacterial STD.

PART II ❖ GYNECOLOGY

14.2.2: Herpetic Lesions in Women

Herpes lesion: found on vagina, vulva, cervix
(female) and around anus (both sexes)

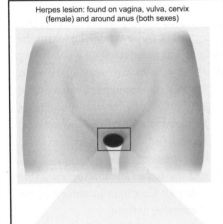

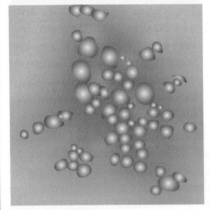

Fig. 14.2.2: Herpetic lesions in women

Genital herpes is a viral infection caused by the herpes simplex virus (most commonly HSV II), which is transmitted through sexual contact. Genital herpes is spread only by direct person-to-person contact. The virus enters through the mucous membrane of the genital tract via microscopic tears. From there the virus travels to the nerve roots near the spinal cord and settles down permanently.

Once exposed to the virus, there is an incubation period, which generally lasts from 3 days to 7 days before development of lesions begin. Prior to this, there are no symptoms and the virus cannot be transmitted to others. The primary infection may be associated with constitutional symptoms like fever, malaise, vulval paresthesia, itching or tingling sensation on the vulva and vagina followed by redness of the skin. Finally, the formation of blisters and vesicles begins, which eventually develop into shallow and painful ulcers within a period of 2–6 weeks. In women, these lesions may appear on the vulva, vagina, cervix, perianal area or inner thigh, and are frequently accompanied by itching and a mucoid vaginal discharge. When the blisters break, they are usually very painful to touch. From the beginning of itching, until the time of complete healing of the ulcer, the infection is definitely contagious.

The Tzanck smear is a rapid, fairly sensitive and inexpensive method for diagnosing HSV infection. Smears are preferably prepared from the base of the lesions and stained with 1% aqueous solution of toluidine blue "O" for 15 seconds. Positive smear is indicated by the presence of multinucleated giant cells with faceted nuclei and homogeneously stained "ground glass" chromatin (Tzanck cells).

Oral antiviral medications, such as acyclovir, (Zovirax), famciclovir (Famvir) or valacyclovir (Valtrex), which prevent the multiplication of the virus, are commonly used for treatment. For the treatment of primary outbreaks, oral acyclovir is prescribed in the dosage of 200 mg five times a day for 5 days. Local application of acyclovir provides relief and accelerates the process of healing. In severe cases, acyclovir can be administered intravenously in the dosage of 5 mg/kg body weight every 8 hourly for 5 days. The couple is advised to abstain from intercourse starting right from time of experiencing prodromal symptoms until total re-epithelization of the lesions occurs. Since the initial infection with HSV tends to be the most severe episode, an antiviral medication is usually recommended.

Couples who want to minimize the risk of transmission should always use condoms if a partner is infected. Such couples must be instructed to avoid all kinds of sexual activity, including kissing, during an outbreak of herpes. Women who have herpes and are pregnant can have a vaginal delivery as long as they are not experiencing symptoms or actually having an active outbreak while in labor. Pregnant women with active herpetic lesion must be preferably delivered by cesarean section.

Picture	Medical/Surgical Description	Management/Clinical Highlights

14.2.3: Gonorrhea (A and B)

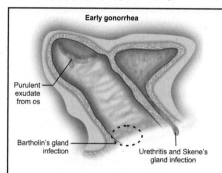

Early gonorrhea

Purulent exudate from os

Bartholin's gland infection

Urethritis and Skene's gland infection

Fig. 14.2.3A: Lesions due to gonorrhea

Gonorrhea is a sexually transmitted disease, which is caused by the bacterium *Neisseria gonorrheae*. Gonorrhea is spread through contact with the penis, vagina, mouth or anus. The disease is characterized by adhesion of the gonococci to the surface of urethra or other mucosal surfaces. The commonest clinical presentation of the disease in men is acute urethritis resulting in dysuria and a purulent penile discharge. The infection may extend along the urethra to the prostate, seminal vesicles and epididymis, resulting in complications such as epididymitis, prostatitis, periurethral abscesses and chronic urethritis. The infection may sometimes spread to the periurethral tissues, resulting in formation of abscesses and multiple discharging sinuses ("watercan perineum").

In women, the primary site of infection due to gonorrhea is the endocervix, and the infection commonly extends to the urethra and vagina, giving rise to mucopurulent discharge. Symptomatic patients commonly experience vaginal discharge, dysuria and abdominal pain. The infection may extend to Bartholin's glands, endometrium and fallopian tubes. Acute salpingitis may be associated with a high probability of sterility, if not treated adequately.

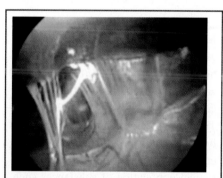

Fig. 14.2.3B: Fitz-Hugh-Curtis syndrome

Peritoneal spread may rarely occur with acute gonococcal/chlamydial infection, producing perihepatic inflammation, resulting in the development of Fitz-Hugh-Curtis syndrome. This syndrome is characterized by the presence of acute onset right quadrant pain in the abdomen. This may increase upon breathing, coughing, sneezing, etc. Symptoms of pelvic infection such as nausea, vomiting, chills, fever, headache, etc. may also be present. The diagnosis is usually confirmed by laparoscopy, which shows presence of typical violin string adhesions between the liver and parietal peritoneum as shown in the adjacent figure.

Due to emerging resistance against most commonly used antibiotics such as penicillin, tetracyclines, etc., third-generation cephalosporins are considered to be most effective form of therapy for this disease. Amongst the various third-generation cephalosporins, ceftriaxone can be considered as safe and effective form of therapy against the gonococcal infection. The CDC recommendations for treatment of gonococcal infection are as follows:

- A single dose of intramuscular ceftriaxone, in the dosage of 250 mg.
- Azithromycin in a single oral dosage of 1 g or doxycycline 100 mg BID for 7 days can be used for chlamydial infection.

Management of this syndrome primarily comprises of the treatment of underlying gonococcal/chlamydial infection. The violin string adhesions may require laparoscopic excision.

14.2.4: Hard Chancre due to Syphilis on the Shaft of Penis in Males

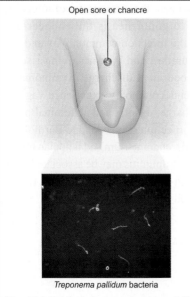

Open sore or chancre

Treponema pallidum bacteria

Fig. 14.2.4: Hard chancre due to syphilis on the shaft of penis in males

Syphilis is a sexually transmitted disease caused by the spirochete *Treponema pallidum*. The disease is typically characterized by three stages: primary, secondary and tertiary. Primary lesions appear approximately 10–90 days after the initial exposure. Primary lesion of syphilis, also known as a hard chancre often appears at the point of contact, usually the external genitalia. The hard chancre of syphilis is a firm, painless, relatively avascular, circumscribed, indurated, superficially ulcerated lesion. The "hard chancre" of syphilis usually persists for about 4–6 weeks and heals spontaneously.

Syphilis is usually diagnosed on the basis of results of serological tests such as Kahn test, venereal disease research laboratory (VDRL) test, rapid plasma reagin test, etc. Single dose of benzathine penicillin G (2.4 million units) intramuscularly is sufficient for the treatment of primary, secondary or latent syphilis of less than 1 year duration. Alternative to penicillin is oral doxycycline 100 mg BID. In case of late syphilis with duration of more than 1 year duration or cardiovascular syphilis, benzathine penicillin G (2.4 million units) intramuscularly weekly is to be given for 3 weeks. Alternatively doxycycline (100 mg BID) can be given daily for 4 weeks.

14.2.5: Condyloma Acunimatum (A and B)

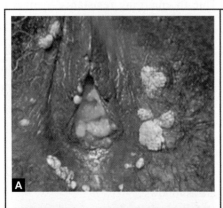

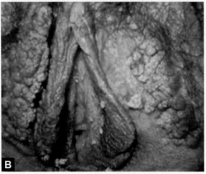

Figs 14.2.5 (A and B): Condyloma acunimatum

Condyloma is proliferation of epithelial tissues resulting from human papilloma virus (HPV) infection, especially that with type 6, 11, 16 and 18. HPV types 16 and 18 are also associated with carcinoma and dysplastic changes. Being a sexually transmitted disease, it commonly develops at the sites of sexual contact or trauma such as urogenital and anogenital regions. The lesions appear as broad based pink masses, whose surface is covered with short blunted projections, resulting in a raspberry or mulberry-like appearance. Condylomas can be multiple and clustered, with the average size of the lesions being about 1–1.5 cm.

Irrespective of the modality of treatment used, the condylomas must be removed because they are contagious and capable of spreading to other surface either through direct or sexual contact. Treatment of large condylomas is mainly by laser ablation, surgical excision, cryotherapy, etc. For small condylomas, topical application of substances such as podophyllin, trichloroacetic acid, bichloroacetic acid, imiquimod, etc. usually is sufficient.

14.3: PELVIC INFLAMMATORY DISEASES

14.3.1: Definition (A to C)

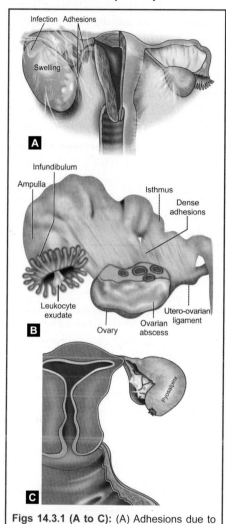

Figs 14.3.1 (A to C): (A) Adhesions due to pelvic inflammatory disease; (B) Dense tubal adhesions; (C) Pyosalpinx

Figures 14.3.1 (A to C) show laparoscopic appearances of various lesions possible as a result of pelvic inflammatory disease (PID). There can be development of tubal adhesions. Fluid collection inside the fallopian tube, which is closed at the fimbrial end due to adhesions, may result in the development of hydrosalpinx. Development of infection inside hydrosalpinx can result in formation of a pyosalpinx.

Pelvic inflammatory disease is a disease of sexually active women and represents a spectrum of infections and inflammatory disorders of the uterus, fallopian tubes and adjacent pelvic structures resulting in endometritis, salpingitis, etc. This spectrum also includes entities such as hydrosalpinx, pyosalpinx tubo-ovarian abscess (TOA), oophoritis, peritonitis, perihepatitis, etc.

14.3.2: Mucopurulent Cervical Discharge

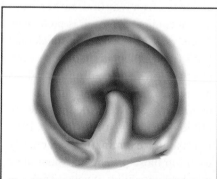

Fig. 14.3.2: Mucopurulent cervical discharge

Presence of mucopurulent discharge as shown in Figure 14.3.2 is a characteristic feature of PID. It is often associated with other symptoms such as lower abdominal pain or tenderness, fever, nausea, vomiting, malaise, back pain, abnormal uterine bleeding, dysuria and dyspareunia, and unusual or foul smelling vaginal discharge.

Minimal diagnostic criteria:
- Cervical motion tenderness
- Uterine or adnexal tenderness
- Lower abdominal or pelvic pain

Additional diagnostic criteria:
- Oral temperature > 101°F (> 38.3°C)
- Abnormal cervical or vaginal mucopurulent discharge
- Leukocytosis on saline microscopic examination of vaginal secretions
- Elevated ESR or C-reactive proteins.

14.3.3: Mechanism of Progression of Pelvic Inflammatory Disease

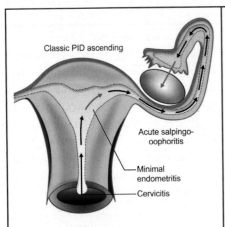

Fig. 14.3.3: Mechanism of progression of pelvic inflammatory disease

Pelvic inflammatory disease occurs as a result of spread of microorganisms from the cervix upward to the superior portion of genital tract such as fallopian tubes, ovaries and other adjacent structures. The initial infection is in form of cervicitis, which spreads to tubes and ovaries resulting in endometritis and salpingo-oophoritis respectively. Treatment with antibiotics usually results in normal pelvis.

Amongst the various microorganisms responsible for causing PID, sexually transmitted organisms such as *C. trachomatis* and *N. gonorrhoeae* are most important. Mixed infection with both aerobic and anaerobic microorganisms (*Bacteroides, Peptostreptococcus, Peptococcus*, etc.) may be also responsible. Risk factors for occurrence of PID include sexual activity with multiple sexual partners, young age, procedures requiring cervical and uterine instrumentation such as IUD insertion, endometrial biopsy, and D & C.

14.3.4: Ultrasound in Case of Chronic Hydrosalpinx

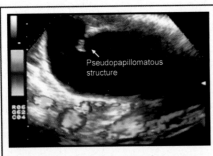

Fig. 14.3.4: Appearance of chronic hydrosalpinx on Doppler ultrasound examination

Figure 14.3.4 shows appearance of hydrosalpinx on Doppler ultrasound examination. There is presence of a dilated fallopian tube with thin-walled incomplete septations. Presence of peripheral vascularization and poor vascularization of septa on Doppler sonography is highly indicative of a hydrosalpinx.

Formation of peritoneal adhesions secondary to PID can compromise the motility of the fallopian tubes. Furthermore, obstruction of the distal end of the fallopian tubes due to adhesions results in accumulation of the normally secreted tubal fluid, creating distension of the tube. This subsequently causes damage to the epithelial cilia and may result in development of hydrosalpinx.

14.3.5: Color Doppler Ultrasound in Case of Tubo-ovarian Abscess

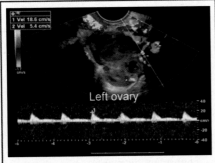

Fig. 14.3.5: Tubo-ovarian mass as visualized on transvaginal sonography

Tubo-ovarian abscess appears as a complex cystic-solid adnexal mass with thick irregular walls and septations. On color flow Doppler, there is prominent vascular perfusion with low-moderate vascular impedance.

For evaluation of cases of tubo-ovarian abscess, transvaginal rather than transabdominal approach is preferable. There may be presence of thickened fluid-filled fallopian tubes. However, absence of such finding also does not reduce the possibility of PID and treatment should be started if there are clinical features suggestive of PID. Ultrasound examination is actually useful in those patients in whom there may be a possibility of pelvic TOA.

14.3.6: Retort-Shaped Tubal Mass Suggestive of Hydrosalpinx

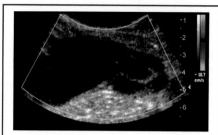

Fig. 14.3.6: Retort-shaped tubal mass suggestive of hydrosalpinx

Presence of a retort-shaped mass arising from the fallopian tubes on transvaginal sonography is suggestive of hydrosalpinx.

The major clinical significance of a hydrosalpinx is its adverse effect on fertility, thereby resulting in a reduced pregnancy rate. A hydrosalpinx, although sterile, can be re-infected at a later date leading to formation of a pyosalpinx.

14.3.7: Laparoscopic Appearance of a Tubo-ovarian Abscess

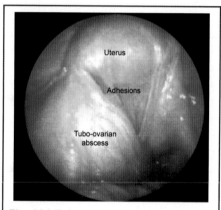

Fig. 14.3.7: Laparoscopic appearance of a tubo-ovarian abscess

Tubo-ovarian abscess can be defined as the collection of pus involving the tubes and the ovary. Figure 14.3.7 demonstrates the laparoscopic appearance of a TOA. Laparoscopy not only helps in the diagnosis of a TOA, it can also be useful for therapeutic purposes. Drainage of a TOA can be done through minimal invasive laparoscopic surgery or posterior colpotomy.

Surgery is rarely required in cases of PID. Indications for surgery in cases of PID are as follows:
- Drainage of a pelvic abscess
- Acute spreading peritonitis resistant to medical treatment
- Presence of a pyoperitoneum
- Intestinal obstruction
- Ruptured TOA
- Suspected intestinal injury
- Removal of septic products of conception from the uterine cavity.

14.3.8: Adhesions Observed Between Omentum and Surface of Uterus on Laparoscopic Examination

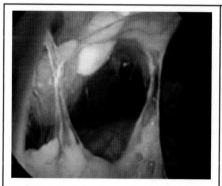

Fig. 14.3.8: Adhesions observed between omentum and surface of uterus on laparoscopic examination

Even though the use of antibiotics is able to clear the infection, there can be formation of adhesions between various pelvic and abdominal structures. Adhesions can be described as bands of scar tissue and can form between the various pelvic and abdominal organs. The scar tissue forms as a result of normal process of healing of the inflamed organs. Figure 14.3.8 shows adhesions between the omentum and surface of uterus.

Pelvic inflammatory disease almost exclusively occurs in sexually active women and amongst adolescents. Symptoms related to PID are usually worse at the end of a menstrual period and for a few days afterward. Abdominal pain, which is usually bilateral, is one of the cardinal symptoms amongst women presenting with PID. Sometimes this pain, which may worsen during sexual intercourse or get aggravated with jarring movements, may be the only presenting symptom. There may be diffuse tenderness in lower abdominal quadrants upon palpation. Formation of adhesions as a result of pelvic infection can serve as an important cause of infertility.

14.3.9: Laparoscopic Aspiration of Fluid-Filled Loculi

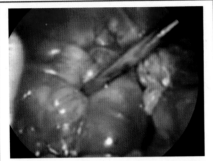

Fig. 14.3.9: Laparoscopic aspiration of fluid-filled loculi formed as a result of infection

As previously described, peritoneal infection and inflammation associated with PID may result in the development of adhesions. This may sometimes initiate the development of individual locules filled with clear or yellow serous or gelatinous fluid.

The fluid present in these locules is usually the exudate, produced as a result of peritoneal inflammation. They may range in size from a few millimeters to a few centimeters. The treatment usually comprises of lysis of the adhesions and aspiration of the fluid filled loculi through laparoscopic route.

14.3.10: Laparoscopic Lysis of Adhesions (A and B)

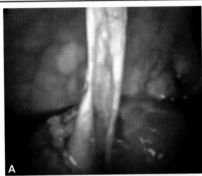

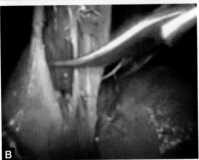

Figs 14.3.10 (A and B): Laparoscopic lysis of adhesions

Figures 14.3.10 (A and B) show cutting of adhesions resulting due to pelvic inflammation. While thin adhesions can be easily lysed at the time of laparoscopy, thick adhesions can also be managed through laparoscopic route and can be cut with help of laparoscopic scissors.

Laparoscopy is not only used for diagnostic purposes in cases of PID, it can be also used for therapeutic purposes, performing minor surgeries such as lysis of adhesions.

| Picture | Medical/Surgical Description | Management/Clinical Highlights |

14.3.11: Recommended Antibiotic Regimens for Treatment of Pelvic Inflammatory Disease

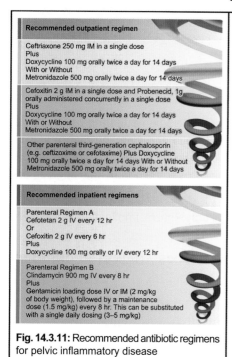

Recommended outpatient regimen

Ceftriaxone 250 mg IM in a single dose
Plus
Doxycycline 100 mg orally twice a day for 14 days
With or Without
Metronidazole 500 mg orally twice a day for 14 days

Cefoxitin 2 g IM in a single dose and Probenecid, 1g
orally administered concurrently in a single dose
Plus
Doxycycline 100 mg orally twice a day for 14 days
With or Without
Metronidazole 500 mg orally twice a day for 14 days

Other parenteral third-generation cephalosporin
(e.g. ceftizoxime or cefotaxime) Plus Doxycycline
100 mg orally twice a day for 14 days With or Without
Metronidazole 500 mg orally twice a day for 14 days

Recommended inpatient regimens

Parenteral Regimen A
Cefotetan 2 g IV every 12 hr
Or
Cefoxitin 2 g IV every 6 hr
Plus
Doxycycline 100 mg orally or IV every 12 hr

Parenteral Regimen B
Clindamycin 900 mg IV every 8 hr
Plus
Gentamicin loading dose IV or IM (2 mg/kg
of body weight), followed by a maintenance
dose (1.5 mg/kg) every 8 hr. This can be substituted
with a single daily dosing (3–5 mg/kg)

Fig. 14.3.11: Recommended antibiotic regimens for pelvic inflammatory disease

The antibiotic regimens for PID as recommended by CDC are described in Figure 14.3.11. If the patient is started on parenteral therapy, change over from parenteral to oral therapy can usually be started, once the patient shows sustained clinical improvement for a period of 24 hours. Such patients must however complete a 14-day course of treatment with oral doxycycline in the dosage of 100 mg, twice daily.

Symptomatic patients may be prescribed antiemetic and/or antipyretic medications depending on the type of symptoms present. Alternative regimen as recommended by CDC comprises of administration of ampicillin-sulbactam intravenously in the dosage of 3 g every 6 hourly along with doxycycline (100 mg twice daily). Amongst the various cephalosporins, ceftriaxone is most effective against gonococcal infection.

14.3.12: Posterior Colpotomy for Drainage of Tubo-ovarian Abscess

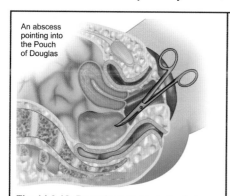

An abscess pointing into the Pouch of Douglas

Fig. 14.3.12: Posterior colpotomy for drainage of tubo-ovarian abscess

Figure 14.3.12 shows the drainage of a TOA with help of an incision given in the Pouch of Douglas. This procedure is known as posterior colpotomy.

For posterior colpotomy, a small transverse incision is made through posterior vaginal fornix and peritoneum with help of an angular blade scissors into the most dependent part of the cul-de-sac. The incision can then be enlarged with help of an artery forceps to permit the drainage of pus. If loculi are present, they can be broken with help of an artery forceps.

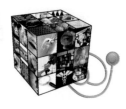

1. EVOLVING PATHOGENS IN VULVOVAGINAL CANDIDIASIS

Over the past 2 decades there has been an increasing trend in the number of women suffering from vaginal candidiasis to be infected by noncandidal infection, particularly Candida tropicalis and Candida glabrata. This could be attributed to the short-term therapy with imidazole agents, which help facilitate the overgrowth of nonalbicans species. The use of broad-spectrum antifungal agents, which also cover the nonalbican species are now advocated.

Source: Horowitz BJ, Giaquinta D, Ito S. Evolving pathogens in vulvovaginal candidiasis: implications for patient care. J Clin Pharmacol. 1992;32(3):248.

2. EFFICACY OF WEEKLY DOSE OF FLUCONAZOLE (150 mg) AS PROPHYLAXIS AGAINST RECURRENT VULVOVAGINAL CANDIDIASIS.

A quantitative systematic review including randomized controlled trials has shown that administration of fluconazole, on 150 mg weekly basis for 6 months as prophylactic treatment against recurrent vulvovaginal candidiasis is more effective than placebo in reducing symptomatic episodes of vulvoginal candidiasis.

Source: Rosa MI, Silva BR, Pires PS, et al. Weekly fluconazole therapy for recurrent vulvovaginal candidiasis: a systematic review and meta-analysis. Eur J Obstet Gynecol Reprod Biol. 2012 Dec 29 S0301-2115(12)00548-9. doi: 10.1016/j.ejogrb.2012.12.001. [Epub ahead of print].

Section 15

Contraception

15.1: CONTRACEPTION

15.1.1: Different Types of Contraception

Picture	Medical/Surgical Description	Management/Clinical Highlights
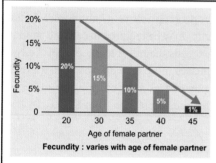 **Fig. 15.1.1:** Different types of contraception	The goal of family planning is to enable couples and individuals to freely choose how many children to have and when to have them. Contraceptive methods may be temporary or permanent. They may be required for following conditions: postponement of first pregnancy; birth spacing; and control and prevention of pregnancy. The detailed use of each contraceptive has been described in each individual Figure.	Various temporary methods of contraception include barrier methods, hormonal contraception (combined hormonal contraception and progestogen only contraception), intrauterine contraceptive devices (IUCDs) and emergency (postcoital) contraception. Permanent methods of contraception include sterilization, which in women can be done using tubal ligation and in men using vasectomy.

15.1.2: Variation in Fecundity with the Age of Female Partner

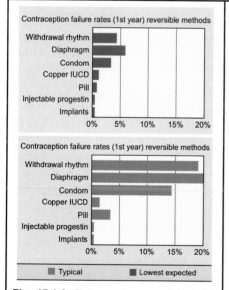 **Fig. 15.1.2:** Variation in fecundity with the age of female partner	Fecundity or reproductive capacity decreases with increasing age of the female partner. As the age of the woman increases, her fecundity decreases and vice versa. This can be related to natural decline in the number of oocytes with aging in women. The decline in fecundity becomes clinically significant when the woman reaches mid-thirties.	This becomes especially important in today's age when women may want to delay childbirth by using some method of contraception due to career, work or family commitments. She must be counseled regarding reduced fecundity in case she has decided to conceive at an older age. Moreover, the woman should be told that even if she does conceive after the age of 40 years, there is likely to be an increase in the complication rate.

15.1.3: Failure Rates Associated with Various Methods of Contraception

Fig. 15.1.3: Failure rates associated with various methods of contraception	Of the various methods of contraception available, some of the most effective methods of contraception include IUCDs, injectable hormones, hormonal implants and sterilization. This is followed by some slightly less effective options such as oral contraceptive pills, hormonal patches and rings. Some of the less effective options include barrier methods (male and female condom, cervical cap, diaphragm, etc.) and natural methods of contraception such as withdrawal method.	The prescription of a contraceptive device must be individualized. The type of contraception, which must be prescribed to a particular patient, is the one that provides effective contraception, acceptable cycle control and is associated with least side effects.

15.2: TEMPORARY METHODS OF CONTRACEPTION

15.2.1: Combined Oral Pills (A and B)

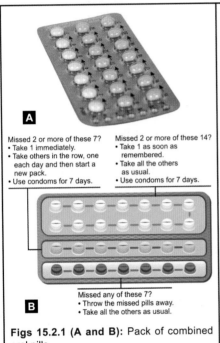

Figs 15.2.1 (A and B): Pack of combined oral pills

The use of combined oral contraceptive pills (COCPs) provides a protective effect against the development of ovarian and endometrial cancer, and probably even colorectal cancer.

Use of COCPs is a highly effective method of reversible contraception, with the failure rate being approximately 0.1 per 100 women years of use. However, COCPs do not provide any protection against sexually transmitted diseases (STD) or human immunodeficiency virus (HIV) infection. Normal menstrual cycles are likely to occur in 99% of the women within 6 months of stopping the pills.

Conventionally, the COCPs must be started during the first 5 days of the menstrual cycle. Once a woman has started taking a COCP, it is important for her to be consistent and take the pill regularly at the same time each day. Women who use a 21-day preparation need to take the pills for 21 days followed by a 7-day pill-free interval. She should be cautioned not to exceed the 7-day pill-free interval between packs. If the woman forgets to take a tablet in a 21-day period, she should take two tablets the following day. Backup method of contraception (e.g. condoms, foam, etc.) may be required in case the woman exceeds the pill-free interval of 7 days; misses more than one tablet in a cycle; experiences a serious adverse effect or requires protection from STDs.

15.2.2: Progesterone Only Modalities

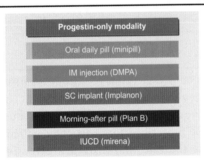

Fig. 15.2.2: Progesterone Only Modalities

Progestogen only containing contraceptive methods are available in various formulations:
- Progestogen only pill (POP) or minipill
- Subdermal contraceptive implants (Norplant I, II and Implanon)
- Progestogen only injectables (POI), e.g. depot-medroxyprogesterone acetate (DMPA)
- Intrauterine system (Mirena and progestasert).

In this Figure, POPs and POIs would be described. Other progestogen only containing contraceptive methods would be described in the subsequent Figures. The POPs may contain 350 µg of norethisterone or 75 µg of norgestrel or 30 µg of levonorgestrel.

Progestogen only pills must be started within 5–7 days of menstruation. Unlike the COCPs, these pills must be taken on a continuous basis without any breaks between packets. These must be consumed in accordance with a strict time schedule everyday (within 3 hours vs 12 hours for COCPs). A backup method should be used for 2 days if a woman is more than 3 hours late in taking a dose. Backup contraception should be considered during the 1st month when the woman first starts taking minipills and then at midcycle every month thereafter (the time when ovulation is likely to occur). The POIs must be injected into the thigh, buttocks or deltoid muscle four times a year (every 11–13 weeks) and provide pregnancy protection starting a week after the first injection.

Picture	Medical/Surgical Description	Management/Clinical Highlights

15.2.3: Subdermal Implants (A and B)

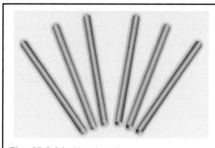 **Fig. 15.2.3A:** Norplant I	Contraceptive implant is a method of birth control, where the device is inserted under the skin. Available subdermal implants are as follows: • Norplant I and Jadelle (Norplant II) • Implanon • Sino-implant II marketed as Zarin, Femplant and Trust. These implants ensure slow, sustained release of progestogens. It is long-acting form of contraception, which is associated with minimal side effects.	With these subdermal implants, return of fertility is almost immediate, following the removal of capsules. It does not harm the quality and quantity of the breast milk, and can be used by nursing mothers starting 6 weeks after childbirth. However, these capsules do not provide protection against STDs. It is an effective form of contraception, with pregnancy rate varying from 0.2 to 1.3 per 100 women years.
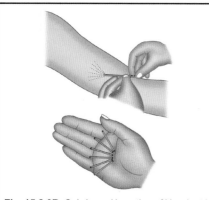 **Fig. 15.2.3B:** Subdermal insertion of Norplant I	Norplant I contains six silastic capsules made up of siloxane of the size 34 mm × 2.4 mm, with each containing about 36 mg of levonorgestrel. Its effects last for approximately 5 years. The implants release 85 mg of levonorgestrel/day in the first 3 months; 50 mg/day for next 18 months and then gradually levels to about 30 mg/day.	The implants are inserted on first day of the menstrual cycle. Following application of a local anesthetic over the upper arm, a needle-like applicator is used to insert the Norplant capsules under the skin (subdermally) on the medial aspect of upper arm. Since the capsules are nonbiodegradable, they need removal at the end of use or earlier if the side effects are intolerable. Both insertion and removal of these implants requires local anesthesia and a small incision.

15.2.4: Intrauterine Devices (A to H)

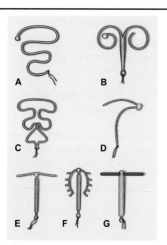 **Fig. 15.2.4A:** Different types of intrauterine contraceptive devices: (A) Lippes-Loop; (B) Saf-T-coil; (C) Dana-Super; (D) Copper-7 (Gravigard); (E) Copper-T (Gyne-T) (F) Multiload; (G) Progesterone IUCD	Each intrauterine device has a nylon thread, which protrudes through the cervical canal into the vagina, where it can be felt by the patient or the doctor. Initially, biologically inert devices such as Lippes loop and Saf-T-coil were introduced, which have now been withdrawn from the market. Newer devices are medicated and contain substances such as copper, progestogens, etc. Copper carrying devices include copper-T 200, copper-7, Multiload, copper-250, copper-T 380, copper-T 220 and Nova T. Their effective life varies from 3 years to 5 years. Recently introduced IUCDs containing progestogen include progestasert, Levonova and Mirena.	Intrauterine devices are flexible plastic devices made up of polyethylene, which are inserted inside the uterine cavity for the purpose of contraception. They are highly effective method of contraception with the pregnancy rate being 2–6 per 100 women years.

Picture	Medical/Surgical Description	Management/Clinical Highlights
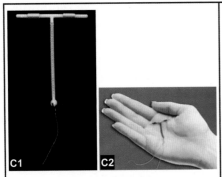 **Fig. 15.2.4B:** Parts of a copper device	Intrauterine devices are flexible plastic devices made up of polyethylene, which are inserted inside the uterine cavity for the purpose of contraception. Each device has a nylon thread, which protrudes through the cervical canal into the vagina, where it can be felt by the patient or the doctor. The IUCD device is preloaded in a sterile hollow tube like inserter, which has an adjustable flange or guard over it. It comes with a solid white plunger, which is used for placing the device inside the uterine cavity.	Though IUCD is commonly inserted in multiparous women, nulliparity is not a contraindication for IUCD use. It can be successfully used in carefully selected nulliparous women. IUCDs per se do not increase the risk of ectopic pregnancy. However, in women who conceive with an IUCD in place, the diagnosis of ectopic pregnancy should be excluded.
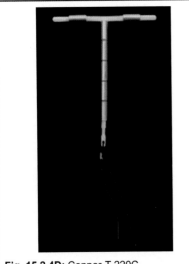 **Figs 15.2.4C (C1 and C2):** Copper-T 380A	Copper-T 380A is a third generation copper device, which is being marketed as ParaGard in the US. Copper wire is wound on its arms and stem, and amounts to a total of 380 mm² of copper. There are two nylon strings attached at one of its end. It has been approved for 10 years of continuous use.	Contraindications for the placement of copper-T 380A are as follows: • Pregnancy or suspicion of pregnancy • Uterine anomalies causing distortion of the uterine cavity • Pelvic inflammatory disease • Postabortal endometritis or postpartum endometritis in past 3 months • Known or suspected uterine/cervical malignancy • Mucopurulent cervicitis • Abnormal uterine bleeding of unknown etiology
Fig. 15.2.4D: Copper-T 220C	The Copper-T 220C is a first generation, T-shaped polyethylene copper device, which has seven solid copper rings (five solid copper sleeves on the vertical arm of the T and two sleeves on the horizontal arm). As a result, it is able to provide an effective surface area of 200 mm². The estimated period of effectiveness of the device is 20 years of continuous use.	The contraindications for the placement of copper-T 220C are same as that of copper-T 380A described in Figure 15.2.4C previously.

Picture	Medical/Surgical Description	Management/Clinical Highlights

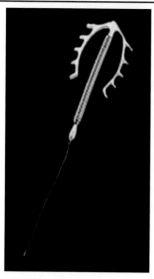

Fig. 15.2.4E: Multiload 375

Multiload is a third generation intrauterine copper device, used for contraception. It has a stem and two small flexible side-arms. The plastic used for making the device is composed of high-density polyethylene, ethylene vinyl acetate copolymer and barium sulfate. A copper wire is wound around the stem. A nylon thread with two ends is attached to the bottom end of the stem. Two types of Multiload devices which are commonly available are:
- Multiload Cu-250 (having a surface area of 250 mm²), whose action lasts for a period of 3 years
- Multiload Cu-375 has a copper wire with surface area of 375 mm² and its action lasts for a period of 5 years. Multiload 375 comes in two sizes, standard and short length, which are used based on the uterine size.

The contraindications for the use of Multiload 375 are same as those described with Cu-T 380A.

Using the Multiload device implies that women should have regular health check-ups especially in the beginning. She should consult her health care prescriber in case she experiences dysmenorrhea, irregular bleeding, infection of lower genital tract or she has sexual contact with multiple partners or has a history of STDs. If in proper place, neither the woman, nor her partner should be able to feel the device at the time of sexual intercourse. The woman must be instructed to check for the presence of thread at regular intervals especially following the menstrual cycles to ensure that it has not been expelled out. In case the woman is unable to feel the thread, she should be instructed to immediately contact her doctor and use an additional method of contraception, until she has an appointment with her doctor.

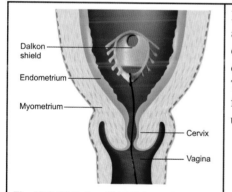

Fig. 15.2.4F: Dalkon Shield intrauterine device

Dalkon Shield was an IUCD in shape of a triangle with five fin-like structures on each of the lower sides. The tail made up of monofilament had wicking properties. The fins acted as a predisposing factor for the IUCD to get embedded inside the uterine walls.

This IUCD was introduced in the US during 1970s and went into dispute due to the numerous problems related to its safety. It was introduced with the aim of having lower rate of infection and expulsion in comparison to other IUCDs. Both the claims were proved false and as a result more than 300,000 lawsuits were filed against AH Robins Company, the manufacturer of Dalkon Shield. This can be considered as one of the largest tort liability cases. This device had caused numerous cases of PID, ectopic pregnancy, infertility and septic abortion, etc. It was eventually withdrawn from the market by 1974. The company had to pay 485 million dollars in settlements and legal costs, following which the company declared bankruptcy in 1986. Due to such complications, other IUCDs at that point of time became a controversial form of contraception.

Picture	Medical/Surgical Description	Management/Clinical Highlights
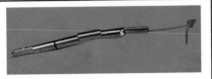 **Fig. 15.2.4G:** Flexiguard 330/gynefix	It is an innovative contraceptive device which is implanted in the wall of the uterus. It comprises of four to six mini copper tubes, threaded on a length of nylon. Knots at the two ends keep the device in place. This is an anchored, frameless and flexible IUCD, which was developed to improve performance and enhance acceptability of intrauterine contraception. Its action lasts for 5 years.	The device is fitted by attaching the anchoring knot to the muscles in the uterine fundus. Being an extremely flexible device, it has a very low incidence of complications. It has a high efficacy, which does not decrease with time and is comparable to that of oral contraceptive pills. It is associated with a low expulsion rate; reduced bleeding and reduced complaints of pain. Presently, it is available in China and Europe. Plans are to market it to USA, Canada and subsequently worldwide.
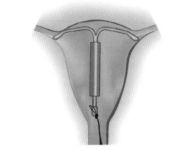 **Fig. 15.2.4H:** The levonorgestrel-intrauterine system (Mirena)	Also known as levonorgestrel-intrauterine system (LNG-IUS), Mirena is a type of progestogen containing IUCD, having 52 mg of levonorgestrel, which is released at the rate of 20 μg/day. The effects of Mirena last for about 5 years.	Mirena is recommended for multiparous women and should be inserted by a trained healthcare provider. Mirena is also indicated for the treatment of menorrhagia in women who want to use IUCD as their method of contraception.

15.2.5: Perforation Caused by Intrauterine Devices (A to D)

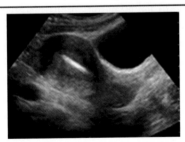 **Fig. 15.2.5A:** Two-dimensional ultrasound showing presence of copper device in the uterine cavity	Uterine perforation is a rare, but serious complication of IUCD insertion, occurring at a rate of 0.6–1.6 per 1,000 insertions. This may occur either at the time of insertion or at a later stage due to the embedment of the device into the myometrium and its subsequent migration into the intra-abdominal cavity.	If the IUCD strings are not seen in the cervical os, the device may have been expelled out or may have perforated the uterine wall. In these cases an ultrasound examination is the investigation of choice to check for the presence of copper device within the uterine cavity.
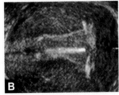 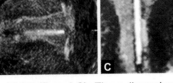 **Figs 15.2.5 (B and C):** Three-dimensional ultrasound showing the presence of an intrauterine copper device	Ultrasound examination, both two-dimensional and three-dimensional, can demonstrate the presence of copper device within the uterine cavity.	While the copper device is seen in form of a bright echogenic shadow on two-dimensional ultrasound, three-dimensional images are able to properly delineate the device.

Picture	Medical/Surgical Description	Management/Clinical Highlights
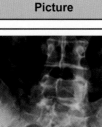 **Fig. 15.2.5D:** X-ray showing intrauterine device inside the abdominal cavity, confirming the diagnosis of uterine perforation	Figure 15.2.5D is X-ray of the lower abdomen showing the presence of copper device outside the uterine cavity. Being a radio-opaque structure due to the presence of impregnated barium sulfate, it can be easily identified on radiological examination.	If the IUCD strings cannot be found, ultrasound is the preferred method to identify the location of the IUCD. If the device is not identified within the uterus or the pelvis, a plain X-ray of the abdomen should be performed to determine whether the device has perforated the uterine wall.

15.2.6: Natural Family Planning Methods

15.2.6.1: Cervical Mucus Method (A to C)

Picture	Medical/Surgical Description	Management/Clinical Highlights
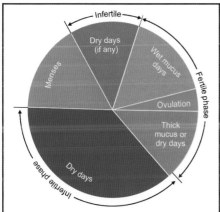 **Fig. 15.2.6.1A:** Cervical mucus method	The cervical mucus method is based on the fact that as the fertile time approaches, the cervical mucus increases in amount, becomes clearer in color, wetter, stretchy and slippery. Following ovulation, the mucus usually becomes sticky, thicker and pasty in character and reduces in amount.	Sexual intercourse is considered safe during the days immediately following the menses until the cervical mucus attains the previously-described characterics. Thereafter, the couple must abstain from having sexual intercourse until the 4th day after the "peak mucus day".
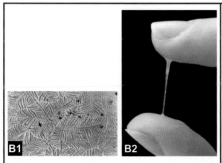 **Figs 15.2.6.1B (B1 and B2):** Estrogen dominant cervical mucus: (B1) Ferning pattern; (B2) Spinnbarkeit test	Under the effect of estrogens, cervical mucus becomes thin, watery, clear and profuse. It has a high content of sodium chloride in it due to which it forms a characteristic pattern of ferning when dried on a glass slide. It has great elasticity and is able to withstand stretching up to 10 cm. This is also known as the spinnbarkeit or the thread test, which is an evidence of estrogenic activity.	Cervical mucus method is one of the natural fertility awareness methods. This method is safe and there are no side effects. However, this method is associated with high failure rate of approximately 20–25 pregnancies per 100 women years of use. The high failure rate associated with this method commonly results due to irregular ovulation or irregular menstrual cycles.

Picture	Medical/Surgical Description	Management/Clinical Highlights
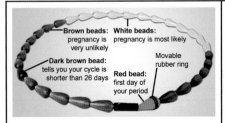 **Fig. 15.2.6.1C:** Progesterone dominant cervical mucus	Figure 15.2.6.1C shows typical pattern of progesterone dominant cervical mucus when smeared on a glass slide and observed under a microscope.	Under the effect of progesterone, the mucus becomes thick, tenacious and highly viscous. It loses its property of spinnbarkeit and easily fractures when put under tension. This property is known as tack.

15.2.6.2: Cyclebeads

Picture	Medical/Surgical Description	Management/Clinical Highlights
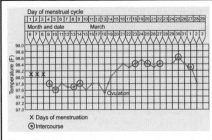 **Fig. 15.2.6.2:** Cyclebeads	This is a natural family planning method, which is designed for women with cycles between 26 to 32 days. The fertile period in these women lasts from 8th to 19th day, which can be identified by the presence of white beads. Brown beads mark the "safe days" or the period during which the woman is likely to be least fertile. During this time, the couple can have unprotected intercourse. A rubber band is moved head to head every day to track the cycle.	This method helps in preventing unwanted pregnancies, using the "Standard Days" method. The users are instructed to avoid unprotected sex by using a condom or abstaining during days 8–19 of the cycle (identified by the white beads)

15.2.6.3: Basal Body Temperature Method

Picture	Medical/Surgical Description	Management/Clinical Highlights
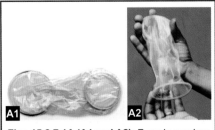 **Fig. 15.2.6.3:** Basal body temperature method	This method is based on the fact that basal body temperature (BBT) increases by 0.2–0.5°C following ovulation under the thermogenic effect of hormone progesterone.	The couple must be instructed that the safest way to use BBT for avoiding pregnancy is to avoid intercourse or use a barrier method during at least the first half of the menstrual cycle until 3 days after there has been a rise in BBT.

15.2.7: Barrier Methods of Female Contraception (A and B)

15.2.7.1: Female Condom (A and B)

Picture	Medical/Surgical Description	Management/Clinical Highlights
Figs 15.2.7.1A (A1 and A2): Female condom (Available under the brand names of Reality, Femidom, Dominique, etc.)	This comprises of strong, soft, transparent polyurethane sheath, which is approximately 15 cm in length and 7 cm in diameter. It has two flexible rings, the inner ring and an outer one. The inner ring at the closed end of the condom eases insertion into the vagina, covering the cervix and holding the condom in place. The outer ring, which is larger than the inner one, stays outside the vagina and covers part of the perineum and labia during intercourse.	The female condom is inserted in the vagina just before sexual intercourse. Similar to the male condom, female condom also helps to prevent pregnancy and STDs as it is impermeable to HIV, cytomegalovirus and hepatitis B virus. The pregnancy rate with a female condom is higher than that with a male condom. Female condoms may be expensive or limited in their availability and may be difficult to insert.

Picture	Medical/Surgical Description	Management/Clinical Highlights
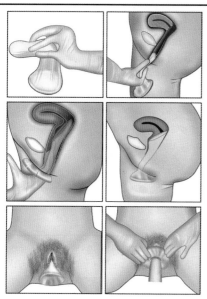 **Fig. 15.2.7.1B:** Method of application of female condom	The female condom is made of polyurethane sheath and comprises of a polyurethane ring at each end. The open ring remains outside the vagina whereas the closed external ring is fitted behind the symphysis and beneath the cervix like a diaphragm. Before inserting the condom through the vagina, the inner ring of the condom must be squeezed with the help of thumb and middle finger so that it becomes long and narrow. The inner ring must be then gently guided with help of fingers through the vaginal opening as far as possible toward the cervical opening. The outer ring should remain on the outside of the vagina, covering the vulva partially. At the time of sexual intercourse, the erect penis must be directed into the condom so that it does not slip into the vagina outside the condom.	At the time of insertion, the woman can be sitting, squatting or be lying down. The condom must be inserted straight and not be twisted inside the vagina. The female condom must be lubricated well prior to use. Female condoms can be safely used with water or silicone-based lubricants. Male and female condoms must not be used together because they are likely to slip, tear or become displaced. Since the female condoms cover part of the vulva, they provide protection against Human Papillomavirus and herpes.

15.2.7.2: Cervical Cap

Picture	Medical/Surgical Description	Management/Clinical Highlights
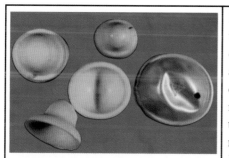 **Fig. 15.2.7.2:** Cervical cap	It is a barrier form of female contraception, which comprises of a small cup-like device made up of silicone, which acts as a physical barrier between the sperm and egg by fitting snugly over the cervix. It must be inserted at least 15 minutes prior to intercourse and must be in place for a minimum of 6–8 hours, but can be left in place for up to 48 hours, following which, it should be removed. Pregnancy rates have been found to vary between 11 to 32%.	A health care professional may be required to fit the cervical cap for a young girl. Prior to insertion, the health care provider must perform a pelvic examination to determine size of the cap that would be right for her. The health care provider can then teach her how to insert and remove the cap. Prior to insertion, hands must be thoroughly washed. Also, after each time of use, the cap must be washed with soap and water, rinsed and dried and then stored in a case.

15.2.7.3: Vaginal Contraceptive Film

Picture	Medical/Surgical Description	Management/Clinical Highlights
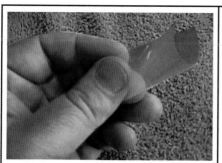 **Fig. 15.2.7.3:** Vaginal contraceptive film	Vaginal contraceptive film (VCF) is a nonhormonal, safe and effective form of barrier contraception, which is in form of a plastic film containing a spermicidal agent. It provides protection within 15 minutes of use and remains active up to 3 hours. It can be used several times in a day. However, it is less effective than other barrier methods of contraception.	The VCF can be inserted deep inside the vagina by either of the partners. First the VCF is held between the index finger and thumb, and then using the fingertip, it is inserted deep inside the vagina over the cervix. Once inside the vagina, it dissolves to form gel like substance, containing a spermicidal agent.

15.2.7.4: Cervical Diaphragm (A to C)

Picture	Medical/Surgical Description	Management/Clinical Highlights
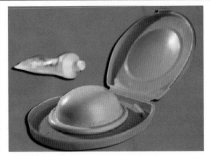 **Fig. 15.2.7.4A:** Cervical diaphragm	A diaphragm is a shallow rubber dome with a firm flexible rim. It is often used in combination with contraceptive jelly, spermicide, etc. Though it is available in many sizes ranging from 50 mm to 105 mm, the most commonly used size in clinical practice is 75 mm.	It is immediately effective and reversible method of contraception, which can be inserted up to 6 hours before intercourse. It should remain in place for at least 6 hours after the intercourse. However, it must not be left inside the vagina for more than 24 hours.
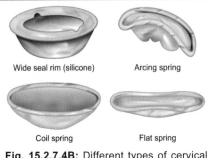 Wide seal rim (silicone) Arcing spring Coil spring Flat spring **Fig. 15.2.7.4B:** Different types of cervical diaphragms	Different types of cervical diaphragms are available. It is made either of latex or silicone, and is available in different sizes ranging from 50 mm to 105 mm. Various types of cervical diaphragms include latex arcing spring, coil spring, flat spring and silicone wide seal rim.	The latex arcing spring diaphragm has a firm rim, which makes its insertion in the posterior fornix easier. The rim of a coil spring diaphragm is soft and flexible, which does not form an arc when folded. This is usually used in women with moderate tone of vaginal muscles. The flat spring diaphragm is similar to coil spring, but has thinner and more delicate rim. It may be used in women with good tone of vaginal muscles.
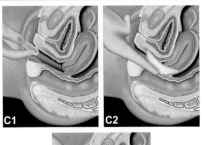 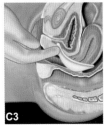 **Figs 15.2.7.4C (C1 to C3):** Method of application of cervical diaphragm: (C1) The lubricated diaphragm is folded and inserted at the introitus; (C2) The cervix should be palpable through the dome of the diaphragm; (C3) The anterior rim of the diaphragm is pushed so that it fits directly behind the pubic bone	The application of a cervical diaphragm involves the following steps: The ring of the diaphragm is lubricated and then folded so that the two sides of ring are touching each other. The vulva is opened with one hand; the other hand is used to gently guide the folded diaphragm inside the vagina and to direct its placement toward the posterior fornix so that the dome of the diaphragm covers the cervical opening. The anterior rim of the diaphragm must be directly behind the pubic bone.	Patient education is an important parameter, which ensures patient compliance and the contraceptive effectiveness of the diaphragm. When the diaphragm is properly fitted, the patient should not be able to feel anything. The patient should be instructed to use spermicidal jelly inside the cup of diaphragm in order to improve its contraceptive efficacy. It should not have any holes or tear. After use, it must be removed, washed with soap and water, rinsed, dried and stored in an airtight container.

15.2.7.5: Today's Sponge (A and B)

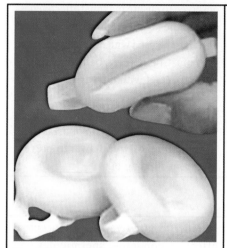

Fig. 15.2.7.5A: Today's sponge

Sponge is a safe, nonhormonal form of contraception, which provides protection for nearly 24 hours. The contraceptive sponge is marketed under the brand name of Today's sponge in the United States, and the brand names of Protectaid and Pharmatex sponges in the UK. Besides acting as a physical barrier, it also contains a spermicidal agent (nonoxynol-9).

The sponges provide contraceptive action by two ways. One is by preventing the sperms from moving inside the cervix. Second is the presence of spermicide in the sponge, which causes immobilization of the sperms. Success rates with the use of Today's sponge have been found to vary between 77 to 91%. Though Today's sponge was first launched in 1983, it was withdrawn from the market in 1994 due to the probable risk of toxic shock syndrome (TSS) and again relaunched in 2009 because the linkage with TSS remained unproven.

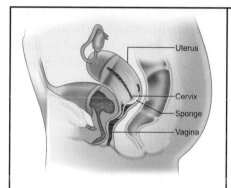

Fig. 15.2.7.5B: Application of Today's sponge

Before insertion, the sponge is soaked in water so that it gets completely wet. This causes activation of the spermicidal agent. Then it is inserted inside the vagina so that it covers the cervix.

It can be inserted up to 24 hours before the sexual intercourse. It should be inserted about 6 hours following sexual intercourse. However, it should not be worn for more than 30 hours in one go.

15.2.8: Barrier Method of Male Contraception (A to C)

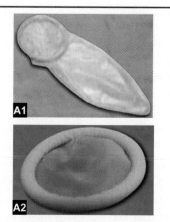

Figs 15.2.8A (A1 and A2): (A1): An unrolled-up male condom made up of latex; (A2): Rolled-up male condom

A male condom is a thin sheath made of latex or other materials. Latex is the most commonly used material. Other less commonly used materials include polyurethane or lamb cecum. They may be available in different sizes.

Condoms are effective form of contraception and when used by motivated couples, failure rates as low as 3–4 per 100 couple years of exposure has been obtained.

However, perfect use rarely occurs and in practical life, high failure rates (10–14 per 100 couple years of use) may be achieved. The main advantage of using condoms is that they provide protection against various STDs. Condoms also help prevent premalignant cervical changes, probably by blocking the transmission of HPV virus.

Picture	Medical/Surgical Description	Management/Clinical Highlights

When putting on a condom, the man must be sure that the rolled up ring is on the outside

Rolled up ring

Correct position   Incorrect position

Fig. 15.2.8B: Correct position of applying male condom

The man must ensure correct application of condom to ensure its maximum efficacy. While putting on a condom, the rolled up ring must be on the outside and not on the inside.

Various precautions, which must be observed to ensure maximal effectiveness of condoms are as follows:
- It must be used with every act of coitus.
- It must be applied before penis has any contact with the vagina.
- Withdrawal must occur with the penis still erect.
- The base of the condom must be held at the time of withdrawal to prevent it from slipping out.

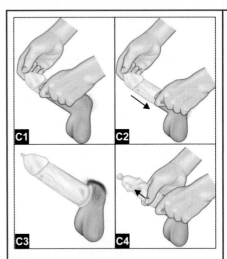

Figs 15.2.8C (C1 to C4): Application of male condom

The man puts the condom on his erected penis, while the condom holds the semen. After having sexual intercourse, the man must carefully take off the condom so that it does not leak. Each condom can be used only once.

In order to improve the contraceptive effect of condoms, spermicides can be used alongside either in form of intravaginal application or in form of condom lubricated with a spermicide. Water-based lubricants can be used while applying a condom. Oil-based products are likely to destroy latex condoms and therefore should not be used.

15.3: METHOD OF COPPER-T INSERTION (A TO I)

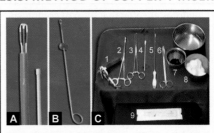

Figs 15.3 (A to C): (A) Copper device is folded and kept inside the inserter; (B) Loaded copper device with the plunger inserted inside; (C) The equipment tray showing various instruments used at the time of Cu-T insertion—(1) Cusco's speculum; (2) Sponge holder; (3) Vulsellum; (4) Uterine sound; (5) Uterine curette; (6) Scissors; (7) Betadine; (8) Gauze; (9) Pack of copper device (380A)

After aseptic preparation of vagina and vulva, cervix is grasped with volsellum or Allis forceps. Length of the uterine cavity is then determined with help of an uterine sound. The copper device with an insertion tube is available in presterilized packs. Prior to insertion, the pack is opened, and the T-arms of the IUCD are folded and mounted into the insertion tube [Figures 15.3 (A to C)].

Prior to insertion, informed consent should be obtained and the patient should be aware of the potential side effects, benefits and alternative methods of contraception. It should be emphasized to the patient that the IUCD does not provide protection against sexually transmitted infections or HIV. The cervix should be carefully inspected for any signs of infection prior to IUCD insertion. If there is any evidence of mucopurulent discharge or pelvic tenderness, cervical swabs should be sent for culture and sensitivity, and IUCD insertion be delayed until the infection (if present) has been treated.

Picture	Medical/Surgical Description	Management/Clinical Highlights
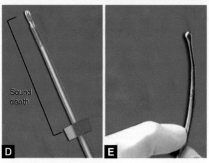 **Figs 15.3 (D and E):** (D) Flange is adjusted based on the uterine size as evaluated by the uterine sound; (E) Calculating uterine size through the uterine sound	Figures 15.3 (D and E) illustrate adjustment of the blue-colored flange/guard on the insertion tube in accordance with the length of the uterine cavity, which had been previously calculated using a uterine sound.	The adjustment of blue flange on the insertion tube in accordance to the length of the uterine cavity is an important step to prevent uterine perforation, a rare but a devastating complication of Copper-T insertion. This step also ensures correct placement of copper device within the uterine cavity depending on the size of uterus.
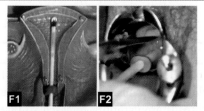 **Figs 15.3F (F1 and F2):** The inserter is introduced inside the uterine cavity till the flange touches the external os	Figures 15.3F (F1 and F2) show how the insertion tube, preloaded with the copper device is passed into the uterine cavity through the cervix.	The insertion tube is gently inserted inside the uterine cavity till the blue flange touches the external os.
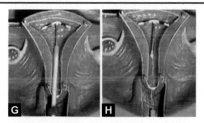 **Figs 15.3 (G and H):** (G) The plunger is pushed inside the inserter to release the device inside the uterine cavity; (H) Copper device inside the uterine cavity	Figure 15.3G shows the plunger being pushed inside the inserter to release the device. Figure 15.3H shows the correct placement of copper device inside the uterine cavity following its release.	Once the insertion tube containing the preloaded copper device is introduced inside the uterus, the solid white rod plunger is put inside the insertion tube so that the IUCD recoils within the uterine cavity.
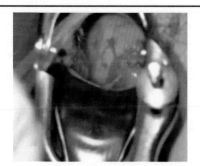 **Fig. 15.3I:** Appearance of cervical os with Cu-T thread protruding out	After withdrawing the plunger, insertion tube is removed and the nylon thread is cut to the required length. The speculum and the forceps are then removed. Figure 15.3I show appearance of the cervical os with Cu-T thread protruding out. A follow-up visit should be scheduled 6 weeks postinsertion, so that the gynecologist can examine the patient, exclude presence of any infection, perform an assessment of any abnormal bleeding and check for the presence of IUCD threads.	Following discharge, the patient is instructed to examine herself and feel for the Cu-T thread every week. An IUCD user should be instructed to contact her health care provider if any of the following occur: IUCD's threads cannot be felt; she or her partner can feel the lower end of the IUCD; she experiences persistent abdominal pain, fever, dyspareunia and/or unusual vaginal discharge, etc.

15.4: INSERTION OF MIRENA (A TO G)

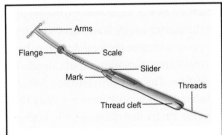

Fig. 15.4A: Parts of Mirena device

Mirena (levonorgestrel-releasing intrauterine system) is in form of a T-shaped polyethylene structure. The T-shaped plane is 32 mm in dimensions (both in horizontal and vertical directions). The polyethylene frame has barium sulfate impregnated in it, which makes the device radio-opaque. The stem is encased by a cylinder, which contains polydimethylsiloxane and levonorgestrel (52 mg). The cylinder contains a permeable membrane, which regulates the rate of release of hormones. At the end of the vertical stem are two threads.

Mirena is packaged in a sterile form within an inserter. The inserter comprises of a body, slider (which is integrated with a flange), prebent insertion tube and plunger. Once Mirena is in place within the uterus, the inserter is discarded. Mirena is inserted with the provided inserter into the uterine cavity within 7 days of the onset of menstruation. Currently, the device has been approved for continuous use for 5 years.

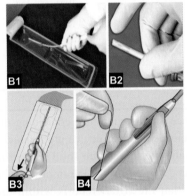

Figs 15.4B (B1 to B4): (B1) By pulling the thread down, arms of the device are pulled inside; (B2) Magnified view showing the device being loaded into the insertion tube; (B3) Diagram showing the slider being pushed in its farthest position; (B4) Diagram showing how the threads are secured into the cleft

Figures 15.4B (B1 to B4) show how by pulling the thread down, arms of the Mirena device are pulled inside the prebent insertion tube.

The clinician picks up the handle of the inserter containing Mirena and the threads are carefully released so that they hang freely. The clinician's thumb or forefinger is then placed on the slider, which is set in the furthest position away from the clinician, i.e. at the top of the handle. While looking at the insertion tube, the arms of the system must be horizontally aligned. Both the threads are pulled on to draw the LNG-IUS into the inserter tube. This action causes the folded device to be drawn up inside the insertion tube. The threads must now be fitted tightly in the cleft at the end of the handle.

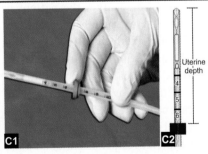

Figs 15.4C (C1 and C2): (C1) Photograph showing how the flange is adjusted in accordance with the uterine size; (C2) Diagram showing how the flange is adjusted in accordance with the uterine size

Figures 15.4C (C1 and C2) show how the flange is set in accordance with the uterine size as determined by sounding the uterus.

The uterine size is estimated by sounding the uterus. A uterine sound is gently inserted to measure the depth of the uterine cavity, confirm its direction and exclude the presence of any uterine anomaly. The uterus should normally sound to a depth of 6–10 cm.

Picture	Medical/Surgical Description	Management/Clinical Highlights
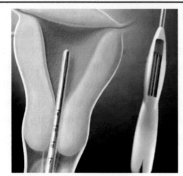 **Fig. 15.4D:** The device is inserted inside the uterine cavity	Figure 15.4D shows the inserter with the loaded device being placed inside the uterus through the cervix to a length 1.5 to 2 cm below the uterine fundus.	The clinician must continue to hold the slider with the thumb or forefinger firmly in its furthermost position. The other hand of clinician must be used for grasping the tenaculum forceps, which holds the anterior lip of cervix. While maintaining traction on the cervix, the insertion tube must be gently advanced through the cervical canal and into the uterine cavity until the flange is 1.5–2 cm away from the external cervical os. This allows sufficient space for the arms of the device to open up, when the device is released within the uterine cavity.
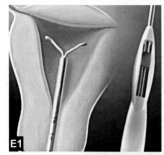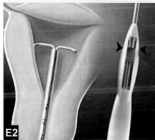 **Figs 15.4E (E1 and E2):** The arms of the device are gradually released by pulling the slider down	Figures 15.4E (E1 and E2) show how the device is gradually released inside the uterine cavity by pulling the slider backward.	While holding the inserter steady, the arms of Mirena are released by pulling the slider back until the top of the slider reaches the mark (raised horizontal line on the handle). The clinician must wait for approximately 10 seconds to allow the horizontal arms of Mirena to open and regain its T-shape.
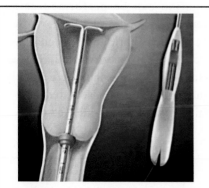 **Fig. 15.4F:** The device is then gradually advanced up to the fundus	Once the device has opened up, it should be carefully pushed up to the fundus.	Once the device has opened up, the inserter containing Mirena device is gradually advanced into the uterine cavity until the flange touches the external cervical os. In order to release the device from the inserter, while holding the inserter steady, the slider must be pulled all the way down to release Mirena. The threads will automatically be released from the cleft and would hang freely. The inserter is then gently withdrawn from the uterus.

Picture	Medical/Surgical Description	Management/Clinical Highlights

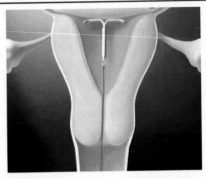

Fig. 15.4G: As the device assumes its correct position inside the uterine cavity, the thread is cut by 3–4 cm

Once the inserter is withdrawn, the hanging threads are cut (Figure 15.4G) perpendicular to the thread length with sterile curved scissors. About 3–4 cm of thread must be visible outside the cervix.

If the clinician suspects that Mirena may not be in the correct position, performing a transvaginal ultrasound can check its proper placement. In case the device has not been properly positioned within the uterus, it must be removed and a new device be placed. A removed Mirena must never be reinserted again.

15.5: PERMANENT METHODS OF CONTRACEPTION

15.5.1: Pomeroy's Technique (A to D)

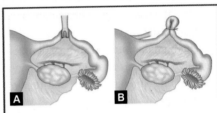

Figs 15.5.1 (A and B): Pomeroy's technique of tubal sterilization: (A) The fallopian tube is grasped with Babcock clamp; (B) A loop is created, which is tied with No. 1 plain catgut sutures

The steps of Pomeroy's technique are described in Figures 15.5.1 (A to D). Figures 15.5.1 (A and B) show how the midportion of the oviduct is grasped with a Babcock clamp, creating a loop, which is then tied with No. 1 plain catgut or No. 0 chromic catgut sutures.

The rationale for this technique is based on the principle that over a period of time, the cut ends of the tube become independently sealed off, thereby retracting from one another. This occurs due to prompt absorption of the suture ligature with subsequent separation of the cut ends of the tube, which then become sealed by spontaneous reperitonealization and fibrosis.

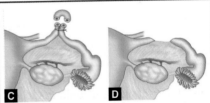

Figs 15.5.1 (C and D): (C) Excision of the loop; (D) Several months later, the ends of the tube get fibrosed, retracting from one another

Figure 15.5.1C shows that segment of the tube having a length of about 1.2–1.5 cm, distal to the ligature is excised. The surgeon must then inspect the segment of the loop that has been removed to ensure that the wall has not been partially resected. The same procedure is then repeated on the other side. Specimen is then submitted for histopathological examination. Figure 15.5.1D shows that after a few months, the ends of the tube get fibrosed, retracting from one another.

Subumbilical minilaparotomy is the most common approach worldwide for postpartum procedures. Tubal ligation can be performed using various techniques such as Pomeroy's Technique, Parkland's Technique, Uchida's Technique, Irving's Technique, etc. Pomeroy's technique is highly successful and is associated with a failure rate of 7.5 per 1,000 cases.

| Picture | Medical/Surgical Description | Management/Clinical Highlights |

15.5.2: Parkland's Technique (A to C)

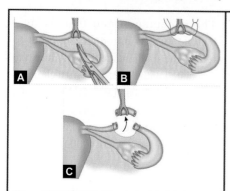

Figs 15.5.2 (A to C): Parkland's technique of tubal sterilization: (A) The fallopian tube is grasped with Babcock's clamp; (B) The mesosalpinx is incised and midsegmental portion of the fallopian tube is ligated at the two ends; (C) The midportion of the tube between the two ligatures is resected

The Parkland's technique is similar to the Pomeroy's technique, except that in this case midsegment resection is performed, involving the excision of 1–2 cm tubal segment, which is then submitted for a histopathological examination. Following this, each limb of the loop is tied separately with a no. 0 chromic catgut sutures.

The Parkland's technique was designed to avoid the intimate approximation of the tubal cut ends, which may occur with the Pomeroy's technique. As a result, the risk of subsequent recanalization is considerably reduced. Failure rates are reported to be 1 case out of 400 patients.

15.5.3: Uchida's Technique (A to D)

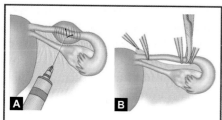

Figs 15.5.3 (A and B): Uchida's technique of tubal sterilization: (A) Mesosalpinx is infiltrated with local anesthetic and is then incised; (B) The midsegment of the fallopian tube is ligated on the two ends

In this technique, a relatively long (5 cm) segment of tubal muscularis is pulled out after giving an incision in the mesosalpinx. This portion of the tube is then ligated proximally and distally with a no. 0 plain catgut sutures. The next steps are described below in Figures 15.5.3 (C and D).

This procedure was introduced by Hajime Uchida in 1940s. This is one of the most complex methods for tubal ligation and therefore takes longer than Pomeroy's or Parkland's technique. The original technique was personally performed by Uchida in nearly 20,000 cases without encountering a single failure.

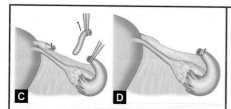

Figs 15.5.3 (C and D): (C) The midportion of the tube between the two ligatures is resected; (D) The medial free end of the tubal stump is then buried in the leaves of broad ligament

Following the ligation of two ends, the portion in between the two ligatures is resected out. The serosal edges are then reapproximated, burying the medial exposed tubal end within the leaves of the broad ligament. The distal end is left exposed.

This sterilization procedure can be performed during the puerperal period. During the puerperium, Uchida modified the sterilization procedure, by including fimbriectomy. The combination of excision of such a large segment of tube along with a fimbriectomy is responsible for a low failure rate of this technique.

15.5.4: Modified Irving's Technique (A to D)

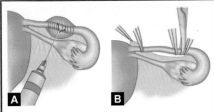

Figs 15.5.4 (A and B): Modified Irving's technique of tubal sterilization: (A) Mesosalpinx is infiltrated with local anesthetic and is then incised; (B) The midsegment of the fallopian tube is ligated on the two ends

In this technique, a small portion of the tube, approximately 1–2 cm in length, about 4 cm from the uterotubal junction, is doubly ligated with No. 0 or 00 absorbable sutures and resected. The sutures on the proximal end are left long. The next steps are described below in Figures 15.5.4 (C and D).

This technique (modified Irving's technique) was introduced in order to reduce the small incidence of failure rate associated with the Pomeroy's technique. This procedure can be considered as one of the most effective procedures for prevention of pregnancy (failure rates of less than 1 case per 1,000 patients).

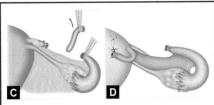

Figs 15.5.4 (C and D): (C) The midportion of the tube between the two ligatures is resected; (D) The medial free end of the tube is then drawn into the myometrial tunnel, following which the sutures are tied

After resection of the midportion of the tube, the surgeon needs to dissect the proximal tube free from the mesosalpinx in order to mobilize it. A small nick is made into the serosa on the posterior (or anterior) uterine wall near the uterotubal junction. This nick is then deepened to a thickness of about 1–2 cm. The free ends of the proximal stump ligature are then brought deep into the myometrium tunnel and out through the uterine serosa. The proximal tubal stump is drawn deep into the myometrial tunnel, following which the sutures are tied. The serosal opening of the tunnel is then closed around the tube with fine absorbable sutures.

According to the original technique described by Irving, the distal end of the tube was also buried between the leaves of the broad ligament. However, in this modified procedure, only the proximal portion of the tube is buried into the myometrium. The distal end of the tube is ligated and left in place. Due to the burying of the proximal portion of the tube into the myometrium, the occurrence of recanalization or development of tuboperitoneal fistula becomes extremely unlikely.

15.5.5: Laparoscopic Sterilization (A to F)

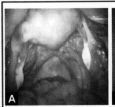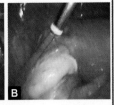

Figs 15.5.5 (A and B): Steps of laparoscopic sterilization using Falope's rings: (A) Laparoscopic visualization of the fallopian tubes of both sides; (B) Application of Falope's rings

Tubal ligation using laparoscopic approach has been practiced since 1970s. Presently, it has become the most commonly used approach for tubal ligation.

Figures 15.5.5 (A to D) illustrate the procedure of laparoscopic sterilization using Falope's rings. Figure 15.5.5A shows normal laparoscopic visualization of the fallopian tubes of both sides. Figure 15.5.5B shows application of Falope's rings over the left fallopian tube.

Laparoscopic tubal ligation is most commonly used as an interval procedures in the United States. This procedure can be carried out using various techniques, such as electrodessication of tubes using electrosurgery or mechanical blockage of tubes using Falope's rings or Filshie's clips. During the procedure of laparoscopic sterilization using Falope's rings, a nonreactive silicone rubber band is applied around the isthmic portion of the fallopian tube.

Picture	Medical/Surgical Description	Management/Clinical Highlights
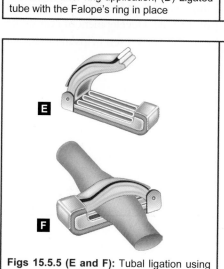 **Figs 15.5.5 (C and D):** (C) Applicator being withdrawn after ring application; (D) Ligated tube with the Falope's ring in place	Figure 15.5.5C shows how the applicator is withdrawn after the Falope's ring has been applied. Figure 15.5.5D shows ligated tube with Falope's ring in place.	The Falope's ring is about 3.6 mm in outer diameter and contains about 5% barium sulfate for radiographic identification. The failure rate with this method has been reported to be 3.3 cases per 1,000 patients.
Figs 15.5.5 (E and F): Tubal ligation using Filshie's clip	The technique of tubal ligation using Filshie's clip is widely used in Canada, the United Kingdom and Australia and was approved for use in the United States in 1997.	This technique involves application of a 12.7 mm long clip of titanium with a silicone rubber lining. The clip is applied laparoscopically with an applicator at right angles to the isthmus approximately, 2–2.5 cm from the uterotubal junction.

15.5.6: Hysteroscopic Sterilization

15.5.6.1: Essure (A to C)

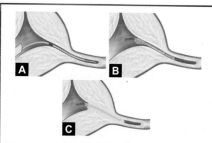

Figs 15.5.6.1 (A to C): Process of Essure hysteroscopic sterilization: (A) Hysteroscopic cannulation of tubal lumen; (B) Microinsert device inserted inside the tubal ostium; (C) Fibrosis develops over the "Essure" Microinsert device over a period of time, resulting in tubal occlusion

Procedure of tubal sterilization using hysteroscopic sterilization is based on using a new device, "Essure", which helps in blocking the fallopian tubes. This device has been approved by "The Food and Drug Administration (FDA)" and consists of using a small metallic implant, called the Essure System. The device consists of polyethylene terephthalate fibers wrapped around a stainless steel core, surrounded by 24 coils of nickel titanium alloy. Out of the 24 coils, at least 3–8 coils must be visible trailing in the uterine cavity, to confirm proper placement of the device.

This is usually performed as an OPD procedure. It involves placing an obstructive device into each of the fallopian tubes at the time of hysteroscopy with help of a special catheter that is inserted through the vagina into the uterus and then into the fallopian tube. While performing hysteroscopy, normal saline is used as the distension medium, because it minimizes the risk of fluid overload and the risk of electrolyte imbalance, which may be associated with the use of isotonic solutions such as glycine and sorbitol. Over a period of time, approximately 3 months, fibrous tissue develops over the implant, blocking the fallopian tube, thereby preventing fertilization of the egg by the sperm.

15.5.6.2: Adiana (A and B)

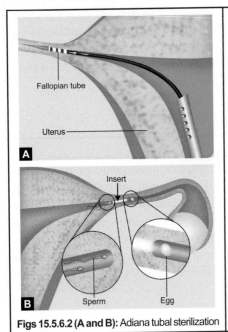

A

B

Figs 15.5.6.2 (A and B): Adiana tubal sterilization

Adiana hysteroscopic tubal sterilization is another new technique for hysteroscopic sterilization, which gained approval by FDA in 2009. In this technique, radiofrequency energy and a polymer microinsert can be used to block the tubes in its interstitial portion.

In this procedure, a catheter is positioned inside the fallopian tube under hysteroscopic guidance. Radiofrequency energy is applied via the catheter to ablate a thin layer of cells lining the fallopian tube. A soft polymer matrix implant is then inserted into this part of the tube. Development of scar tissue over the microinsert helps in producing tubal blockage.

15.5.7: Vasectomy (A to C)

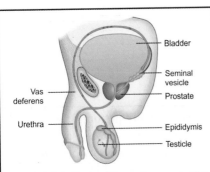

Fig. 15.5.7 A: Parts of the male reproductive system

The two main male sex organs include penis (which is located externally) and the testes (located inside the scrotal sac), which produce sperms and semen. Epididymis is a coiled tube like structure, which is present against the testicles. Here the sperms undergo maturation and are stored before they pass out to the vas deferens. Vas deferens, also known as ductus deferens are tube like structures (about 30-40 cm) in length, which carry sperms from epididymis to the ejaculatory ducts. During ejaculation, the smooth muscles of vas deferens contract, thereby propelling the sperms forward through the ejaculatory ducts into the urethra. Other accessory sex glands such as seminal vesicles, prostate and bulbourethral glands also contribute their secretions and form bulk of the semen.

Vasectomy is a procedure in which the vas deferens (tubes carrying sperms from the testicles and epididymis to the urinary tract and urethra) are surgically blocked to prevent the sperms from passing through and fertilizing the egg at the time of sexual intercourse. For couples who do not want to have any more children, vasectomy is the safest and easiest form of permanent sterilization. Following vasectomy, fertility can sometimes be restored either through surgical reanastomosis techniques or by sperm retrieval from the testes.

Picture	Medical/Surgical Description	Management/Clinical Highlights

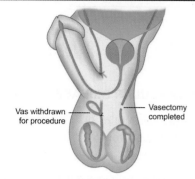

Fig. 15.5.7B: The procedure of vasectomy

Vasectomy is a highly effective procedure, having a failure rate as low as 0.02–0.2%, which is less than that of tubal sterilization. Except for complete abstinence, no method can be considered to be more effective than vasectomy in preventing pregnancy. Vasectomy does not cause loss of masculinity. Even though vasectomy has been performed, until there has been complete expulsion of sperms stored distal to the vas (which requires nearly 20 ejaculations or 3 months), another method of contraception should be used. This must be continued until laboratory and microscopic examination of the patient's semen reveals azoospermia.

The procedure of vasectomy comprises of the following steps:
- A scalpel is used to make two small incisions on each side of the scrotum at a location that allows the surgeon to bring out each vas deferens to the surface.
- The vas deferentia are cut (sometimes a piece removed), separated and then at least one side is sealed by suture ligation, cauterization or clamping, before being dropped back into the scrotum.

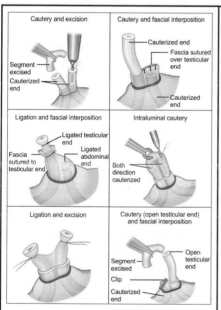

Fig. 15.5.7C: Different methods used for blocking the vas

The blockage of vas through the process of vasectomy blocks the flow of sperms, thereby resulting in sterility. Some variations in the vasectomy techniques can be employed to improve the results of surgery. Some such variations, which are used for blocking the cut ends of vas have been shown in Figure 15.5.7C. These include excision followed by cautery, cautery followed by interpositioning of fascia or intraluminal cautery.

Some of the newer methods for blocking the vas deferens include use of mesh intravas device, plug intravas device, polymer gel, application of clips, etc.

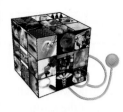

1. COMBINED HORMONAL CONTRACEPTIVES AND THE RISK OF CARDIOVASCULAR DISEASE

Women using combined contraceptive pills containing progestins, such as drospirenone, norelgestromin or eltonorgestrel has been found to be associated with significantly increased risk of venous thrombosis in comparison to low-estrogen standard combined hormonal contraceptive agents.

Source: FDA Office of Surveillance and Epidemiology. Combined Hormonal Contraceptives (CHCs) and the Risk of Cardiovascular Disease Endpoints. [online] Available from www.fda.gov/downloads/Drugs/DrugSafety/ UCM277384.pdf. [Accessed on February, 2012.

2. USE OF INTRAUTERINE CONTRACEPTIVE DEVICES IN ADOLESCENTS

According to new guidelines issued by the American College of Obstetricians and Gynecologists, long-acting, reversible contraceptive methods such as intrauterine devices and implants can be considered as the best methods to prevent unintended pregnancy amongst adolescent girls. These contraceptive methods are associated with low pregnancy rate and higher patient satisfaction rate. Moreover the use of IUCDs is not associated with an increased risk for pelvic inflammatory disease or infertility.

Source: American College of Obstetrics and gynecology. Committee Opinion No. 539: Adolescents and long-acting reversible contraception: implants and intrauterine devices. Obstet Gynecol. 2012;120(4):983-8.

3. MAKING ORAL CONTRACEPTIVES AVAILABLE OVER THE COUNTER

Oral contraceptives should be available to women over the counter (OTC) in the US because the benefit of reducing unwanted pregnancies outweighs the risks of dispensing the drugs without a prescription, the American Congress of Obstetricians and Gynecologists (ACOG) has announced.

According to ACOG, making the oral contraceptives available over the counter would be helpful in reducing the "unacceptably high" rate of unintended pregnancies. The FDA however, has yet not given its approval for making oral contraceptives available over the counter.

Source: The American College of Obstetricians and gynaecologists. Over-the-Counter Access to Oral Contraceptives. Committee opinion, No 544, Dec 2012. Obstet Gynecol. 2012:120;1527-1531.

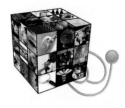

BIBLIOGRAPHY

1. Abbott J, Emmans LS, Lowenstein SR. Ectopic pregnancy: ten common pitfalls in diagnosis. Am J Emerg Med. 1990;8(6):515-22.
2. Abbott J, Hawe J, Hunter D, et al. Laparoscopic excision of endometriosis: a randomized, placebo-controlled trial. Fertil Steril. 2004;82: 878-84.
3. Abbott JA, Hawe J, Clayton RD, et al. The effects and effectiveness of laparoscopic excision of endometriosis: a prospective study with 2–5 year follow-up. Hum Reprod. 2003;18:1922-7.
4. ACC/AHA 2006 guidelines for management of patients with valvular heart disease. A report of the American College of Cardiology/ American Heart Association. Task Force on Practice Guidelines (Writing Committee to Revise the 1998 Guidelines for the Management of Patients With Valvular Heart Disease). J Am Coll Cardiol. 2006;48:e1-e148.
5. Acien P, Acien M, Sanchez-Ferrer M. Complex malformations of the female genital tract. New types and revision of classification. Hum Reprod. 2004;19:2377-84.
6. Acien P. Uterine anomalies and recurrent miscarriage. Infertil Reprod Med Clin N Am. 1996;7:689-720.
7. Acker DB, Sachs BP, Friedman EA. Risk factors for shoulder dystocia. Obstet Gynecol. 1985;66:762-8.
8. ACOG Committee on Gynecologic Practice. The role of the generalist obstetrician-gynecologist in the early detection of ovarian cancer. Gynecol Oncol. 2002;87:237-9.
9. ACOG committee opinion. Delivery by vacuum extraction. Number 208, September 1998. Committee on Obstetric Practice. American College of Obstetricians and Gynecologists. Int J Gynecol Obstet. 1999;64(1):96.
10. ACOG practice bulletin on diagnosing and managing preeclampsia and eclampsia. American Academy of Family Physicians website. Available at: http://www.aafp.org/afp/20020715/practice.html [Accessed April 2009].
11. ACOG Practice Bulletin: Clinical Management Guidelines for Obstetrician-Gynecologists Number 76, October 2006: postpartum hemorrhage. Obstet Gynecol. 2006;108:1039-47.
12. ACOG. American College of Obstetricians and Gynecologists Practice Bulletin. Intrapartum Fetal Heart Rate Monitoring. Clinical Management Guidelines for Obstetricians Gynecologists. No 36. American College of Obstetricians and Gynecologists:Washington, DC; December 2005.
13. ACOG. American College of Obstetricians and Gynecologists Practice Bulletin. Dystocia and augmentation of labor. Clinical management guidelines for obstetricians gynecologists. No 49. American College of Obstetricians and Gynecologists: Washington, DC; December 2003.
14. ACOG. American College of Obstetricians and Gynecologists Practice Bulletin. Obstetric Analgesia and Anesthesia. Clinical Management Guidelines for Obstetricians Gynecologists. No 36. American College of Obstetricians and Gynecologist: Washington, DC; July 2002.
15. Advincula AP. Surgical techniques: robot-assisted laparoscopic hysterectomy with the da Vinci surgical system. Int J Med Robot. 2006;2:305-11.
16. Afolabi BB, Lesi FE, Merah NA. Regional vesus general anesthesia for cesarean section. Cochrane Database Syst Rev. 2006;(4):CD 004350.
17. Agostini A, Cravello L, Bretelle F, et al. Risk of uterine perforation during hysteroscopic surgery. J Am Assoc Gynecol Laparosc. 2002;9:264-7.
18. Aguero O, Alvarez H. Fetal injury due to the vacuum extractor. Obstet Gynecol. 1962;19:212.
19. Ahuja GL, Willoughby MLN, Kerr MM, et al. Massive subaponeurotic hemorrhage in infants born by vacuum extraction. Br Med J. 1969;3:743.
20. Aitken AGF, Godden OJ. Real time ultrasound diagnosis of deep vein thrombosis: a comparison with venography. Clin Radiol. 1987;38:309.
21. Alderdice F, McKenna D, Dornan J. Techniques and materials for skin closure in cesarean section. Cochrane database syst Rev. 2003;(2):CD 003577.
22. Alfirevic Z, Sundberg K, Brigham S. Amniocentesis and chorionic villus sampling for prenatal diagnosis. Cochrane Database Syst Rev. 2004;CD003252.
23. Allahbadia G. Hypogastric artery ligation: a new perspective. Obstet Gynecol Surv. 1993;48:613-5.
24. Allan A, Williams JT, Bolton JP, et al. The use of graduated compression stockings in the prevention of postoperative deep vein thrombosis. Br J Surg. 1983;70:172.
25. Al-Sunaidi M, Tulandi T. Surgical treatment of ectopic pregnancy. Semin Reprod Med. 2007;25(2):117-22.
26. Althuisius SM, Dekker GA, Hummel P, et al. Final results of the cervical incompetence prevention randomized cerclage trial (CIPRACT): therapeutic cerclage with bed rest versus bed rest alone. Am J Obstet Gynecol. 2001;185:1106-12.
27. Alvarez M, Lockwood CJ, Ghidini A, et al. Prophylactic and emergent arterial catheterization for selective embolization in obstetric hemorrhage. Am J Perinatol. 1992;9:441-4.

28. Amer SA, Banu Z, Li TC, et al. Long-term follow-up of patient with polysystic ovarian syndrome after laparoscopic drilling: Endocrine and ultrasonographic outcomes. Hum Reprod. 2002;17:2851-7.

29. American Academy of Pediatrics and American College of Obstetricians and gynecologists. Guidelines for Perinatal care, 6th edition. Washington DC; 2007, p. 158.

30. American Academy of Pediatrics and American College of Obstetrics and Gynecology. Guidelines for perinatal care. 6th edition. Elk Grove III:American Academy of Pediatrics;2007.

31. American College of Cardiology/American Heart Association Task Force on Practice Guidelines. ACC/AHA 2006 Guidelines for the Management of Patients With Valvular Heart Disease A Report of the American College of Cardiology/American Heart Association Task Force on Practice Guidelines. JACC. 2006;48(3).

32. American College of Obsterians and Gynecologists:Gestational Diabetes: Practice Bulletin No 22, November 2000.

33. American College of Obstetricians and Gynecologists (2002, reaffirmed 2006). Management of infertility caused by ovulatory dysfunction. ACOG Practice Bulletin No. 34. Obs and Gynecol. 2002;99(2):347-58.

34. American College of Obstetricians and Gynecologists (ACOG). Medical management of ectopic pregnancy. Washington (DC): American College of Obstetricians and Gynecologists (ACOG); 2008. p. 7 (ACOG practice bulletin; no. 94).

35. American College of Obstetricians and Gynecologists. ACOG technical bulletin. Sterilization. No. 222—April 1996 (replaces no. 113, February 1988). American College of Obstetricians and Gynecologists. Int J Gynaecol Obstet. 1996;53(3):281-8.

36. American College of Obstetricians and Gynecologists. Operative vaginal delivery. Clinical management guidelines for obstetrician-gynecologists. Int J Gynaecol Obstet. 2001;74(1):69-76.

37. American College of Obstetricians and Gynecologists. Placenta accreta. ACOG Committee Opinion #266. American College of Obstetricians and Gynecologists, Washington, DC 2002.

38. American College of Obstetricians and Gynecologists. Postpartum hemorrhage. ACOG educational bulletin 1998; Number 243. In 2001 Compendium of selected publications, Washington DC: ACOG.

39. American College of Obstetricians and Gynecologists. Vaginal birth after previous cesarean delivery Practice Bulletin No 2. Washington, D.C: ACOG;1998.

40. American College of Obstetricians and Gynecologists: Operative vaginal deliveries.ACOG, Technical Bulletin No. 196. Washington; 1994.

41. American College of Obstetricians and Gynecologists: Operative Vaginal Deliveries. Technical Bulletin No. 196. Washington, DC: ACOG; 1994.

42. American College of Obstetricians and Gynecologists:Gestational Diabetes. Practice Bulletin No 30, September 2001.

43. American College of Obstetricians-Gynecologists. Episiotomy. Clinical Management Guidelines for Obstetrician-Gynecologists. ACOG Practice Bulletin. 2006:71.

44. American Diabetes Association: Clinical practice recommendations. Diabetes Care. 1999;23:S10.

45. American Diabetes Association: Gestational Diabetes Mellitus. Diabetes Care. 2003;26:S103.

46. American Diabetes Association: Report of the Expert Committee on the diagnosis and classifi cation of diabetes mellitus. Diabetes Care. 2004; 27 (suppl): 5.

47. American fertility Society. Classification of Müllerian anomalies. Fertil Steril. 1988;49:944.

48. Anderson DO, Ferris BC. Role of tobacco smoking in the causation of chronic respiratory disease. N Engl J Med. 1962;267:787.

49. Angioli R, Gómez-Marín O, Cantuaria G, et al. Severe perineal lacerations during vaginal delivery: the University of Miami experience. Am J Obstet Gynecol. 2000;182(5):1083-5.

50. Angstmann T, Gard G, Harrington T, et al. Surgical management of placenta accreta: a cohort series and suggested approach. Am J Obstet Gynecol. 2010;202:38e1-e9.

51. Ankum WM, Mol BW, Van der Veen F, et al. Risk factors for ectopic pregnancy: a meta-analysis. Fertility & Sterility. 1996;65(6):1093-9.

52. Api M, Api O, Yayla M. Fertility after B-Lynch suture and hypogastric artery ligation. Fertil Steril. 2005;84(2):509.

53. Arjona JE, Miño M, Cordón J, et al. Satisfaction and tolerance with office hysteroscopic tubal sterilization. Fertil Steril. 2008;90(4):1182-6.

54. Attilakos G, Sibanda T, Winter C, et al. A randomised controlled trial of a new handheld vacuum extraction device. BJOG. 2005;112(11):1510-5.

55. Baggish MS, Brill AI, Rosenwig B, et al. Fatal acute glycine and sorbitol toxicity during operative hysteroscopy. J Gynecol Surg. 1993;9:137-43.

56. Bailey PE. The disappearing art of instrumental delivery: time to reverse the trend. Int J Gynaecol Obstet. 2005;91(1):89-96.

57. Bajekal N, Li TC. Fibroids, infertility and pregnancy wastage. Hum Reprod Update. 2000;6(6):614-20.

58. Baker R, Caplan A, Emanuel LL, et al. Crisis, ethics, and the American Medical Association 1847 and 1997. JAMA. 1997;278:163-4.

59. Balen AH, Jacobs HS. A prospective study comparing unilateral and bilateral laparoscopic ovarian diathermy in women with the polycystic ovarian syndrome. Fertil Steril. 1994;62:921-5.

60. Baskett TF, Allen AC. Perinatal implications of shoulder dystocia. Obstet Gynecol. 1995;86:14-7.

61. Bates B. A guide to physical examination and history taking, 6th edition. Philadelphia: J.B. Lippincott Company.

62. Baxley EG, Gobbo RW. Shoulder dystocia. Am Fam Physician. 2004;69:1707-14.

63. Beer E, Folghera MG. Time for resolving shoulder dystocia. Am J Obstet Gynecol. 1998;179:1376-7.

64. Benson J, et al. Clinical Management of Abortion Complications: A Practical Guide. WHO;1994.

65. Berek JS, Stubblefield PG: Anatomic and clinical correlates of uterine perforation. Am J Obstet Gynecol. 1979;135:181.

66. Berek JS. Abnormal bleeding. In: Berek JS, Olive DL (Eds). Novak's Gynecology—Self-Assessment and Review, 12th edition. Philadelphia: Lippincott Williams & Wilkins; 1996. pp. 331-98.

67. Bettocchi S, Nappi L, Ceci O, et al. What does 'diagnostic hysteroscopy' mean today? The role of the new techniques. Curr Opin Obstet Gynecol. 2003;15:303-8.

68. Bhide A, Guven M, Prefumo F, et al. Maternal and neonatal outcome after failed ventouse delivery: comparison of forceps versus cesarean section. J Matern Fetal Neonatal Med. 2007;20(7):541-5.

69. Bishop E, Nelms WF. A simple method of tubal sterilization. NY State J Med. 1930;30:214-6.

70. B-Lynch C, Coker A, Lawal AH, et al. The B-Lynch surgical technique for the control of massive postpartum hemorrhage: an alternative to hysterectomy? Five cases reported. Br J Obstet Gynaecol. 1997;104(3):372-5.

71. Boer-Meisel ME, teVelde ER, Habbema JDF, et al. Predicting the pregnancy outcome in patients treated for hydrosalpinx: a prospective study. Fertil Steril. 1986;45(1):23-9.

72. Bofill JA, Rust OA, Perry KG, et al. Operative vaginal delivery: a survey of fellows of ACOG. Obstet Gynecol. 1996;88(6):1007-10.

73. Bofill JA, Vincent RD, Ross EL, et al. Nulliparous active labor, epidural analgesia and cesarean delivery for dystocia. Am J Obstet Gynecol. 1997;177(6):1465-70.

74. Boggess JF. Robotic Surgery in Gynecologic Oncology: Evolution of a New Surgical Paradigm. J Robotic Surg. 2007;1:31-3.

75. Bonnar J. Venous thromboembolism and gynecologic surgery. Clin Obstet Gynecol. 1985;28(2):432-46.

76. Bonney V. The technique and results of myomectomy. Lancet. 1931;220:171-7.

77. Boronow RC. Therapeutic alternative to primary exenteration for advanced vulvo-vaginal cancer. Gynecol Oncol. 1973;1:223-30.

78. Bosteels J, Van Herendael B, Weyers S, et al. The position of diagnostic laparoscopy in current fertility practice. Hum Reprod Update. 11 2007.

79. Bradley LD. Complications in hysteroscopy: prevention, treatment and legal risk. Curr Opin Obstet Gynecol. 2002;14:409-15.

80. Brambati B, Terzian E, Tognoni G. Randomized clinical trial of transabdominal vs transcervical chorionic villus sampling methods. Prenat Diagn. 1991;11:285-93.

81. Brown JS, Waetjen LE, Subak LL, et al. Pelvic organ prolapse surgery in the United States, 1997. Am J Obstet and Gynecol. 2002;186(4):712-6.

82. Bruhat MA, Mahnes H, Mage G, et al. Treatment of ectopic pregnancy by means of laparoscopy. Fertil Steril. 1980;33:411-4.

83. Bruner JP, Drummond SB, Meenan AL, et al. All-fours maneuver for reducing shoulder dystocia during labor. J Reprod Med. 1998;43:439-43.

84. Bulletti C, DE Ziegler D, Levi Setti P, et al. Myomas, pregnancy outcome, and in vitro fertilization. Ann NY Acad Sci. 2004;1034:84-92.

85. Bump RG, Mattiasson A, Bo K, et al. The standardization of terminology of female pelvic organ prolapse and pelvic floor function. Am J Obstet Gynecol. 1996;175:10.

86. Burns DL, Mascioli EA, Bistrian BR. Parenteral iron dextran therapy: A review. Nutrition. 1995;11(2):163-8.

87. Buttram VC, Reiter RC. Uterine leiomyomata: etiology, symptomatology, and management. Fertil Steril. 1981;36:433-45.

88. Buttram VC, Gibbons WE. Müllerian anomalies: a proposed classification. Fertil Steril. 1979;32:40-6.

89. Buttram VC, Vaquero C. Post-ovarian wedge resection adhesive disease. Fertil Steril. 1975;26:874.

90. Caldwell WE, Moloy HC. Anatomical variations in the female pelvis and their effect in labor with a suggested classification. Am J Obstet Gynecol. 1933;26:479.

91. Campbell DM. Multiple pregnancy. Baillieres Clin Obstet Gynaecol. 1990;4(1):109-27.

92. Campo S, Felli A, Lamanna MA, et al. Endocrine changes and clinical outcome after Laparoscopic ovarian resection in with polycystic ovaries. Hum reprod. 1993;8(3):359-63.

93. Carbonell JL, Velazco A, Rodriguez Y, et al. Oral versus vaginal misoprostol for cervical priming in first trimester abortion. A randomized trial. Eur J Contracept Reprod Health Care. 2001;6(3):134-40.

94. Carmona F, Martinez-Roman S, Manau D, et al. Immediate maternal and neonatal effects of low-forceps delivery according to the new criteria of The American College of Obstetricians and Gynecologists compared with spontaneous vaginal delivery in term pregnancies. Am J Obstet Gynecol. 1995;173(1):55-9.

95. Carpenter MW, Coustan DR. Criteria for screening tests for gestational diabetes. Am J Obstet Gynecol. 1982;144:768-73.

96. Carroli G, Mignini L. Episiotomy for vaginal birth. Cochrane Database of Systematic Reviews 2009, Issue 1, Art. No.: CD000081. DOI: 10.1002/14651858 CD000081.pub2.

97. Caspi E, Halperin V, Bukovsky I. The importance of periadnexal adhesions in tubal reconstructive surgery for infertility. Fertil Steril. 1979;31(3):296-300.

98. Caspi E, Schneider DF, Mor Z, et al. Cervical internal os cerclage. Description of new technique and comparison with Shirodkar operation. Am J Perinatol. 1990;7:347-9.

99. Castadot RG. Pregnancy termination: Techniques, risks, and complications and their management. Fertil Steril. 1986;45:5.

100. Castaneda S, Karrison T, Cibils LA. Peripartum hysterectomy. J Perinat Med. 2000;28(6):472-81.

101. Caughey AB, Hopkins LM, Norton ME. Chorionic villus sampling compared with amniocentesis and the difference in the rate of pregnancy loss. Obstet Gynecol. 2006;108(3 Pt 1):612-6.

102. Caughey AB, Sandberg PL, Zlatnik MG, et al. Forceps compared with vacuum: rates of neonatal and maternal morbidity. Obstet Gynecol. 2005;106(5 pt 1):908-912.

103. Center for disease control. Recommendations to prevent and control iron deficiency in the United States. MMWR 1998; 47(No. RR-3) p. 51 [online] Available from http://www.cdc.gov/[Accessed April 2009]

104. Chamberlain G, Wraight A, Steer P. Pain and its relief in labor: Report of the 1990 NBT survey. Churchill Livingstone, Edinburgh 1993.

105. Chan YK, Ng KP. Regional Analgesia in Obstetrics in the Far East. In Felicity Reynolds (Ed): Regional Analgesia in Obstetrics—a millenium update. London: Springer-Verlag; 2000. pp. 73-8.

106. Chapron C, Vercellini P, Barakat H, et al. Management of ovarian endometriomas. Hum Reprod Update. 2002;8(6):591-7.

107. Chemotherapy for advanced ovarian cancer. Advanced ovarian cancer triallists group. The Cochrane Database of Systematic Reviews. 2006. Issue 1.

108. Chen LH, Lai SF, Lee WH, et al. Uterine perforation during elective first-trimester abortions: A 13-year review. Singapore Med J. 1995;36:63.

109. Cheng YW, Hopkins LM, Caughey AB. How long is too long: does a prolonged second stage of labor in nulliparous women affect maternal and neonatal outcomes? Am J Obstet Gynecol. 2004;191(3):933-8.

110. Cheong Y, Ledger WL. Hysteroscopy and hysteroscopic surgery. Obstet Gynecol Reprod Med. 2007;17:99-104.

111. Cherney LS. A modified transverse incision for low abdominal operations. Surg Gynecol Obstet. 1941;72:92.

112. Chou MM, Ho ES, Lee YH. Prenatal diagnosis of placenta previa accreta by transabdominal color Doppler ultrasound. Ultrasound Obstet Gynecol. 2000;15:28-35.

113. Chou MM, Hwang JI, Tseng JJ, et al. Internal iliac artery embolization before hysterectomy for placenta accreta. J Vasc Interv Radiol. 2003;14:1195-9.

114. Christianson LM, Bovbjerg VE, McDavitt EC, et al. Risk factors for perineal injury during delivery. Am J Obstet Gynecol. 2003;189(1): 255-60.

115. Clark SL, Koonings PP, Phelan JP. Placenta previa/accreta and prior cesarean section. Obstet Gynecol. 1985;66:89-92.

116. Clark SL, Phelan JP, Yeh SY, et al. Hypogastric artery ligation for obstetric hemorrhage. Obstet Gynecol. 1985;66:353-6.

117. Clark SL. Rupture of the scarred uterus. Obstet Gynecol Clin North Am. 1988;15(4):737-44.

118. Clarke-Pearson DL, Creasman WT, Coleman ER, et al. Perioperative external pneumatic compression as thromboembolism prophylaxis in gynecologic oncology: Report of a randomized clinical trial. Gynecol Oncol. 1984;18:226.

119. CLASP (Collaborative Lowdose Aspirin Study in Pregnancy). A randomized trial of lowdose aspirin for prevention and treatment of preeclampsia among 9364 pregnant women. Lancet. 1994;343(8898):619-29.

120. Coco AS, Silverman SD. External Cephalic Version. Am Fam Physician. 1998;58(3):731-8, 742-4.

121. Cohen J. Laparoscopic procedures for treatment of infertility related to polycystic ovarian syndrome. Hum Reprod Update. 1996;2(4): 337-44.

122. Combs CA, Murphy EL, Laros RK. Factors associated with postpartum hemorrhage in cesarean birth. Obstet Gynecol. 1991;77:77-82.

123. Combs CA. Murphy EL. Factors associated with postpartum hemorrhage with vaginal birth. Obstet Gynecol. 1991;77:69-76.

124. Comstock CH, Love JJ, Bronsteen RA, et al. Sonographic detection of placenta accreta in the second and third trimesters of pregnancy. Am J Obstet Gynecol. 2004;190:1135-40.

125. Comstock CH. Antenatal diagnosis of placenta accreta: a review. Ultrasound Obstet Gynecol. 2005;26:89-96.

126. Crandon AJ, Peel KR. Amniocentesis with and without ultrasound guidance. Br J Obstet Gynaecol. 1979;86(1):1-3.

127. Crawshaw R, Link C. Evolution of form and circumstance in medical oaths. West J Med. 1996;164:452-6.

128. Creasy RK, Resnik R, Iams JD. Maternal Fetal Medicine. In: Principles and Practice. 5th ed. Philadelphia, Pa: WB Saunders; 2004.

129. Cruikshank DP, White CA. Obstetric malpresentations: Twenty years' experience. Am J Obstet Gynecol. 1973;116(8): 1097-104.

130. Cruikshank DP. Breech presentation. Clin Obstet Gynecol. 1986;29:255-63.

131. Cunanan RG, Courey NG, Lippes J. Complications of laparoscopic tubal sterilization. Obstet Gynecol. 1980;55(4):501-6.

132. Cunningham FG, Gant NF, Leveno KJ. Williams Obstetrics. 22nd ed. New York, NY: McGraw-Hill; 2005.

133. DA Grimes, IG Ray, CJ Middleeton. Lamicel versus laminaria for cervical dialation before early second trimester abortion a randomized clinical trial. Obstetrics and Gynecology. 1987;69:887-90.

134. Dabirashrafi H. Complications of laparoscopic ovarian cauterization. Fertil Steril. 1989;52:878.

135. Damos JR, Bassett R. Chapter H: assisted vaginal delivery. In: Advanced Life Support in Obstetrics (ALSO) Provider Syllabus. 4th edition. Leawood, Kan.: American Academy of Family Physicians; 2003:3-8.

136. Daniell JF, Miller W. Polycystic ovaries treated by laparoscopic laser vaporization. Fertil Steril. 1989;51:232.

137. Darai E, Deval B, Darles C, et al. Myomectomy: laparoscopy or laparotomy. Contracept Fertil. 1996;24:751-6.

138. Dauphin-McKenzie N, Celestin MJ, Brown D, et al. The advanced life support in obstetrics course as an orientation tool for obstetrics and gynecology residents. Am J Obstet Gynecol. 2007;196(5):e27-e8.

139. De Maeyer EM et al. Preventing and controlling iron deficiency anaemia through primary health care. Geneva, World Health Organization, 1989.

140. De Swiet M. Cardiac disease. In: Lewis G, Drife J, (eds). Why mothers die 1997–1999. The Confidential enquiries intomaternal deaths in the United Kingdom. London: Royal College of Obstetricians and Gynaecologists. 2001;153-64.

141. DeCherney AH, et al. Current Obstetric and Gynecologic Diagnosis and Treatment, 9th edition. New York: McGraw-Hill Medical; 2003.

142. Dell DL, Sightler SE, Plauche WC. Soft cup vacuum extraction: a comparison of outlet delivery. Obstet Gynecol. 1985;66(5):624-8.

143. Deng L, Yan X, Zhang J, et al. Combination chemotherapy for high-risk gestational trophoblastic tumor. Cochrane Database of Systematic Reviews 2006, Issue 3. Art. No.: CD005196. DOI:10.1002/14651858.CD005196.pub2

144. Dennen EH, Dennen PC: Dennen's forceps deliveries, 3rd edition. Philadelphia:FA Davis;1989.

145. Department of Health. National Service Framework for Diabetes: Standards. London: Department of Health; 2002.

146. Derman RJ, et al. Oral misoprostol in preventing postpartum hemorrhage in resource-poor communities: a randomised controlled trial. Lancet. 2006;368:1248-53.

147. Di Renzo GC, Luzietti R, Gerli S, et al. The ten commandments in multiple pregnancies. Twin Res. 2001;4(3):159-64.

148. Di Spiezio Sardo A, Mazzon I, Bramante S, et al. Hysteroscopic myomectomy: a comprehensive review of surgical techniques. Hum Reprod Update. 2008;14(2):101-19.

149. Dodd JM, Crowther CA. Evidence based care for women with a multiple pregnancy. Best Pract Res Clin Obstet Gynaecol. 2005;19(1):131-53.

150. Donald I (Ed): Practical Obstetric Problems. London: Lloyd-Luke; 1969. p. 608.

151. Druzin ML. Packing of lower uterine segment for control of post cesarean bleeding in instances of placenta previa. Surg Gynecol Obstet. 1989;169:543-5.

152. Dubuisson JB, Chavet X, Chapron C, et al. Uterine rupture during pregnancy after laparoscopic myomectomy. Hum Reproduct. 1995;10:1475-7.

153. Dubuisson JB, Morice P, Chapron C, et al. Salpingectomy: the laparoscopic surgical choice for ectopic pregnancy. Hum Reprod. 1996;11(6):1199-203.

154. Duley L, Gulmezoglu AM, Henderson-Smart DJ. Magnesium sulfate and other anticonvulsants for women with preeclampsia (Cochrane Review). The Cochrane Library. 2003:CD000025.

155. Dyer SJ, Tregoning SK. Laparoscopic reconstructive tubal surgery in a tertiary referral centre. A review of 177 cases. S Afr Med J. 2000;90:1015-9.

156. Dysfunctional uterine bleeding. In: Speroff L, Glass RH, Kase NG, (Eds). Clinical gynecologic endocrinology and infertility. 5th edition. Baltimore: Williams and Wilkins; 1994:531-46.

157. Edwards JE, Darney PD, Paul M. Surgical abortion in the first trimester. In: Paul M, Lichtenberg ES, Borgatta L, et al (Eds). A Clinician's Guide to Medical and Surgical Abortion. New York: Churchill Livingstone;1999. pp. 107–21.

158. Elancey JO. Anatomy and biomechanics of genital prolapse. Clin Obstet Gynecol. 1993;36(4):897-909.

159. Ellis H, Bucknail T, Cox P. Abdominal incisions and their closure: current problems in surgery. Chicago: Year Book Medical Publishers; 1985.

160. Emanuel MH, Wamsteker K, Hart AA, et al. Long-term results of hysteroscopic myomectomy for abnormal uterine bleeding. Obstet Gynecol. 1999;93(5 Pt 1):743-8.

161. Emanuel MH, Wamsteker K. Uterine leiomymas. In: Brosens I, Wamsteker K (Eds). Diagnostic Imaging and Endoscopy in Gynecology. London: WB Saunders; 1997. pp. 185-98.

162. Enkin MW, Wilkinson C. Single vesus two layer suturing for closing the uterine incision at cesarean section. Cochrane Database Syst Rev. 2000;(2):CD 000192.

163. Fanning J, Pruett A, Flora RF. Feasibility of the Maylard transverse incision for ovarian cancer cytoreductive surgery. J Minim Invasive Gynecol. 2007;14(3):352-5.

164. Farhi J S, et al. Effect of Laparoscopic ovarian electrocautery on ovarian response and outcome of treatment with gonadotrophins in clomphene citrate resistant patients with PCOS. Fertil Steril. 1995;64:930-5.

165. Farmer RM, Kirschbaum T, Potter D, et al. Uterine rupture during trial of labor after previous cesarean section. Am J Obstet Gynecol. 1991;165:996-1001.

166. Farmer RM, Kirschbaum T, Potter D, et al. Uterine rupture during trial of labor after previous cesarean section. Am J Obstet Gynecol. 1991;165(4 Pt 1):996-1001.

167. Farquhar CM. Ectopic pregnancy. Lancet. 2005;366(9485):583-91.

168. Figge DC, Gaudenz R. Invasive carcinoma of the vulva. Am J Obstet Gynecol. 1974;119:382-95.

169. Filshie GM, Casey D, Pogmore JR, et al. The titanium/silicone rubber clip for female sterilization. Br J Obstet Gynaecol. 1981;88(6):655-62.

170. Flamm BL. Once a cesarean, always a controversy. Obstet Gynecol. 1997;90:312.

171. Franchi M, Ghezzi F, Raio L, et al. Joel-Cohen or Pfannenstiel incision at cesarean delivery: does it make a difference? Acta Obstet Gynecol Scand. 2002;81(11):1040-6.

172. Frank RT. Formation of an artificial vagina without operation. Am J Obstet Gynecol. 1938;35:1053.

173. Frenckner B, Euler CV. Influence of pudendal block on the function of the anal sphincters. Gut. 1975;16:482-9.

174. Friedman EA. Labor. In: Clinical evaluation and management. New York, NY: Appleton-Century-Crofts; 1967:34.

175. Friedman EA. Midforceps delivery: no? Clin Obstet Gynecol. 1987;30(1):93-105.

176. Friedman EA. Patterns of labor as indicators of risk. Clin Obstet Gynecol. 1973;16(1):172-83.

177. Friedman W, Maier RF, Luttkus A, et al. Uterine rupture after laparoscopic myomectomy. Acta Obstet Gynecol Scand. 1996;75:683-4.

178. Gabbe SG, Niebyl JR, Simpson JL. Obstetrics Normal and Problem Pregnancies. 5th ed. New York: Churchill Livingstone; 2007.

179. Gamlins FMC, Lyons G. Spinal analgesia in labor. International Journal of Obstetric Anesthesia 1997; 6:161-72.

180. Garry R. Towards evidence-based hysterectomy. Gynaecological Endoscopy. 1998;7:225-33

181. Geary M, McParland P, Johnson H, et al. Shoulder dystocia—is it predictable? Eur J Obstet Gynecol Reprod Biol. 1995;62:15-8.

182. Gehlbach DL, Sousa RC, Carpenter SE, et al. Abdominal myomectomy in the treatment of infertility. Int J Gynecol Obstet. 1993;40:45-50.

183. Geisthovel L. A Comment on European Society of Human Reproduction and Embryology/American Society of Reproductive Medicine, Consensus of the Polycystic Ovarian Syndrome. Reprod Biomed Online. 2003;7(6):602-5.

184. Gemer O, Segal S. Incidence and contribution of predisposing factors to transverse lie presentation. Int J Gynaecol Obstet. 1994;44: 219-21.

185. Gestational trophoblastic diseases: Report of a WHO scientific group. WHO Tech Rep Ser. 1983;692:51.

186. Gherman RB, Goodwin TM, Souter I, et al. The McRobert's maneuver for the alleviation of shoulder dystocia: how successful is it? Am J Obstet Gynecol. 1997;176:656-61.

187. Gherman RB, Ouzounian JG, Goodwin TM. Obstetric maneuvers for shoulder dystocia and associated fetal morbidity. Am J Obstet Gynecol. 1998;178:1126-30.

188. Gherman RB, Ouzounian JG, Miller DA, et al. Spontaneous vaginal delivery: a risk factor for Erb's palsy? Am J Obstet Gynecol. 1998;178:423-7.

189. Gherman RB, Tramont J, Muffley P, et al. Analysis of McRobert's maneuver by x-ray pelvimetry. Obstet Gynecol. 2000;95:43-7.

190. Gielchinsky Y, Mankuta D, Rojansky N, et al. Perinatal outcome of pregnancies complicated by placenta accreta. Obstet Gynecol. 2004;104:527-30.

191. Giorlandino C, Mobili L, Bilancioni E, et al. Transplacental amniocentesis: is it really a high-risk procedure? Prenat Diagn. 1994;14: 803-6.

192. Gjonnaess H. Polycystic ovarian syndrome treated by ovarian cautery through the laparoscope. Fertil Steril. 1984;41:20-5.

193. Gleeson R, Farrell J, Doyle M, et al. HELLP syndrome: A condition of varied. presentation. Ir J Med Sci. 1996;165:265-7.

194. Goldberg J, Pereira L, Berghella V. Pregnancy after uterine artery embolization. Obstet Gynecol. 2002;100:869-72.

195. Goldberg, J, Holtz D, Hyslop T, et al. "Has the use of routine episiotomy decreased? Examination of episiotomy rates from 1983 to 2000." Obstetrics and Gynecology. 2002;99:395-400.

196. Gomel V, Swolin K. Salpingostomy: microsurgical techniques and results. Clin Obstet Gynecol. 1980;23:1243-58.

197. Gomel V. Clinical results of infertility microsurgery. In: Crosignani PG, Rubin BL (Eds). Microsurgery in Female Infertility. London: Academic Press; 1980. pp. 1269.

198. Gomel V. From microsurgery to laparoscopic surgery: a progress. Fertil Steril. 1995;43(3):464-8.

199. Gomel V. Microsurgery in Female Infertility. Boston: Lottle, Brown; 1983.

200. Gomel V. Reconstructive surgery of the oviduct. J Reprod Med. 1977;18:181-90.

201. Gomel V. Salpingostomy by microsurgery. Fertil Steril. 1978;29:380-7.

202. Gordon MC, Narula K, O'Shaughnessy R, et al. Complications of third-trimester amniocentesis using continuous ultrasound guidance. Obstet Gynecol 2002 Feb; 99(2):255–59.

203. Graczykowski JW, Mishell DR. Methotrexate prophylaxis for persistant ectopic pregnancy after conservative treatment by salpingostomy. Obstet Gynecol. 1997;89(1):118-22.

204. Greenberg JI, Suliman A, Iranpour P, et al. Prophylactic balloon occlusion of the internal iliac arteries to treat abnormal placentation: a cautionary case. Am J Obstet Gynecol. 2007;197:470e1-e4.

205. Greenblatt EM, Casper RF. Adhesion formation after laparoscopic ovarian cautery for polycystic ovarian syndrome: lack of correlation with pregnancy rate. Fertil Steril. 1993;60:766-9.

206. Greenwall MJ, Evans M, Pollock AV. Midline or transverse laparotomy? A random controlled clinical trial. Br J Surg. 1980;67(3):191-4.

207. Greis JB, Bieniarz J, Scommegna A: Comparison of maternal and fetal effects of vacuum extraction with forceps or cesarean deliveries. Obstet Gynecol. 1981;57:571.

208. Grimbizis GF, Camus M, Tarlatzis BC, et al. Clinical implications of uterine malformations and hysteroscopic treatment results. Hum Reprod Update. 2001;7:161-74.

209. Grimes DA, Schulz KF, Cates WJ. Prevention of uterine perforation during curettage abortion. JAMA. 1984;251:2108.

210. Grimes DA, Wallach M. Female sterilization. In: Grimes DA, Wallach M, (Eds). Modern Contraception: Updates from the Contraception Report. Totowa, NJ: Emron; 1997:167-90.

211. Grimes DA. Management of abortion in TeLinde's Operative Gynecology, 9th edition. Philadelphia: Lippincot Williams & Wilkins;1997. p. 8.

212. Gross SJ, Shime J, Farine D. Shoulder dystocia: predictors and outcome. A five-year review. Am J Obstet Gynecol. 1987;156:334-6.

213. Grosvenor A, Silver R, Porter TF, et al. Optimal management of placenta accreta. Am J Obste Gynecol. 2007;195:S82.

214. Gupta D, Sinha R. Management of placenta accreta with oral methotrexate. Int J Gynaecol Obstet. 1998;60:171-3.

215. Gurewitsch ED, Johnson TL, Allen RH. After shoulder dystocia: managing the subsequent pregnancy and delivery. Semin Perinatol. 2007;31(3):185-95.

216. Gyamfi C, Juhasz G, Gyamfi P, et al. Single versus double–layer uterine incision closure and uterine rupture. J Mater Fetal Neonatal Med. 2006;19:639-43.

217. Habek D, Vranjes M, Bobic Vukovic M, et al. Successful term pregnancy after B-Lynch compression suture in a previous pregnancy on account of massive primary postpartum hemorrhage. Fetal Diagn Ther. 2006;21(5):475-6.

218. Hahnemann N, Mohr J. Genetic diagnosis in the embryo by means of biopsy from extra-embryonic membrane. Bull Eur Soc Hum Genet. 1968;2:23-9.

219. Hajenius PJ, Mol F, Mol BW, et al. Interventions for tubal ectopic pregnancy. Cochrane Database Syst Rev. 2007;(1):CD000324.

220. Hale R. Dennen's Forceps Deliveries. 4th edition. Philadelphia:FA Davis; 2001.

221. Hallez JP. Single stage total hysteroscopic myomectomies: indications, techniques and results. Fertil Steril. 1995;63:703-8.

222. Hammond, Charles B. Gynecology: The Female Reproductive Organs. In: Sabiston Textbook of Surgery. Philadelphia: W. B. Saunders Company; 2001.

223. Hankins GD, Clark SL. Brachial plexus palsy involving the posterior shoulder at spontaneous vaginal delivery. Am J Perinatol. 1995;12: 44-5.

224. Hannah ME, Hannah WJ, Hewson SA, et al. Planned cesarean section versus planned vaginal birth for breech presentation at term: A randomised multicentre trial. Lancet. 2000;356:1375-83.

225. Harkki-Siren P, Kurki T. A nationwide analysis of laparoscopic complications. Obstet Gynecol. 1997;89:108-12.

226. Harley JM. Cesarean section. Clin Obstet Gynaecol. 1980;7(3):529-59 (Review).

227. Harris WJ. Uterine dehiscence following laparoscopic myomectomy. Obstet and Gynecol. 1992;80(3):545-6.

228. Hartmann K, Vishwanathan M, Palmieri R, et al. Outcomes of routine episiotomy. JAMA. 2005;293:2141-8.

229. Hawkins, Joy L, David H. Obstetric Anesthesia. Obstetrics: Normal & Problem Pregnancies. In: Chestnut, Charles P. Gibbs. (Eds). Philadelphia: Churchill Livingstone; 2002.

230. Haxton H. The influence of suture materials and methods on the healing of abdominal wounds. Br J Surg. 1965;52:372.

231. Hayashi RH. Midforceps delivery: yes? Clin Obstet Gynecol. 1987;30(1):90-2.

232. Healy DL, Laufe LE. Survey of obstetric forceps training in North America in 1981. Am J Obstet Gynecol. 1985;151(1):54.

233. Helmkamp BF, Krebs HB. The Maylard incision in gynecologic surgery. Am J Obstet Gynecol. 1990;163(5 Pt 1):1554-7.

234. Hendrix SL, Schimp V, Martin J, et al. The legendary superior strength of the Pfannenstiel incision: a myth? Am J Obstet Gynecol. 2000;182(6):1446-51.

235. Herman JB. Tensile strength and knot security of surgical suture materials. Am Surg. 1971;37:209.

236. Herrmann JB. Changes in tensile strength and knot security of surgical sutures in vivo. Arch Surg. 1973;106:707.

237. Hillis SD, Marchbanks PA, Peterson HB. Uterine size and risk of complications among women undergoing abdominal hysterectomy for leiomyomas. Obstet Gynecol. 1996;87:539-43.

238. Hofmeyr GJ, Walraven G, Gulmesoglu AM, et al. Misoprostol to treat postpartum hemorrhage: A systemic review. Br J Obstet Gynecol. 2005;112:547-53.

239. Holland Brew's Textbook of Obstetrics, 14th edition. Churchill Livingstone.

240. Homer HA, Li TC, Cooke ID. The septate uterus: a review of management and reproductive outcome. Fertil Steril. 2000;73:1-14.

241. Hong TM, Tseng HS, Lee RC, et al. Uterine artery embolization: an effective treatment for intractable obstetric haemorrhage. Clin Radiol. 2004;59:96-101.

242. Hope E, Frith P, Craze J, et al. Developing guidelines for medical students about the examination of patients under 18 years old. BMI. 2007;331:1384-6.

243. Howes EL, Harvey SC. The strength of the healing wound in relation to the holding strength of the chromic catgut suture. N Engl J Med. 1929;200:1285.

244. Hsu S, Mitwally MF, Aly A, et al. Laparoscopic management of tubal ectopic pregnancy in obese women. Fertil Steril. 2004;81(1): 198-202.

245. Hsu S, Rodgers B, Lele A, et al. Use of packing in obstetric hemorrhage of uterine origin. J Reprod Med. 2003;48:69-71.

246. Hung TH, Shau WY, Hsieh CC, et al. Risk factors for placenta accreta. Obstet Gynecol. 1999;93:545.

247. Hurd WW, Pearl ML, DeLancey JO, et al. Laparoscopic injury of abdominal wall blood vessels: a report of three cases. Obstet Gynecol. 1993;82(4 Pt 2 Suppl):673-6.

248. International Classification of Diseases (ICD version 2007). Pregnancy, childbirth and the puerperium: Complications of labour and delivery. World Health Organization website [online] Available from http://www.who.int/classifications/apps/icd/icd10online/?go60. htm+o68 [accessed September 2008].

249. International Confederation of Midwives (ICM) and the International Federation of Gynecology and Obstetrics (FIGO). Management of the third stage of labour to prevent postpartum hemorrhage. J Obstet Gynaecol Can. 2003;25(11):952-3.

250. Iversen T, Abeler V, Aalders J. Individualization of treatment for stage 1 squamous cell vulvar carcinoma. Obstet Gynecol. 1981;57:85-9.

251. Jacinto MS, Madan S. Iron deficiency anemia. Pharmacist. 2000;HS39-HS48.

252. Jackson LG, Zachary JM, Fowler SE, et al. A randomized comparison of transcervical and transabdominal chorionic-villus sampling. The U.S. National Institute of Child Health and Human Development Chorionic Villus Sampling Amniocentesis Study Group. N Engl J Med. 1992;327(9):594-8.

253. Jamieson DJ, Hillis SD, Duerr A, et al. Complications of interval laparoscopic tubal sterilization: findings from the United States Collaborative Review of Sterilization. Obstet Gynecol. 2000;96(6):997-1002.

254. Janni W, Schiessl B, Peschers U, et al. The prognostic impact of a prolonged second stage of labor on maternal and fetal outcome. Acta Obstet Gynecol Scand. 2002;81(3):214-21.

255. Jansen FW, Vredevoogd CB, van Ulzen K, et al. Complications of hysteroscopy: a prospective, multicenter study. Obstet Gynecol. 2000;96:266-70.

256. Jeanty P, Rodesch F, Romero R, et al. How to improve your amniocentesis technique? Am J Obstet Gynecol. 1983;146(6):593-6.

257. Jeffcoate N. Hysterectomy and its aftermath. In: Kumar P, Malhotra N (Eds). Jeffcoate's Principles of gynaecology, 7th edition. New Delhi: Jaypee brothers; 2008.

258. Johanson R, Menon V. Soft versus rigid vacuum extractor cups for assisted vaginal delivery. Cochrane Database Syst Rev. 2000;(2):CD000446.

259. Johanson R. Choice of instrument for vaginal delivery. Curr Opin Obstet Gynecol. 1997;9:361-5.

260. Johanson RB, Menon BK. Vacuum extraction versus forceps for assisted vaginal delivery. Cochrane DatabaseSyst Rev.

2000;(2):CD000224.

261. John OL DeLancy. Surgical anatomy of female pelvis. In: John A Rock, Howard W Jones II (Eds). Telinde Operative Gynecology. Philladelphia: Lippincott William ana Wilkins; 2009. pp. 82-112.

262. Johnson JH, Figueroa R, Garry D, et al. Immediate maternal and neonatal effects of forceps and vacuum-assisted deliveries. Obstet Gynecol. 2004;103(3):513-8.

263. Johnson N, Barlow D, Lethaby A, et al. Methods of hysterectomy: systematic review and meta-analysis of randomised controlled trials. BMJ. 25 2005;330(7506):1478.

264. Jones HW, Rock JA (Eds). Surgery for correction of defects in pelvic support and pelvic fistulas. Te Linde's Operative Gynecology. 10th edition. Philadelphia: JB Lippincott; 2008. pp. 720-3.

265. Jones HW. Abdominal hysterectomy. In: Rock JA, Jones HW (Eds). Te Linde's Operative Gynecology 10th edition. Philadelphia: Lippincott Williams & Wilkin; 2008.

266. Joshi VM, Shrivastava M. Partial ischemic necrosis of the uterus following a uterine brace compression suture. BJOG. 2004;111(3): 279-80.

267. Kadar N. A laparoscopic technique for dissecting the pelvic retroperitoneum and identifying the ureters. J Reprod Med. 1995;40:116-22.

268. Kalogiannidis I, Lambrechts S, Amant F,et al. Laparoscopy-assisted vaginal hysterectomy compared with abdominal hysterectomy in clinical stage I endometrial cancer: safety, recurrence, and long-term outcome. Am J Obstet Gynecol. 2007;196:248.1-8.

269. Kane-Low, Lisa, Seng J, et al. "Clinician-specific episiotomy rates: impact on perineal outcomes." Journal of Midwifery and Women's Health. 2000;45:87-93.

270. Kaser O, Ikg FA, Hirsch HA. Atlas of Gynecologic Surgery, 2nd edition. New York, Thieme-Stratton; 1985. pp. 6.1-6.9

271. Kayem G, Davy C, Goffinet F, et al. Conservative versus extirpative management in cases of placenta accreta. Obstet Gynecol. 2004;104:531-6.

272. Keder LM. Best practices in surgical abortion. Am J Obstet Gynecol. 2003;189(2):418-22.

273. Kelly H. Ligation of both internal iliac arteties for haemorrhage in hysterectomy for carcinoma uterus. John Hopkins Med J. 1894;5:53-4.

274. Kennedy S, Bergqvist A, Chapron C, et al. ESHRE guideline for the diagnosis and treatment of endometriosis. Human Reprod. 2005;20(10):2698-704.

275. Kerin JF, Munday DN, Ritossa MG, et al. Essure hysteroscopic sterilization: results based on utilizing a new coil catheter delivery system. J Am Assoc Gynecol Laparosc. 2004;11(3):388-93.

276. Kerr JN. The lower uterine segment incision in conservative cesarean section. J Obstet Gynecol Br Emp. 1921;28:475.

277. Khamashta MA, Hughes GR. ACP Broadsheet no 136: February 1993. Detection and importance of anticardiolipin antibodies. J Clin Pathol. 1993;46:104-7.

278. Khan KS, Rizvi A. The partograph in the management of labor following cesarean section. Int J Gynaecol Obstet. 1995;50(2):151-7.

279. Khan KS, Wojdyla D, Say L, et al. WHO analysis of causes of maternal death: a systematic review. Lancet. 2006;367(9516):1066-74.

280. Khong TY, Healy DL, McCloud PI. Pregnancies complicated by abnormally adherent placenta and sex ratio at birth. BMJ. 1991;302: 625-6.

281. Kilpatrick SJ, Laros RK. Characteristics of normal labor. Obstet Gynecol. 1989;74(1):857.

282. Kim AH, Adamson GD. Surgical treatment options for endometriosis. Clin Obstet Gynecol. 1999;42(3):633-44.

283. Kirkinen P, Helin-Martikainen HL, Vanninen R, et al. Placenta accreta: imaging by gray-scale and contrast-enhanced color Doppler sonography and magnetic resonance imaging. J Clin Ultrasound. 1998;26:90-4.

284. Korttila K. Recovery from outpatient anesthesia. Anesthesia. 1995;50(suppl):22-8.

285. Kovacs G, Buckler H, Bangah M, et al. Treatment of anovulation due to PCOS by laparoscopic ovarian cautery. Br J Obstet. Gynaecol. 1991;98(1):30-5.

286. Kripalaani A, Manchanda R, et al. Laparoscopic ovarian drilling in clomiphene resistant women with polycystic ovarian syndrome. J Am Assoc. Gynaecol laprosc. 2001;8(4):511-8.

287. Kumpf VJ, Holland EG. Parenteral iron dextran therapy. DICP. 1990;24(2):162-6.

288. Kupferminc MJ, Tamura RK, Wigton TR, et al. Placenta accreta is associated with elevated maternal serum alpha fetoprotein. Obstet Gynecol. 1993;82:266-9.

289. Labor: clinical evaluation and management. New York (NY): Appleton Century Crofts; 1978

290. lbers LL, Schiff M, Gorwoda JG. The length of active labor in normal pregnancies. Obstet Gynecol. 1996;87(3):355-9.

291. Leach RE, Ory SJ. Modern management of ectopic pregnancy. J Reprod Med. 1989;34(5):324-38.

292. Lemons JA, Vargas P, Delaney JJ. Infant of the diabetic mother. Review of 225 cases. Obstet Gynecol. 1981;57:187-92.

293. Lentz GM. Anatomic defects of the abdominal wall and pelvic floor: abdominal and inguinal hernias, cystocele, urethrocele, enterocele, rectocele, uterine and vaginal prolapse and rectal incontinence: Diagnosis and Management. In: Katz VL, LentzGM, Lobo RA, Gershenson DM (Eds). Comprehensive Gynecology. 5th edition. Philadelphia: Mosby Elsevier; 2007.

294. Letterie GS. Structural abnormalities and reproductive failure: Effective techniques of diagnosis and management. New York: Blackwell Science; 1998.

295. Levallois P, Rioux JE. Prophylactic antibiotics for suction curettage abortion: Results of a clinical controlled trial. Am J Obstet Gynecol. 1988;158:100.

296. Leveno KJ. Controversies in ob-gyn: Should we rethink the criteria for VBAC? Contemporary OB/GYN;1999.

297. Levgur M, Duvivier R. Pelvic inflammatory disease after tubal sterilization: a review. Obstet Gynecol Surv. 2000;55(1):41-50.

298. Levine D, Hulka CA, Ludmir J, et al. Placenta accreta: evaluation with color Doppler US, and MR imaging. Radiology. 1997;205:773-6.

299. Levine JS, Branch DW, Rauch J. The antiphospholipid syndrome. N Engl J Med. 2002;346:752-63.

300. Li TC, Mortimer R, Cooke ID. Myomectomy: a retrospective study to examine reproductive performance before and after surgery. Hum Reprod. 1999;14(7):1735-40.

301. Lichtenberg ES, Grimes DA, Paul M. Abortion complications: Prevention and management. In: Paul M, Lichtenberg ES, Borgatta L, et al (Eds). A Clinician's Guide to Medical and Surgical Abortion. New York: Churchill Livingstone;1999. p.197.

302. Lijoi, AF, Brady J. Vasa Previa Diagnosis and Management. J Am Board Fam Pract. 2003;16:543-8.

303. Lipscomb GH, Stovall TG, Ramanathan JA, et al. Comparison of silastic rings and electrocoagulation for laparoscopic tubal ligation under local anesthesia. Obstet Gynecol. 1992;80(4):645-9.

304. Long CA, Gast MJ. Menorrhagia. Obstet Gynecol Clin North Am. 1990;17(2):343-59.

305. Loret de Mola JR, Carpenter SE. Management of genital prolapse in neonates and young women. Obstet Gynecol Surv. 1996;51(4):253-60.

306. Lucas MJ. The role of vacuum extraction in modern obstetrics. Clin Obstet Gynecol. 1994;37:794-805.

307. Lundorff P, Hahlin M, Sjoblom P, et al. Persistent trophoblast after conservative treatment of tubal pregnancy: prediction and detection. Obstel Gynecol. 1991;77(1):1129-33.

308. Lyell DJ, Caughey AB, Hu E, et al. Peritoneal closure at primary cesarean delivery and adhesions. Obstet Gynecol. 2005;106:275-80.

309. Mac Naughton MC, Chalmers IG, Dubovitz V, et al. Final report of the medical Royal Committee and Royal College of Obstetrics and Gynecology multicentric randomized trial of cervical cerclage. Br J Obstet Gynecol. 1993;100:156.

310. Magann EF, Evans S, Hutchinson, et al. Postpartum hemorrhage after vaginal birth: An analysis of risk factors. South Med J. 2005;98(4):419-22.

311. Magpie Trial Collaboration Group. Do women with preeclampsia, and their babies, benefit from magnesium sulfate? The Magpie Trial: A randomised placebo controlled trial. Lancet. 2002;359(9321):1877-90.

312. Mais V, Ajossa S, Guerriero S, et al. Laparoscopic versus abdominal myomectomy: a prospective, randomized trial to evaluate benefits in early outcome. Am J Obstet Gynecol. 1996;174(2):654-8.

313. Maldjian C, Adam R, Pelosi M, et al. MRI appearance of placenta percreta and placenta accreta. Magn Reson Imaging. 1999;17:965-71.

314. Mammer EF. Venous thromboeblism. Semin Thrombo Hemost. 1976;2:4.

315. Management of Early Pregnancy Loss. ACOG Practice Bulletin (American College of Obstetricians and Gynecologists) 24 (February), 2001.

316. Marcoux S, Maheux R, Berube S, et al. Laparoscopic surgery in infertile women with minimal and mild endometriosis. New Engl J Med. 1997;97:212-22.

317. Mathai M, Hofmeyr G. Abdominal surgical incisions for cesarean section. Cochrane Database Syst Rev. 2007;24:CD 004453.

318. Mathai M, Sanghvi H, Guidotti RJ, et al. Paracervical block in MCPC (P1). WHO;2000.

319. McIndoe AH, Banister JB. An operation for the case of congenital absence of vagina. BJOG. 1938;45:490

320. McIndoe AH. Treatment of congenital absence and obliterative conditions of vagina. Br J Plast Surg. 1950;2:254.

321. McKee RF, Scott EM. The value of routine preoperative investigations. Annals of the Royal College of Surgeons of England. 1987;69:160-2.

322. Mcpherson K, Metcalfe MA, Herbert A, et al. Severe complications of hysterectomy: the VALUE study. BJOG. 2004;111:688.

323. McQuivey RW. Vacuum assisted delivery: a review. J Matern Fetal Neonatal Med. 2004;16(3):171-80.

324. Meeks GR, Harris RL. Surgical approach to hysterectomy: abdominal, laparoscopy-assisted, or vaginal. Clin Obstet Gynecol. 1997;40(4):886-94.

325. Meeks GR, Trenhaile TR. Management of abdominal incisions. J Pelvic Surg. 2002;8:295-300.

326. Mettler L, Semm K, Shive K. Endoscopic management of adnexal masses. J Soc Laparoendosc Surg. 1997;1(2):103-12.

327. Mettlin C, Jones G, Averette H, et al. Defining and updating the American Cancer Society Guidelines for the cancer-related checkup: Prostate and endometrial cancers. CA Cancer J Clin. 1993;43:42-6.

328. Metzger BE, Coustan DR. Summary and recommendations of the fourth internal workshop-conference on gestational diabetes mellitus. Diabetes Care. 1998;21(2):B161.

329. Mikolajczyk RT, Zhang J, Troendle J, et al. Risk factors for birth canal lacerations in primiparous women. Am J Perinatol. 2008;25(5):259-64.

330. Miller CE, Johnston M, Rundell M. Laparoscopic myomectomy in the infertile woman. J Am Assoc Gynecol Laparosc. 1996;3:525-9.

331. Miller DA, Chollet JA, Goodwin TM. Clinical risk factors for placenta previa-placenta accreta. Am J Obstet Gynecol. 1997;177:210-4.

332. Mintz M. Risks and prophylaxis in laparoscopy: a survey of 100,000 cases. J Reprod Med. 1977;18(5):269-72.

333. Mittleman JS, Edwards WS, McDonald JB. Effectiveness of leg compression in preventing venous stasis. Am J Surg. 1982;144:611.

334. Miyakis S, Lockshin MD, Atsumi T, et al. International consensus statement on an update of the classifi cation criteria for definite antiphospholipid syndrome (APS). Journal of Thrombosis and Haemostasis. 2006;4:295-306.

335. Modlin IM, Kidd M, Lye KD. From the lumen to the laparoscope. Arch Surg. 2004;139:1110-26.

336. Montan S. Medical prevention of pre-eclampsia. Acta Obstet Gynecol Scand Suppl. 1997;164:111-5.

337. Moore CL, Vasquez NF, Lin H, et al. Major vascular injury after laparoscopic tubal ligation. J Emerg Med. 2005;29(1):67-71.

338. Morley GW. Treatment of uterine and vaginal prolapse. Clin Obstet Gynecol. 1996;39(4):959-69.

339. Mozukewich EL, Hutton EK. Elective repeat cesarean delivery versus trial of labour: A metaanalysis of literature from 1989 to 1999. Am J Obstet Gynecol. 2000;183:1187.

340. Munrokerr's Operative Obstetrics,10th edition. Bailliere Tindall.

341. Munshi A, Munshi S. Abdominal hysterectomy. In: Puri R, Malhotra N (Eds). Operative obstetrics and gynecology. New Delhi: Jaypee

Brothers; 2009.

342. Mussalli GM, Shah J, Berck DJ, et al. Placenta accreta and methotrexate therapy: three case reports. J Perinatol. 2000;20:331-4.

343. National high blood pressure education programme: Working group report on high blood pressure in pregnancy. Am J Obstet Gynecol. 2000;183:51.

344. National Institute for Health and Clinical Excellence (March 2008). Diabetes in pregnancy: Management of diabetes and its complications from preconception to the postnatal period. RCOG Press: London.

345. National Institute for Health and Clinical Excellence. Diabetes in Pregnancy: Management of Diabetes and Its Complications from Preconception to the Postnatal Period. London: RCOG Press; 2008.

346. National Institutes of Health: Cesarean childbirth. NIH Publication No. 82–2067. Bethesda MD: US Department of Health and Human Services;1981.

347. Nehzat C, Nehzat F, Silfen S. Laparoscopic myomectomy. Int J Fertil. 1991;36:275-80.

348. Neuwirth RS, Amin HK. Excision of submucous fibroids with hysteroscopic control. Am J Obstet Gynecol. 1976;126:95-9.

349. Neuwirth RS. Hysteroscopic management of symptomatic submucous fibroids. Obstet Gynecol. 1983;62:509-11.

350. Newlands ES, Paradinas FJ, Fisher RA. Recent advances in gestational trophoblastic diseases. Hematol Oncol Clin North Am. 1999;13: 225-42.

351. Nezhat C. The "cons" of laparoscopic myomectomy in women who may reproduce in the future. Int J Fertil Menopausal Stud. 1996;41: 280-3.

352. NICE technology appraisal guidance 156 (2008). Routine antenatal anti-D prophylaxis for women who are rhesus D negative. Review of NICE technology appraisal guidance 41.

353. Nichols DH, Milley PS, Randall CL. Significance of restoration of normal vaginal depth and axis. Obstet Gynecol. 1970;36:251.

354. Nicholson JM. Noncephalic presentation in late pregnancy. BMJ. 2006;333(7568):562-3.

355. Nicolaides K, Brizot M de L, Patel F, et al. Comparison of chorionic villus sampling and amniocentesis for foetal karyotyping at 10-13 weeks' gestation. Lancet. 1994;344:435-9.

356. Norwitz ER, Robinson JN, Repke JT. Labor and delivery. In: Gabbe SG, Niebyl JR, Simpson JL, (Eds). Obstetrics: Normal and problem pregnancies. 3rd edition. New York: Churchill Livingstone;2003.

357. Nouri K, Ott J, Huber JC, et al. Reproductive outcome after hysteroscopic septoplasty in patients with septate uterus—a retrospective cohort study and systematic review of the literature. Reprod Biol Endocrinol. 2010;8(1):52.

358. Nygaard IE, Squatrito RC. Abdominal incisions from creation to closure. Obstet Gynecol Surv. 1996;51(7):429-36.

359. O'Driscoll K, Meagher D. Introduction. In: O'Driscoll K, Meagher D, (Eds). Active Management of Labor. 2nd edition Eastbourne, United Kingdom: Balliere Tindall; 1986.

360. O'Grady JP. Modern instrumental delivery. Baltimore: Williams & Wilkins;1988. pp. 155-85.

361. O'Leary JA. Hemorrhage with uterine artery ligation. Contemp Ob/Gyn Update Surg. 1986;27:13-6.

362. Oakeshott P, Hay P. Best practice in primary care. BMJ. 2006;333:173-4.

363. Ojala K, Perala J, Kariniemi J, et al. Arterial embolization and prophylactic catheterization for the treatment for severe obstetric hemorrhage. Acta Obstet Gynecol Scand. 2005;84:1075-80.

364. Olive DL, Lee KL. Analysis of sequential treatment protocols for endometriosis-associated infertility. Am J Obstet Gynecol. 1986;154: 613-9.

365. Operative vaginal delivery. ACOG Technical Bulletin Number 196—August 1994 (replaces No. 152, February 1991). Int J Gynaecol Obstet. 1994;47(2):179-85.

366. Oppelt P, von Have M, Paulsen M, et al. Female genital malformations and their associated abnormalities. Fertil Steril. 2007;87:335-42.

367. Ory SJ, Nnadi E, Herrmann R. Fertility after ectopic pregnancy. Fertil Steril. 1993;60(2):231-5.

368. Owen J, Iams JD, Hauth JC. Vaginal sonography and cervical incompetence. Am J Obstet Gynecol. 2003;188:586-96.

369. Palmer R. Safety in laparoscopy. J Reprod Med. 1974;13(1):1-5.

370. Papadopoulos NP, Magos A. First-generation endometrial ablation: roller-ball vs loop vs laser. Best Pract Res Clin Obstet Gynaecol. 2007;21(6):915-29.

371. Parikh MN. Emergency Contraception, editorial. J Obs & Gyn Ind. 2002;52:27-9.

372. Park RC, Duff WP. Role of cesarean hysterectomy in modern obstetric practice. Clin Obstet Gynecol. 1980;23(2):601-20.

373. Parker J, Bistis A. Laparoscopic surgical treatment of ectopic pregnancy: salpingectomy or salpingostomy? Aus NZ J Obstet Gynaecol. 1997;37(1):115-7.

374. Parsnezhad ME, et al. Hyperprolactinemia after Laparoscopic ovarian drilling: an unknown phenomenon. Rep Endocrin. 2005;3:3.

375. Pati S, Cullins V. Female sterilization. Evidence. Obstet Gynecol Clin North Am. 2000;27(4):859-99.

376. Patterson RH. A code of ethics. J Neurosurg. 1986;65:271-7.

377. Patton PE. Anatomic uterine defects. Clin Obstet Gynecol. 1994;37:705-21.

378. Paull J. Epidural analgesia for labor. In: Drs David J Birbach, Stephen Gatt, Sanjay Datta (Eds). Textbook of Obstetric Anesthesia. Churchill Livingstone, Philadelphia 2000;145-56.

379. Peacock EE. Wound healing. In: Schwartz SI, Shires GT, Spenser FC (Eds.) Principles of surgery. 3rd edition. New York: Mc Graw-Hill; 1979. pp. 303.

380. Pelage JP, Le Dref O, Mateo J, et al. Life-threatening primary postpartum hemorrhage: treatment with emergency selective arterial embolization. Radiology. 1998;208(2):359-62.

381. Pellegrino ED. The metamorphosis of medical ethics: A 30-year retrospective. JAMA. 1993;269:1158-62.

382. Pennes DR, Bowerman RA, Silver TM, et al. Failed first-trimester pregnancy termination: Uterine anomaly as etiologic factor. J Clin

Ultrasound. 1987;15:165.

383. Peterson CE, Kwann HC. Current concepts of warfarin therapy. Arch Intern Med. 1986;146:581.

384. Peterson HB, Pollack AE, Warshaw JS. Tubal sterilization. In: Rock JA, Thompson JD, (Eds). Te Linde's Op Gynecol. 74(1). 8th edition. Philadelphia: Lippincott-Raven; 1997:529-47.

385. Peterson HB, Xia Z, Hughes JM, et al. The risk of ectopic pregnancy after tubal sterilization. U.S. Collaborative Review of Sterilization Working Group. N Engl J Med. 1997;336(11):762-7.

386. Peterson HB, Xia Z, Hughes JM, et al. The risk of pregnancy after tubal sterilization: findings from the U.S. Collaborative Review of Sterilization. Am J Obstet Gynecol. 1996;174:1161–70.

387. Phelan JP, Boucher M, Mueller E, et al. The nonlaboring transverse lie. A management dilemma. J Reprod Med. 1986;31(3):184-6.

388. Plauché WC. Cesarean hysterectomy: indications, technique and complications. Clin Obstet Gynecol. 1986;29(2):318-28.

389. Plauche WC. Fetal cranial injuries related to delivery with the Malstrom vacuum extractor (review). Obstet Gynecol. 1979;53:750.

390. Podymow T, Phyllis A.Update on the use of antihypertensive drugs in pregnancy. Hypertension. 2008;51:960-69.

391. Polena V, Mergui JL, Perrot N, et al. Long-term results of hysteroscopic myomectomy in 235 patients. Eur J Obstet Gynecol Reprod Biol. 2007;130:232-7.

392. Pollock A. Surgical prophylaxis: The emerging picture. Lancet. 1988;1:225-30.

393. Polyzos NP, Mauri D, Tsioras S, et al. Intraperitoneal dissemination of endometrial cancer cells after hysteroscopy: a systematic review and meta-analysis. Int J Gynecol Cancer. 2010;20(2):261-7.

394. Pouly JL, Mahnes H, Mage G, et al. Conservative laparoscopic treatment of 321 ectopic pregnancies. Fertil Steril. 1986;46:1093-7.

395. Powell J, Gilo N, Foote M, et al. Vacuum and forceps training in residency: experience and self-reported competency. J Perinatol. 2007;27(6):343-6.

396. Prendiville WJ, Elbourne D, McDonald S. Active versus expectant management in the third stage of labor. Cochrane Database Syst Rev. 2000;CD000007.

397. Pritts EA. Fibroids and infertility: a systematic review of the evidence. Obstet Gynecol Surv. 2001;56:483-91.

398. Propst AM, Liberman RF, Harlow BL, et al. Complications of hysteroscopic surgery: predicting patients at risk. Obstet Gynecol. 2000;96:517-20.

399. Randomised trial to assess safety and fetal outcome of early and midtrimester amniocentesis. The Canadian Early and Mid-trimester Amniocentesis Trial (CEMAT) Group. Lancet. 1998;351(9098):242-7.

400. Ranney B, Frederick I. The occasional need for myomectomy. Obstet Gynecol. 1979;53:437-41.

401. Ravina JH, Herbreteau D, Ciraru-Vigneron N, et al. Arterial embololization to treat uterine myomas. Lancet. 1995;46:671-2.

402. Ray JA, Doddi N, Regula D, et al. Polydioxanone (PDS), a novel monofilament synthetic absorbable suture. Surg Gynecol Obstet. 1981;151:497.

403. Ray P, Murphy GJ, Shutt LE. Recognition and management of maternal cardiac disease in pregnancy. British Journal of Anesthesia. 2004;93(3):428-39.

404. Raziel A, Golan A, Ariely S, et al. Repeated ultrasonography and intramuscular methotrexate in the conservative management of residual adherent placenta. J Clin Ultrasound. 1992;20:288-90.

405. RCOG (2004). The management of tubal pregnancy. Guideline No. 21.

406. RCOG. Placenta previa and placenta previa accreta: diagnosis and management. Guideline No. 27. Revised October 2005.

407. Read JA, Cotton DB, Miller FC. Placenta accreta: changing clinical aspects and outcome. Obstet Gynecol. 1980;56:31-4.

408. Reagan MA, Isaacs JH. Office diagnosis of endometrial carcinoma. Prim Care Cancer. 1992;12:49-52.

409. Reich H, DeCaprio J, McGlynn F. Laparoscopic hysterectomy. J Gynecol Surg. 1989;5:213-6.

410. Reich H. Laparoscopic hysterectomy. Surgical Laparoscopy & Endoscopy. Raven Press: New York; 1992;2: pp. 85-8.

411. Reich WT (Ed). Encyclopedia of Bioethics, 2nd edition. New York: Macmillan Publishing Co Inc;1995:2605-30.

412. Devi R, Sreenivas N, Rajangam S. Bad Obstetric History and Infectious Causes. Int J Hum Genet. 2002;2(4):269-71.

413. Reveiz L, Gyte GML, Cuervo LG. Treatments for iron deficiency anemia in pregnancy. Cochrane Database of Systematic Reviews 2007, Issue 1. Art. No.: CD003094. DOI:10.1002/14651858.CD003094.pub2

414. Reynolds F. Pain relief in labor. British Journal of Obstetrics and Gynecology 1993;100:979-83.

415. Ricci JV. Sterilization. In: One Hundred Years of Gynaecology, 1800-1900. Philadelphia: Blakiston Co; 1945:539-40.

416. Rinne KM, Kirkinen PP. What predisposes young women to genital prolapse? Eur J Obstet Gynecol Reprod Biol. 1999;84(1):23-5.

417. Roberts WE. Emergent obstetric management of postpartum hemorrhage. Obstet Gynecol Clin North Am. 1995;22(2):283-302.

418. Roberts, Joyce E. "The 'push' for evidence: management of the second stage." Journal of Midwifery and Women's Health. 2002;47:2-15.

419. Robinson N, Hall G. Preoperative assessment. How to survive in anesthesia? 2nd edition. London: BMJ Publishing group;1977. p. 98.

420. Robinson P, Hall G. Preoperative assessment. How to survive in anesthesia? London: BMJ publishing group; 1997. p. 98.

421. Rock JA, Jones HM. TeLinde's Operative Gynecology, 10th Edition. Philadelphia: Lippincott Williams Wilikins; 2003.

422. Rock JA, Katayama KP, Martin EJ, et al. Factors influencing the success of salpingostomy techniques for distal fimbrial obstruction. Obstet Gynecol. 1978;52(5):591-6.

423. Roemer T, Straube W. Operative Hysteroscopy: A Practical Guide. Berlin: Walter de Gryuter; 1997. pp. 84-9.

424. Roizen MF. Pre-operative Testing. In: Handbook of Preoperative Assessment and Management. Sweitzer B-J (Ed). Lippincott Williams & Wilkins; 2000.

425. Romero R, Jeanty P, Reece EA, et al. Sonographically monitored amniocentesis to decrease intraoperative complications. Obstet Gynaecol. 1985;65(3):426-30.

426. Rosen DM. Learning curve for hysteroscopic sterilisation: lessons from the first 80 cases. Aust N Z J Obstet Gynaecol. 2004;44(1):62-4.

427. Ross MG. Vacuum delivery by soft cup extraction. Contemp Ob Gyn. 1994;39:48-53.

428. Rothman DJ. Strangers at the Bedside. New York: Basic books, 1991.

429. Royal College of Clinicians and Gynaecologists (RCOG). External cephalic version and reducing the incidence of breech presentation. London (UK): Royal College of Clinicians and Gynaecologists; 2006 (Green-top guideline; no. 20a).

430. Royal College of Clinicians and Gynaecologists (RCOG). The management of breech presentation. London: Royal College of Clinicians and Gynaecologists;2006. p. (Green-top guideline; no. 20b).

431. Royal College of Obstericians and Gynecologists (2002). The investigation and management of the small-for-gestational-age fetus. Guideline No. 31

432. Royal College of Obstericians and Gynecologists (2007). A difficult birth: What is shoulder dystocia? [online] Available from http://www.rcog.org.uk/womens-health/clinical-guidance/difficult-birth-what-shoulder-dystocia [Accessed March 2010].

433. Royal College of Obstetricians and Gynecologists (2005). Amniocentesis and chorionic villus sampling. RCOG Website [online] Available from http://www.rcog.org.uk/resources/Public/pdf/aminiocentesis_chorionicjan2005. pdf [accessed August 2008].

434. Royal College of Obstetricians and Gynecologists. The initial management of menorrhagia. Evidence-Based Guidelines No. 1. London, UK: RCOG Press; 1998.

435. Rulin MC. Is salpingostomy the surgical treatment of choice for unruptured tubal pregnancy? Obstet Gynecol. 1995;86(6):1010-3.

436. Rush CB, Entman SS. Pelvic organ prolapse and stress urinary incontinence. Med Clin North Am. 1995;79(6):1473-9.

437. Ryan KJ, Berkowitz RS, Barbieri RL (Eds). Kistner's Gynecology and Women's Health, 7th edition. St. Louis, MO: Mosby, Inc; 1999.

438. Ryder RM, Vaughan MC. Laparoscopic tubal sterilization. Methods, effectiveness, and sequelae. Obstet Gynecol Clin North Am. 1999;26(1):83-97.

439. Sanders B. Uterine factors and infertility. J Reprod Med. 2006;51:169-76.

440. Sanders RJ, Di Ciemente D. Principles of abdominal wound closure: II. Prevention of wound dehiscence. Arch Surg. 1977;112:1188.

441. Sandmire HF, DeMott RK. Erb's palsy: concepts of causation. Obstet Gynecol. 2000;956(pt 1):941-2.

442. Sanz LE. Wound management: technique and suture material. In: Gynecologic surgery. Sanz LE. (Ed). Ordell, NJ: Medical Economic Books; 1988: pp. 21.

443. Sartore A, De Seta F, Maso G, et al. The effects of mediolateral episiotomy on pelvic floor function after vaginal delivery. Obstet Gynecol. 2004;103:669-73.

444. Savare J. Hetrotopic pregnancies after in-vitro fertilization and embryo tranfer. A Danish survey. Human Reproduction. 1993;8:116.

445. Sawin SW, Pilevsky ND, Berlin JA, et al. Comparability of perioperative morbidity between abdominal myomectomy and hysterectomy for women with uterine leiomyomas. Am J Obstet Gynecol. 2000;183:1448-55.

446. Sawin SW, Pilevsky ND, Berlin JA, et al. Comparability of perioperative morbidity between abdominal myomectomy and hysterectomy for women with uterine leiomyomas. Am J Obstet Gynecol. 2000;183(6):1448-55.

447. Schecter WP, Bongard FS, Gainor BJ, et al. Pain control in outpatient surgery. J Am Coll Surg. 2002;195:95-104.

448. Schemmel M, Haefner HK, Selvaggi SM, et al. Comparison of the ultrasonic scalpel to CO2 laser and electrosurgery in terms of tissue injury and adhesion formation in a rabbit model. Fertil Steril. 1997;67(2):382-6.

449. Schifrin BS. Polemics in perinatology: disengaging forceps. J Perinatol. 1988;8(3):242-5.

450. Schlaff WD, Hassiakos DK, Damewood MD, et al. Neosalpingostomy and distal tubal obstruction: prognostic factors and impact of surgical technique. Fertil Steril. 1990;54:984-90.

451. Schlueter DP. High-risk Gynecology: pulmonary risks. Clin Obstet Gynecol. 1973;16:91.

452. Schnorr JA, Singer JS, Udoff EJ, et al. Late uterine wedge resection of placenta increta. Obstet Gynecol. 1999;94:823-5.

453. Schorge JO, Schaffer JI, Halvorson LM, et al. Hysterectomy. In: William's gynecology. New York: McGraw Hill; 2008.

454. Schroder W, Heyl W. HELLP-syndrome. Diffi culties in diagnosis and therapy of a severe form of preeclampsia. Clin Exp Obstet Gynecol. 1993;20:88-94.

455. Scott JS. Antepartum Hemorrhage-1. BMJ. 1964:1163-65.

456. Scottish Executive Committee of the RCOG (2000). Scottish Obstetric Guidelines and Audit Project. The Management of Postpartum Hemorrhage. [online]. Available from http://www.nhshealthquality.org/nhsqis/files/MATERNITYSERVICES_ Postpartum Haemorrage_ SPCERH6_JUN98.pdf. [Accessed March 2009].

457. Scully RE. Classification, pathology and biologic behavior of ovarian tumors. Meadowbrook Staff Journal. 1968;1:148-63.

458. Sebire NJ, Seckl MJ. Gestational trophoblastic disease: Current management of hydatidiform mole. BMJ. 2008;337:453-58.

459. Seeds JW. Diagnostic mid-trimester amniocentesis: how safe? Am J Obstet Gynecol. 2004; 191(2):607-15.

460. Sehgal N, Haskins AL. The mechanism of uterine bleeding in the presence of fibromyomas. Am Surg. 1960;26:21-3.

461. Selby M. Please don't touch me there: The ethics of intimate examinations: Informed consent failed to protect me. BMJ. 2003;326:1326.

462. Semm K. New methods of pelviscopy (gynecologic laparoscopy) for myomectomy, ovariectomy, tubectomy, and adenectomy. Endoscopy. 1997;11:85-93.

463. Seth SS. Vaginal hysterectomy. In: Puri R, Malhotra N (Eds). Operative obstetrics and gynecology. New Delhi: Jaypee Brothers; 2009.

464. Sheiner E, Levy A, Feinstein U, et al. Risk factors and outcome of failure to progress during the fi rst stage of labor: A population based study. Acta Obstet Gynecol Scand. 2002;81(3): 22-26.

465. Shellhaas C. National institute of child health and human development maternal-fetal medicine unit network: the MFMU cesarean registry: cesarean hysterectomy-its indications, morbidities and mortality. Am J Obstet Gynecol. 2001;185:5123.

466. Shibli KU, Russell IF. A survey of anesthetic techniques used for cesarean section in the UK in 1997. Int J Obstet Anesth. 2000;9(3): 160-7.

467. Shiono P, Klebanoff MA, Carey JC. Midline episiotomies: more harm than good? Obstet Gynecol. 1990;75:765-70.

468. Shrivastava V, Nageotte M, Major C, et al. Case-control comparison of cesarean hysterectomy with and without prophylactic placement of intravascular balloon catheters for placenta accreta. Am J Obstet Gynecol. 2007;197:402e1-e5.

469. Shuster E. The Nuremberg Code: Hippocratic ethics and human rights. Lancet. 1998;351:974-7.

470. Sibai BM, Frangieh AY. Management of severe preeclampsia. Curr Opin Obstet Gynecol. 1996;8:110-3.

471. Sibai BM, lipshitz J, Anderson GD, et al. Reassessment of intravenous MgSO4 therapy in preeclampsia-eclampsia. Obstet Gynecol. 1981;57:199-202.

472. Siegler AM, Kemmann E. Location and removal of misplaced or embedded intrauterine devices by hysteroscopy. J Reprod Med. 1976;16(3):139-44.

473. Silber SJ, Cohen R. Microsurgical reversal of tubal sterilization: factors affecting pregnancy rate with long-term follow-up. Obstet Gynecol. 1984;64(5):679-82.

474. Silver AL. Tubal ligation, hysterectomy, and risk of ovarian cancer. JAMA. 1994;271(16):1235; author reply 1236-7.

475. Silver LE, Hobel CJ, Lagasse L, et al. Placenta previa percreta with bladder involvement: new consideration and a review of the literature. Ultrasound Obstet Gynecol. 1997;9:131-8.

476. Silver R, Depp R, Sabbagha RE, et al. Placenta previa: Aggressive expectant management. Am J Obstet Gynecol. 1984;150(1):15-22.

477. Silversides CK, Colman JM, Sermer M, et al. Cardiac risk in pregnant women with rheumatic mitral stenosis. Am J Cardiol. 2003;91:1382-85.

478. Slotnick, Robert N. "Isoimmunization." In: Niswander K, Evans A (Eds). Manual of Obstetrics. Philadelphia: Lippincott, Wilkins & Wilkins, 2000.

479. Smidt-Jensen S, Philip J. Comparison of transabdominal and transcervical CVS and amniocentesis: sampling success and risk. Prenat Diagn. 1991;11:529-37.

480. Smith GC, Pell JC, Cameron AD, et al. Risk of perinatal death associated with labor after previous cesarean delivery in uncomplicated term pregnancies. JAMA. 2000;287:2684.

481. Smorgick N, Barel O, Halperin R, et al. Laparoscopic removal of adnexal cysts: is it possible to decrease inadvertent intraoperative rupture rate? Am J Obstet Gynecol. 2009;200(3):237.e1-3.

482. Snells RA. Snell's Clinical Anatomy for Regions, 8th Edition. Philadelphia: Lippincott Williams Wilikins; 2008.

483. Snooks SJ, Swash M, Henry MM, et al. Risk factors in childbirth causing damage to the pelvic floor innervation. Int J Colorectal Dis. 1986;1(1):20-4.

484. Society of Obstetricians and Gynaecologists of Canada. Guidelines for operative vaginal birth. Number 148;2004. Int J Gynaecol Obstet. 2005;88(2):229-36.

485. SOGC clinical practice guideline. Diagnosis and Management of Placenta Previa. No. 189, March 2007.

486. Sokol RJ, Blackwell SC. American College of Obstetricians and Gynecologists. Committee on Practice Bulletins–Gynecology. ACOG practice bulletin no. 40: shoulder dystocia. Int J Gynaecol Obstet. 2003;80:87-92.

487. Song SH, Oh MJ, Kim T, et al. Finger-assisted stretching technique for cesarean section. Int J Gynecol Obstet. 2006;92:212-6.

488. Sophie CM, Philippe B, Irving MS. Medical Termination of pregnancy. N Engl J Med. 2000;342:946-55.

489. Souhami R, Tobias J. Cancer and its Management, 5th edition. Oxford: Blackwell Scientific Publications; 2005.

490. Sowter MC, Farquhar CM. Ectopic pregnancy: an update. Curr Opin Obstet Gynecol. 2004;16(4):289-93.

491. Speroff L, Fritz M. Clinical Gynecologic Endocrinology and Infertility, 7th edition. Philadelphia, PA: Lippincott Williams & Wilkins; 2005.

492. Stallings SP, Edwards RK, Johnson JW. Correlation of head-to-body delivery intervals in shoulder dystocia and umbilical artery acidosis. Am J Obstet Gynecol. 2001;185:268-74.

493. Stamatellos I, Bontis J. Hysteroscopic myomectomy. Eur Clinics Obstet Gynecol. 2007;3:17-23.

494. Stanco LM, Schrimmer DB, Paul RH, et al. Emergency peripartum hysterectomy and associated risk factors. Am J Obstet Gynecol. 1993;168:879-83.

495. Stanco LM, Schrimmer DB, Paul RH, et al. Emergency peripartum hysterectomy and associated risk factors. Am J Obstet Gynecol. 1993;168:879-83.

496. Stedman CM, Kline RC. Intraoperative complications and unexpected pathology at the time of cesarean section. Obstet Gynecol Clin North Am. 1988;15(4):745-69.

497. Steer P, Flint C. ABC of labour care: Physiology and management of normal labor. BMJ 1999;318:793-96.

498. Stegmann BJ, Craig HR, Bay RC, et al. Characteristics predictive of response to ovarian diathermy in women with polycystic ovarian syndrome. Am J Obstet and Gynecol. 2003; 188(5):1171-73.

499. Stein FI, Levanthal ML. Amenorrhoea associated with bilateral polycystic ovaries. American Journal of Obstetrics and Gynecology. 1935;29:181-91.

500. Stiller KR, Munday RM. Chest physiotherapy for the surgical patient. Br J Surg. 1992;79:745.

501. Stirrat GM. Recurrent miscarriage. Lancet. 1990;336:673-5.

502. Stock RJ. Persistant tubal pregnancy. Obstet Gynecol. 1991;77(2):267-70.

503. Stone HH, Hoefling SJ, Strom PR, et al. Abdominal incisions: transverse vs vertical placement and continuous vs interrupted closure. South Med J. 1983;76(9):1106-8.

504. Stovall TG, Kellerman AL, Ling FW, et al. Emergency department diagnosis of ectopic pregnancy. Ann Emerg Med. 1990;19(10): 1098-103.

505. Stovall TG, Ling FW, Gray LA. Single-dose methotrexate for treatment of ectopic pregnancy. Obstet Gynecol. 1991;77(5):754-7.

506. Stubblefield PG. Control of pain for women undergoing abortion. Int J Gynaecol Obstet Suppl. 1989;3:131.

507. Sudik R, Husch K, Steller J, et al. Fertility and pregnancy outcome after myomectomy in sterility patients. Eur J Obstet Gynecol Reprod Biol. 1996;65(2):209-14.

508. Stubblefield PG. Surgical techniques of uterine evacuation in first- and second-trimester abortion. Clin Obstet Gynecol. 1986;13:53-70.

509. Sweeny WJ, Gepfert R. The fallopian tube. Clin Obstet Gynecol. 1965;8:32-47.

510. Tan CH, Tay KH, Sheah K, et al. Perioperative endovascular internal iliac artery occlusion balloon placement in management of placenta accreta. Am J Roentgenol. 2007;189:1158-63.

511. Taylor MS. Managing postoperative pain. Hosp Med. 2001;62:560-3.

512. Tharker SB, Stroup D, Chang M. Electronic fetal heart rate monitoring for fetal assessment during labor. Cochrane Database of Systemic Reviews II. 2001;CD00063.

513. The Medical Termination of Pregnancy Act, 1971 (Act No 34 of 1971, 10th August 1971).

514. The Royal College of Obstetricians and Gynecologists (2007). Birth after previous caesarean birth. Green top Guideline No 45.

515. The Royal College of Obstetricians and Gynecologists. Birth after previous caesarean birth. Green top Guideline No 45. London: Royal College of Obstetricians and Gynaecologists; 2007.

516. The Royal College of Obstetricians and Gynecologists. The management of gestational trophoblastic neoplasia. Guideline No. 38, February 2004.

517. Tho PT, Byrd JR, McDonough PG. Etiologies and subsequent reproductive performance of 100 couples with recurrent abortion. Fertil Steril.1979;32:389-95.

518. Towner D, Castro MA, Eby-Wilkens E, et al. Effect of mode of delivery in nulliparous women on neonatal intracranial injury. N Engl J Med. 1999;341(23):1709-14.

519. Towner DR, Ciotti MC. Operative vaginal delivery: a cause of birth injury or is it? Clin Obstet Gynecol. 2007;50(3):563-81.

520. Traina E, Mattar R, Moron AF, et al. Diagnostic accuracy of hysterosalpingography and transvaginal sonography to evaluate uterine cavity diseases in patients with recurrent miscarriage. RBGO. 2004;26:527-33.

521. Trew GH. Hysteroscopy and hysteroscopic surgery. Curr Obstet Gynaecol. 2004;14:183-90.

522. Trimbos JB. Security of various knots commonly used in surgical practice. Obstet Gynecol. 1984;64:274.

523. Troiano RN, McCarthy SM. Müllerian duct anomalies: imaging and clinical issues. Radiology. 2004;233:19-34.

524. Tsuji S, Takahashi K, Yomo H, et al. Effectiveness of antiadhesion barriers in preventing adhesion after myomectomy in patients with uterine leiomyoma. Eur J Obstet Gynecol Reprod Biol. 2005;123(2):244-8.

525. Tulandi T, Arronet GH, McInnes RA. Arcuate and bicornuate uterine anomalies and infertility. Fertil Steril. 1980;34:362-4.

526. Tulandi T, Murray C, Guralnick M. Adhesion formation and reproductive outcome after myomectomy and second-look laparoscopy. Obstet Gynecol. 1993;82(2):213-5.

527. Tulandi T, Saleh A. Surgical management of ectopic pregnancy. Clin Obstet Gynecol. 1999;42(1):31-8.

528. Tulandi T, Watkin K, Tan SL. Reproductive performance and three dimensional ultrasound volume determination of polycystic ovaries following laparoscopic ovarian drilling. Int J Fertil Womens Med. 1997;42:436-40.

529. Tulandi T. Modern surgical approaches to female reproductive tract. Hum Reprod Update. 1996;2:419-27.

530. Tulandi T. Tubal sterilization. N Engl J Med. 1997;336(11):796-7.

531. Tuomivaara l, Kauppila A. Radical or conservative surgery for ectopic pregnancy? A follow-up study of fertility of 323 patients. Fertil Steril. 1988;50(4):580-3.

532. Twersky RS, Singleton G. Preoperative pregnancy testing: justice and testing for all. Anesth Analg. 1996;83(2):438-9.

533. Uchida H. Uchida tubal sterilization. Am J Obstet Gynecol. 1975;121(2):153-8.

534. Uchil D, Arulkumaran S. Neonatal subgaleal hemorrhage and its relationship to delivery by vacuum extraction. Obstet Gynecol Surv. 2003;58(10):687-93.

535. Ugur M, Turan C, Mungan T, et al. Laparoscopy for adhesion prevention following myomectomy. Int J Gynecol Obstet. 1996;53:145-9.

536. Urman B, Gomel V, McComb P, et al. Midtubal occlusion: etiology, management and outcome. Fertil Steril. 1992;57(4):747-50.

537. Vacca A. Handbook of Vacuum Extraction in Obstetric Practice. 1st edition. London, UK: E. Arnold; 1992. p. 32.

538. Valenti C, Schutta EJ, Kehaty T. Prenatal diagnosis of Down's syndrome. Lancet. 1968;2(7561):220.

539. Valenzano MM, Mistrangelo E, Lijoi D, et al. Transvaginal sonohysterographic evaluation of uterine malformations. Eur J Obstet Gynecol Reprod Biol. 2006;124:246-9.

540. Valle RF, Sabbagha. Management of first-trimester pregnancy termination failures. Obstet Gynecol. 1980;55:625.

541. Van Rijssel EJ, Trimbos JB, Booster MH. Mechanical performance of square knots and sliding knots in surgery: A comparative study. Am J Obstet Gynecol. 1990;162:93.

542. Veatch RM (Ed). Medical ethics. Boston: Jones and Bartlett Publishers;1989.

543. Vercellini P, Chapron C, De Giorgi O, et al. Coagulation or excision of ovarian endometriomas? Am J Obstet Gynecol. 2003b;188: 606-10.

544. Vermesh M, Silva PD, Rosen GF, et al. Management of unruptured ectopic gestation by linear salpingostomy: a propective, randomized clinical trial of laprascopy versus lapratomy. Obstet Gnecol. 1989;73(3 Pt 1):400-4.

545. Viswanathan M, Hartmann K, Palmieri R, et al. The use of episiotomy in obstetric care: a systematic review. Agency for Healthcare Research and Quality. Rockville, MD: Evidence Report/Technology Assessment 112. AHRQ Publication; 2005. pp. 05-E009-2 [online] Available from http://www.ncbi.nlm.nih.gov/books bv.fcgi?rid= hstat1a.section. 88924 [Accessed March 2010].

546. Vloka JD, Hadzic A, Drobnik L. Nerve blocks in the pregnant patient. In Drs David J Birbach, Stephen Gatt and Sanjay Datta (Eds). Textbook of Obstetric Anesthesia. Churchill Livingstone, Philadelphia, 2000;693-706.

547. Wadstrom J, Getdin B. Closure of the abdominal wall: How and why? Acta Chir Scand. 1990;156:75.

548. Wai CY, Zekam N, Sanz LE. Septate uterus with double cervix and longitudinal vaginal septum. A case report. J Reprod Med. 2001;46: 613-7.

549. Wallace D, Hernandez W, Schlaerth JB, et al. Prevention of abdominal wound disruption utilizing the Smead-Jones closure technique. Obstet Gynecol. 1980;56(2):226-30.

550. Wallach EE. Myomectomy: a guide to indications and technique. Contemp Obstet Gynecol. 1988;31:74.

551. Walsh, Patrick C, et al. Campbell's Urology. 8th edition. Philadelphia: Elsevier Science; 2002.

552. Wamsteker K, Emanuel MH, de Kruif JH. Transcervical hysteroscopic resection of submucous fibroids for abnormal uterine bleeding: results regarding the degree of intramural extension. Obstet Gynecol. 1993;82(5):736-40.

553. Wamsteker K, Emanuel MH. Uterine leiomyomas. In: Brosens I, Wamsteker K (Eds). Diagnostic Imaging and Endoscopy in Gynecology. London: WB Saunders; 1997. pp. 185-98.

554. Way S. Carcinoma of the vulva. Am J Obstet Gynecol. 1960;79:692-7.

555. Weber AM, Walters MD, Piedmonte MR. Sexual function and vaginal anatomy in women before and after surgery for pelvic organ prolapse and urinary incontinence. Am J Obstet Gynecol. 2000;182(6):1610-5.

556. Weiland DE, Bay RC, Del Sordi S. Choosing the best abdominal closure by meta-analysis. Am J Surg. 1998;176(6):666-70.

557. Wen SW, Liu S, Kramer MS, et al. Comparison of maternal and infant outcomes between vacuum extraction and forceps deliveries. Am J Epidemiol. 2001;153(2):103-7.

558. West JH, Robinson DA. Endometrial resection and fluid absorption. Lancet. 1989;2:1387-8.

559. Wester C, Brubaker L. Normal pelvic floor physiology. Obstet Gynecol Clin North Am. 1998;25(4):707-22.

560. Westrom L. Effect of acute pelvic inflammatory disease on fertility. Am J Obstet Gynecol. 1975; 121(5):1707-13.

561. Wilcox LS, Chu SY, Eaker ED, et al. Risk factors for regret after tubal sterilization: 5 years of follow-up in a prospective study. Fertil seril. 1991;55(5):927-33.

562. Wilkinson C, Enkin MW. Manual removal of placenta at cesarean section. Cochrane Database Syst Rev. 2000;(2):CD 000130.

563. William's Obstetrics. Dystocia and Abnormal Labor. In: Cunnigham FG, Leveno KJ, Bloom SL, Hauth JC, Gilstrap LC, & Wenstrom KD (Eds). 23rd edition. US: Mc Graw Hill; 2009. pp. 513-7.

564. Williams MC. Vacuum-assisted delivery. Clin Perinatol. 1995;22:933-52.

565. Winston RML, Margara RA. Microsurgical salpingostomy is not an obsolete procedure. Br J Obstet Gynecol. 1991;98:637-42.

566. Winston RML. Reversal of sterilization. Clin Obstet Gynecol. 1980;23(4):1261-8.

567. Woelfer B, Salim R, Banerjee S, et al. Reproductive outcomes in women with congenital uterine anomalies detected by three-dimensional ultrasound screening. Obstet Gynecol. 2001;98:1099-103.

568. Wood C, Ng KH, Hounslow D, et al. Time—an important variable in normal delivery. J Obstet Gynaecol Br Commonw. 1973;80: 295-300.

569. Woodland MB. Ureter injury during laparoscopy-assisted vaginal hysterectomy with the endoscopic linear stapler. Am J Obstet Gynecol. 1992;167:756-7.

570. World Health Organization (2006). WHO Recommendations for the Prevention of Postpartum Haemorrhage. [online]. Available from http://www.who.int/making_pregnancy_safer/publications/WHO Recommendations for PP Haemorrhage.pdf [Accessed May 2010].

571. Wortman M, Dagget A. Hysteroscopy myomectomy. J Am Assoc Gynecol Laparosc. 1995;3:39-46.

572. Wu MH, Hsu CC, Huang KE. Detection of congenital Müllerian duct anomalies using three-dimensional ultrasound. J Clin Ultrasound. 1997;25:487-92.

573. Xue P, Fa Y-Y. Microsurgical reversal of female sterilization. J Reprod Med. 1939;34:451.

574. Yang J, Yin TL, Xu WM, et al. Reproductive outcome of septate uterus after hysteroscopic treatment with neodymium: YAG laser. Photomed Laser Surg. 2006;24(5):625.

575. Yao M, Tulandi T. Current status of surgical and non-surgical management of ectopic pregnancy. Fertility and Sterility. 1997;67(3): 421-33.

576. Yildirim G, Beji NK. Effects of pushing techniques in birth on mother and fetus: a randomized study. Birth. 2008;35(1):25-30.

577. Yiostalo P, Cacciatore B, Sjoberg J, et al. Expectant management of ectopic pregnancy. Obstet Gynecol. 1992;80(3 Pt 1);345-8.

578. Zelop CM, Harlow BL, Frigoletto FD, et al. Emergency peripartum hysterectomy. Am J Obstet Gynecol. 1993;168:1443-8.

579. Zilber U, Pansky M, Bukovsky I, et al. Laparoscopic salpingostomy versus laparoscopic methotrexate injection in the management of unruptured ectopic gestation. Am J Obstet Gynecol.1996;175(3):600-2.

Index